Diagnostic Histopathology
of the Lymph Node

Diagnostic Histopathology of the Lymph Node

James A. Strauchen, M.D.

Professor of Pathology
Professor of Medicine
Derald H. Ruttenberg Cancer Center
Mount Sinai School of Medicine
New York, New York

New York   Oxford
Oxford University Press
1998

Oxford University Press

Oxford   New York
Athens   Auckland   Bangkok   Bogota   Bombay
Buenos Aires   Calcutta   Cape Town   Dar es Salaam
Delhi   Florence   Hong Kong   Istanbul   Karachi
Kuala Lumpur   Madras   Madrid   Melbourne
Mexico City   Nairobi   Paris   Singapore
Taipei   Tokyo   Toronto   Warsaw

and associated companies in
Berlin   Ibadan

Copyright © 1998 by Oxford University Press, Inc.

Published by Oxford University Press, Inc.,
198 Madison Avenue, New York, New York 10016

Oxford is a registered trademark of Oxford University Press

Library of Congress Cataloging-in-Publication Data
Strauchen, James A.
Diagnostic histopathology of the lymph node /
James A. Strauchen.
p.   cm.   Includes bibliographical references and index.
ISBN 0-19-511860-X
1. Lymph nodes—Histopathology.   2. Lymph nodes—Biopsy.
3. Lymphnodes—Diseases—diagnosis.
4. Lymphoproliferative disorders—Diagnosis.
I. Title.   [DNLM: 1. Lymph Nodes—pathology.   2. Biopsy—methods.
3. Lympatic Diseases—diagnosis.   4. Immunophenotyping—methods.
WH 700 S912d   1988]   RC646.S825   1998
616.4′207583—dc21   DNLM/DLC   for Library of Congress   97-33563

9 8 7 6 5 4 3 2 1

Printed in Hong Kong
on acid-free paper

To Helen
To Vivienne, Jennifer, and Katherine
In memory of Murray

Preface

This book is written as an introduction and guide to the interpretation of the lymph node biopsy. It is intended primarily for pathologists, pathologists-in-training, and fellows in hematologic pathology, but may be of some interest to hematologists and medical oncologists interested in the pathology of their patients. The format and approach will be familiar to readers of the author's previous volume, *Diagnostic Histopathology of the Bone Marrow* (New York, Oxford University Press, 1996). Although an emphasis has been placed on interpretation of the routinely stained hematoxylin and eosin section, no consideration of lymph node pathology could be considered complete without consideration of the immunologic and molecular biologic advances which have revolutionized hematopathology. An effort has been made, therefore, to integrate the classic approach to biopsy interpretation, including histopathology and clinical features, with the newer immunophenotypic and molecular biologic techniques. The Revised European-American Lymphoma (REAL) classification for lymphoid neoplasms, which is coming into increasingly wide clinical use, is utilized in the discussion of the malignant lymphomas. Although the clinical superiority of any one classification has yet to be established, the REAL classification provides a logical framework for consideration of these neoplasms. Because many pathologists and clinicians continue to use the Working Formulation in day-to-day practice, the equivalent terms in that classification are also utilized.

The illustrative material used in the book was gathered from the pathology files at the Mount Sinai Medical Center and from consultation material received over the years by the author. I would like to thank the clinicians and pathologists who permitted me to participate in the care of their patients and provided the material upon which this book is based. I am also indebted to my mentors in hematology and hematopathology, Drs. Robert Silber and Costan Berard, to whom I express my gratitude, and also to Drs. Alan Schiller and James F. Holland for their continued encouragement and support.

<table>
<tr><td>New York, NY</td><td style="text-align:right">JAS</td></tr>
<tr><td>September 1997</td><td></td></tr>
</table>

Contents

IV Proliferations of Other Elements   **319**

I

General Considerations

1

The Lymph Node Biopsy

Indications for Lymph Node Biopsy

Lymphadenopathy is an extremely common sign in clinical medicine which may accompany a wide variety of conditions. The diagnosis of the etiology of lymphadenopathy will not infrequently require biopsy of an enlarged lymph node for pathologic examination and study. Selection of patients requiring lymph node biopsy requires a good deal of clinical judgment. The significance of palpably enlarged lymph nodes ranges from the trivial (e.g., cervical lymph node enlargement accompanying an upper respiratory infection) to the life threatening (e.g., lymph node enlargement as a manifestation of acquired immunodeficiency syndrome [AIDS] or malignant lymphoma). Lymph node enlargement may be localized or generalized but will usually have been persistent and unexplained before lymph node biopsy is considered. The differential diagnosis of lymph node enlargement will vary with the age of the patient. Reactive lymphadenopathies are, in general, more common in childhood and young adulthood, whereas malignant neoplasms, both primary (i.e., malignant lymphoma) and secondary (i.e., metastatic carcinoma), are more common in adults. Similarly, clinical findings also affect the differential diagnosis. A lymph node which is tender to palpation and soft in consistency is most likely reactive, whereas a lymph node which is rock hard is most commonly malignant. The lymph nodes in malignant lymphoma typically have a firm or "rubbery" consistency on palpation. The size of the lymph nodes is also of significance. The largest lymph nodes are typically seen in neoplastic conditions, such as Hodgkin's disease and non-Hodgkin's lymphomas; however, striking lymph node enlargement may be seen in some reactive conditions, for example Rosai-Dorfman disease (sinus histiocytosis with massive lymphadenopathy). Similarly, lymph nodes which are only slightly enlarged may harbor malignant lymphoma, particularly if other suggestive clinical signs (i.e., hepatosplenomegaly) are evident. Selection of patients for lymph node biopsy therefore requires consideration of all the clinical signs and symptoms. Laboratory evaluation may also be helpful prior to lymph node biopsy. For example, examination of the peripheral blood smear may reveal the characteristic changes of infectious mononucleosis in the young adult, or chronic lymphocytic leukemia in the older adult, obviating the need for lymph node biopsy.

Selection of a Lymph Node for Biopsy

In general, the largest, deepest lymph node is the one most likely to yield diagnostic information. It is not uncommon for overlying superficial lymph nodes to show only nonspecific reactive changes while a deeper lymph node contains malignant lymphoma. In patients with generalized lymphadenopathy no particular lymph node group is more or less likely to yield diagnostic material than any other, and biopsy should be directed to the largest lymph node. Although it has been commonly stated that inguinal lymph nodes should be avoided for biopsy because they frequently show nonspecific changes, in practice these lymph node are as frequently diagnostic as any other if pathologically enlarged.

In patients with regional lymphadenopathy, the distribution of enlarged lymph node may be of differential diagnostic value. For example, posterior cervical lymphadenopathy is common in viral infections and toxoplasmic lymphadenitis, whereas supraclavicular lymphadenopathy is frequently due to malignant lymphoma, granulomatous disease, or metastatic carcinoma. Similarly, epitrochlear lymphadenopathy is distinctly uncommon in Hodgkin's disease but relatively frequent in non-Hodgkin's lymphoma and sarcoidosis. Although enlargement of superficial lymph nodes is frequently due to reactive hyperplasia, this is seldom the case for retroperitoneal or mediastinal lymph nodes, enlargement of which is frequently due to neoplasia.

Choice of Biopsy Technique

Several techniques are available to obtain biopsy material of enlarged lymph nodes for pathological investigation. These include fine needle aspiration, core needle biopsy, and excisional or incisional surgical biopsy. The choice of technique will depend on the clinical situation as well as the locally available expertise and experience.

Fine Needle Aspiration

Fine needle aspiration has emerged in recent years as a valuable minimally invasive technique for obtaining diagnostic material from lymph nodes and other organs. Fine needle aspiration of superficial lymph nodes is readily performed in the physician's office, outpatient department, or pathology suite. Fine needle aspiration of clinically inaccessible nodes (e.g., retroperitoneal or mesenteric) may be performed with radiologic or ultrasonographic guidance. The presence of the pathologist at the procedure is optimal to insure adequacy and proper handling of the material obtained. Fine needle aspiration material is smeared on slides for rapid-fixation Papanicolaou-stained preparations and for air-dried Giemsa-stained preparations; material is also fixed in ethanol for paraffin-embedded cell block preparations. Material for immunophenotypic studies can also be obtained with multiple needle passes and studied by flow cytometry or immuno-peroxidase on cytospin preparations. The major limitation of fine needle aspiration is the lack of architecture in the cytologic specimen obtained.

Fine needle aspiration of lymph nodes can provide diagnostically meaningful informa-tion (Steel et al, 1995). For enlarged superficial lymph nodes, especially cervical lymph nodes in which metastatic squamous carcinoma of the head and neck is a diagnostic consideration, fine needle aspiration is an important screening tool which directs the subsequent workup of the patient. If metastatic squamous carcinoma is found, the pa-tient can be referred for appropriate otolaryngologic evaluation and definitive therapy without surgical lymph node biopsy. Similarly, if fine needle aspiration reveals reactive lymphoid hyperplasia in a young patient with cervical lymphadenopathy, cautious clini-cal follow-up in lieu of surgical biopsy may be recommended. The role of fine needle aspiration biopsy in the diagnosis of hematologic neoplasms is, however, more limited. Although Hodgkin's disease and many non-Hodgkin's lymphomas can be reliably diag-nosed by fine needle aspiration in experienced hands, subclassification based on archi-tectural details (e.g., nodular versus diffuse) is often difficult. Since excisional biopsy of a superficial lymph node has minimal morbidity, surgical biopsy for confirmation of a diagnosis of malignant lymphoma is usually warranted. For lesions involving retroperi-toneal, mesenteric, or other surgically inaccessible lymph nodes, however, the added information provided by surgical biopsy may not outweigh the morbidity of surgical exploration, and therapy based on the results of fine needle aspiration is reasonable. Similarly, although excision biopsy of a superficial lymph node is recommended for the initial diagnosis of malignant lymphoma, fine needle aspiration biopsy may suffice for the diagnosis of recurrent disease, or disease at other sites, in patients with a previously established diagnosis of malignant lymphoma.

Core Needle Biopsy

Core needle lymph node biopsy, performed with any one of a variety of needles specifi-cally designed for this purpose, may also be used to provide diagnostic material in lieu of surgical biopsy. Core needle biopsy provides a larger specimen than fine needle aspi-ration and can be used for routine histopathology as well as to provide material for immunohistochemical studies. Core needle biopsy can be satisfactorily performed on palpably enlarged superficial lymph nodes as well as on deeply situated lymph nodes by radiographic or ultrasonographic guidance, provided vital structures are not at risk. The larger specimen obtained by core needle biopsy provides limited architectural informa-tion which is not provided by fine needle aspiration cytology. Core needle biopsy is a useful technique when excisional biopsy would be hazardous or inconvenient. The pathologist, however, should not hesitate to defer diagnosis on a core needle biopsy if the tissue is insufficient and request an excisional biopsy.

Excisional Biopsy

Excisional biopsy of an intact lymph node is the procedure of choice for lymph node biopsy. Excisional biopsy of a superficial lymph node may be performed in the physi-cian's office, outpatient department, outpatient surgery center, or hospital operating room. The procedure is usually performed with local anesthesia unless unusually extensive or deep dissection is anticipated, in which case regional or general anesthesia may be used. The largest, deepest lymph node should generally be the one excised, since smaller, more superficial lymph nodes, although technically easier to reach, may not show diagnostic changes. It is a surgical truism that lymph nodes are frequently found to be much deeper than appreciated on palpation, and biopsy of even the most superficial of lymph nodes should be undertaken only by an experienced surgeon. The lymph node should ideally be excised intact, with an intact capsule, avoiding fragmentation of the specimen.

Incisional Biopsy

Occasionally patients present with very large, matted, or deeply fixed lymph nodes, excisional biopsy of which is impractical or would cause undue morbidity. In these cases, incisional biopsy of the lymph node may be performed. Ideally, a portion of capsule and surrounding tissue should be included in the specimen submitted.

Processing the Lymph Node Specimen

The lymph node should be received fresh and unfixed in the pathology laboratory. The lymph node must be handled carefully to avoid artifactual distortion caused by crushing during handling or by drying out as a result of being placed on dry gauze or paper toweling. Transportation in a petri dish in saline solution or in wet gauze is satisfactory. The lymph node must be carefully divided to insure that maximal diagnostic information is obtained and that adequate tissue is preserved for special studies. Many laboratories have established protocols for handling lymph node specimens. The types of studies that may be provided for include routine paraffin embedding for histology, special stains, and immunohistochemical studies on deparaffinized sections; imprint and touch preparations for Giemsa and cytochemical staining; "snap frozen" tissue for frozen section immunohistochemistry and immunophenotyping; frozen cells or tissue for molecular studies; fresh tissue for cell suspensions for immunophenotyping by flow cytometry; fresh tissue handled with sterile technique for microbiologic culture; fresh tissue for cytogenetic studies; and tissue for electron microscopy fixed in glutaraldehyde.

Frozen Section Examination

Frozen section examination plays a limited role in the diagnostic evaluation of the lymph node biopsy and will rarely result in a definitive hematopathologic diagnosis. Frozen section examination may be performed to "triage" the lymph node biopsy and insure that tissue is preserved for all the appropriate studies; frozen section may also be used to confirm that diagnostic material has been obtained. Frozen section examination will seldom result in the definitive diagnosis of malignant lymphoma; however, a diagnosis of metastatic carcinoma or granulomatous disease may be established. In our laboratory, we utilize the frozen section examination as an opportunity to preserve fresh tissue for immunophenotypic and molecular studies and to obtain tissue for additional studies such as microbiologic cultures, and electron microscopy, as indicated. The surgeon should appreciate, however, that the tissue used to prepare a frozen section of a lymph node may be useless for subsequent definitive diagnosis. If diagnostic material is limited, therefore, the pathologist should not hesitate to decline to perform a frozen section, preserving the tissue necessary for special studies and deferring diagnosis to permanent sections.

Choice of Fixative

Lymph nodes are unforgiving of poor histologic technique and must be well fixed prior to processing. The choice of fixative varies widely from laboratory to laboratory; 10% neutral buffered formalin is widely used. Formalin provides reasonably good histology and adequate preservation of antigenicity for immunohistochemical studies. Formalin is a relatively slow fixative and overnight fixation of even small specimens is recommended. Lymph node specimens should be sliced to approximately 2-mm thickness before being placed in formalin to insure adequate penetration. An intact lymph node simply "dropped" into a jar of formalin will remain unfixed in the center. Tissue fixed in formalin frequent exhibits a characteristic artifact consisting of enlarged vesicular "bubbly" nuclei. This artifact is familiar to most pathologists. A variety of other fixatives may be used which provide better nuclear detail, including Bouin's solution and Zenker's solution. These fixatives, however, may cause a shrinkage artifact, can result in "overfixation," and may require altered histologic processing. B-5 solution is an excellent fixative which provides exceptional nuclear detail and excellent preservation of antigenicity for immunohistochemical studies, but it must be prepared fresh, can cause overfixation, and requires altered histologic processing. Because of environmental and occupational health concern about formaldehyde, a number of commercial alcohol-based fixatives have recently been made available. These, however, are relatively expensive and unsuited for large specimens. For these reasons, we prefer 10% neutral buffered formalin as an all-around fixative despite its acknowledged disadvantages.

Routine Histology

Lymph nodes fixed in 10% neutral buffered formalin are processed overnight on an automated tissue processor. Care should be taken not to overheat the paraffin, which results in artifactually distorted, homogenous, basophilic nuclear staining. Lymph nodes embedded in paraffin should be cut on a microtome by an experienced histotechnologist at no more than 4-μm thickness. Lymph node sections are stained routinely with hematoxylin and eosin. Other special stains are obtained as necessary.

Imprints and Touch Preparations

Imprints or touch preparations of lymph nodes can be a valuable adjunct to histology (Koo et al, 1989). Imprints are prepared from the unfixed lymph node by making a fresh slice through the lymph node with a scalpel blade or razor, blotting the surface of the node against a paper towel to remove excess fluid, and then touching the surface of the node to a clean glass slide at several places. The touch should be brief and perpendicular to the slide; shearing or smearing should be avoided. The touch preparation is air dried and stained with Giemsa or another hematologic Romanowsky-based stain. Air-dried touch preparations are also suitable for cytochemical or immunocytochemical studies, such as might be used on blood or bone marrow smears (e.g., peroxidase, non-specific esterase, and tartrate-resistant acid phosphatase).

Immunophenotypic Studies

Immunophenotypic studies on fresh tissue are a valuable adjunct to histologic examination of the lymph node and offer advantages over immunohistochemical studies on formalin-fixed, paraffin-embedded tissue. Immunophenotypic studies are performed by immunoperoxidase immunohistochemistry on frozen sections or by immunofluorescence flow cytometry on cell suspensions. In either case, tissue must be preserved prior to fixation. Tissue for immunophenotypic studies on frozen sections is snap frozen in isopentane and dry ice and stored in the $-70°$ C freezer. The tissue may be embedded in a commercially available frozen section embedding medium to facilitate the cutting of frozen sections and to protect the tissue from desiccation in the freezer. If freezing facilities are not available, tissue may be frozen and stored in the cryostat (the automatic defrost cycle must be turned off). The snap-frozen tissue is also suitable for molecular genetic and DNA studies.

Cell suspensions for immunofluorescence flow cytometry are prepared from fresh, unfixed tissue. The tissue is minced with a scalpel blade or razor in tissue culture medium and tissue fragments are removed by straining through a wire mesh. The cell suspension may be stained immediately or frozen in dimethylsulfoxide for future use.

Microbiologic Cultures

If the clinical features or results of frozen section examination suggest an infectious etiology of lymphadenopathy, tissue for microbiologic cultures should be taken. This will usually include cultures for aerobic and anaerobic bacteria, acid fast bacteria, and fungi. Cultures for organisms requiring special conditions or media (e.g., cat scratch bacilli, leishmania) may be requested if indicated. Tissue for microbiologic cultures should be handled sterilely. If sterile instruments are not available in the pathology laboratory, the tissue may be divided in the operating room. Direct smears of lymph node material for Gram stain, acid fast stain, and fungal stains may also be useful in selected cases.

Cytogenetic Studies

Cytogenetic studies have been employed in the diagnosis and classification of malignant lymphomas in which specific cytogenetic abnormalities and chromosomal translocation have been characterized. Cytogenetic study of malignant lymphomas by karyotyping of metaphase cells has been challenging in the past because of the difficulties of growing lymphoma cells in culture. This has been in part obviated by the technique of fluorescence in situ hybridization (or FISH) which detects chromosomal abnormalities in interphase cells (Wolman, 1994). Tissue for karyotyping must be viable and handle aseptically; FISH may be performed on lymph node imprints or cell suspensions.

REFERENCES

Koo CH, Rappaport H, Sheibani K, Pangalis GA, Nathwani BN, Winberg C. Imprint cytology of non-Hodgkin's lymphomas based on a study of 212 immunologically characterized cases: Correlation of touch imprints with tissue sections. Hum Pathol 20:1–138 (suppl 1), 1989.

Steel BL, Schwartz MR, Ramzy I. Fine needle aspiration biopsy in the diagnosis of lymphadenopathy in 1,103 patients. Role, limitations and analysis of diagnostic pitfalls. Acta Cytol 39:76–81, 1995.

Wolman SR. Fluorescence in situ hybridization: A new tool for the pathologist. Hum Pathol 6:586–590, 1994.

2

Immunologic and Molecular Techniques

Immunologic and molecular techniques have had major impact on hematopathological diagnosis. The diagnosis and classification of the malignant lymphomas has evolved from an essentially morphologic descriptive level in the 1960s to the immunophenotypic level in the 1970s and to the genotypic level in the 1980s and 1990s. Immunologic and molecular techniques are routinely applied to the diagnosis of lymph node biopsies. The development of monoclonal antibody technology has vastly expanded the availability of diagnostic reagents for the recognition of lymphoid differentiation antigens (Kishimoto et al, 1997). The development of monoclonal antibodies suitable for immunohistochemical studies on deparaffinized sections has broadened the applicability of immunophenotypic studies to routinely processed tissue and permitted the use of archival material (Perkins and Kjeldsberg, 1993). Similarly, the development of the polymerase chain reaction (PCR) for amplifying small sequences of deoxyribonucleic acid (DNA) has permitted molecular studies on DNA extracted from routinely processed paraffin embedded tissue (Mies, 1994). The diagnostic techniques reviewed in this chapter are an adjunct to histopathologic diagnosis and no one of these techniques can be considered a "gold standard" for hematopathologic diagnosis. The information gleaned from these techniques must be integrated with the histopathologic and clinical findings.

Immunophenotypic Studies

Immunophenotypic studies on fresh tissue can be performed by immunohistochemistry on frozen sections or by immunofluorescence flow cytometry on cell suspensions. Each technique has advantages and disadvantages. Immunohistochemistry on frozen sections permits direct visualization of the cells stained and permits correlation with the morphologic features (i.e., the "immunoarchitecture" of the lymph node). Interpretation is, however, nonquantitative and may be subjective. Immunofluorescence flow cytometry, in contrast, is quantitative, but dependent on the representativeness of the cell suspension (which may vary considerably in lymph nodes with fibrosis or focal lesions) and on the ability to selectively "gate" on the cells of interest. In our laboratory, we generally employ immunohistochemistry on frozen sections for the immunophenotyping of lymph node specimens and immunofluorescence flow cytometry for the immunophenotyping of blood and bone marrow specimens.

Immunophenotypic Studies on Frozen Sections

Immunophenotypic studies on lymph nodes (and other tissue) are conveniently performed by immunohistochemistry on frozen sections prepared from snap-frozen tissue set aside prior to fixation. The frozen tissue may be stored in the $-70°$ C freezer for future use for molecular or other studies. Frozen sections are cut in the cryostat at 5-μm thickness, air dried, and fixed in cold acetone for 10 minutes at 4° C prior to staining. The air dried frozen sections may be stored at $-20°$ C for up to 1 week before staining. Frozen sections are stained with monoclonal antibodies utilizing the avidin-biotin-complex (ABC) technique, or immunoalkaline phosphatase, or a related immunoenzymatic method (Hsu et al, 1981).

Immunophenotypic Studies by Flow Cytometry

Immunophenotypic studies are performed on cell suspensions by flow cytometry. Cell suspensions are readily prepared from lymph nodes, peripheral blood, or fresh bone marrow aspirate. The cells may be separated with Ficoll-Hypaque or other separation medium prior to study. The cells are stained with monoclonal antibodies tagged with a fluorescent label. Most current flow cytometers are equipped for two-color analysis, permitting simultaneous staining with two different monoclonal antibodies tagged with different labels (e.g., fluorescein and rhodamine or fluorescein and phycoerythrin). Some newer machines are capable of three- or four-color analysis, permitting simultaneous staining with multiple antibodies. Flow cytometry is based on analysis of single cells as they pass through a laser light beam. The cells are examined for fluorescence at the wavelengths characteristic of the fluorescent labels utilized and for optical light scatter at 0 and 90°, which are characteristic of cell size and granularity, respectively (Fig. 2.1). Use of the latter two parameters permits the operator to "gate" on the cells of interest. When the "gates" are set, the flow cytometer records the fluorescence only of cells of specified size and granularity. For immunophenotyping of lymphoid cells, the "gate" would be set for small and large nongranular cells, corresponding to small and large lymphocytes. Other, potentially confounding cells (e.g., granulocytes, monocytes, cell debris) are excluded from the analysis. The ability to "gate" on specific cell populations (e.g., small lymphocytes, large lymphocytes) is one of the more powerful aspects of flow cytometric analysis, but also a potential pitfall, since it is possible to unintentionally "gate out" the cells of interest altogether. The fluorescence data is presented as a histogram or "bitmap" and also as a percentage of positive cells. Interpretation should be based on the histogram or bitmap, since the percentage of positive cells is determined by an arbitrary threshold and subtle shifts in fluorescence may be missed. Appro-

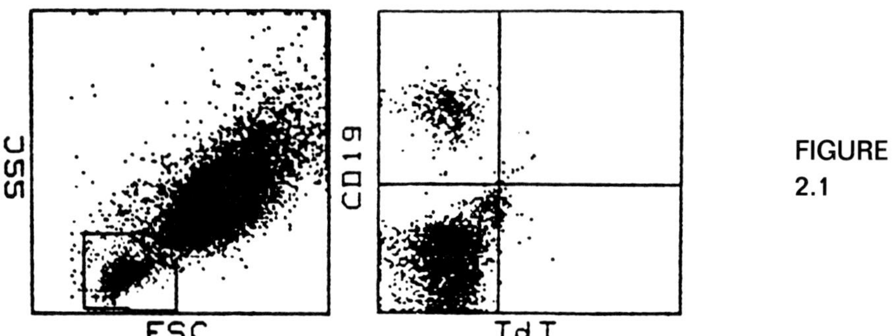

FIGURE
2.1

Immunophenotypic studies by immunofluorescence flow cytometry. Left, gating by optical light scatter: optical light scatter at 0° (forward scatter, FSC), a measure of cell size, on the horizontal axis and optical light scatter at 90° (side scatter, SSC), a measure of cell granularity, on the vertical axis. Gated cells, indicated by box, are small lymphocytes. Right, two color immunofluorescence analysis of gated cells for terminal deoxynucleotidyl transferase (TdT), on the horizontal axis, and CD19, a B cell antigen, on the vertical axis. CD19-positive B cells, in this case, are negative for TdT.

priate controls for nonspecific antibody binding ("isotype" controls) must always be included. The role of flow cytometry in the diagnosis of hematologic neoplasms has recently been reviewed (Jennings and Foon, 1997).

Monoclonal Antibodies

A large number of mouse monoclonal antibodies to human lymphoid antigens have become commercially available for use in immunophenotyping. Antibodies are available in purified form for immunohistochemistry or labeled with a fluorescent tag for immunofluorescence flow cytometry. Antibodies are designated by specificity using the CD (Cluster of Differentiation) nomenclature established by the International Workshop on Leukocyte Differentiation Antigens (Kishimoto et al, 1997; Kishimoto and Kikutani, 1997). At present, 190 antibodies to leucocyte differentiation antigens are recognized and classified by CD number; however, approximately 30 are used routinely for immunophenotyping. These are divided into T and NK cell antigens, B cell antigens, myeloid antigens, and nonlineage-specific antigens.

T and NK Cell Antigens

CD1a CD1a is an antigen expressed on immature (thymic) T cells at the "common" thymocyte stage of development and on dendritic cells of Langerhans' type. CD1a is not expressed on mature peripheral T cells. CD1a is positive in some cases of T cell lymphoblastic lymphoma and in Langerhans' cell histiocytosis.

CD2 CD2 is a leukocyte function antigen (LFA) which corresponds to the "E-rosette" receptor for sheep erythrocytes. CD2 is expressed on T cells and on some NK cells.

CD3 CD3 is an antigen which is expressed on polypeptides linked to the T cell antigen receptor complex. CD3 is expressed in the cytoplasm of immature T cells and on the cell surface of mature T cells. Polyclonal antibodies to CD3 are reactive with T cells in paraffin-embedded tissue and also stain NK cells.

CD4 CD4 is the T helper cell antigen, which is expressed on helper-inducer T cells. CD4 is coexpressed with CD8 on immature (thymic) T cells at the "common" thymocyte stage of T cell development. CD4 is also expressed on monocyte-macrophages and Langerhans' cells. CD4 is expressed on many peripheral T cell lymphomas and on most cutaneous T cell lymphomas. The CD4 molecule is a receptor for the human immunodeficiency virus (HIV).

CD5 CD5 is expressed on T cells and on a subset (approximately 20%) of mature peripheral B cells. The CD5-positive B cell subset is increased in autoimmune diseases and may be related to autoantibody production. CD5 is coexpressed with B cell antigens on the cells of some B cell neoplasms including B cell chronic lymphocytic leukemia, B cell small lymphocytic lymphoma, and mantle cell lymphoma.

CD7 CD7 is expressed on mature and immature T cells. CD7 is frequently deleted in peripheral T cell lymphomas and cutaneous T cell lymphomas. CD7 may also be absent in some benign cutaneous T lymphoid infiltrations.

CD8 CD8 is the T suppressor cell antigen which is expressed on cytotoxic-suppressor T cells. CD8 is coexpressed with CD4 on immature (thymic) T cells at the "common" thymocyte stage of T cell development. CD8 is also expressed on some NK cells. CD8 is positive on the cells of some peripheral T cell lymphomas and on the cells of large granular lymphocyte leukemia.

CD16 AND CD56 CD16 and CD56 are markers of NK cells and are also expressed on subsets of T cells. CD16 and CD56 are expressed on the cells of NK cell neoplasms and NK-like T cell lymphomas and on the cells of large granular lymphocyte leukemia.

CD57 CD57 is a marker of NK cells and is also expressed on subsets of T cells. CD57 (also known as Leu 7 or HNK-1) is frequently expressed on the cells of large granular lymphocyte leukemia. CD57-positive T cells are prominent in the nodules of nodular lymphocyte predominance Hodgkin's disease.

B Cell Antigens

CD19 CD19 is a B cell antigen which is expressed on mature and immature B cells. CD19 is expressed at the earliest stages of B cell development. CD19 is positive on virtually all B cell leukemias and lymphomas.

CD20 CD20 is a B cell antigen which is expressed on mature B cells. CD20 is positive on most B cell leukemias and lymphomas. An epitope of CD20 (L26) is reactive in paraffin embedded tissue.

CD21 CD21 is expressed on mature B cells and is the C3d complement receptor and is also the receptor for Epstein-Barr virus. CD21 is strongly expressed on follicular dendritic cells.

CD22 CD22 is expressed in the cytoplasm of immature B cells and on the cell surface of mature B cells. CD22 is strongly expressed on the cells of hairy cell leukemia and dimly expressed on the cells of chronic lymphocytic leukemia.

CD23 CD23 is a B cell activation antigen. It is expressed on the cells of B cell chronic lymphocytic leukemia and small lymphocytic lymphoma, but not on the cells of mantle cell lymphoma. It is therefore of value in the differential diagnosis of CD5-positive B cell neoplasms.

IMMUNOGLOBULINS Immunoglobulins are present at the pre-B cell stage of development as cytoplasmic μ chains and on mature B cells as cell surface IgM and/or IgD. Cell surface immunoglobulin is lost with plasma cell differentiation. Cell surface immunoglobulin is present on many B cell lymphomas and exhibits clonal light chain restriction. Plasma cells express cytoplasmic immunoglobulin.

Myeloid Antigens

CD11c CD11c is expressed on granulocytes and monocytes. It is also expressed on NK cells and the cells of hairy cell leukemia and some marginal-zone and monocytoid B cell lymphomas.

CD13 CD13 is expressed on mature granulocytes and monocytes. CD13 is positive on some myeloid leukemias and granulocytic sarcomas. It is also expressed on a subset of B cell chronic lymphocytic leukemia.

CD14 CD14 is expressed on monocyte-macrophages. CD14 is positive on the cells of monocytic leukemias and "true" histiocytic lymphomas. Langerhans' cells and Langerhans' cell histiocytosis also express CD14.

CD15 CD15 is a granulocyte antigen which is expressed on mature granulocytes. CD15 is also expressed on the Reed-Sternberg cells of classical Hodgkin's disease and on some peripheral T cell lymphomas.

CD33 CD33 is a granulocyte antigen which is expressed on immature granulocytes and monocytes. CD33 is positive on myeloid leukemias and granulocytic sarcomas.

Nonlineage-Specific Antigens

TERMINAL DEOXYNUCLEOTIDYL TRANSFERASE Terminal deoxynucleotidyl transferase (TdT) is a template-independent DNA polymerase expressed in precursor B and T lymphoid cells. TdT is a nuclear enzyme which is demonstrated by immunocytochemistry or by flow cytometry on fixed, permeabilized cells. TdT is expressed in precursor B and T cell neoplasms, including acute lymphocytic leukemia and lymphoblastic lymphoma. Some cases of acute granulocytic leukemia are also positive. TdT is not expressed in non-Hodgkin's lymphomas other than lymphoblastic lymphoma.

CD10 CD10 is the common acute lymphocytic leukemia antigen (CALLA). It is a neutral endopeptidase which is widely expressed on immature B cells, some immature T cells, follicular center B cells, and mature granulocytes. CD10 is positive on the cells of B lineage acute lymphocytic leukemia, some T cell lymphoblastic lymphomas, Burkitt's lymphoma, and follicular lymphomas.

HLA-DR HLA-DR is a class II histocompatibility antigen. It is expressed on mature and immature B cells, monocyte-macrophages, and activated T cells, but not on precursor T cells. It is expressed on B lineage acute lymphocytic leukemia and most non-Hodgkin's lymphomas.

CD25 CD25 is an antigen which corresponds to the α chain of the interleukin-2 (IL-2) receptor. CD25 is expressed on activated T cells, B cells, and macrophages. CD25 is expressed at high levels on the cells of adult T cell lymphoma/leukemia associated with the human T lymphocytotrophic virus (HTLV) and on the cells of hairy cell leukemia. It is also expressed on some peripheral T cell lymphomas, B cell lymphomas, and Hodgkin's disease (Strauchen and Breakstone, 1987).

CD30 CD30 is the lymphocyte activation antigen Ki-1. It is expressed on activated T cells, B cells, and macrophages. CD30 is strongly expressed on the Reed-Sternberg cells of classical Hodgkin's disease and on some non-Hodgkins lymphomas (anaplastic large cell lymphomas). CD30 belongs to the tumor necrosis factor (TNF) receptor family of proteins. An epitope of CD30 (BerH2) is reactive in paraffin-embedded tissue.

CD34 CD34 is the human progenitor cell antigen. It is expressed on hematopoietic stem cells, precursor B and T cells, and endothelial cells. CD34 is expressed on the cells of a subset of acute lymphocytic leukemia and acute granulocytic leukemia and on the cells of some lymphoblastic lymphomas and granulocytic sarcomas.

CD38 CD38 is an antigen that is expressed on precursor and activated T and B lymphocytes and on plasma cells. CD38 is frequently used as a marker for plasma cells, which are characteristically CD38-positive and CD45-negative.

CD45 CD45 is a group of proteins which constititute the leukocyte common antigen (LCA). CD45RB is the isoform commonly stained for which is expressed on most hematopoietic cells including B cells, T cells, monocyte-macrophages, and granulocytes, but not on nonhematopoietic cells. CD45 is useful in the differential diagnosis of malignant lymphoma versus nonhematopoietic neoplasms, particularly metastatic carcinoma and melanoma. Plasmacytomas and some large cell anaplastic lymphomas, however, may be CD45-negative. CD45 staining is also applicable to paraffin-embedded tissue.

Interpretation of Immunophenotypic Studies

Immunophenotypic studies are interpreted with regard to determination of lineage, determination of abnormal phenotypes, and determination of B cell clonality by light chain restriction.

Determination of Lineage

Lineage is determined by expression of one or more lineage-specific antigens. CD19, CD20, and CD22 define B cell lineage. Clonally restricted surface or cytoplasmic immunoglobulin is also a definitive B cell marker. CD2, CD3, CD5, and CD7 define T cell lineage. CD3 and CD7 are definitive T cell markers. (Polyclonal CD3 may also stain NK cells in paraffin-embedded tissue, vide infra.) CD5 is coexpressed on some B cell neoplasms (B cell chronic lymphocytic leukemia, B cell small lymphocytic lymphoma, and mantle cell lymphoma). CD2 and CD8 are frequently expressed on NK cells. Polyclonal CD3 may also stain NK cells in paraffin embedded tissue due to cytoplasmic expression of the ϵ chain of CD3. Definitive identification of NK cell lineage is often difficult since the NK-associated antigens CD16, CD56, and CD57 are also expressed on some T cells. NK cells, however, lack the T antigen receptor rearrangement.

Determination of Abnormal Phenotype

Demonstration of an abnormal lymphoid phenotype may aid in the diagnosis of malignant lymphoma. T cell lymphomas frequently demonstrate clonal deletion of one or more pan T cell antigens, most commonly CD7. Demonstration of an abnormal T cell phenotype is presumptive evidence of a clonal T cell proliferation; however, loss of CD7 may also be seen in some benign cutaneous T cell infiltrates. Loss of pan B cell antigens in a B cell lymphoma may correlate with poor prognosis (Spier et al, 1988).

Determination of B Cell Clonality by Light Chain Restriction

Determination of B cell clonality by light chain restriction is one of the most important applications of immunophenotyping. During B cell development, each B cell undergoes a unique rearrangement of the immunoglobulin heavy and light chain genes. As a result of this rearrangement each B cell produces either κ, or λ light chains but not both. In a monoclonal proliferation, in which all the cells are derived from a single clone, all of the lymphocytes will, therefore, produce either κ, or λ light chains but not both. This phenomenon is referred to as light chain restriction (Fig. 2.2). In a polyclonal proliferation, in contrast, in which the cells are derived from a number of different clones, both κ and λ light chains will be produced. Demonstration of light chain restriction is strong evidence of a clonal B cell lymphoproliferative disorder. There are some pitfalls to interpretation, however. Background or interstitial immunoglobulin may obscure cell surface staining in immunohistochemical preparations. Similarly, apparent staining of B cells for both κ and λ light chains may be due to nonspecific binding of immunoglobulin by Fc receptors which are expressed on B cells and B cell lymphomas. The cells of some B cell lymphoproliferative disorders (e.g., chronic lymphocytic leukemia and small lymphocytic lymphoma) express surface immunoglobulin only dimly; other B cell lymphomas (most commonly B large cell lymphomas) may not express surface immunoglobulin at all (Strauchen and Mandeli, 1991). In these cases demonstration of clonality by light chain restriction may not be possible. Similarly, normal follicular center B cells may not express immunoglobulin (Picker et al, 1987). In equivocal or immunoglobulin-negative cases, determination of clonality by immunoglobulin gene rearrangement studies may be necessary (Wu et al, 1990; Cossman et al, 1991).

Immunohistochemistry on Paraffin-Embedded Tissue

Immunohistochemistry on paraffin-embedded tissue is widely utilized since it permits the use of routinely processed tissue and the study of archival material. In recent years

FIGURE 2.2

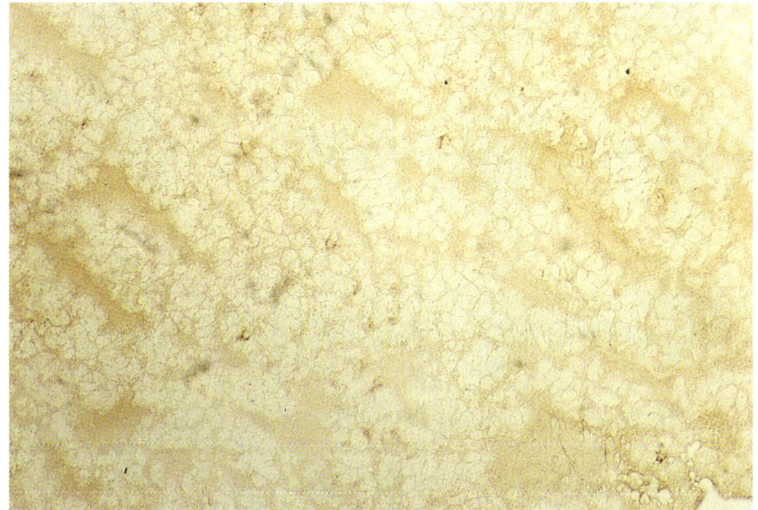

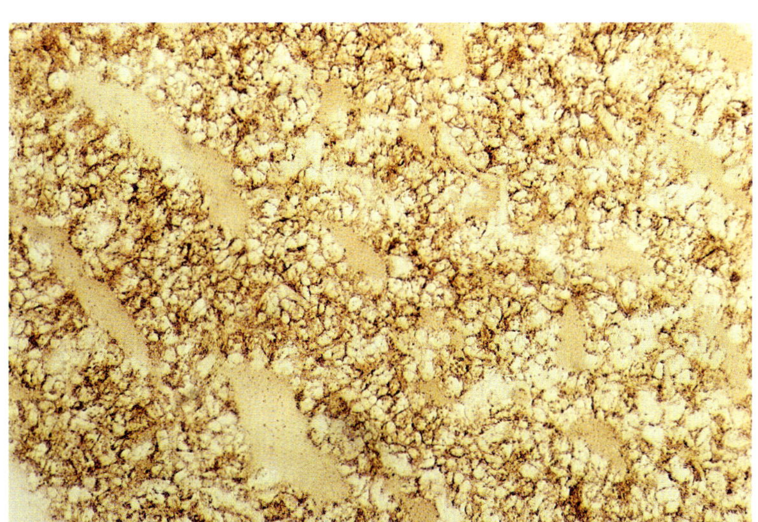

Determination of clonality by immunoglobulin light chain restriction. A. Frozen section of a B cell lymphoma stained for κ light chain. B. Frozen section of a B cell lymphoma stained for λ light chain. The demonstration of expression of single immunoglobulin light chain type indicates a monoclonal B cell proliferation.

a number of monoclonal antibodies to lymphoid antigens have become available which are suitable for use on paraffin-embedded tissue (Perkins and Kjeldsberg, 1993). In general, studies with these antibodies are less sensitive and specific than comparable studies on frozen tissue or cell suspensions and the inability to consistently stain surface immunoglobulin in paraffin-embedded tissue remains a major limitation. Nevertheless, studies on paraffin-embedded tissue can provide useful immunophenotypic information from routinely processed material. For some problems requiring detailed cytologic study (e.g., immunophenotyping of Hodgkin's disease or T-cell-rich B cell lymphomas) studies on paraffin-embedded tissue are preferred because of the improved histologic detail afforded by paraffin processing. For other problems requiring definitive determination of B cell clonality (e.g., evaluation of extranodal small lymphocytic proliferations) studies on paraffin-embedded tissue are less useful.

Antigens Detected in Paraffin-Embedded Tissue

T and NK Cell Antigens

CD3(P) Polyclonal antibodies to CD3 are reactive with T cells in paraffin-embedded tissue. Some NK cells and NK cell neoplasms also stain.

CD45RO Antibodies to CD45RO (UCHL1) detect a subset of T cells in paraffin-embedded tissue which correspond to "memory" T cells. CD45RO is expressed on the majority of peripheral T cell lymphomas. Some B cell lymphomas also stain.

CD43 CD43 (Leu 22, MT-1)) is widely distributed on T cells, granulocytes, and plasma cells but is not expressed on normal B cells. Antibodies to CD43 stain T cells in paraffin-embedded tissue and are particularly useful in the identification of some low-grade B cell lymphomas when only paraffin-embedded tissue is available. CD43 is expressed on CD5–positive B cell lymphomas (small lymphocytic lymphoma and mantle cell lymphoma) and on some cases of extranodal lymphomas of mucosa associated lymphoid tissue (MALT lymphomas), but not on normal or reactive B cells. Demonstration of CD43-positive B cells in paraffin-embedded tissue may, therefore, substitute for the demonstration of monoclonality by immunoglobulin light chain restriction in the diagnosis of some low grade B cell lymphomas. CD43 is not expressed on the B cells of follicular lymphomas, however, and CD43 is not useful in the differential diagnosis of follicular lymphoid proliferations. CD43 is also positive on the cells of almost all cases of granulocytic sarcoma.

CD57 Leu 7 stains CD57-positive NK cells and a subset of T cells in paraffin-embedded tissue.

B Cell Antigens

CD20 L26 stains an epitope of CD20 which is preserved in paraffin-embedded tissue. L26 is positive on most B cell non-Hodgkin's lymphomas and in nodular lymphocyte predominance Hodgkin's disease. L26 is a sensitive and specific antibody for B cells in paraffin-embedded tissue. Plasma cells and plasmacytomas are frequently negative, however.

CD45R 4KB5 stains an isoform of CD45 with restricted B cell expression, which is preserved in paraffin-embedded tissue. Most B cell non-Hodgkin's lymphomas are positive; occasional T cell non-Hodgkin's lymphomas are also positive.

CDw75 AND CD74 CDw75 and CD74 are antigens detected in paraffin-embedded tissue by the monoclonal antibodies LN1 and LN2, respectively. LN1 stains predominantly follicular center B lymphocytes; LN2 stains follicular center and other B lymphocytes. LN1 and LN2 are positive in most B cell non-Hodgkin's lymphomas; some T cell non-

Hodgkin's lymphomas also stain. LN2 stains the Reed-Sternberg cells in most cases of classical Hodgkin's disease.

CD79a CD79a is a component of the cell surface immunoglobulin antigen receptor complex, which is detected in paraffin-embedded tissue from most B cell neoplasms including B lineage acute lymphocytic leukemias and some plasmacytomas.

IMMUNOGLOBULINS Cell surface immunoglobulin is not consistently stained in paraffin-embedded tissue, a significant limitation compared with frozen tissue or cell suspensions. Predigestion of deparaffinized sections with trypsin has been reported to improve staining of cell surface immunoglobulin (Perkins and Kjeldsberg, 1993); however, determination of clonality by cell surface light chain restriction in paraffin-embedded tissue remains problematic. Cytoplasmic immunoglobulin, by contrast, is well stained in paraffin-embedded sections, permitting determination of clonality by light chain restriction of plasma cells, plasmacytomas, and some plasmacytoid lymphomas.

Myeloid Antigens

CD68 KP1 stains CD68, a granule-associated antigen preserved in paraffin-embedded tissue, which is expressed in granulocytes, monocyte-macrophages, and mast cells. KP1 stains the cells of some granulocytic leukemias, granulocytic sarcomas, Langerhans' cell histiocytosis, "true" histiocytic lymphoma, and mastocytosis.

MYELOPEROXIDASE Monoclonal antibodies to myeloperoxidase are the most sensitive and specific stain for granulocytes in paraffin-embedded tissue. The cells of most granulocytic leukemias and granulocytic sarcomas are stained.

LYSOZYME, α-1–ANTITRYPSIN, α-1–ANTICHYMOTRYPSIN Antibodies to these lysosomal enzymes stain granulocytes and monocyte-macrophages in paraffin-embedded tissue.

CD15 Leu M1 stains CD15, an antigen expressed in mature granulocytes, which is also expressed on the Reed-Sternberg cells of classical Hodgkin's disease, and on some peripheral T cell lymphomas. Reed-Sternberg cells exhibit characteristic membranous and Golgi staining for CD15.

Nonlineage-Specific Antigens

CD45RB Leukocyte common antigen (LCA) is recognized in paraffin-embedded tissues by antibodies to the CD45RB isoform. The great majority of non-Hodgkin's lymphomas of B and T cell types are stained. Anaplastic large cell lymphomas and plasmacytomas are frequently negative. The Reed-Sternberg cells of classical Hodgkin's disease are usually negative; however the "L&H" cells of nodular lymphocyte predominance Hodgkin's disease are positive. Staining in paraffin-embedded tissue is less sensitive than staining in frozen tissue or cell suspensions.

EMA Epithelial membrane antigen is expressed on epithelial and glandular cells, plasma cells, some anaplastic large cell lymphomas, and the "L&H" cells of nodular lymphocyte predominance Hodgkin's disease.

CD30   Epitopes of CD30 preserved in paraffin-embedded tissue are stained by the monoclonal antibody Ber H2. CD30 is an activation antigen expressed on activated T cells, B cells, and macrophages. Ber H2 also stains plasma cells. CD30 is positive on the Reed-Sternberg cells of classical Hodgkin's disease and on the cells of anaplastic large cell lymphomas. Amongst nonhematopoietic neoplasms, germ cell tumors and embryonal carcinomas are frequently positive, a potential source of diagnostic confusion.

BCL-2 ONCOPROTEIN   BCL-2 oncoprotein is overexpressed in follicular B cell lymphomas as a result of the t(14;18) chromosome translocation. BCL-2 is a mitochondrial "antiapoptosis" protein which is normally expressed in mantle B cells and other lymphoid cells. BCL-2 is not expressed in normal follicular centers and is therefore useful in the differential diagnosis of follicular lymphoma. BCL-2 is also positive in a variety of other non-Hodgkin's lymphomas. BCL-2 is stained in paraffin-embedded as well as frozen tissue. Normal positive-staining mantle cells are a convenient internal positive control.

BCL-1 ONCOPROTEIN   BCL-1 oncoprotein (PRAD-1, Cyclin D1) is overexpressed in mantle cell lymphomas as a result of the t(11;14) chromosome translocation. BCL-1 is a nuclear protein involved in regulation of the cell cycle. Expression of BCL-1 is specific for mantle cell lymphoma. BCL-1 is stained in paraffin-embedded as well as frozen tissue. Specific staining is nuclear.

Molecular Studies

Molecular studies have revolutionized hematopathologic diagnosis. Identification of lineage-specific antigen receptor gene rearrangements allows determination of B or T cell clonality at the molecular level using Southern blotting or polymerase chain reaction (PCR) techniques (Cossman et al, 1991; Sklar and Longtine, 1992). Identification of oncogene rearrangements, which correspond to specific chromosomal translocations, allows the molecular diagnosis of specific types of lymphoma and a molecular approach to lymphoma classification (Lo Coco et al, 1994; Hill et al, 1996). The two major molecular techniques which are utilized to identify gene rearrangements in DNA extracted from lymphoid lesions are Southern blotting and PCR.

Southern Blotting

Southern blotting is performed on high molecular weight DNA extracted from snap-frozen tissue or frozen cell suspensions. DNA may also be extracted from paraffin-embedded tissue, but degradation of the DNA is a major problem (Mies et al, 1991). The extracted, purified, high molecular weight DNA is digested with a restriction endonuclease, which breaks the DNA into fragments of characteristic length. For antigen receptor gene rearrangement analysis three endonucleases are typically studied: *Eco*RI, *Hind*III, and *Bam*HI. The restriction fragments are separated by electrophoresis in agarose gel and then transferred onto nitrocellulose or nylon membranes. The restriction fragments are then hybridized with a radiolabeled (phosphorus 32) or biotinylated DNA probe for the gene of interest. For antigen receptor gene rearrangement analysis, probes to the joining region of the immunoglobulin heavy chain gene (JH), the joining region of the

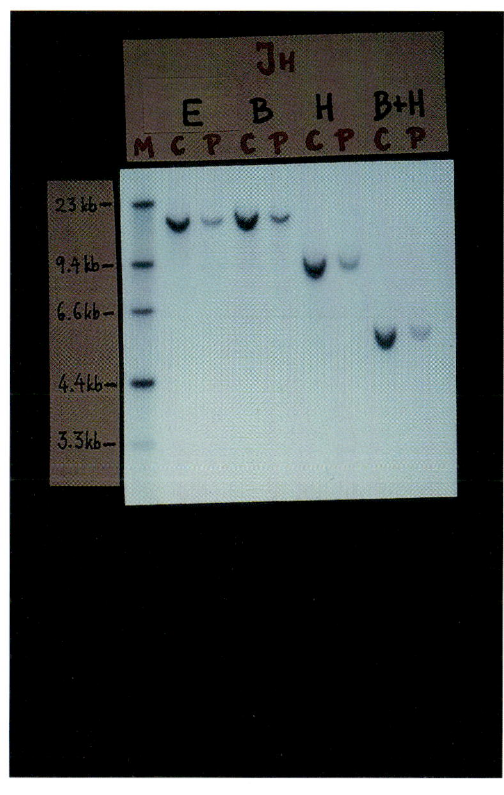

A

FIGURE 2.3

Immunoglobulin gene rearrangement study by Southern blotting with a probe to the joining region of the immunoglobulin heavy chain gene (JH). DNA size markers, at far left, are indicated by "M"; control lanes, consisting of placental DNA, are indicated by "C"; patient lanes by "P." Each pair of lanes corresponds to a different restriction endonuclease: *Eco*RI ("E"), *Bam*HI ("B"), *Hind*III ("H"), or a combination of *Bam*HI and *Hind*III ("B+H"). A. Polyclonal B cell proliferation, showing germline configuration of the JH gene. B. Monoclonal B cell proliferation, showing clonal rearrangement of the JH gene, indicated by the presence of rearranged bands in the patient lanes (P) compared to the control lanes (C).

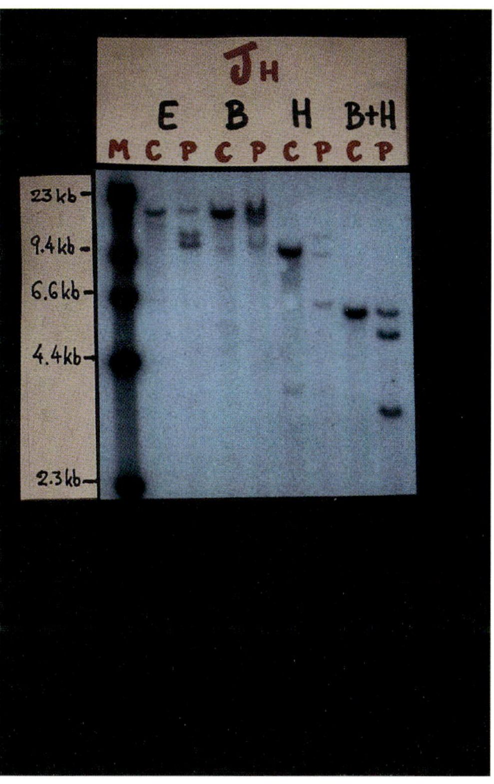

B

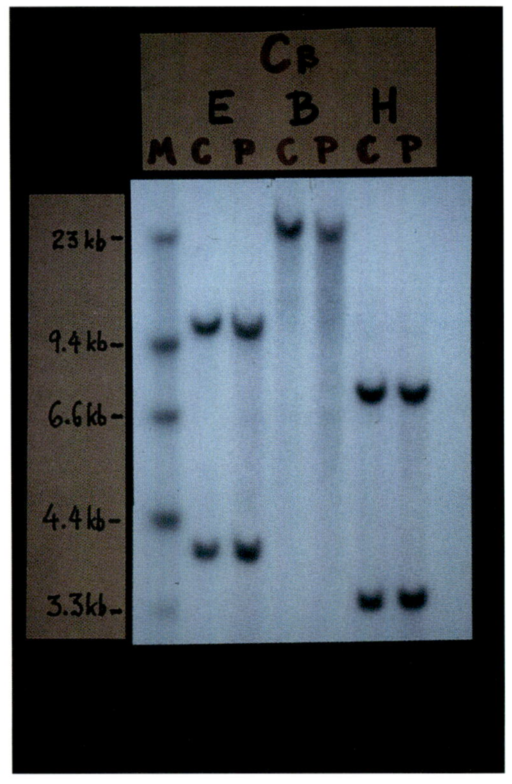

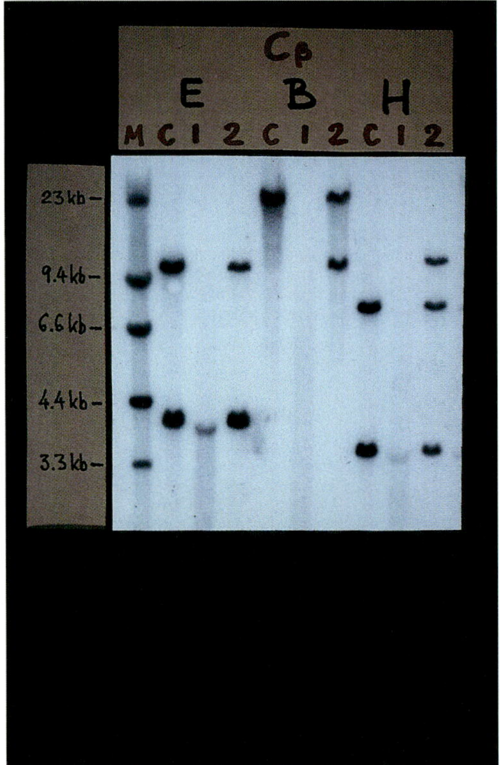

FIGURE 2.4

T cell antigen receptor rearrangement study by Southern blotting with a probe to the constant region of the T cell antigen receptor beta chain (CTBeta). DNA size markers, at far left, are indicated by "M"; control lanes, consisting of placental DNA, are indicated by "C"; patient lanes by "P" or numeral. Each pair of lanes corresponds to a different restriction endonuclease: *Eco*RI ("E"), *Bam*HI ("B"), or *Hind*III ("H"). A. Polyclonal T cell proliferation, showing germline configuration of the CTBeta gene. B. Monoclonal T cell proliferation, showing clonal rearrangement of the CTBeta gene, indicated by the presence of rearranged bands in the patient lanes "2," compared to the control lane (C).

kappa light chain gene (JK), and the constant region of the β chain of the T cell antigen receptor (CTBeta) are commonly used (Figs. 2.3 and 2.4). Following hybridization and washing to remove unhybridized probe, the membranes are developed by autoradiography on X-ray film for radiolabeled probe or by avidin-biotin for biotinylated probe. The result is a radioautograph showing one or more bands indicating the position of the gene of interest on the restriction fragments. A control of placental DNA is run on each gel to indicate the position of the germline configuration of the gene. A gene rearrangement is indicated by the presence of rearranged bands, not detected in the placental (germline) DNA. For antigen receptor gene rearrangements, formal criteria have been established (Cossman et al, 1991). The presence of one rearranged band with two or more restriction enzymes, or the presence of two rearranged bands with one restriction enzyme, is considered a positive result. Care must be taken not to interpret partial digest bands (due to incomplete digestion with the restriction endonuclease) as rearrangements. Partial digest bands occur at predictable locations. (A partial digest band of 8.5 kb is commonly seen in *Eco*RI digests with the CTBeta probe.) The presence of a partial digest band can be confirmed by disappearance of the band with more prolonged incubation.

Polymerase Chain Reaction

PCR is a technique for amplifying small segments of DNA. The major advantages are speed (the procedure can be completed in 1–2 days as opposed to Southern blotting which can take 7–10 days), the small quantity of DNA required (allowing use of DNA extracted from paraffin blocks and archival material), and extreme sensitivity (allowing detection of minimal numbers of positive cells). The PCR reaction employs a pair of DNA primers which bracket the segment of DNA to be amplified and a thermally resistant DNA polymerase (Taq polymerase). The reaction is carried out by repetitively heating and cooling the reactants, allowing amplification to proceed. For detection of gene rearrangements, primers are selected such that a product is formed in the presence of a rearrangement of the gene of interest. The reaction products are analyzed by gel electrophoresis. The amount of DNA produced in the reaction is sufficiently great such that the reaction products can be visualized directly by ethidium bromide staining and viewing with ultraviolet light. Up to 90% of immunoglobulin gene rearrangements can be identified by PCR with selection of optimal primers (Medeiros and Weiss, 1994). Quantitative PCR techniques can detect as few as one rearranged genome in 200,000 normal cells (Roberts et al, 1997).

Antigen Receptor Gene Rearrangements

During development, B cells undergo rearrangement of the variable (V), diversity (D), joining (J), and constant (C) regions of the immunoglobulin heavy and light chain genes and T cells undergo rearrangement of the α-β and γ-δ T cell antigen receptor genes. These antigen receptor gene rearrangements result in the generation of immunologic diversity and the ability to produce a nearly unlimited number of immunoglobulin and T cell antigen receptor specificities from a finite number of antigen receptor genes. Additional diversity is generated by the enzyme terminal deoxynucleotidyl transferase

(TdT), a template-independent DNA polymerase expressed in precursor lymphoid cells, which adds bases to the ends of DNA at random. This phase of B and T cell development occurs in the absence of antigenic stimulation and is antigen independent. B cells undergo additional genetic modification as a result of somatic mutations during proliferation in the follicular centers. This phase of B cell development requires antigenic stimulation and is antigen dependent. The end result is a unique configuration of the V, D, J, and C regions of the immunoglobulin heavy and light chain genes in each B cell and a similarly unique configuration of the T cell antigen receptor α and β genes in each T cell (the T cell antigen receptor γ and δ genes having a more limited repertoire). The rearranged antigen receptor genes are a unique marker for each individual B and T cell and for clonal proliferations arising from it. Thus, detection of a clonal rearrangement of the immunoglobulin heavy or light chain genes, or of the T antigen receptor gene, in a lymphoid lesion, by Southern blotting or PCR, indicates the presence of a B or T cell monoclonal proliferation. In practice, clonal rearrangements of the immunoglobulin heavy and light chain genes or of the T cell antigen receptor genes are detected in greater than 90% of cases of lymphoproliferative disorders studied by Southern blotting (Cossman et al, 1991).

Gene rearrangement studies must, however, be interpreted with some caution and in light of the clinical and histopathologic findings. Antigen receptor gene rearrangements indicating the presence of clonal populations of B or T cells are regularly detected in a number of conditions which are not considered lymphoid malignancies (Medeiros and Weiss, 1994). For example, clonal T cell receptor rearrangements are regularly found in cases of lymphomatoid papulosis and pityriasis lichenoides et varioliformis acuta (Mucha-Haberman disease), clinically benign skin disorders (Weiss et al, 1986; Weiss et al 1987). Similarly, clonal immunoglobulin gene rearrangements, indicating the presence of monoclonal B cell populations, are frequently found in benign lymphoepithelial lesions (Fishleder et al, 1987). Thus, the strong correlation of monoclonality with malignancy at the phenotypic level breaks down at the genotypic level. The detection of clonal populations of lymphoid cells in these lesions may represent an oligoclonal immune response, as has been reported in cases of chronic Epstein–Barr virus (EBV) infection (Cossman et al, 1991) or true clonal proliferations with limited biological potential. The latter interpretation is consistent with the observation that cutaneous lymphoid hyperplasias containing clonal immunoglobulin gene rearrangements are more likely to progress to overt malignant lymphoma than hyperplasias lacking gene rearrangements (Wood et al, 1989). Conversely, bona fide malignant lymphomas may not exhibit clonal antigen receptor rearrangements (Kneba et al, 1991). These receptor rearrangement-negative lymphomas are high-grade lymphomas with poor prognosis and include precursor cell lymphomas, lymphomas of NK or "true" histiocytic type, and lymphomas with deletions of the antigen receptor genes. Gene rearrangement studies, therefore, must always be considered in relation to the clinical and histopathologic features.

Oncogene Rearrangements

Non-Hodgkin's lymphomas frequently contain nonrandom chromosomal translocations which result in rearrangements of specific oncogenes (Table 2.1). These oncogene re-

Table 2.1 Oncogene Rearrangements in Non-Hodgkins Lymphoma

Oncogene	Translocation	Non-Hodgkin's Lymphoma
C-MYC	t(8;14)	Burkitt's lymphoma
	t(8;22)	
	t(2;8)	
BCL-2	t(14;18)	Follicular lymphoma
		B large cell lymphoma
BCL-1	t(11;14)	Mantle cell lymphoma
BCL-6	t(3;x)	B large cell lymphoma
PAX-5	t(9;14)	Lymphoplasmacytoid lymphoma
NPM/ALK	t(2;5)	Anaplastic large cell lymphoma

arrangements are of both diagnostic and pathophysiologic interest. The oncogene rearrangements are specific to different types of lymphoma and activation of specific oncogenes may play a role in lymphomagenesis. The prototypical example is Burkitt's lymphoma, which is regularly associated with rearrangement of the C-MYC oncogene. The C-MYC rearrangement results from a t(8;14) chromosomal translocation in which the C-MYC gene is transposed from its usual location on chromosome 8 to a new location in juxtaposition to the immunoglobulin heavy chain gene on chromosome 14. Since the immunoglobulin heavy chain gene is activated in B lymphocytes, the juxtaposition results in B cell specific dysregulation and overexpression of C-MYC, a growth-promoting gene. A number of specific human lymphomas are now recognized to be associated with specific oncogenes, including C-MYC in Burkitt's and AIDS-related lymphomas, BCL-2 in follicular lymphomas and some B large cell lymphomas, BCL-1 in mantle cell lymphoma, BCL-6 in B large cell lymphomas, NPM/ALK in anaplastic large cell lymphomas, and, most recently, PAX-5 in lymphoplasmacytic lymphoma.

C-MYC

C-MYC rearrangements are detected in virtually all cases of Burkitt's lymphoma and in a high percentage of AIDS-related lymphomas (Ballerini et al, 1993). C-MYC rearrangements in Burkitt's lymphoma are associated with the t(8;14) chromosome translocation involving the immunoglobulin heavy chain gene and C-MYC; or, less frequently with the t(2;8) or t(8;22) chromosome translocations involving the immunoglobulin light chain genes and C-MYC.

BCL-2

BCL-2 rearrangements are detected in 85% of follicular lymphomas and 20% of diffuse large B cell lymphomas as a result of the t(14;18) chromosome translocation (Hill et al, 1996). The t(14;18) translocation places the BCL-2 gene in juxtaposition to the immunoglobulin heavy chain gene on chromosome 14 and results in dysregulation and overexpression of BCL-2. BCL-2 protein normally blocks apoptosis (programmed cell death); dysregulation of BCL-2 expression in follicular center B cells, therefore, results in "immortalization" of the cells. Demonstration of the BCL-2 rearrangement by Southern blotting or PCR, or demonstration of overexpression of BCL-2 protein in follicular center cells by immunohistochemistry, is helpful in the differential diagnosis of follicular lymphomas. BCL-2 expression in diffuse large B cell lymphomas has been associated with a poorer prognosis (Hill et al, 1996). Small numbers of cells with the BCL-2 rearrangement may be detected in the blood of apparently normal individuals by sensitive PCR techniques (Limpens et al, 1995).

BCL-1

BCL-1 rearrangements are detected in the majority of cases of mantle cell lymphoma. BCL-1 (also known as PRAD-1) is the gene for Cyclin D1, a protein involved in regulation of the cell cycle. In mantle cell lymphoma BCL-1 is rearranged as a result of the t(11;14) chromosome translocation. BCL-1 is transposed in juxtaposition to the immunoglobulin heavy chain gene on chromosome 14, resulting in overexpression of Cyclin D1. Demonstration of the BCL-1 rearrangement by Southern blotting or PCR, or demonstration of Cyclin D1 overexpression by immunohistochemistry is of value in the differential diagnosis of mantle cell lymphoma.

BCL-6

BCL-6 rearrangements are detected in 20–40% of cases of diffuse large B cell lymphomas and rarely in other B cell lymphomas (Lo Coco et al, 1994). BCL-6 rearrangements involve a breakpoint at chromosome 3q27. BCL-6 protein is normally expressed in follicular center B cells, suggesting a role in the follicular stage of B cell development (Chen et al, 1998). Large B cell lymphomas expressing BCL-6 are frequently extranodal, have a low incidence of bone marrow involvement and may have an improved prognosis (Offit et al, 1994).

PAX-5

PAX-5 rearrangements have recently been detected in association with the t(9;14) chromosome translocation which is found in 50% of cases of lymphoplasmacytoid lymphoma, a form of low-grade B cell lymphoma associated with plasmacytoid differentiation and paraprotein production (plasmacytoid small lymphocytic lymphoma). The PAX-5 rearrangement results in juxtaposition of the PAX-5 gene with the immunoglobulin heavy chain gene on chromosome 14. PAX-5 appears to encode a B-cell-specific transcription factor which is involved in the regulation of B cell proliferation and differentiation, and dysregulation of which may play a role in lymphomagenesis (Iada et al, 1996).

NPM/ALK

NPM/ALK is a fusion gene resulting from the t(2;5) translocation found in a high proportion of CD30-positive anaplastic large cell lymphomas of T and null cell type (Morris et al, 1994). NPM/ALK results from fusion of a nucleolar phosphoprotein gene (NPM) on chromosome 5 with a previously unrecognized protein kinase gene, now designated ALK (for anaplastic lymphoma kinase) on chromosome 2. The resultant fusion gene results in a hybrid protein with kinase activity, dysregulated expression of which in lymphoid cells may play a role in lymphomagenesis. Detection of the NPM/ALK rearrangement may have value in the differential diagnosis of anaplastic large cell lymphoma, since NPM/ALK appears not to be rearranged in related lymphoproliferative disorders, including Hodgkin's disease and cutaneous CD30–positive lymphoproliferative disorders (Wood et al, 1996).

REFERENCES

Ballerini P, Gatineau G, Gong J, Tarsi V, Saglio G, Knowles DM, Della-Favera R. Multiple genetic lesions in acquired immunodeficiency syndrome-related non-Hodgkin's lymphoma. Blood 81:166–176, 1993.

Chen W, Iida S, Louie DC, Dalla-Favera R, Chaganti RSK. Heterologous promotors fused to BCL6 by chromosomal translocations affecting band 3q27 cause its deregulated expression during B-cell differentiation. Blood 91:603–607, 1998.

Cossman J, Zehnbauer B, Garrett CT, Smith LJ, Williams M, Jaffe ES, Hanson LO, Love J. Gene rearrangements in the diagnosis of lymphoma/leukemia. Guidelines for use based on a multiinstitutional study. Am J Clin Pathol 95:347–354, 1991.

Fishleder A, Tubbs R, Hesse B, Levine H. Uniform detection of immunoglobulin-gene rearrangements in benign lymphoepithelial lesions. N Engl J Med 316:1118–1126, 1987.

Hill ME, MacLennan KA, Cunningham DC, Hudson BV, Burke M, Clarke P, Di Stefano F, Anderson Lee, Hudson GV, Mason D, Selby P, Linch DC. Prognostic significance of BCL-2 expression and bcl-2 major breakpoint region rearrangement in diffuse large cell non-Hodgkin's lymphoma: A British National Lymphoma Investigation Study. Blood 88:1046–1051, 1996.

Hsu SM, Raine L, Fanger H. Use of avidin-biotin-peroxidase complex (ABC) in immunoperoxidase techniques: A comparison between ABC and unlabelled antibody (PAP) procedures. J Histochem Cytochem 29:577–580, 1981.

Iada S, Rao PH, Nallasivam P, Hibshoosh H, Butler M, Louie DC, Dyomin V, Ohno H, Chaganti RSK, Dalla-Favera R. The t(9;14)(p13;q32) chromosome translocation associated with lymphoplasmacytoid lymphoma involve the PAX-5 gene. Blood 88:4110–4117, 1996.

Jennings CD, Foon KA. Recent advances in flow cytometry: Application to the diagnosis of hematologic malignancy. Blood 90:2863–2892, 1997.

Kishimoto T, Goyert S, Kikutani H, Mason D, Miyasaka M, Moretta L, et al. CD antigens 1996. Blood 89:3502, 1997.

Kishimoto T, Kikutani H (eds): Leukocyte Typing VI White cell differentiation antigens. New York, Garland, 1997.

Kneba M, Bolz I, Bergholz M, Batge R, Nauk M, Nitsche R, Krieger G. Clinical characteristics of high-grade lymphomas with immune genes in germline configuration. Cancer 67:603–609, 1991.

Limpens J, Stad R, Vos C, de Vlaam C, de Jong D, van Ommen G-JB, Schuuring E, Kluin PM. Lymphoma-associated translocation of t(14;18) in blood B cells of normal individuals. Blood 85:2528–2536, 1995.

Lo Coco F, Ye BH, Lista F, Corradini P, Offit K, Knowles DM, Chaganti RSK, Dalla-Favera R. Rearrangements of the BCL6 gene in diffuse large cell non-Hodgkin's lymphoma. Blood 83:1757–1759, 1994.

Medeiros LJ, Weiss LM. The utility of the polymerase chain reaction as a screening method for the detection of antigen receptor gene rearrangements. Hum Pathol 25:1261–1263, 1994.

Mies C. Molecular biological analysis of paraffin-embedded tissue. Hum Pathol 25:555–560, 1994.

Mies C, Houldsworth J, Chaganti RSK. Extraction of DNA from paraffin blocks for Southern blot analysis. Am J Surg Pathol 15:169–174, 1991.

Morris SW, Kirstein MN, Valentine MB, Dittmer KG, Shapiro DN, Saltman DL, Look AT. Fusion of a kinase gene, ALK, to a nucleolar protein gene, NPM, in non-Hodgkin's lymphoma. Science 263:1281–1284, 1994.

Offit K, Lo Coco F, Louie DC, Parsa NZ, Leung D, Portlock C, Bihui HY, Lista F, Filippa DA, Rosenbaum A, Ladanyi M, Jhanwar S, Dalla-Favera R, Chaganti RSK. Rearrangements of the bcl-6 gene as a prognostic marker in diffuse large-cell lymphoma. N Engl J Med 331:74–80, 1994.

Perkins SL, Kjeldsberg CR. Immunophenotyping of lymphomas and leukemias in paraffin-embedded tissues. Am J Clin Pathol 99:362–373, 1993.

Picker LJ, Weiss LM, Medeiros JJ, Wood GS, Warnke RA. Immunophenotypic criteria for the diagnosis of non-Hodgkin's lymphoma. Am J Pathol 128:181–201, 1987.

Roberts WM, Estrov Z, Ouspenskaia MV, Johnston DA, McClain KL, Zipf TF. Measurement of residual leukemia during remission in childhood acute lymphoblastic leukemia. N Engl J Med 336:317–323, 1997.

Sklar J, Longtine J. The clinical significance of antigen receptor gene rearrangements in lymphoid neoplasia. Cancer 70(suppl):1710–1718, 1992.

Spier CM, Grogan TM, Lippman SM, Slyman DJ, Rybak JA, Miller TP. The aberrancy of immunophenotype and immunoglobulin status as indicators of prognosis in B cell diffuse large cell lymphoma. Am J Pathol 133:118–126, 1988.

Strauchen JA, Breakstone BA. Il-2 receptor expression in human lymphoid lesions. Immunohistochemical study of 166 cases. Am J Pathol 126:506–512, 1987.

Strauchen JA, Mandeli JP. Immunoglobulin expression in B-cell lymphoma. Immunohistochemical study of 345 cases. Am J Clin Pathol 95:692–695, 1991.

Weiss LM, Wood GS, Trela MJ et al. Clonal T cell populations in lymphomatoid papulosis: Evidence for a lymphoproliferative etiology in a clinically benign disease. N Engl J Med 315:475–479, 1986.

Weiss LM, Wood GS, Ellisen L, et al. Clonal populations in pityriasis lichenoides et varioliformis acuta (Mucha-Haberman disease). Am J Pathol 126:417–421, 1987.

Wood GS, Ngan B-Y, Tung R, Hoffman TE, Abel EA, Hoppe RT, Warnke RA, Cleary ML, Sklar J. Clonal rearrangements of immunoglobulin genes and progression to B cell lymphoma in cutaneous lymphoid hyperplasia. Am J Pathol 135:13–19, 1989.

Wood GS, Hardman DL, Boni R, Dummer R, Kim Y-H, Smoller BR, Takeshita M, Kikuchi M, Burg G. Lack of the t(2;5) or other mutations resulting in expression of the anaplastic lymphoma kinase catalytic domain in CD30+ primary cutaneous lymphoproliferative disorders and Hodgkin's disease. Blood 88:1765–1770, 1996.

Wu AM, Winberg CD, Sheibani K, Colombero AM, Wallace RB, Rappaport H. Genotype and phenotype: A practical approach to the immunogenetic analysis of lymphoproliferative disorders. Hum Pathol 21:1132–1141, 1990.

3

The Normal Lymph Node

The lymph node is an integral component of the immune system. The lymph node facilitates the processing of antigens from lymph and the presentation of processed antigen to immunocompetent cells (T and B lymphocytes), which mediate the immune response. The lymph node is the major site of antigen-dependent lymphocyte proliferation and differentiation (Stewart and Schwartz, 1994).

The Immune System

The immune system consists of central and peripheral organs. The central organs (bone marrow and thymus) are the sites of antigen-independent proliferation and differentiation of immunocompetent cells (precursor T and B lymphocytes). The peripheral organs (lymph nodes, mucosa-associated lymphoid tissue, and spleen) are the sites of antigen-dependent proliferation and further differentiation of immunocompetent cells (T and B lymphocytes). T and B precursor cells develop from pluripotential hematopoietic stem cells in the bone marrow. T precursor cells migrate to the thymus where they undergo proliferation, differentiation, and selection under the influence of the thymic epithelium (Acuto and Reinherz, 1985). Two species of T cells are recognized. Alpha-beta T cells have rearranged α and β T cell receptor genes, express CD4 or CD8, are the predominant peripheral T cell population, and mediate most of the functions of cellular immunity. Gamma-delta T cells have rearranged γ and δ T cell receptor genes, are usually "double negative" for CD4 and CD8, account for a minor population of peripheral T cells, and have an unclear cytotoxic function. Gamma-delta T cells appear earlier in development than α-β T cells and may represent a more primitive T cell type. Immunocompetent T cells leave the thymus and migrate to the peripheral lymphoid organs where they take up residence in the paracortex of the lymph nodes and periarteriolar sheaths of the spleen. T cells proliferate in response to antigen presented on dendritic cells (interdigitating reticulum cells) and undergo transformation to T immunoblasts. T immunoblasts differentiate into effector T cells and long-lived recirculating memory T cells.

B cells, in contrast, undergo maturation in the bone marrow (Cooper, 1987). (In birds, the B or "bursal" lymphocytes undergo maturation in the bursa of Fabricius, a lympho-epithelial organ near the cloaca. In mammals, however, no bursal equivalent has been identified; the B cells mature in the bone marrow.) Immunocompetent B cells emerge from the bone marrow and migrate to the peripheral lymphoid organs where they take up residence in the primary follicles of the lymph nodes, mucosa-associated lymphoid tissue, and splenic white pulp. B cells undergo proliferation in response to antigen presented on dendritic cells (follicular dendritic cells) resulting in formation of secondary follicles containing follicular centers (or germinal centers). The function of the follicular center was, until recently, unknown. It is now evident that the follicular center is the major site of antigen-dependent B cell selection and "maturation" of the immune response (Stewart and Schwartz, 1994). The B cells, which have already undergone antigen-independent rearrangement of their immunoglobulin genes in the bone marrow, undergo additional somatic mutation at specific loci ("hot spots") in the hypervariable region of the immunoglobulin gene during antigen-dependent proliferation in the follicular center. This results in the generation of B cells with additional immunologic diversity and "fine tuning" of the B cell response. B cells producing antibody binding avidly to antigen are selected for; B cells producing less avid antibody are eliminated by apoptosis. Secondary immunoglobulin gene rearrangements may also occur (Han et al, 1997). The apoptotic debris is ingested by follicular center macrophages, becoming the familiar "tingible body macrophages" characteristic of reactive follicular centers. The transformed B cell emerges from the follicular center as a B immunoblast, the immediate precursor of the immunoglobulin-secreting plasma cell.

Lymph Node Architecture

Lymph nodes are ovoid encapsulated structures distributed at intervals along the lymphatic chains which accompany the vascular trunks (Fig. 3.1). Lymph flows into the lymph nodes via afferent lymphatics at the lymph node periphery and leaves the lymph node via the efferent lymphatics at the lymph node hilum, ultimately returning to the venous circulation through the thoracic duct. The lymph node contains specialized anatomic structures which facilitate the functions of the lymph node, including the processing of antigen, the presentation of antigen to immunocompetent cells, and the antigen-dependent proliferation and differentiation of immunocompetent cells. The functional compartments of the lymph node include the sinuses, the cortex, the paracortex, and the medulla. The functional compartments are organized by a supporting skeleton including the capsule, fibrous trabeculae, and hilum.

Sinuses

The sinuses of the lymph node consist of the subcapsular sinus, trabecular sinuses, and medullary sinuses. The sinuses conduct the lymph through the lymph node. The afferent lymphatics enter the lymph node at the subcapsular sinus (Fig. 3.2). The lymph flows through the subcapsular, trabecular, and medullary sinuses, leaving via the efferent lymphatics at the hilum. The sinuses contain phagocytic macrophages which remove and process antigen in the lymph for presentation to immunocompetent cells. The macrophages are also effector cells, phagocytosing and destroying microorganisms in the lymph. Plasma cells in the medullary cords secrete immunoglobulin into the medullary sinuses, resulting in opsonization of microorganisms in the lymph and facilitating phagocytosis. The lymph node sinuses are, likely, also the first line of defense against meta-

FIGURE 3.1

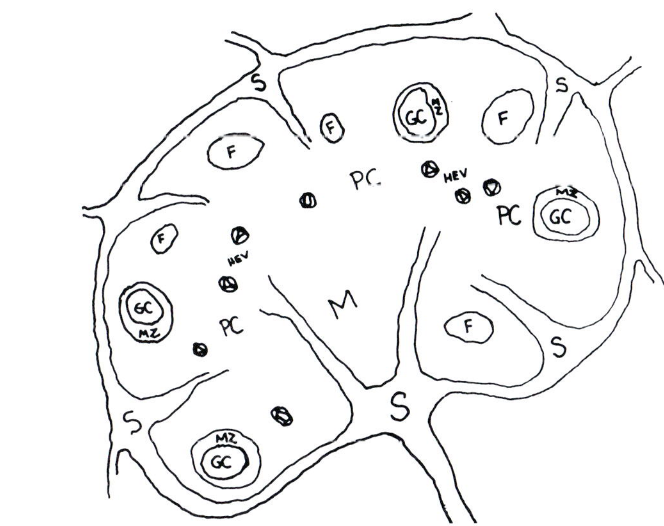

Schematic representation of lymph node architecture. S = sinus, PC = paracortex, M = medulla, F = follicle, GC = germinal center, MZ = mantle zone, HEV = high endothelial venule.

FIGURE 3.2

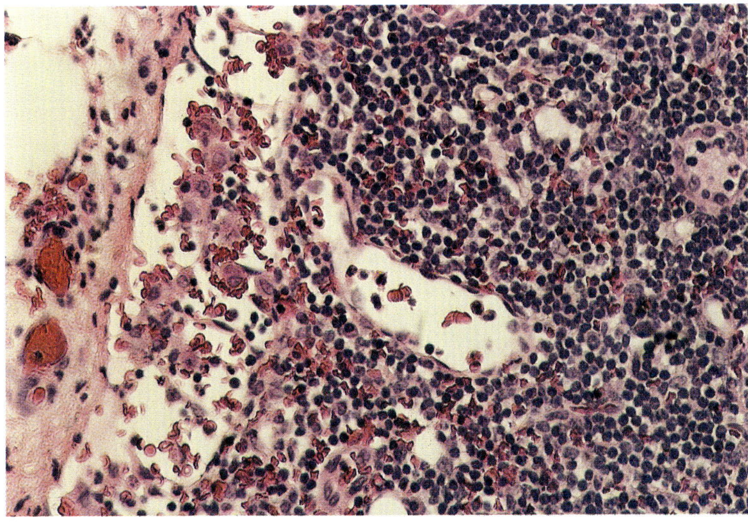

Subcapsular lymph node sinus containing sinus macrophages.

static tumor cells, as it has long been recognized that metastases to lymph nodes are usually first evident in the subcapsular sinus.

Cortex

The cortex of the lymph node includes the primary and secondary follicles. The cortex is the major site of B cell proliferation in the lymph node in response to antigen. The primary follicles are found in unstimulated lymph nodes and consist of rounded aggregates of darkly staining small B lymphocytes beneath the lymph node capsule (Fig. 3.3). Following antigen stimulation, secondary follicles appear in the lymph node (Fig. 3.4).

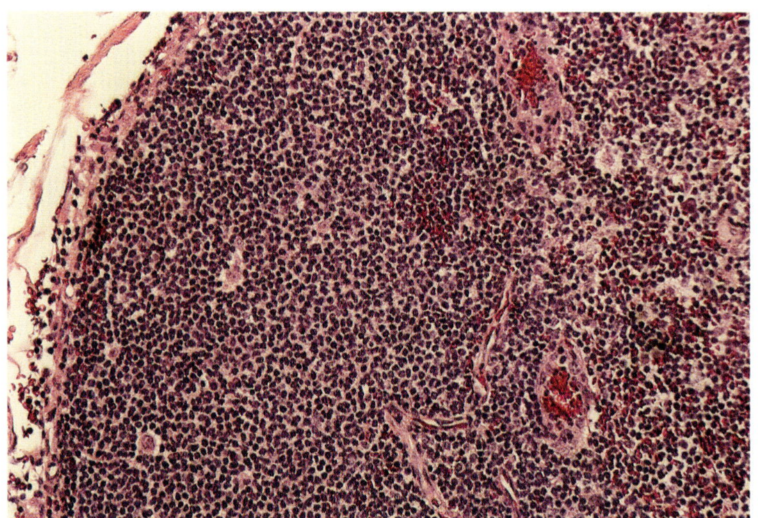

FIGURE 3.3

Primary B cell follicle.

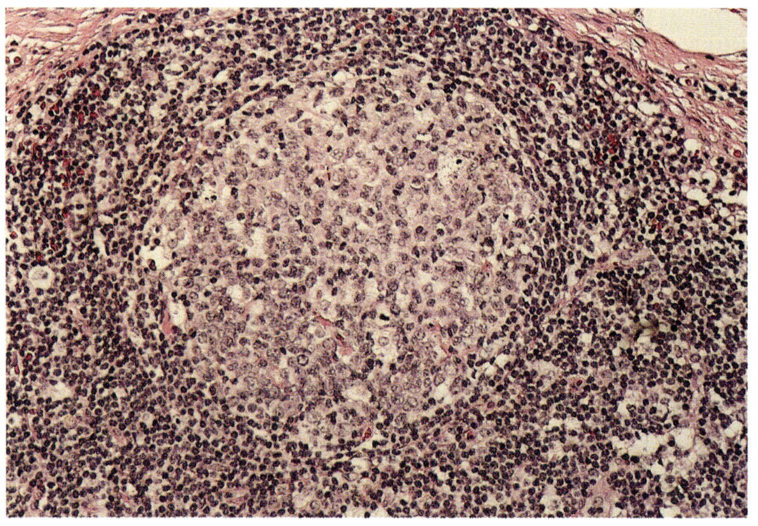

FIGURE 3.4

Secondary B cell follicle containing paler follicular center.

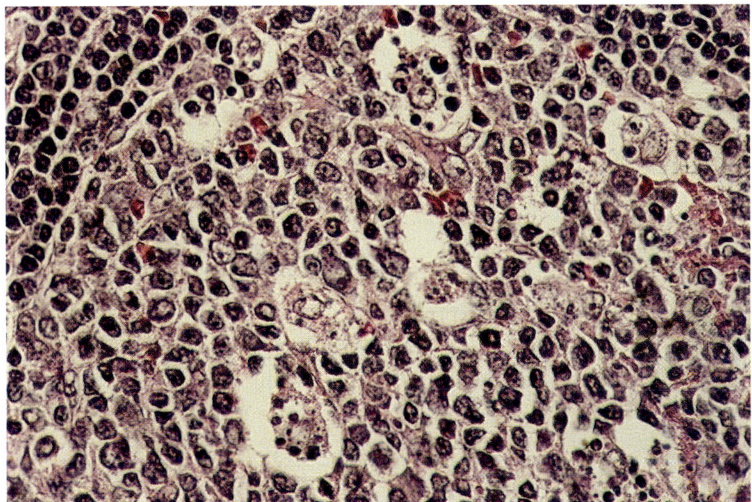

FIGURE
3.5

Follicular center containing large, transformed B cells undergoing antigen-dependent proliferation and "tingible body" macrophages. Phagocytosed material is derived from apoptotic follicular center cells.

These consist of a pale follicular center (germinal center), a darker mantle zone, and a lighter outer marginal zone. The follicular center is composed of transformed follicular B lymphocytes (follicular center cells), follicular dendritic cells, macrophages ("tingible body cells"), and helper T cells. The follicular center cells have a complex morphology, consisting of small and large cleaved cells and small and large noncleaved cells with numerous mitoses and abundant apoptotic debris. The latter is phagocytosed by follicular center macrophages ("tingible body cells") (Fig. 3.5). The follicular centers appear pale because of the large size and relatively abundant cytoplasm of the cells. The mantle zone is composed of the residual primary follicle and consists of a dark zone of small, slightly irregular lymphocytes which surround the follicular center. The marginal zone is difficult to appreciate in lymph nodes. but is readily observable in the splenic follicles, and consists of an outermost zone of slightly larger, paler lymphocytes (Fig. 3.6). The physiologic events occurring in the follicle are reflected in its morphology. The mantle zone consists of unstimulated, resting B lymphocytes. The follicular centers consist of large transformed B cells undergoing antigen-dependent proliferation, somatic mutation of the immunoglobulin variable region genes, and selection, in response to antigen presented on follicular dendritic cells. The B cells not selected for are lost by the process of apoptosis; the apoptotic fragments are ingested by follicular center macrophages, the so called "tingible body cells."

Paracortex

The paracortex is the major T cell domain in the lymph node and consists of the region between the follicles (interfollicular zone) (Fig. 3.7). The paracortex consists of T cells, dendritic cells of interdigitating reticulum and Langerhans' cell type, and the specialized vascular structures referred to as "high endothelial venules" or "postcapillary venules"

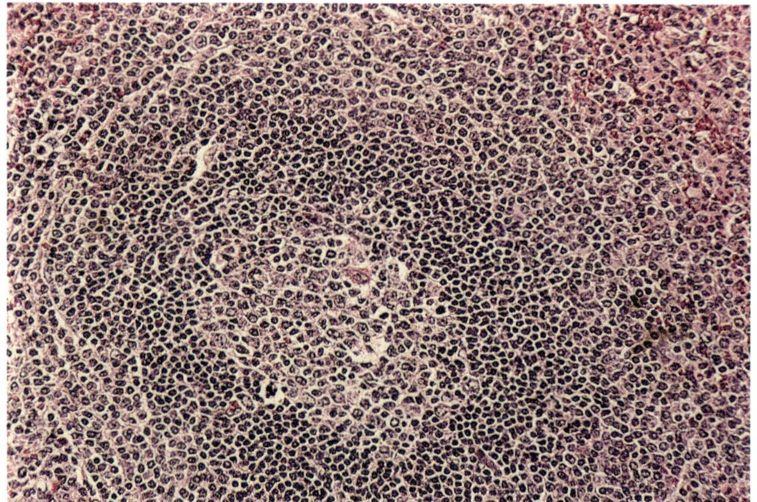

Splenic B cell follicle showing dark mantle zone and outer marginal zone composed of larger lymphocytes.

which contain specialized endothelial cells which permit the recognition and entry of peripheral blood lymphocytes into the lymph node (Fig 3.8). These specialized endothelial cells, which are recognized morphologically by their tall, cuboidal configuration, express a human peripheral lymph node vascular addressin which functions as a ligand for lymphocyte L-selectin, permitting selective recognition and entry of lymphocytes into the lymph node (Michie et al, 1993). Other addressins likely direct lymphocytes to mucosa-associated lymphoid tissue, skin, and other sites. The paracortex is the major site of antigen-dependent T cell proliferation in response to antigens presented on interdigitating reticulum cells. The latter cell is a type of dendritic cell closely associated with T lymphocytes. Activated T cells and T immunoblasts, and cells recruited by cytokines produced by activated T cells, including eosinophils and epithelioid histiocytes, are commonly found in the paracortex.

Medulla

The medulla of the lymph node consists of cords and sinuses, the latter in continuity with the trabecular and subcapsular sinuses. The cords of the medulla contain plasma cells and small B lymphocytes, the cord and sinus architecture facilitating immunoglobulin secretion.

Supporting Structures

The supporting structures of the lymph node consist of the lymph node capsule, fibrous trabeculae, and hilum. The capsule is a thin fibrous structure which surrounds and delimits the lymph node. The capsule is penetrated by the afferent lymphatics which enter the subcapsular sinus immediately beneath the capsule. The fibrous trabeculae are fibrous bands which extend from the capsule into the lymph node parenchyma and are

FIGURE
3.7

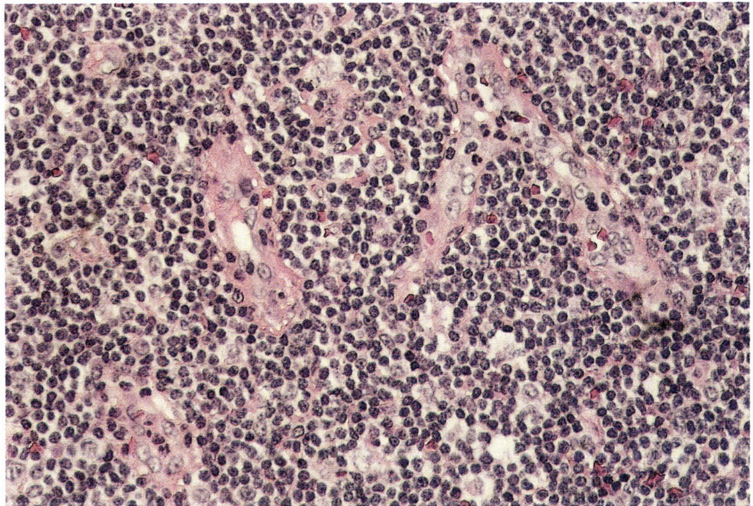

Paracortex contains T cells, interdigitating reticulum cells, and specialized high endothelial venules.

FIGURE
3.8

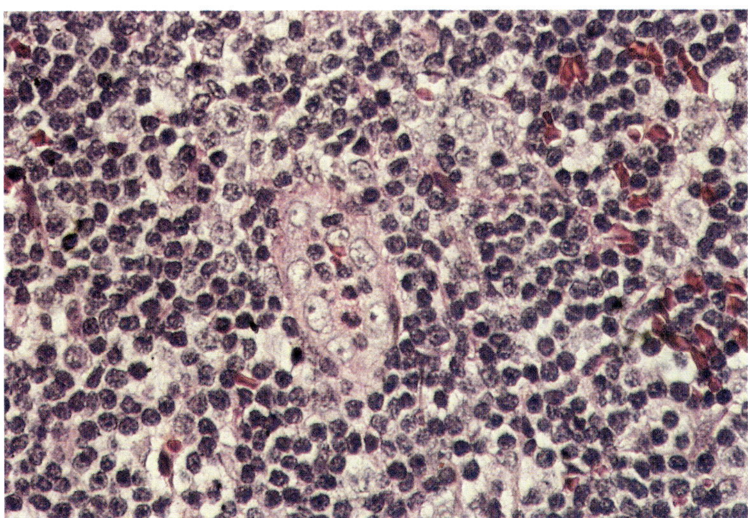

High endothelial venule contains specialized endothelial cells which express an addressin, human peripheral lymph node vascular addressin, which is the ligand for lymphocyte L-selectin, permitting selective entry of lymphocytes into the lymph node.

accompanied by the trabecular sinuses. The hilum of the lymph node contains the draining efferent lymphatics and major vascular structures. The lymph node stroma is composed of a network of supporting cells and reticulin fibers. The supporting stroma of the lymph node is difficult to appreciate in normal lymph nodes but becomes evident in lymph nodes depleted of lymphoid elements, as occurs in the advanced stages of HIV infection (Reichert et al, 1983).

Lymph Node Cells

Some of the types of cells which may be found in the normal lymph node have been mentioned above. The cell types found in the lymph node include B and T lymphocytes in varying stages of antigen-dependent proliferation, plasma cells, macrophages (sinus histiocytes and follicular macrophages or "tingible body cells"), dendritic cells (follicular dendritic cells, interdigitating reticulum cells, Langerhans' cells), and supporting cells (fibroblastic reticulum cells).

B Cells

The B cells of the lymph node consist of follicular B cells (follicular center cells, mantle cells, and marginal zone cells), monocytoid B cells, B immunoblasts, plasma cells and medullary B cells.

FOLLICULAR CENTER CELLS The follicular center cells consist of small and large cleaved cells (sometimes referred to as "centrocytes") and small and large noncleaved cells (referred to as "centroblasts"). Follicular center cells are transformed B lymphocytes, proliferating in response to antigen presented by follicular dendritic cells. Follicular center cells express pan B cell antigens (CD19, CD20, CD22), are positive for CD10, are negative for CD5, and are frequently negative for surface immunoglobulin. Immunoglobulin staining of follicular centers is often difficult to interpret because of extracellular interstitial immunoglobulin and immunoglobulin bound to the surface of follicular dendritic cells by Fc receptors.

MANTLE CELLS Mantle cells are small compact B cells distributed in a mantle or "corona" around the follicular center. Mantle cells express pan B cell antigens (CD19, CD20, CD22) and surface immunoglobulin and are negative for CD10. Mantle cells in adults are predominantly negative for CD5; however, mantle cell lymphomas, fetal mantle cells, and a subset of normal mantle cells express CD5 (Weisenberger and Armitage, 1996). Mantle cells are believed to be the precursor cells of follicular center cells and related to the immunologically "naive" cells of the primary lymphoid follicle.

MARGINAL ZONE CELLS Marginal zone cells are difficult to identify in normal lymph nodes but are readily identified in the spleen as a pale zone of slightly larger lymphocytes surrounding the mantle zone of splenic follicles. Marginal zone cells are larger and have more abundant cytoplasm than mantle cells. Marginal zone cells express pan B cell antigens and surface immunoglobulin and are negative for CD5 and CD10.

MONOCYTOID B CELLS Monocytoid B cells are seen in lymph nodes in some pathologic conditions, particularly toxoplasmic lymphadenitis and HIV infection (Sheibani et al, 1984). Monocytoid B cells are believed to be derived from the marginal zone. Monocytoid B cells have an ovoid or indented nucleus and abundant clear-to-eosinophilic cytoplasm and are found in the lymph node sinuses, frequently admixed with neutrophils. Monocytoid B cells express pan B cell antigens and surface immunoglobulin, are negative for CD5 and CD10, and are frequently positive for CD11c (Sheibani et al, 1988).

B IMMUNOBLASTS B immunoblasts are fully transformed B cells and the immediate precursors of plasma cells. B immunoblasts are large cells with prominent central nucleoli, abundant amphophilic cytoplasm, eccentric nucleus, and prominent Golgi zone. B immunoblasts are morphologically indistinguishable from "plasmablasts." B immunoblasts express pan B cell antigens (CD19, CD20, CD22) and may express cytoplasmic or cell surface immunoglobulin. B immunoblasts are believed to derive from follicular center cells and are found outside the follicles in the paracortex.

PLASMA CELLS Plasma cells are the terminally differentiated cells of the B cell lineage which secrete immunoglobulin. Plasma cells in the lymph nodes are found predominantly in the medullary cords but may also be found in the paracortex and follicular centers. Plasma cells are readily recognized by their characteristic morphology with eccentric nucleus, "cart wheel" chromatin, and prominent Golgi zone. Plasma cells lose their B cell markers and are negative for pan B cell antigens (CD19, CD20, CD22) and frequently for CD45. Plasma cells are negative for surface immunoglobulin but contain abundant cytoplasmic immunoglobulin which is readily detected by immunohistochemical staining in deparaffinized sections. Plasma cells are frequently positive for "secretory" antigens such as epithelial membrane antigen (EMA) and plasma cell antigens such as CD38 and PCA-1. Plasma cells are intensely pyroninophilic on staining with methyl green–pyronine due to high cytoplasmic content of ribonucleic acid.

MEDULLARY B CELLS Medullary B cells are the small B lymphocytes of the medullary cords. Medullary B cells express pan B cell antigens (CD19, CD20, CD22) and surface immunoglobulin.

T Cells

T cells are found predominantly in the paracortex of the lymph node and consist of both CD4 (helper-inducer) and CD8 (cytotoxic-suppressor) T cells. A population of T cells is also found in the follicular centers and consists preferentially of CD4 (helper-inducer) T cells which play a role in B cell differentiation. Paracortical T cells undergo antigen-dependent proliferation in response to antigens presented on interdigitating reticulum cells, a class of antigen presenting dendritic cell found in close association with T cells in the paracortex.

T IMMUNOBLASTS T immunoblasts are transformed T lymphocytes which are large cells with prominent nucleoli and abundant clear cytoplasm. T immunoblasts are found in the paracortex, frequently in association with cells recruited by cytokines produced by activated T cells, including eosinophils and epithelioid histiocytes, and vascular proliferation. T immunoblasts mature into effector T cells and memory T cells.

PLASMACYTOID T CELLS "Plasmacytoid T cells" are small mononuclear cells with ovoid nucleus and eccentric amphophilic cytoplasm which are found in clusters in the paracortex in some pathologic conditions (most prominently in Kikuchi's necrotizing lymphadenitis) (Fig. 3.9). Plasmacytoid T cells stain for some T cell associated antigens (CD4, CD43) but are strongly positive for CD68 and are now considered to be of myelomonocytic derivation (plasmacytoid monocytes).

Dendritic Cells

Dendritic cells are the antigen-presenting cells of the immune system (Hart, 1997). Dendritic cells in the lymph node consist of follicular dendritic cells (dendritic reticulum cells) found in the follicular centers which present antigen to B cells and interdigitating

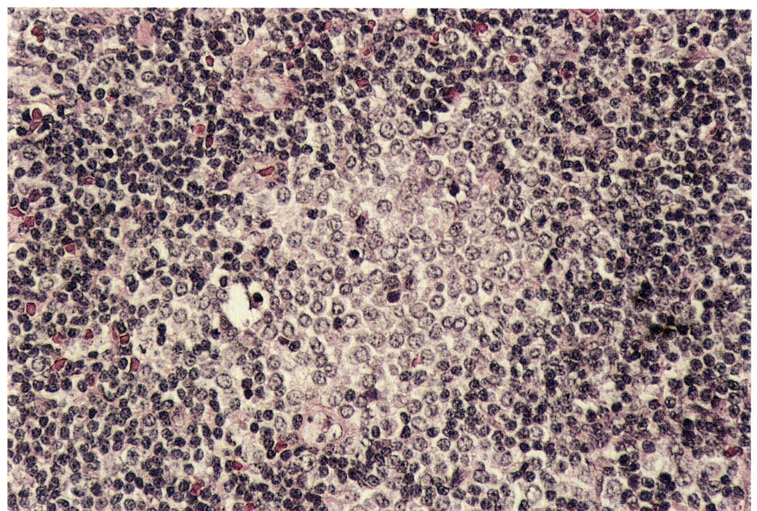

Plasmacytoid "T cells" (plasmacytoid monocytes) occur in clusters in the paracortex in reactive lymph nodes and express myelomonocytic markers.

reticulum cells and Langerhans' cells found in the paracortex which present antigen to T cells (Weiss et al, 1990). Dendritic cells are nonphagocytic, HLA-DR–positive, histiocyte-like cells (Van Voorhis et al, 1983). Dendritic cells are difficult to recognize morphologically in normal lymph nodes but are readily recognized immunologically and immunohistochemically. The derivation of dendritic cells was previously unsettled; however, dendritic cells appear to be bone marrow derived cells which share a common precursor with monocyte-macrophages (Santiago-Schwartz et al, 1994).

FOLLICULAR DENDRITIC CELLS   Follicular dendritic cells (dendritic reticulum cells) are the principal antigen presenting cells of the follicular center. Follicular dendritic cells are strongly positive for CD21 and CD35, which are the receptors for the C3d and C3b components of complement, respectively, and readily demonstrated in frozen or paraffin-embedded tissue, by immunohistochemistry, providing a sensitive and specific marker (Fig 3.10). Follicular dendritic cells have a characteristic ultrastructure with long, branching cell processes and desmosomal attachments.

INTERDIGITATING RETICULUM CELLS   Interdigitating reticulum cells are the principal antigen presenting cells of the paracortex. Interdigitating reticulum cells are negative for CD21 and CD35 but are positive for S-100 protein. Interdigitating reticulum cells are closely associated with T lymphocytes.

LANGERHANS' CELLS   Langerhans' cells are also found in the paracortex. Langerhans' cells are the principal antigen-presenting cells of the skin. Langerhans' cells resemble interdigitating reticulum cells and are also positive for S-100 protein but in addition are positive for CD1a and have characteristic Birbeck granules ultrastructurally. Langerhans' cells are increased in some pathological conditions, particularly dermatopathic lymphadenopathy.

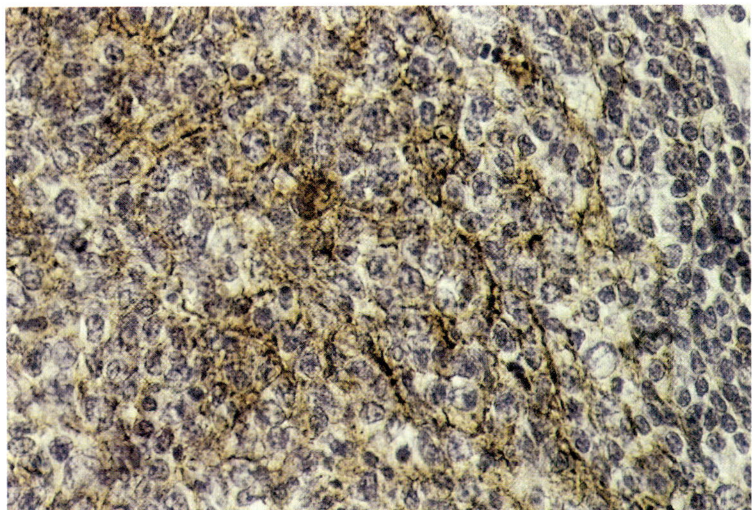

Follicular dendritic cells in a follicular center stained by monoclonal antibodies to CD21. Follicular dendritic cells are the principal antigen-presenting cells to B lymphocytes.

Macrophages

Macrophages are antigen processing cells. Macrophages are HLA-DR–positive and differ from dendritic cells in being actively phagocytic and rich in lysosomal enzymes (Van Voorhis et al, 1983). Macrophages phagocytose and destroy microorganisms and immunoglobulin-coated cells. In pathologic conditions, the interaction of CD4 helper T cells and macrophages leads to granuloma formation. The normal macrophages of the lymph node consist of the follicular center macrophages ("tingible body cells") and the sinus histiocytes. As noted previously plamacytoid T cells are also of myelomonocytic derivation (plasmacytoid monocytes).

FOLLICULAR CENTER MACROPHAGES   The follicular center macrophages ("tingible body cells") phagocytose apoptotic debris from proliferating follicular center cells and may also play a role in processing antigen for follicular B cells. The "tingible bodies" are apoptotic bodies derived from follicular center cells undergoing apoptosis. Follicular center macrophages are evident morphologically as large cells with abundant vacuolated cytoplasm containing phagocytosed basophilic debris ("tingible bodies"). At low magnification they may appear as "holes" in the follicular center because of their abundant vacuolated cytoplasm. Follicular center macrophages are positive for monocyte-macrophage antigens CD14 and CD68.

SINUS HISTIOCYTES   Sinus histiocytes are found within the subcapsular, trabecular, and medullary sinuses of the lymph node. The sinus histiocytes phagocytose and process antigen from lymph. Sinus histiocytes have abundant eosinophilic cytoplasm and delicate, round-to-ovoid vesicular nuclei. Sinus histiocytes are positive for the monocyte-macrophage antigens CD14 and CD68.

Supporting Cells

The supporting structure of the lymph node includes mesenchymal cells of the usual types (endothelial cells, fibroblasts) and fibroblastic reticulum cells, specialized fibroblast-like cells of uncertain function (Gould et al, 1995).

FIBROBLASTIC RETICULUM CELLS Fibroblastic reticulum cells are fibroblast-like cells which occur in the lymph node and are increased in reactive conditions, forming a network around follicles, sinuses, and vessels (Gould et al, 1995). Fibroblastic reticulum cells appear to play a role as supporting cells in the lymph node. Fibroblastic reticulum cells express vimentin, cytokeratins 8 and 18, and α smooth muscle actin (Gould et al, 1995). The presence of cytokeratin-positive cells in normal and reactive lymph nodes is a potential source of diagnostic confusion (Domagala et al, 1992).

REFERENCES

Acuto O, Reinherz EL. The human T-cell receptor. Structure and function. N Engl J Med 312:1100–1111, 1985.

Cooper MD. B lymphocytes. Normal development and function. N Engl J Med 317:1452–1456, 1987.

Domagala W, Bedner E, Chosia M, Weber K, Osborn M. Keratin-positive reticulum cells in fine needle aspirates and touch imprints of hyperplastic lymph nodes. A possible pitfall in the immunocytochemical diagnosis of metastatic carcinoma. Acta Cytol 36:241–245, 1992.

Gould VE, Bloom KJ, Franke WW, Warren WH, Moll R. Increased numbers of cytokeratin-positive interstitial reticulum cells (CIRC) in reactive, inflammatory and neoplastic lymphadenopathies: hyperplasia or induced expression. Virchows Arch 426:617–629, 1995.

Han S, Dillon SR, Zheng B, Shimoda M, Schlissel MS, Kelsoe G. V(D)J recombinase activity in a subset of germinal center B lymphocytes. Science 278:301–305, 1997.

Hart DNJ. Dendritic cells: Unique leukocyte populations which control the primary immune response. Blood 90:3245–3287, 1997.

Michie SA, Streeter PR, Bolt PA, Butcher EC, Picker LJ. The human peripheral lymph node vascular addressin. An inducible endothelial antigen involved in lymphocyte homing. Am J Pathol 143:1688–1698, 1993.

Reichert CM, O'Leary TJ, Levens DL, Simrell CR, Macher AM. Autopsy pathology in the acquired immune deficiency syndrome. Am J Pathol 112:357–382, 1983.

Santiago-Schwartz F, Coppock DL, Hindenburg AA, Kern J. Identification of a malignant counterpart of the monocyte-dendritic cell progenitor in acute myeloid leukemia. Blood 84:3054–3062, 1994.

Sheibani K, Fritz RM, Winberg CD, Burke JS, Rappaport H. "Monocytoid" cells in reactive follicular hyperplasia with and without multifocal histiocytic reactions: An immunohistochemical study of 21 cases including suspected cases of toxoplasmic lymphadenitis. Am J Clin Pathol 81:453–458, 1984.

Sheibani K, Burke JS, Swartz WG, Nademanee A, Winberg C. Monocytoid B cell lymphoma. Clinicopathologic study of 21 cases of a unique type of low-grade lymphoma. Cancer 62:1531–1538, 1988.

Stewart AK, Schwartz RS. Immunoglobulin V Regions and the B cell. Blood 83:1717–1730, 1994.

Van Voorhis WC, Witmer MD, Steinman RM. The phenotype of dendritic cells and macrophages. Fed Proc 42:3114–3118, 1983.

Weisenberger DD, Armitage JO. Mantle cell lymphoma—an entity comes of age. Blood 87:4483–4494, 1996.

Weiss LM, Berry GJ, Dorfman RF, Banks P, Kaiserling E, Curtis J, Rosai J, Warnke RA. Spindle cell neoplasms of lymph nodes of probable reticulum cell lineage. True reticulum cell sarcoma? Am J Surg Pathol 14:405–414, 1990.

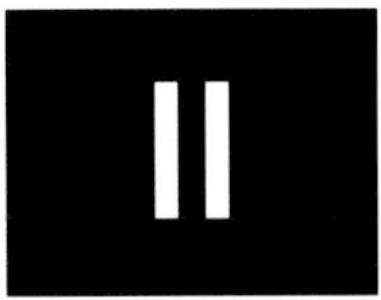

Reactive and Infectious Lymphadenopathies

4

Reactive Lymph Node Hyperplasia

General Features of Reactive Lymph Node Hyperplasia

Reactive hyperplasias of the lymph node result from expansion of one or more of the lymph node compartments by proliferation of lymphoid cells in response to antigenic or other stimulus. Reactive hyperplasias differ from the malignant lymphomas in being benign, self-limited responses to a physiologic stimulus rather than an autonomous proliferation; however, the nature of the stimulus in some cases may remain obscure. Reactive hyperplasias are, by definition, polyclonal lymphoid proliferations, in which different clones respond to a common stimulus. Some reactive hyperlasias are oligoclonal, as result of a restricted immune response, particularly in the setting of immunosuppression and/or Epstein-Barr virus infection. In general, reactive hyperplasias are polymorphous in appearance, reflecting the proliferation of a variety of cells, in contrast to the monomorphous appearance of many malignant lymphomas. Reactive hyperplasias are nondestructive proliferations in which the architecture of the lymph node is, in most cases, at least partially, preserved.

Diagnosis by Pattern

The pattern of reactive hyperplasia is frequently a clue to the likely etiology and a useful feature in differential diagnosis (Dorfman and Warnke, 1974) (Table 4.1). The pattern of reactive hyperplasia in lymph nodes varies with the nature of the stimulus. Antigens stimulating a predominantly B cell response result in follicular lymphoid hyperplasia. Antigens stimulating a predominantly T cell response result in paracortical (diffuse) hyperplasia. Materials stimulating a predominantly macrophage response (e.g., lymphangiogram contrast material) result in changes affecting the lymph node sinuses. In some cases, more than one pattern may be evident in a lymph node (e.g., follicular and paracortical hyperplasia); however, usually one pattern is predominant.

Table 4.1 Differential Diagnosis of Reactive Lymph Node Hyperplasias

Follicular Pattern
  HIV infection (follicular phase)
  Rheumatoid arthritis
  Syphilis
  Toxoplasmic lymphadenitis
  Castleman's disease
  Nonspecific follicular lymphoid hyperplasia
Diffuse Pattern
  HIV infection (involuted phase)
  Postvaccinial lymphadenopathy
  Viral lymphadenitis
  Infectious mononucleosis
  Drug-induced and hypersensitivity lymphadenopathy
  Dermatopathic lymphadenopathy
Sinus Patterns
  Lymphangiogram effect
  Sinus histiocytosis with massive lymphadenopathy
  Sinus hyperplasia
  Vascular transformation of lymph node sinuses

Follicular Patterns

Follicular patterns predominate in pathologic processes characterized by B cell proliferation. These include the early response to HIV infection (follicular phase of persistent generalized lymphadenopathy), rheumatoid arthritis, toxoplasmic lymphadenitis, luetic lymphadenitis, and Castleman's disease (angiofollicular lymph node hyperplasia).

Diffuse Patterns

Diffuse patterns result from paracortical expansion and predominate in processes characterized by T cell proliferation. These include postvaccinial lymphadenopathy, viral

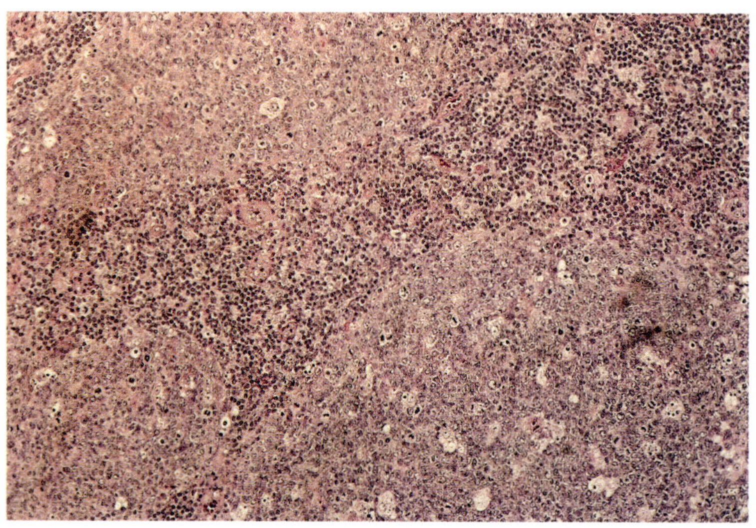

**FIGURE
4.1**

Follicular lymphoid hyperplasia showing increase in size and number of follicular centers.

lymphadenitis, infectious mononucleosis, drug-induced and hypersensitivity lymphadenopathy, and dermatopathic lymphadenopathy. The advanced stage of HIV infection (involuted phase of persistent generalized lymphadenopathy) may also present with a diffuse pattern.

Sinus Patterns

Sinus patterns result from pathologic processes affecting the sinus marophages. These
include lymphangiogram effect and sinus histiocytosis with massive lymphadenopathy
(Rosai-Dorfman disease). Vascular proliferations may also have a predominantly sinusoidal distribution, including vascular transformation of lymph node sinuses and Kaposi's
sarcoma.

Histopathology of Reactive Lymph Node Hyperplasia

Follicular Lymphoid Hyperplasia

In follicular lymphoid hyperplasia the follicles are increased in number and size with
numerous secondary follicles with prominent follicular centers (Fig. 4.1). In florid follicular lymphoid hyperplasia, follicles are found throughout the lymph node, in the medulla, and occasionally outside the lymph node capsule. The follicles in follicular
lymphoid hyperplasia exhibit considerable variation in size and shape, and unusual
"dumbbell"-shaped forms may be present (Fig. 4.2). In follicular lymphoid hyperplasia
associated with HIV infection (persistent generalized lymphadenopathy) the follicles are
particularly large and irregular with a geographic or "map-like" configuration. The hyperplastic follicular centers contain numerous mitoses and frequent "tingible body" macrophages, resulting from phagocytosis of apoptotic debris (Fig. 4.3). The follicles frequently demonstrate the phenomenon of "polarity," with light- and dark-staining zones

FIGURE
4.2

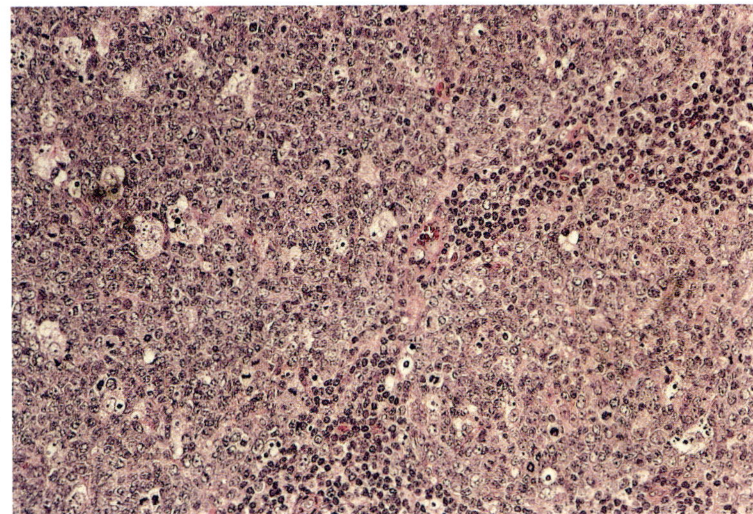

Follicular lymphoid hyperplasia showing variation in size and shape of
follicular centers.

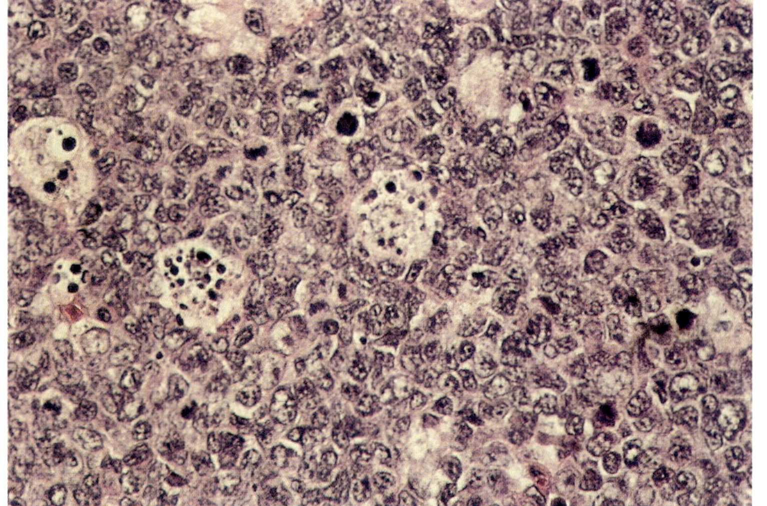

FIGURE 4.3

Follicular lymphoid hyperplasia showing follicular center with numerous mitoses and tingible body macrophages.

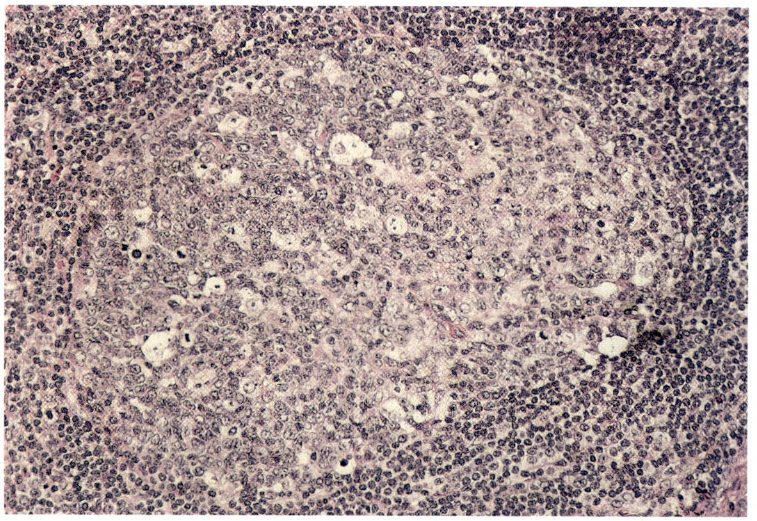

FIGURE 4.4

Follicular center exhibiting phenomenon of polarity with "light" and "dark" zones, due to segregation of pale staining "centrocytes" (small and large cleaved cells) from more darkly staining "centroblasts" (small and large noncleaved cells). "Light" zone is polarized toward the lymph node periphery.

at the opposite poles of the follicle (Fig. 4.4). Polarity is due to segregation of light staining "centrocytes" (small and large cleaved cells) from the more darkly staining "centroblasts" (small and large noncleaved cells) at opposite poles of the follicle. The follicles tend to be polarized with the light zone oriented toward the periphery of the lymph node. The mantle zone is also frequently thickened eccentrically, with the "bulge" toward the periphery of the lymph nodes. It is hypothesized that the polarization of the follicular center and mantle zone reflects the direction from which antigen is coming,

FIGURE
4.5

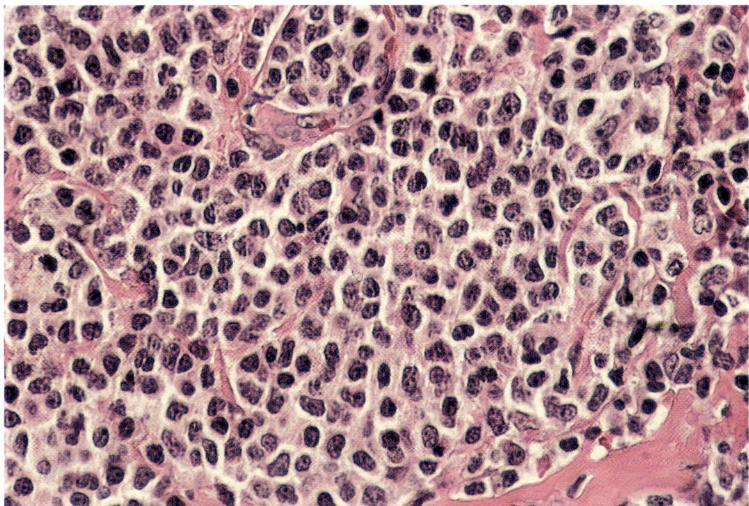

Hyperplasia of marginal zone cells (monocytoid B cells) frequently accompanies follicular lymphoid hyperplasia.

FIGURE
4.6

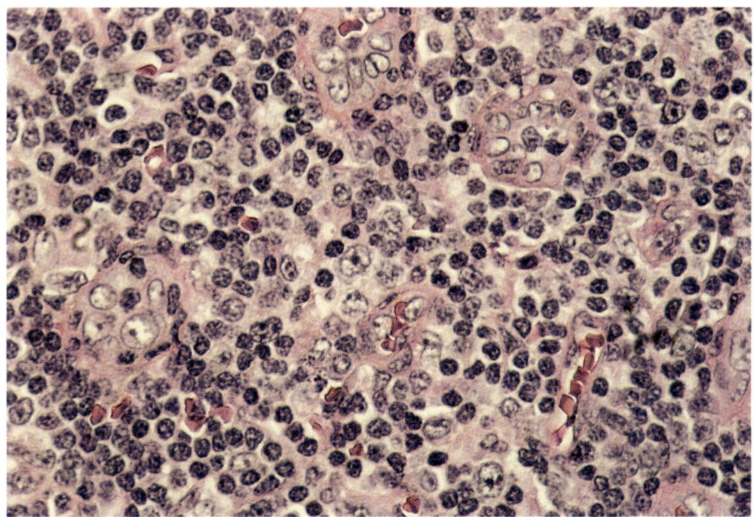

Paracortical lymphoid hyperplasia showing expansion of the paracortex by a mixed population of small and large lymphocytes and high endothelial venules.

usually the subcapsular sinus. In follicular lymphoid hyperplasia associated with HIV infection, the mantle zone may be thinned or absent, giving rise to "naked" follicular centers. Hyperplasia of marginal zone cells (monocytoid B cells) frequently accompanies follicular lymphoid hyperplasia (Fig. 4.5).

Paracortical (Diffuse) Lymphoid Hyperplasia

In paracortical (diffuse) lymphoid hyperplasia the paracortex (interfollicular zone) is expanded by proliferation of lymphocytes admixed with other cells including plasma cells, eosinophils, and histiocytes (Fig. 4.6). Immunoblasts, large transformed lymphocytes, are a frequent feature and when prominent give a "moth-eaten" or "mottled" appearance to the paracortex at low magnification (Figs. 4.7 and 4.8). Paracortical hyperplasia is frequently associated with vascular proliferation and high endothelial venules are often prominent.

Sinus Hyperplasia

Sinus hyperplasia (formerly sinus histiocytosis) is a common reaction pattern in lymph nodes removed for other reasons (e.g., lymph node dissections for cancer). The sinuses

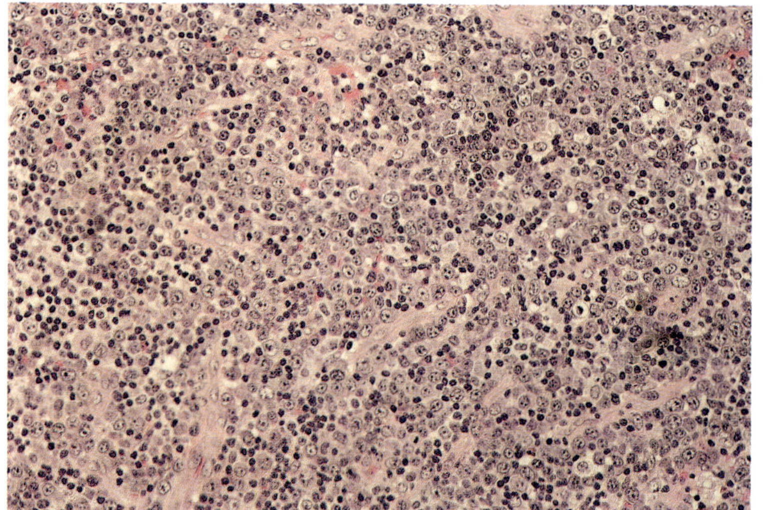

FIGURE 4.7

Paracortical lymphoid hyperplasia with numerous immunoblasts, resulting in a "moth-eaten" or "mottled" appearance of the paracortex at low magnification.

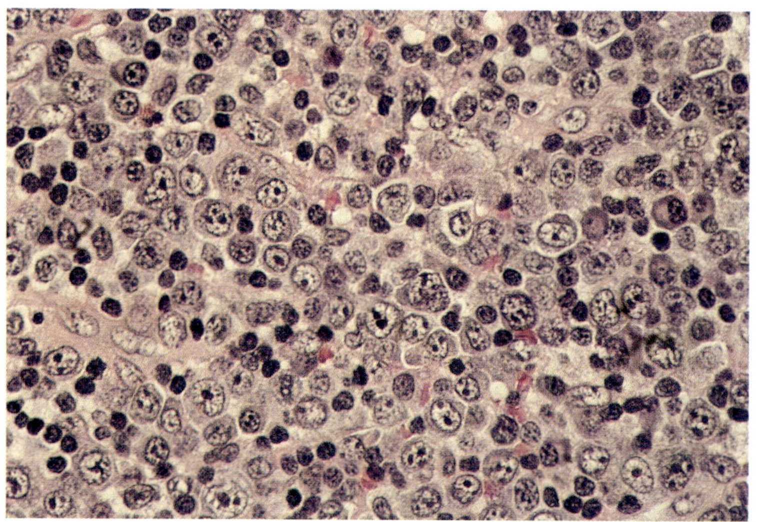

FIGURE 4.8

Paracortical lymphoid hyperplasia with numerous immunoblasts with prominent nucleoli and amphophilic cytoplasm.

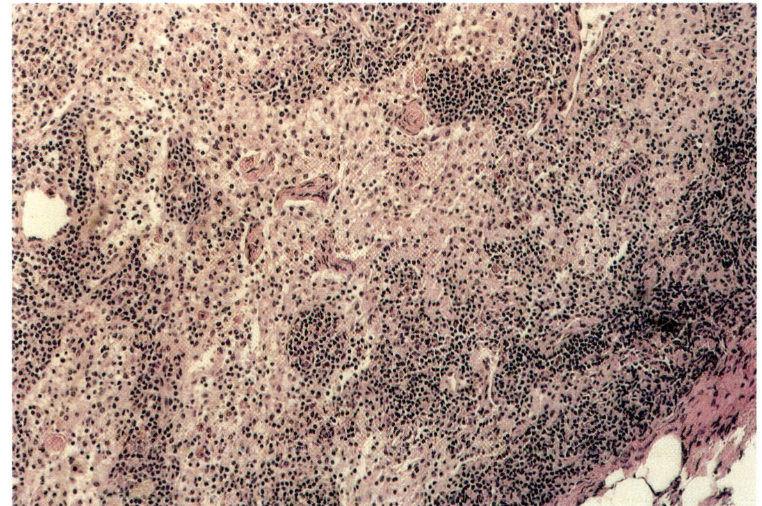

FIGURE 4.9

Sinus hyperplasia showing dilated sinuses filled with sinus histiocytes.

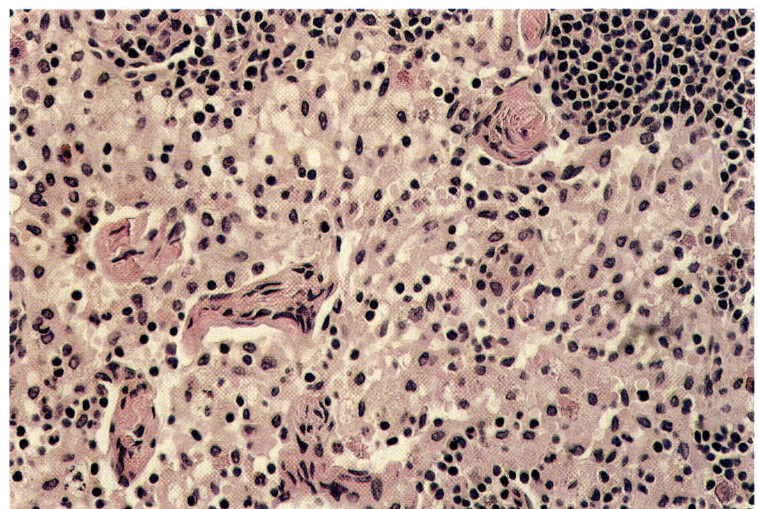

FIGURE 4.10

Sinus hyperplasia showing sinus histiocytes with cytologically bland nuclei and abundant pale eosinophilic cytoplasm.

are dilated and filled with bland-appearing sinus histiocytes (Figs. 4.9 and 4.10). Foreign material deposited in the lymph node sinuses also frequently elicits a macrophage response, as typified by lymphangiogram effect.

Nonspecific Reactive Lymph Node Hyperplasia

Enlarged lymph nodes removed at surgery will not infrequently show reactive lymph node hyperplasia for which no specific etiology is identified. The diagnosis of nonspecific reactive lymph node hyperplasia is then made. Typically the patient is young and presents with a single enlarged cervical lymph node. The lymph node may show any of the patterns described above; however, follicular lymphoid hyperplasia usually predominates. The relatively high frequency of cervical lymph node involvement suggests a possible role of oropharyngeal or viral upper respiratory infection. The course of nonspecific reactive lymph node hyperplasia is benign and self-limited and lymphadenopathy seldom recurs. It should be recalled that nonspecific changes in a superficial lymph node may be secondary to more significant pathology in deeper lymph nodes. Retroperitoneal or mediastinal lymphadenopathy is rarely due to nonspecific reactive lymph node hyperplasia.

Atypical Lymphoid Hyperplasia

Atypical lymphoid hyperplasia is not a disease entity but a diagnostic category applied to lymph nodes which show an atypical lymphoid proliferation, which shows some, but not all, of the features of malignant lymphoma. The proliferation may be of any of the patterns described above; however, diffuse lymphoid proliferations with prominent immunoblasts predominate. The application of immunophenotyping and molecular studies should minimize the number of cases in this category. The diagnosis of atypical lymphoid hyperplasia is a signal to the clinician that the eventual development of malignant lymphoma cannot be ruled out and that further workup, including biopsy of persistent or recurrent lymphadenopathy, is indicated. Of patients with lymph node biopsies showing atypical lymphoid hyperplasia, 20–40% will have a subsequent biopsy showing malignant lymphoma, usually within 1 year. Most of these cases are malignant lymphomas from the outset, in which the lymphoma cells are obscured by reactive hyperplasia or partial lymph node involvement. Rarely, however, such cases may represent examples of malignant lymphoma arising in a lymphoid hyperplasia (i.e., lymphoma-in-evolution).

REFERENCES

Dorfman RF, Warnke R. Lymphadenopathy simulating the malignant lymphomas. Hum Pathol 5:519–550, 1974.

5

Human Immunodeficiency Virus Infection and the Acquired Immunodeficiency Syndrome

Infection with the human immunodeficiency virus (HIV) cause a complex disorder resulting in the acquired immunodeficiency syndrome (AIDS). The lymph nodes are an important site of HIV replication and of the pathophysiologic events leading to immunodeficiency. The lymph nodes are also a major site of involvement of the opportunistic infections and neoplasms which characterize the acquired immunodeficiency syndrome.

General Features of HIV Infection

HIV infection is acquired from infected blood or secretions. Seroconversion to HIV is frequently accompanied by an acute retroviral syndrome with fever and lymphadenopathy, clinically resembling infectious mononucleosis (Cooper et al, 1985). Acute infection is characterized by a viremic phase with widespread dissemination of the virus to lymphoid tissue, followed by an immune response, and a latent, or asymptomatic interval, which may last up to 10 years (Fauci et al, 1996). Recent evidence indicates, however, that during this latent interval there is active replication of HIV in lymph nodes (Pantaleo et al, 1993). HIV infects cells by binding to the CD4 receptor. Several cell types within the lymph node are capable of being infected with HIV. These include CD4 T cells, monocyte-macrophages, Langerhans' cells, and follicular dendritic cells. The last cell type has emerged as an important reservoir of HIV which likely plays a major role in disseminating HIV to CD4 T cells (Fox et al, 1991). There is also evidence that HIV infects hematopoietic precursor cells in the bone marrow (Folks et al, 1988) and thymus (Stanley et al, 1993). As a result of these effects of HIV on T cells and T cell lymphopoiesis, eventually CD4 cell production can no longer keep up with CD4 cell destruction, and the phase of full-blown AIDS ensues, characterized by recurrent opportunistic infections and AIDS-related neoplasms.

The Syndrome of Persistent Generalized Lymphadenopathy

Persistent generalized lymphadenopathy (PGL) is a frequent manifestation of HIV infection and is a manifestation of HIV lymphadenitis (Metroka et al, 1983). Persistent generalized lymphadenopathy is defined clinically as lymph node enlargement exceeding 1.0 cm, at two or more noninguinal sites, and persisting for 3 or more months without other etiology. PGL is the clinical manifestation of HIV lymph node infection. HIV infects several cell types in the lymph node, including CD4 T cells, monocyte-macrophages, Langerhans' cells, and follicular dendritic cells. The follicular dendritic cell has emerged as the major reservoir of HIV in lymph nodes and plays a major role in the pathogenesis of PGL. PGL progresses histopathologically through phases of florid follicular lymphoid hyperplasia, follicular involution, and lymphoid depletion (Metroka et al, 1983). In the first phase, florid follicular lymphoid hyperplasia results from antigen-dependent follicular B cell proliferation induced by HIV trapped on follicular dendritic cells. In the second phase, follicular involution results from HIV-induced follicular dendritic cell injury and/or loss of helper T cells, the follicular lymphoid hyperplasia becoming unsustainable. In the third phase, lymphoid depletion results from the progressive depletion of T cells as the immune system is destroyed. The last phase is seen frequently at autopsy (Reichert et al, 1983).

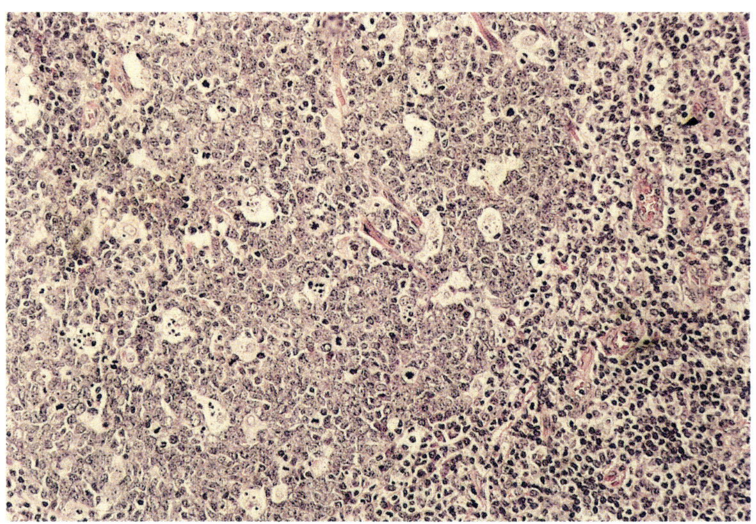

**FIGURE
5.1**

Persistent generalized lymphadenopathy showing a hyperplastic follicular center with numerous tingible body macrophages and an attenuated mantle zone, resulting in a so called "naked" follicular center.

Histopathology of Persistent Generalized Lymphadenopathy

Follicular Hyperplasia

The florid follicular hyperplasia phase of PGL is characterized by greatly expanded follicular centers with irregular, bizarre "map-like" or geographic shapes, a pattern aptly termed "explosive follicular hyperplasia" (Metroka et al, 1983). The follicular centers contain numerous mitoses and tingible body macrophages (Fig. 5.1). The mantle zones

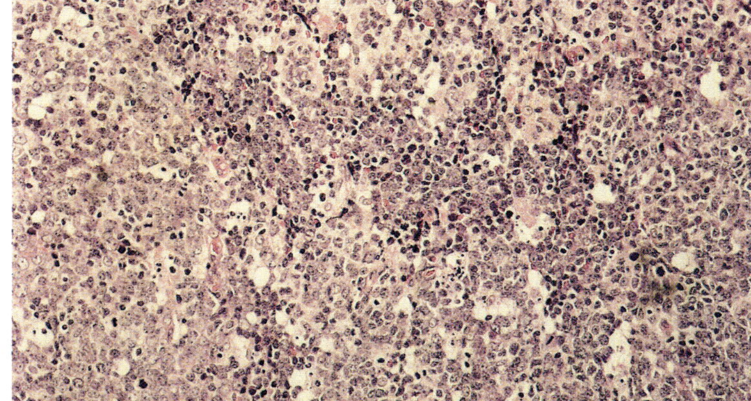

FIGURE 5.2

Persistent generalized lymphadenopathy showing folliculolysis. The follicular center is invaded by mantle-zone lymphocytes.

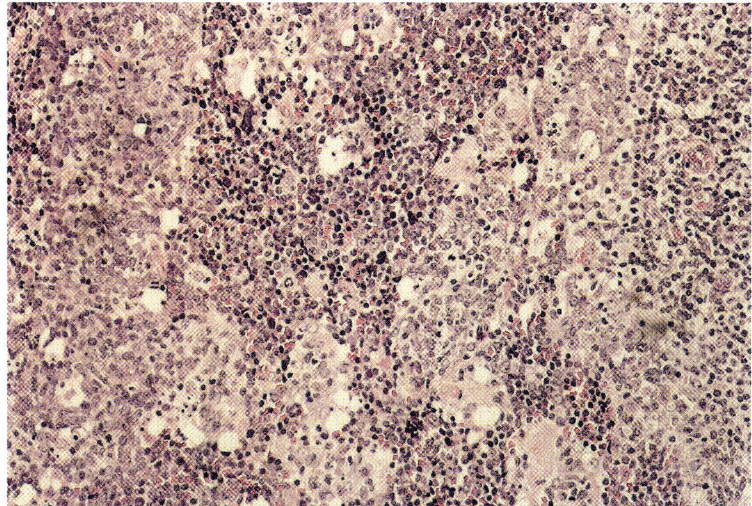

FIGURE 5.3

Persistent generalized lymphadenopathy showing folliculolysis with invasion and dissolution of the follicular center by mantle-zone lymphocytes.

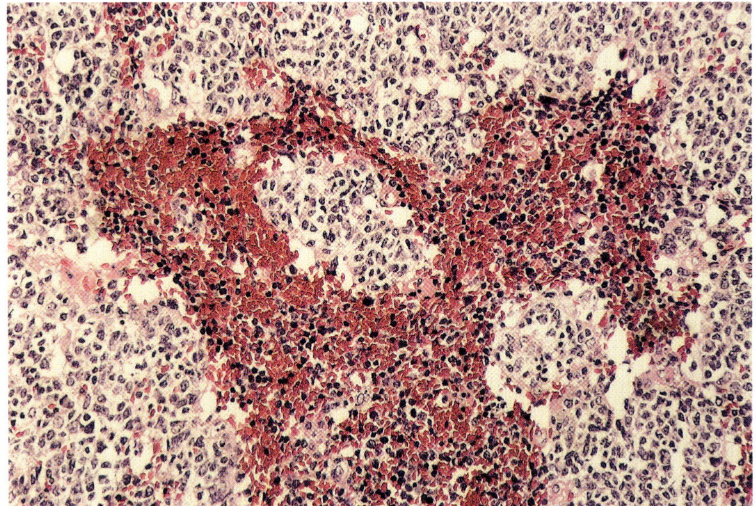

FIGURE 5.4

Persistent generalized lymphadenopathy showing folliculolysis with hemorrhage into the follicular center.

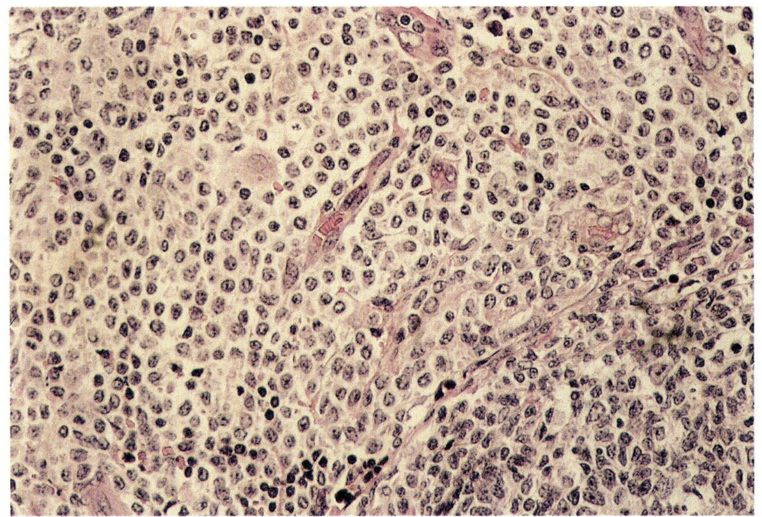

FIGURE 5.5

Persistent generalized lymphadenopathy showing clusters of monocytoid B cells in the sinuses.

are attenuated and frequently are found to invade and fragment the follicular centers, a phenomenon referred to as "folliculolysis" (Figs. 5.2 and 5.3). Folliculolysis may be associated with hemorrhage into the follicular centers (Fig 5.4). The lymph node sinuses frequently contain clusters of monocytoid B cells (reactive B lymphocytes with ovoid nuclei and abundant clear to eosinophilic cytoplasm) and neutrophils (Fig. 5.5). The paracortex contains variable numbers of endothelial cells, plasma cells, eosinophils, and immunoblasts (Fig. 5.6). Multinucleate giant cells, resembling the Warthin-Finkeldey cells of measles, may be present in the follicles or paracortex (Fig. 5.7). Immunohistochemical studies show expansion and disruption of the follicular dendritic cell network

FIGURE
5.6

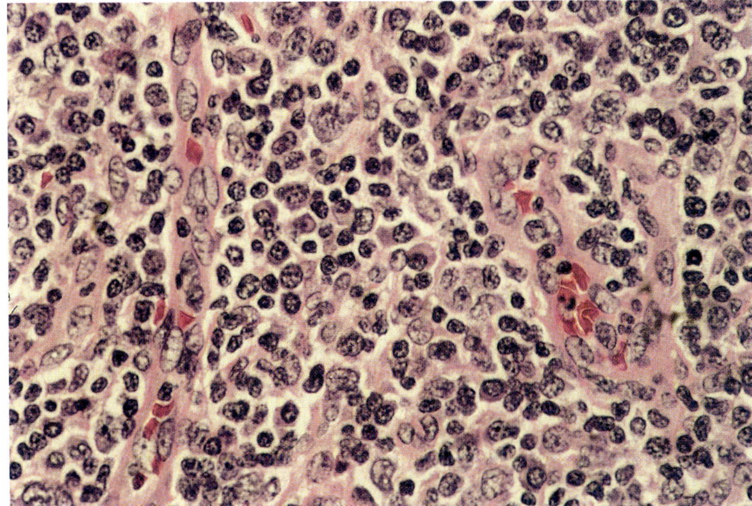

Persistent generalized lymphadenopathy showing paracortical vascular proliferation, lymphocytes, and plasma cells.

FIGURE
5.7

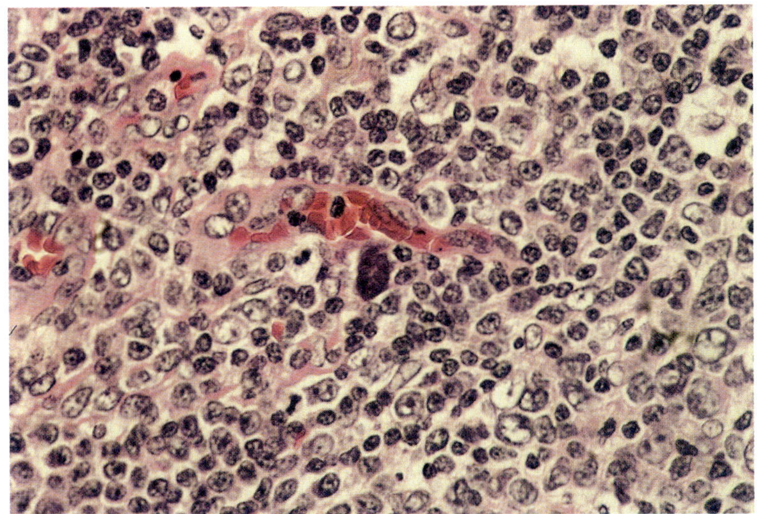

Persistent generalized lymphadenopathy showing a paracortical multinucleate giant cell.

(Piris et al, 1987). The ratio of CD4 to CD8 T cells in the lymph node is decreased and the decrease may precede the decrease in the peripheral blood (Raphael et al, 1985).

Follicular Involution

The follicular involution phase of PGL is characterized by follicles which are involuted and atrophic, resembling the hyalinized follicles of the hyaline-vascular form of Castleman's disease (Figs. 5.8 and 5.9). Follicular involution may be mixed with areas of residual follicular hyperplasia or may predominate in the lymph node (Metroka et al,

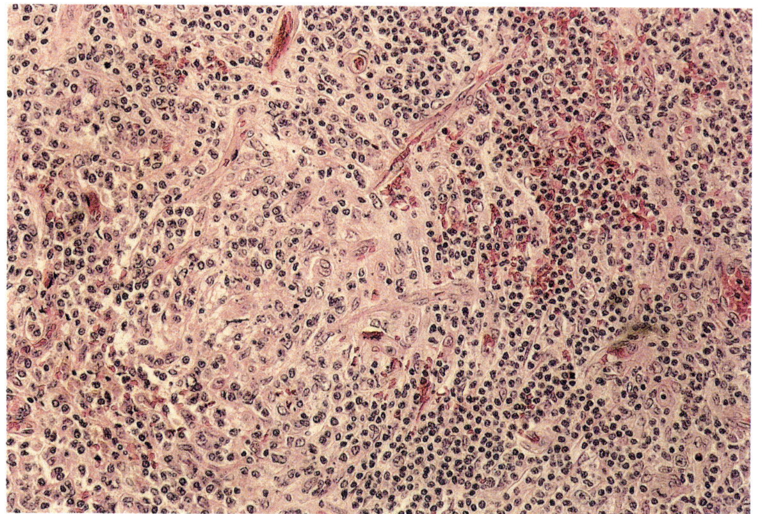

Persistent generalized lymphadenopathy showing follicular involution
with depletion of follicular center and vascular proliferation.

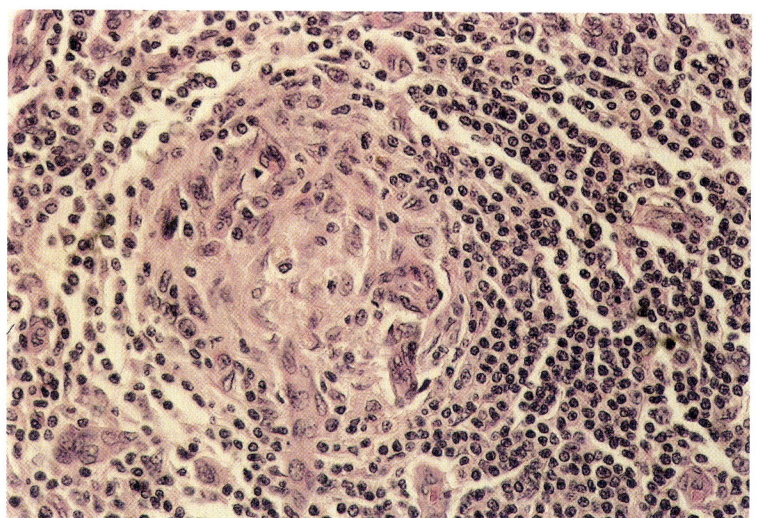

Persistent generalized lymphadenopathy showing follicular involution
with an atrophic, hyalinized follicular center, resembling the hyaline-
vascular form of Castleman's disease.

1983). The follicles in follicular involution are small and hypocellular, depleted of
lymphocytes, and consist of concentric rings of "naked" follicular dendritic cells and
hyaline material, surrounding a central blood vessel. The paracortex is expanded and
hypervascular, with numerous plasma cells, histiocytes, and immunoblasts. Warthin-
Finkeldey-like multinucleate giant cells may be present in the paracortex, resembling
the syncytia observed in cultured T cells infected with HIV (Popovic et al, 1984).

The histopathologic findings in the follicular involution phase of PGL may resemble
other disorders, including Castleman's disease and angioimmunoblastic lymphadenopa-

thy with dyspsroteinemia (AILD). The follicular involution phase of PGL may be morphologically indistinguishable from the multicentric form of Castleman's disease, and multicentric Castleman's disease has been reported in association with HIV infection (Lowenthal et al, 1987; Oksenhendler et al, 1996). Recent reports of Kaposi's sarcoma–associated herpesvirus (KSHV) DNA in both HIV-positive and HIV-negative cases of multicentric Castleman's disease suggest both forms may be related to KSHV (Soulier et al, 1995). The hypervascular paracortex and numerous immunoblasts and plasma cells in the follicular involution phase of PGL may resemble angioimmunoblastic lymphadenopathy with dysproteinemia (AILD).

Lymphoid Depletion

The lymphoid depletion phase of PGL is usually seen at autopsy (Reichert et al, 1983). The lymph nodes are small, depleted of lymphocytes, and consist of little more than "naked" stroma with fibrosis and vascular proliferation (Figs. 5.10 and 5.11). Scattered residual plasma cells and macrophages may be present. Erythrophagocytosis has been prominent in some autopsy cases (Reichert et al, 1983).

Differential Diagnosis of Persistent Generalized Lymphadenopathy

The follicular hyperplasia phase of PGL must be distinguished from follicular lymphoma and other causes of follicular lymphoid hyperplasia. Distinction from follicular lymphoma is usually not difficult. The extreme variation in follicular size and shape, folliculolysis, and prominent tingible body macrophages are not a feature of follicular lymphoma. Immunophenotypic studies for light chain restriction and BCL-2 oncoprotein expression will permit definitive distinction but should seldom be necessary. Needle

FIGURE 5.10

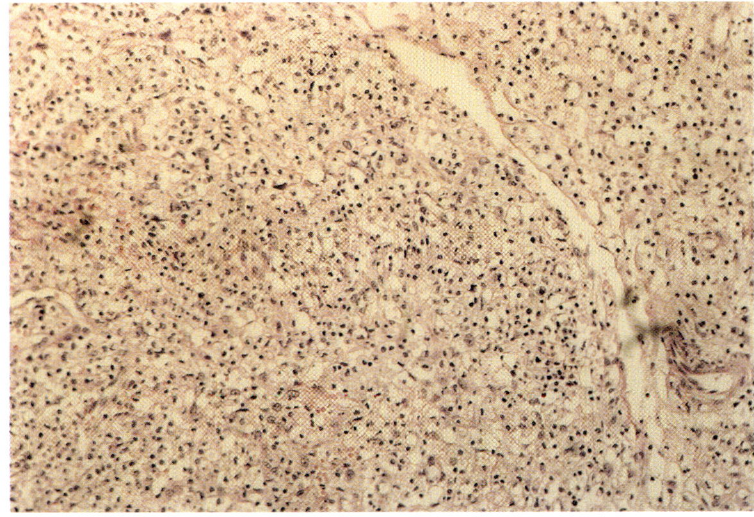

Persistent generalized lymphadenopathy showing lymphoid depletion. The lymph node is nearly devoid of lymphocytes.

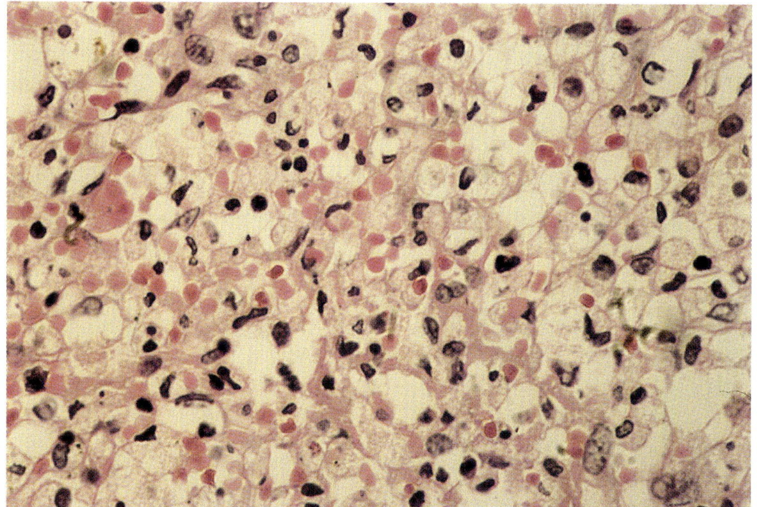

FIGURE 5.11

Persistent generalized lymphadenopathy showing lymphoid depletion. The lymph node consists of "naked" stroma containing scattered macrophages and erythrocytes.

biopsies from these lymph nodes must be interpreted with caution; a small needle biopsy specimen may be unrepresentative, consisting only of a greatly enlarged follicular center, and be confused with a large cell lymphoma.

The "explosiveness" of the follicular hyperplasia and the presence of folliculolysis help to distinguish PGL from other causes of follicular lymphoid hyperplasia. None of these features is, however, diagnostic of HIV infection. Therefore, although the histopathologic findings may strongly suggest a diagnosis of PGL in a patient whose HIV status is unknown, serologic confirmation of HIV infection is always required.

The follicular involution phase of PGL must be distinguished from multicentric Castleman's disease and from angioimmunoblastic lymphadenopathy with dysproteinemia (AILD). Distinction from multicentric Castleman's disease may be impossible on morphologic grounds alone. Serological testing for HIV is therefore recommended in cases of apparent multicentric Castleman's disease if the HIV status is unknown. Distinction from AILD will usually be possible on clinical grounds, since these patients are typically elderly with fever and skin rash.

The lymphoid depletion phase of PGL is usually seen in autopsy material and is seldom a problem in differential diagnosis. The "naked" stroma of the lymph node may be confused with a vascular or spindle cell lesion, including Kaposi's sarcoma; however, attention to the preservation of the underlying architecture will usually permit distinction.

Opportunistic Infections

The lymph nodes may be the site of involvement of a variety of opportunistic infections in patients with AIDS (Figs. 5.12 and 5.13). These include mycobacteria *(Mycobacterium tuberculosis, Mycobacterium avium-intracellulare)*, fungi *(Histoplasma capsula-*

FIGURE 5.12

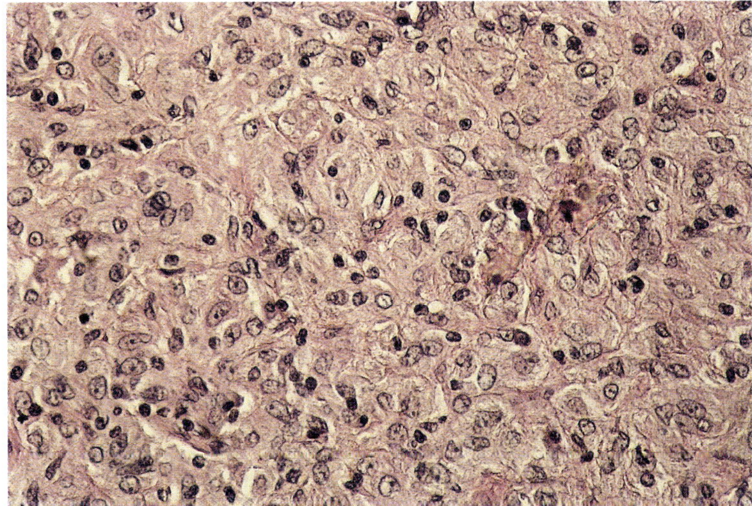

Mycobacterium avium-intracellulare infection in a patient with AIDS. The lymph node is infiltrated by macrophage-histiocytes.

FIGURE 5.13

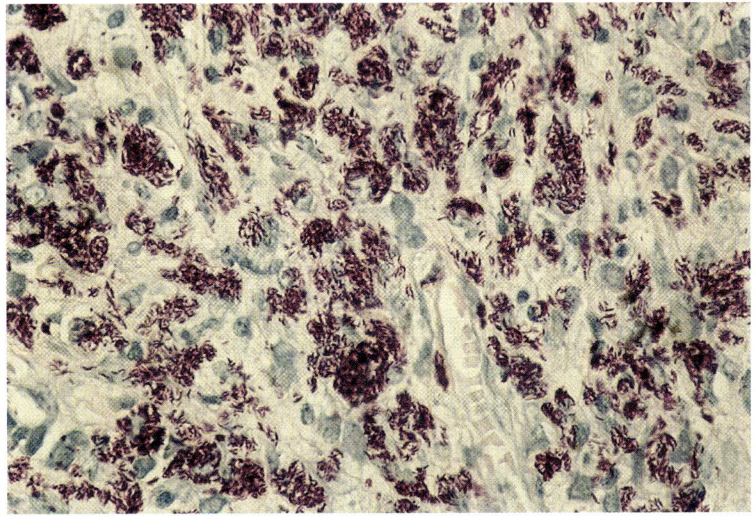

Mycobacterium avium-intracellulare infection in a patient with AIDS. Acid fast stain showing numerous intracellular acid fast bacilli.

tum, Cryptococcus neoformans), protozoans *(Toxoplasma gondii)* and organisms of uncertain classification *(Pneumocystis carinii)*. The pathology of specific infections is considered in Chapters 8 and 9.

Lymphoproliferative Disorders

Lymphoproliferative disorders are a feature of AIDS and include non-Hodgkin's lymphomas, Hodgkin's disease, and other lymphoproliferative disorders.

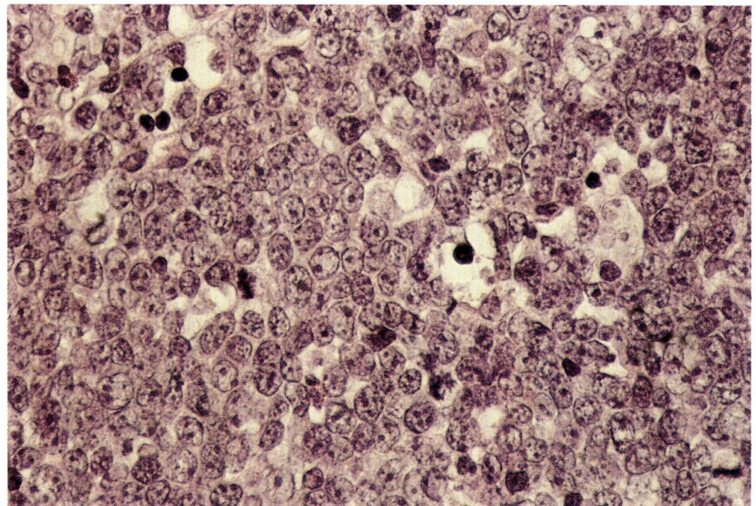

Malignant lymphoma, small noncleaved cell in a patient with AIDS.

Non-Hodgkin's Lymphomas

Non-Hodgkin's lymphomas occur with increased incidence in patients with AIDS and may be the first clinical manifestation of HIV infection (Ziegler et al, 1984). Although central nervous system and other extranodal presentations are frequent, lymph node involvement is not uncommon (Fig. 5.14). The lymphomas are predominantly of aggressive B cell types, including diffuse large cell lymphoma (large noncleaved cell and B immunoblastic) and Burkitt's-like lymphomas (small noncleaved cell) (Knowles et al, 1988). Molecular genetic alterations, including C-MYC rearrangements in small noncleaved cell lymphoma and Epstein-Barr virus in B immunoblastic lymphomas, are not uncommon (Ballerini et al, 1993). Other, less common forms of non-Hodgkin's lymphomas have also been reported in association with AIDS and include primary effusion lymphomas associated with the Kaposi's sarcoma–associated herpesvirus (Nador et al, 1996), CD30-positive large cell anaplastic lymphomas (Chadburn et al, 1993), peripheral T cell lymphoma (Nasr et al, 1988), and T lymphoblastic lymphoma (Ruff et al, 1989).

Hodgkin's Disease

Hodgkin's disease occurs in HIV-positive patients with distinctive clinical and pathologic features, although it is not established that the incidence is increased (Ree et al, 1991). HIV-associated Hodgkin's disease presents as a distinctive disorder with high frequency of constitutional "B" symptoms, advanced stage at presentation, and bone marrow involvement in greater than 50% of the patients. The cases are predominantly of mixed cellularity type and may show unusual histopathologic features, including lymphoid depletion and prominent fibrohistiocytoid stromal cells (Ree et al, 1991). In contrast to Hodgkin's disease in normal hosts, the CD4:CD8 ratio of the lymphocyte population is reversed (Unger and Strauchen, 1986). Epstein-Barr virus in present in the Reed-Sternberg cells of nearly all cases (Herndier et al, 1993).

Other Lymphoproliferative Disorders

Other lymphoproliferative disorders have been reported in association with HIV infection. These include lymphomatoid granulomatosis (Mittal et al, 1990), chronic CD8 lymphocytosis (Knowles et al, 1988), acute B cell lymphocytic leukemia (Flanagan et al, 1988), and plasmacytoma (Gold et al, 1990).

Kaposi's Sarcoma

Kaposi's sarcoma is a frequent manifestation of HIV infection. Kaposi's sarcoma occurs in classical, post-transplantation, endemic, and epidemic forms, the latter in association with HIV infection. Kaposi's sarcoma involves the skin, mucosal surfaces, and visceral organs. Lymph node involvement ("lymphadenopathic Kaposi's sarcoma") is frequently associated with HIV infection. Kaposi's sarcoma is highly associated with the Kaposi's sarcoma–associated herpesvirus (KSHV), a recently discovered herpesvirus of the Gammaherpesvirinae family, which shares sequence homology with Epstein-Barr virus and herpesvirus saimiri, two oncogenic herpesviruses (Moore and Chang, 1996). KSHV is found regularly in HIV-associated and non–HIV-associated cases of Kaposi's sarcoma, and in cases of multicentric Castleman's disease (Soulier et al, 1995) and primary effusion lymphomas (Nador et al, 1996). HIV-related Kaposi's sarcoma occurs predominantly in male homosexuals, suggesting sexual transmission of KSHV (Monini et al, 1996).

Other Neoplasms

A variety of other neoplasms have been reported in association with HIV infection and may involve lymph nodes. Leiomyosarcomas and other smooth muscle tumors have been reported with greater than expected frequency in children and young adults with HIV infection and frequently contain Epstein-Barr virus (McClain et al 1995). These tumors have been predominantly of the gastrointestinal tract and lung and strongly express CD21, the Epstein-Barr virus receptor. We have seen one additional case involving kidney, which was misdiagnosed as a Wilms' tumor in a child. An intranodal leiomyoma has been described in an adult patient with AIDS (Starasoler et al, 1991). Immunohistochemical studies for smooth muscle antigens are helpful in the recognition of these tumors and in distinction from other spindle cell proliferations in AIDS, including Kaposi's sarcoma and pseudosarcomatous *Mycobacterium avium-intracellulare* infection (Brandwein et al, 1990).

Squamous carcinomas of the oral and anogenital regions and cervical intraepithelial neoplasia (CIN) have been reported with increased frequency in HIV infection and likely result from infection with the human papilloma virus (HPV). Germ cell tumors of the testes have also been reported in association with HIV infection (Tessler and Catanese, 1987).

REFERENCES

Ballerini P, Gaidano G, Gong JZ, Tassi V, Saglio G, Knowles DM, Dalla-Favera R. Multiple genetic lesions in acquired immunodeficiency syndrome-related non-Hodgkin's lymphoma. Blood 81:166–176, 1993.

Brandwein M, Choi HH, Strauchen JA, Stoler M, Jagirdar J. Spindle cell reaction to nontuberculous mycobacteriosis in AIDS mimicking a spindle cell neoplasm. Virchows Archiv A Pathol Anat 416:281–286, 1990.

Chadburn A, Cesarman E, Jagirdar J, Subar M, Mir RN, Knowles DM. CD30 (Ki1) positive anaplastic large cell lymphomas in individuals infected with the human immunodeficiency virus. Cancer 72:3078–3090, 1993.

Cooper DA, et al. Acute AIDS retrovirus infection: Delineation of a clinical illness associated with seroconversion. Lancet 1:537, 1985.

Fauci AS, Pantaleo G, Stanley S, Wissman D. Immunopathogenic mechanisms of HIV infection. Ann Intern Med 124:654–663, 1996.

Flanagan P, Chowdhury V, Costello C. HIV-associated B-cell ALL. Br J Haematol 69:287, 1988.

Folks TM, Kessler SW, Orenstein JM, Justement JS, Jaffe ES, Fauci AS. Infection and replication of HIV-1 in purified progenitor cells of normal human bone marrow. Science 242:919–922, 1988.

Fox CH, Tenner-Racz K, Pacz P, Firpo A, Pizzo PA, Fauci AS. Lymphoid germinal centers are reservoirs of human immunodefciency virus type 1 RNA. J Infect Dis 164:1051–1057, 1991.

Gold JE, Schwam L, Castella A, Pike SB, Opfell R, Zalusky R. Malignant plasma cell tumors in HIV-infected patients. Cancer 66:363–368, 1990.

Herndier BG, Sanchez HC, Chang KL, Chen YY, Weiss LM. High prevalence of Epstein-Barr virus in the Reed-Stenberg cells of HIV-associated Hodgkin's disease. Am J Pathol 142:1073–1079, 1993.

Knowles DM, Chamulak GA, Subar M, Burke JS, Dugan M, Wernz J, Slywotzy C, Pelicci P-G, Dalla-Favera R, Raphael B. Lymphoid neoplasia associated with the acquired immunodeficiency syndrome (AIDS). The New York University Medical Center Experience with 105 patients (1981–1986), Ann Intern Med 108:744–753, 1988.

Lowenthal DA, Filippa DA, Richardson ME, Bertoni M, Straus DJ. Generalized lymphadenopathy with morphologic features of Castleman's disease in an HIV-positive man. Cancer 60:2454–2458, 1987.

McClain KL, Leach CT, Jenson HB, Joshi VV, Pollock BH, Parmley RT, DiCarlo FJ, Chadwick EG, Murphy SB. Association of Epstein-Barr virus with leiomyosarcomas in young people with AIDS. N Engl J Med 332:12–18, 1995.

Metroka CE, Cunningham-Rundles S, Pollack MS, Sonnabend JA, Davis JM, Fordon B, Fernandez RD, Mouradian J. Generalized lymphadenopathy in homosexual man. Ann Intern Med 99:585–591, 1883.

Mittal K, Neri A, Feiner H, Schinella R, Alfonso F. Lymphomatoid granulomatosis in the acquired immunodeficiency syndrome. Caner 65:1345–1349, 1990.

Monini P, De Lellis L, Fabris M, Rigolin F, Cassai E. Kaposi's sarcoma-associated herpesvirus DNA sequences in prostate tissue and human semen. N Engl J Med 334:1168–1172, 1996.

Moore PS, Chang Y. Detection of herpesvirus-like DNA sequences in Kaposi"s sarcoma in patients with and without HIV infection. N Engl J Med 332:1181–1185, 1996.

Nador RG, Cesarman E, Chadburn A, Dawson DB, Ansari MQ, Said J, Knowles DM. Primary effusion lymphoma: A distinct clinicopathologic entitiy associated with the Kaposi's sarcoma-associated herpesvirus. Blood 88:645–656, 1996.

Nasr SA, Brynes RK, Garrison CP, Chan WC. Peripheral T-cell lymphoma in a patient with acquired immune deficiency syndrome. Cancer 61:947–951, 1988.

Oksenhendler E, Duarte M, Soulier J, Cacoub P Welker Y, Cadranel J, et al. Multicentric Castleman's disease in HIV infection: a clinical and pathological study of 20 patients. AIDS 10:61–67, 1996.

Pantaleo G, Graziosi C, Demarest JF, Butini L, Montroni M, Fox CH et al. HIV infection is acitve and progressive in lymphoid tissue during the clinically latent stage of disease. Nature 362:355–358, 1993.

Piris MA, Rivas C, Morente M, Rubio C, Martin C, Olivia H. Persistent and generalized lymphadenopathy: A lesion of follicular dendritic cells? An immunohistologic and ultrastructural study. Am J Clin Pathol 87:716–724, 1987.

Popovic M, Sarngadharan MG, Read E, Gallo RC. Detection, isolation, and continuous production of cytopathic retroviruses (HTLV-III) from patients with AIDS and pre-AIDS. Science 224:497–500, 1984.

Raphael M, Pouletty P, Cavaille-Coll M, Rozenbaum W, Homond A, Nonnenmacher L, Delcourt A, Gluckman JC, Debre P. Lymphadenopathy in patients at risk for acquired immunodeficiency syndrome. Histopathology and histochemistry. Arch Pathol Lab Med 109:128–132, 1985.

Ree HJ, Strauchen JA, Khan AA, Gold JE, Crowley JP, Kahn H, Zalusky R. Human immunodeficiency virus-associated Hodgkin's disease: Clinicopathologic studies of 24 cases and preponderance of mixed cellularity type characterized by the occurrence of fibrohistiocytoid stromal cells. Cancer 67:1614–1621, 1991.

Reichert CM, O'Leary TJ, Levens DL, Simrell CR, Macher AM. Autopsy pathology in the acquired immunodeficiency syndrome. Am J Pathol 112:357–382, 1983.

Ruff P, Bagg A, Papadopoulos K. Precursor T-cell lymphoma association with human immunodeficiency virus type 1 (HIV-1) infection: First reported case. Cancer 64:39–42, 1989.

Soulier J, Grollet L, Oksenhendle E, Cacoub P, Cazals-Hatem D, Babinet P, et al. Kaposi's sarcoma-associated herpesvirus-like DNA sequences in multicentric Castleman's disease. Blood 86:1276–1280, 1995.

Stanley SK, McCune JM, Kaneshima H, Justement JS, Sullivan M, Boone E, et al. Human immunodeficiency virus infection of the human thymus and disruption of the thymic microenvironment in the SCID-hu mouse. J Exp Med 178:1151–1163, 1993.

Starasoler L, Vuitch F, Albores-Saavedra J. Intranodal leiomyoma: Another distinctive primary spindle cell neoplasm of lymph node. Am J Clin Pathol 95:858–862, 1991,

Tessler AN, Catanese A. AIDS and germ cell tumors of the testis. Urology 30:203–204, 1987.

Unger PD, Strauchen JA. Hodgkin's disease in AIDS-complex patients. Report of four cases and tissue immunologic marker studies. Cancer 589:821–825, 1986.

Ziegler JL, Beckstead JA, Volberding PA, Abrams DI, Levine AM, Lukes RJ, et al. Non-Hodgkin's lymphoma in 90 homosexual men. Relation to generalized lymphadenopathy and the acquired immunodeficiency syndrome. N Engl J Med 311:565–570, 1984.

Drug Induced, Hypersensitivity, and Dermatopathic Lymphadenopathies

Drug induced, hypersensitivity, and dermatopathic lymphadenopathies are frequent causes of paracortical ("T-zone") lymph node hyperplasia.

Drug Induced and Hypersensitivity Lymphadenopathy

Reactions to drugs are a frequent cause of hypersensitivity lymphadenopathy. Most reported cases have been to anticonvulsant drugs of the Dilantin (diphenylhydantoin) class, including related drugs, such as Mesantoin, Mysoline, and Celontin; however similar reactions to other drugs, such as carbamazepine (Tegretol), have also been reported (De Vriese et al, 1995; Gordon and Ferry, 1996). Because of their frequent association with anticonvulsant drugs, these reactions are sometimes referred to as "anticonvulsant lymphadenopathy" (Saltzstein and Ackerman, 1959).

Clinical Features

Drug hypersensitivity lymphadenopathy in reaction to Dilantin has been reported to occur from 1 week to 30 years after the start of the drug (Abbondanzo et al, 1995); however, most cases occur in the first months of treatment. Drug hypersensitivity lymphadenopathy is frequently associated with a "pseudolymphoma" syndrome, with fever, skin rash, hepatosplenomegaly, and peripheral eosinophilia. An infectious mononucleosis-like syndrome with atypical lymphocytosis may also occur (Siegal and Berkowitz, 1961). Lymphadenopathy is generalized in most cases. The lymphadenopathy

FIGURE
6.1

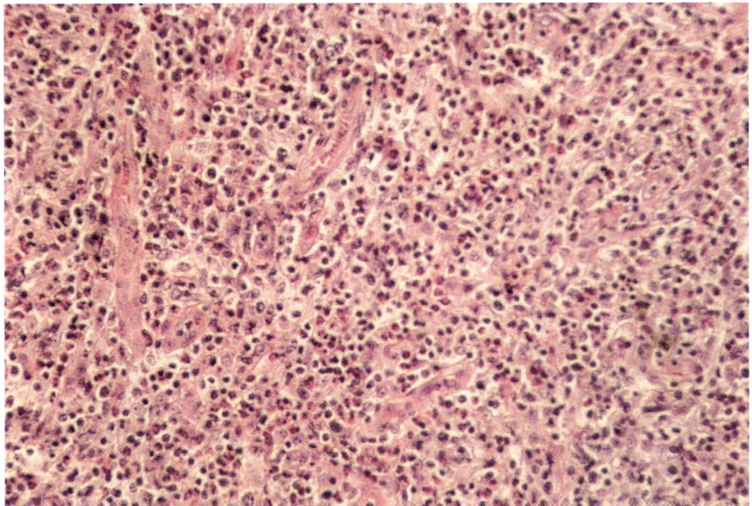

Drug-induced hypersensitivity lymphadenopathy associated with ampicillin. The paracortex is expanded and hypervascular.

FIGURE
6.2

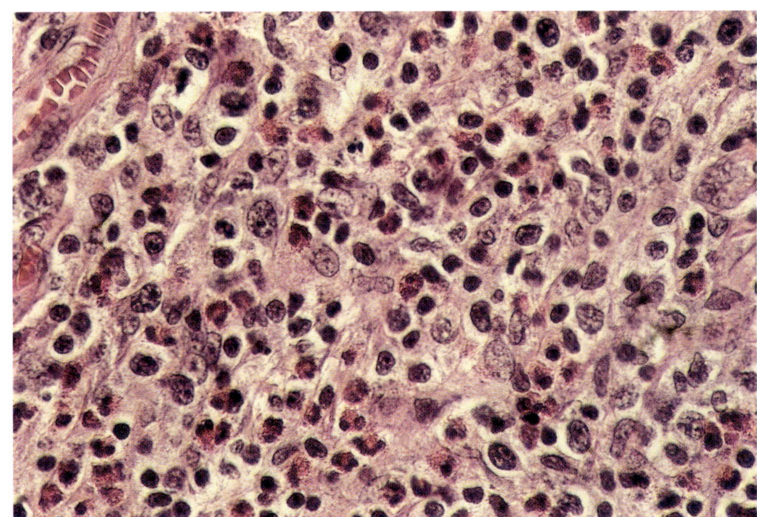

Drug-induced hypersensitivity lymphadenopathy associated with ampicillin. The paracortex contains immunoblasts and numerous eosinophils.

characteristically regresses with discontinuation of the drug. In a few reported cases malignant lymphoma has later developed ("pseudo-pseudolymphoma") (Gams et al, 1968); however, a causal relation is unproven.

Histopathology

Drug induced and hypersensitivity lymphadenopathy is predominantly a paracortical ("T-zone") process. The paracortex is expanded, hypervascular, and contains a mixed population of cells with numerous immunoblasts and, frequently, eosinophils (Figs. 6.1,

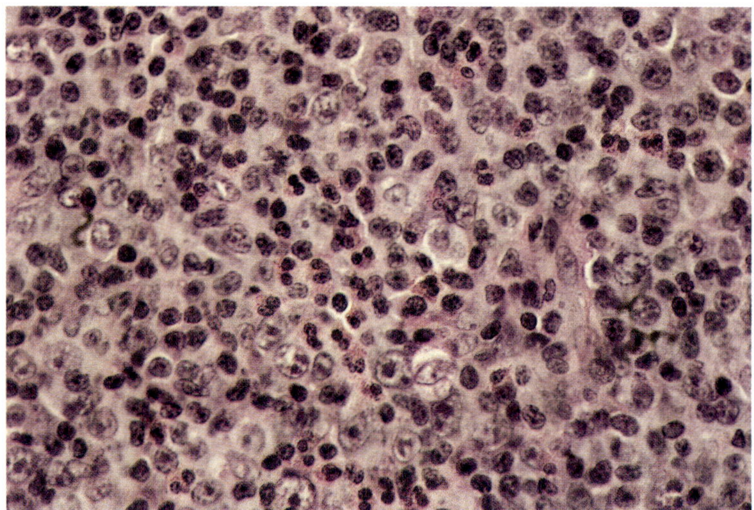

Drug-induced hypersensitivity lymphadenopathy associated with diphen-ylhydantoin (Dilantin). Paracortical immunoblasts and eosinophils.

6.2, and 6.3). The follicles may be hyperplastic or involuted; in some cases disruption of the follicles may be identified with immunohistochemical staining for follicular dendritic cells. Foci of necrosis and vasculitis are present in some cases. Abbondanzo and colleagues, in their review of 25 cases associated with Dilantin (Abbondanzo et al, 1995), identified three patterns: paracortical immunoblastic hyperplasia with hyperplastic follicular centers, paracortical immunoblastic hyperplasia with atrophic follicular centers, and a miscellaneous group. The first group all had onset within the first 15 months of therapy and were considered to represent a hypersensitivity reaction. The second group had onset from 15 months to many years after the initiation of therapy and were considered to represent late effects. The third group had onset 10 or more years after the initiation of therapy and had a variety of lesions, including dermatopathic lymphadenopathy, necrotizing lymphadenitis, and other lymphoid hyperplasias. Some of these reactions may be coincidental.

Development of Malignant Lymphoma

Bona fide malignant lymphomas have been reported in patients taking anticonvulsant drugs (Hyman and Sommers, 1966); however, a causal relationship has not been established. The lymphomas have been of no specific type; both Hodgkin's disease and non-Hodgkin's lymphomas have been described. Most of the patients have been on anticonvulsants for many years at the time lymphoma is diagnosed. Lymphoma may be present in the initial biopsy or may develop following benign lymphadenopathy (the "pseudo-pseudolymphoma syndrome"). Progression from paracortical hyperplasia to malignant lymphoma in sequential biopsies has been reported (Abbondanzo et al, 1995).

Differential Diagnosis

Drug-induced and hypersensitivity lymphadenopathy must be distinguished from other causes of paracortical hyperplasia and from malignant lymphoma. Distinction from other causes of paracortical hyperplasia, principally postvaccinial and viral lymphadenitis, requires correlation with the clinical history. A history of drug administration may be overlooked or simply may not be provided to the pathologist. Angioimmunoblastic lymphadenopathy with dysproteinemia (AILD) shares clinical and histopathologic features with drug-induced and hypersensitivity lymphadenopathy, and a history of drug exposure is obtained in up to one third of cases (Steinberg et al, 1988). Most workers, however, now consider AILD to be a type of T cell lymphoma, based on the frequent presence of clonal rearrangements of the T cell antigen receptor genes (Weiss et al, 1986). Nevertheless, the possibility of drug-induced or hypersensitivity lymphadenopathy should be considered in patients presenting with AILD-like findings. In questionable cases, withdrawing the offending drug and/or T cell antigen receptor gene rearrangement studies may be helpful.

Distinction from malignant lymphoma, particularly peripheral T cell lymphoma, may be difficult. The polymorphous cellular composition, lack of atypia of the small lymphocytes, and preservation of architecture are features favoring a reactive process. In questionable cases, immunophenotypic studies and antigen receptor gene rearrangement studies may be helpful. The presence of eosinophils may suggest a diagnosis of Hodgkin's disease; however, diagnostic Reed-Sternberg cells will be lacking. Immunohistochemical studies may also be helpful, since the immunoblasts in drug-induced and hypersensitivity lymphadenopathy are typically negative for CD30, in contrast to the cells of Hodgkin's disease (Abbondanzo et al, 1995).

Course and Prognosis

Drug-induced and hypersensitivity lymphadenopathy regresses with withdrawal of the offending drug. The possible development of malignant lymphoma in rare cases has been discussed.

Dermatopathic Lymphadenopathy

Dermatopathic lymphadenopathy is a reaction pattern seen in lymph nodes draining areas of dermatitis and also in association with cutaneous T cell lymphoma (mycosis fungoides or Sezary's syndrome).

Clinical Features

Dermatopathic lymphadenopathy exhibits no consistent clinical features. The associated skin disease may be a chronic dermatitis, exfoliative dermatitis, or cutaneous T cell lymphoma (mycosis fungoides or Sezary's syndrome); occasional patients exhibit no identifiable skin disease. Lymph node changes indistinguishable from dermatopathic lymphadenopathy are seen in some patients with AIDS (Burns et al, 1985).

Histopathology

Dermatopathic lymphadenopathy is predominantly a paracortical ("T-zone") process. The paracortex is expanded and at low magnification has a characteristic "pale" appearance (Fig. 6.4). At higher magnification, the pallor is seen to be due to infiltration with pale-staining histiocytes, dendritic cells, and Langerhans' cells (Fig. 6.5). The histiocytes (monocyte-macrophages) have ovoid nuclei and abundant clear to eosinophilic cytoplasm, which frequently contains melanin pigment (Figs. 6.6 and 6.7). Depositon of lipid may also be present ("lipomelanotic reticulosis"). The Langerhans' cells have delicately folded or "grooved" nuclei and abundant pale cytoplasm. Scattered lymphocytes, plasma cells, and eosinophils are admixed. The follicles may be hyperplastic or involuted. In cases of dermatopathic lymphadenopathy associated with cutaneous T cell lymphoma, collections of Sezary's-like cells, with irregular cerebriform nuclei, may be noted in the paracortex (Figs. 6.8 and 6.9). Small numbers of similar-appearing cells, however, may be seen in dermatopathic lymphadenopathy unassociated with cutaneous T cell

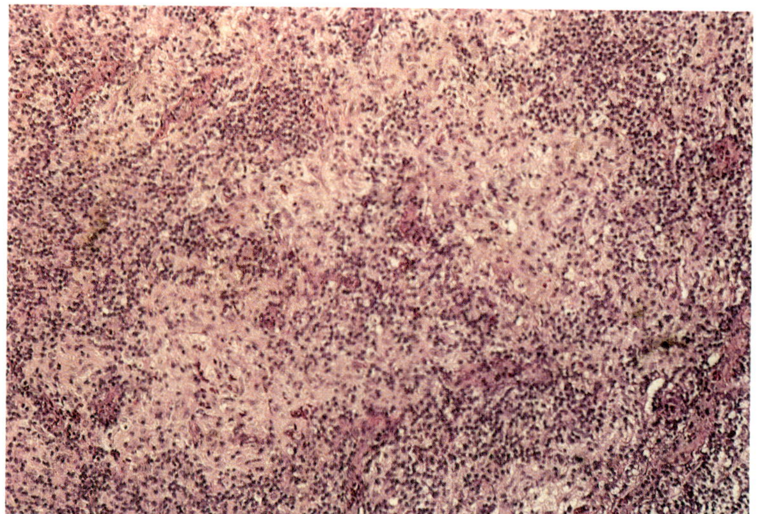

FIGURE 6.4

Dermatopathic lymphadenopathy showing pale appearance of paracortex at low magnification.

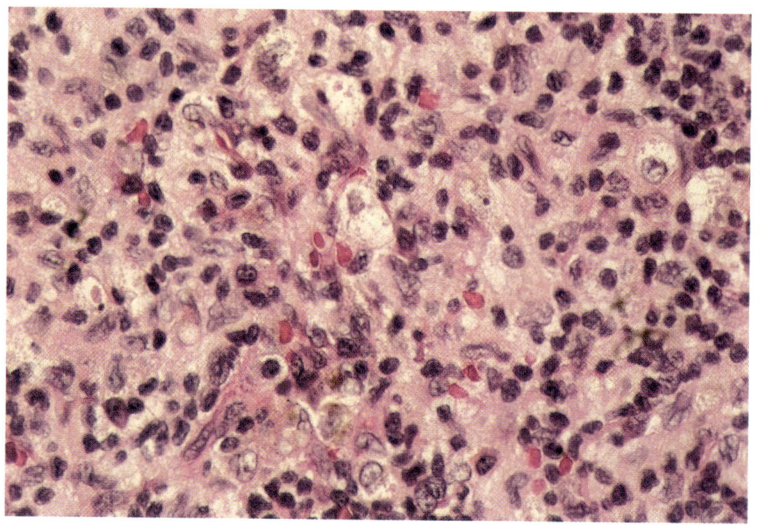

FIGURE 6.5

Dermatopathic lymphadenopathy. Pallor of paracortex is due to infiltration with pale-staining histiocytes, dendritic cells, and Langerhans' cells.

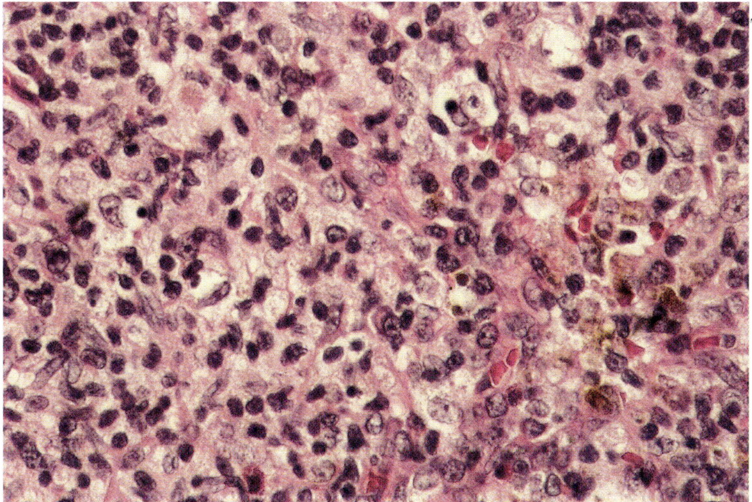

FIGURE 6.6

Dermatopathic lymphadenopathy showing deposition of melanin pigment in macrophage-histiocytes. Deposition of lipid may also be present ("lipomelanotic reticulosis").

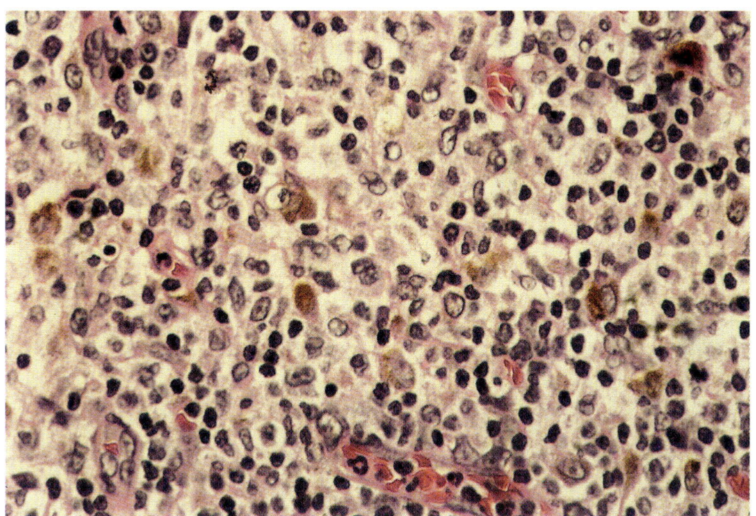

FIGURE 6.7

Dermatopathic lymphadenopathy in a patient with AIDS. Melanin pigment is prominent.

lymphoma (Burke and Colby, 1981). Immunohistochemical studies in dermatopathic lymphadenopathy demonstrate large numbers of Langerhans' cells (HLA-DR positive, S-100 positive, CD1a positive) and interdigitating reticulum cells (HLA-DR positive, S-100 positive, CD1a negative).

Differential Diagnosis

Dermatopathic lymphadenopathy must be distinguished from other paracortical lymphoid hyperplasia, particularly drug induced and hypersensitivity lymphadenopathy

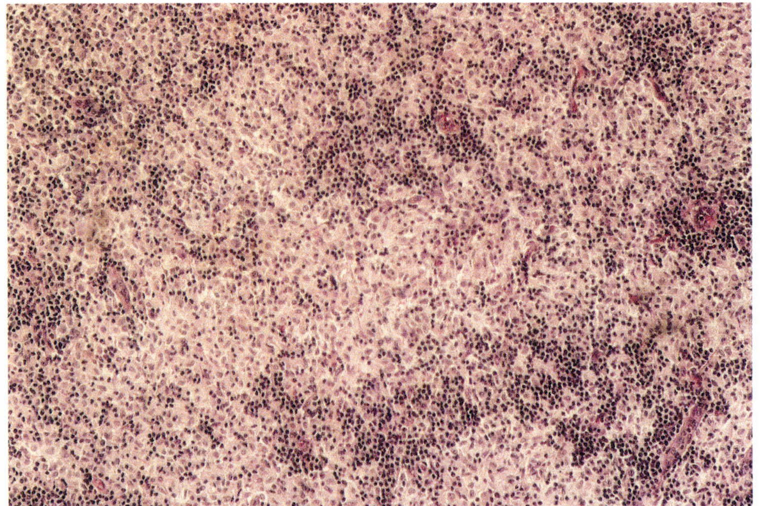

FIGURE 6.8

Dermatopathic lymphadenopathy in cutaneous T cell lymphoma.

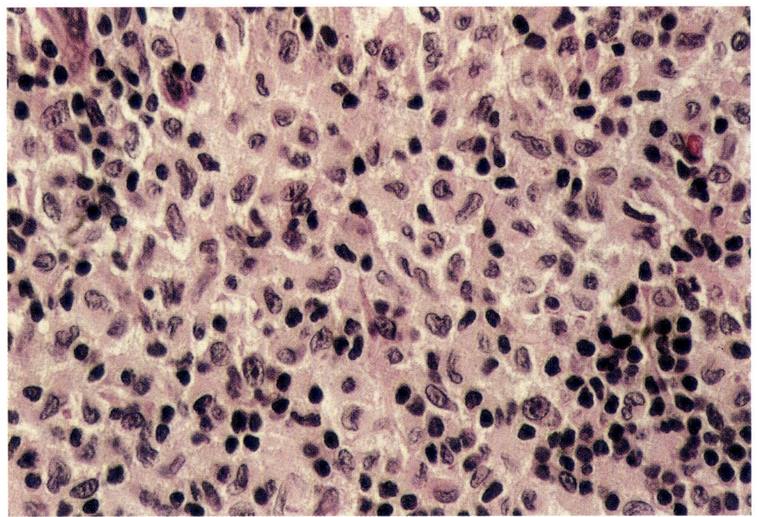

FIGURE 6.9

Dermatopathic lymphadenopathy in cutaneous T cell lymphoma. Small clusters of irregular, hyperchromatic lymphocytes may be seen in some cases of dermatopathic lymphadenopathy with or without associated cutaneous T cell lymphoma.

and postvaccinial and viral lymphadenitis. The characteristic "pallor" of the paracortex in dermatopathic lymphadenopathy, prominence of Langerhans' cells and melanin-containing macrophages, and paucity of immunoblasts usually permit ready distinction. A particular problem in the setting of cutaneous T cell lymphoma is distinguishing dermatopathic lymphadenopathy from lymph node involvement with cutaneous T cell lymphoma (Burke and Colby, 1981). Frequently the two coexist. Small numbers of irregular lymphocytes may be seen in cases of dermatopathic lymphadenopathy, both with and without associated cutaneous T cell lymphoma. T cell antigen receptor gene rearrangement studies, however, demonstrate clonal T cell antigen receptor gene rearrangements in the majority of lymph nodes from patients with cutaneous T cell lymphoma and dermatopathic lymphadenopathy (Weiss et al, 1985). The detection of neoplastic T cells in lymph nodes showing only dermatopathic lymphadenopathy morphologically explains the adverse prognostic significance of dermatopathic lymphadenopathy in patients with cutaneous T cell lymphoma.

REFERENCES

Abbondanzo SL, Irey NS, Frizzera G. Dilantin-associated lymphadenopathy. Spectrum of histopathologic patterns. Am J Surg Pathol 19:675–686, 1995.

Burke JS, Colby TV. Dermatopathic lymphadenopathy. Comparison of cases associated and unassociated with mycosis fungoides. Am J Surg Pathol 5:343–352, 1981.

Burns BF, Wood GS, Dorfman RF. The varied histopathology of lymphadenopathy in the homosexual male. Am J Surg Pathol 9:287–297, 1985.

De Vriese AS, Phillipe J, Van Renterghem DM, et al. Carbamazepine hypersensitivity syndrome: Report of 4 cases and review of the literature. Medicine (Baltimore) 74:144–151, 1995.

Gams RA, Neal JA, Conrad FG. Hydantoin-induced pseudo-pseudolymphoma. Ann Intern Med 69:557–568, 1968.

Gordon JB, Ferry JA. Case records of the Massachusetts General Hospital. Case 26–1996. N Engl J Med 335:577–584, 1996.

Hyman GA, Sommers SC. The development of Hodgkin's disease and lymphoma during anticonvulsant therapy. Blood 28:416–427, 1966.

Saltzstein SL, Ackerman LV. Lymphadenopathy induced by anti-convulsant drugs and mimicking clinically and pathologically malignant lymphoma. Cancer 12:164–182, 1959.

Siegal S, Berkowitz J. Diphenylhydantoin (Dilantin) hypersensitivity with infectious mononucleosis-like syndrome and jaundice. J Allergy 32:447–451, 1961.

Steinberg AD, Seldin MF, Jaffe ES, Smith HR, Klinman DM, Krieg AM, Cossman J. Angioimmunoblastic lymphadenopathy with dysproteinemia. NIH Conference. Ann Intern Med 108:575–584, 1988.

Weiss LM, Hu E, Wood GS, Moulds C, Cleary ML, Warnke R, Sklar J. Clonal rearrangements of the T cell receptor genes in mycosis fungoides and dermatopathic lymphadenopathy. N Engl J Med 313:539–544, 1985.

Weiss LM, Strickler JG, Dorfman RF, Horning SJ, Warnke RA, Sklar J. Clonal T-cell populations in angioimmunoblastic lymphadenopathy and angioimmunoblastic lymphadenopathy-like lymphoma. Am J Pathol 122:392–397, 1986.

7

Postvaccinial and Viral Lymphadenitis and Infectious Mononucleosis

Postvaccinial lymphadenitis, viral lymphadenitis, and infectious mononucleosis are lymph node responses to viral infections which are characterized by striking immunoblastic hyperplasia which may mimic malignant lymphoma.

Postvaccinial Lymphadenitis

Postvaccinial lymphadenitis classically follows immunization for smallpox (Hartsock, 1968) but may also follow other vaccines (Dorfman and Herweg, 1966). We have seen one case following immunization for hepatitis B.

Clinical Features

Postvaccinial lymphadenitis typically follows immunization by 1 to several weeks and is characterized by tender, regional lymphadenopathy, most frequently involving unilateral axillary or supraclavicular lymph nodes. The history of recent immunization may not be appreciated (Hartsock, 1968).

Histopathology

Postvaccinial lymphadenitis is predominantly a paracortical process. At low magnification, the paracortex is expanded and has a mottled or "moth-eaten" appearance (Fig. 7.1). At higher magnification the mottled appearance is seen to be due to a striking

FIGURE
7.1

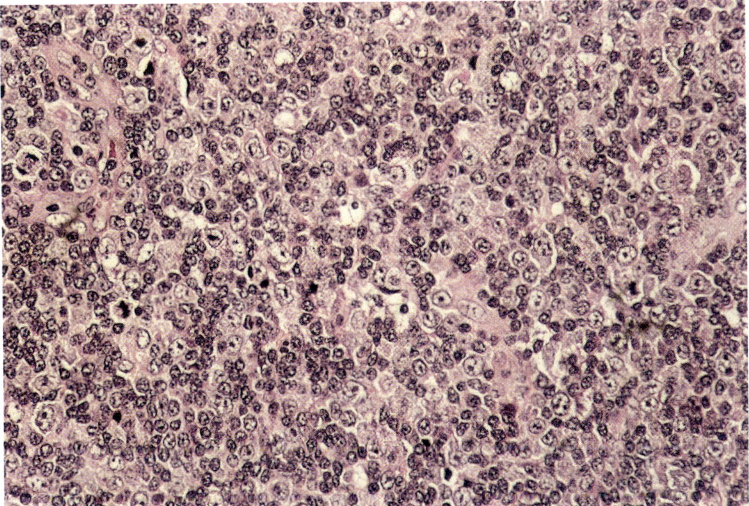

Postvaccinial lymphadenitis showing "mottled" or "moth-eaten" appearance of the paracortex at low magnification.

FIGURE
7.2

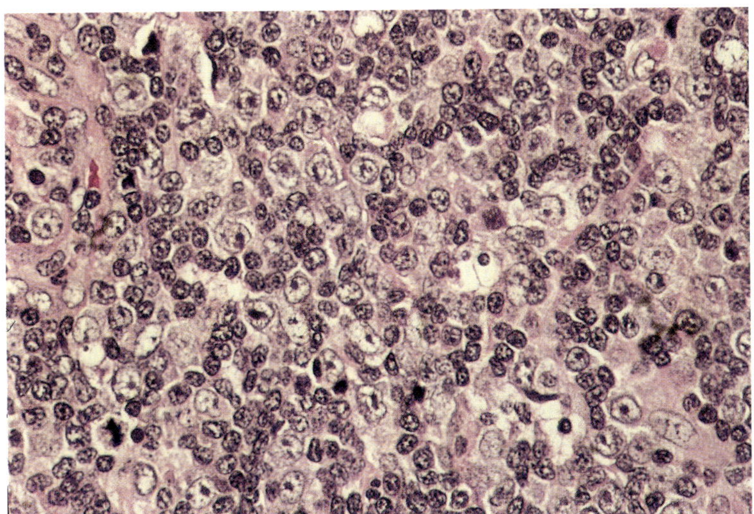

Postvaccinial lymphadenitis showing numerous paracortical immunoblasts.

proliferation of immunoblasts (Fig. 7.2). The latter are large cells, with prominent central nucleoli and abundant amphophilic cytoplasm. Admixed lymphocytes in varying stages of transformation, plasma cells, and eosinophils are frequently present. Vascular proliferation, with prominent endothelial cells, may be pronounced. Follicles are inconspicuous in early lymph node biopsies; follicular hyperplasia is frequent in later biopsies. In postvaccinial lymphadenitis following live attenuated measle vaccine, Warthin-Finkeldey giant cells may be present (Dorfman and Herweg, 1966).

Differential Diagnosis

Postvaccinial lymphadenitis must be distinguished from other paracortical lymph node hyperplasias and from malignant lymphoma. The history of recent immunization is frequently overlooked (Hartsock, 1968). The striking immunoblastic hyperplasia may be confused with non-Hodgkin's lymphoma, or the pleomorphic immunoblasts may be confused with the Reed-Sternberg cells of Hodgkin's disease. The mottled or "moth-eaten" appearance of the paracortex, partial preservation of architecture, and presence of lymphocytes at varying stages of transformation are features in favor of a reactive process.

Viral Lymphadenitis

Viral lymphadenitis is seen in lymph nodes draining sites of cutaneous viral infections (herpes simplex lymphadenitis, herpes zoster lymphadenitis) and in systemic viral infections (measles lymphadenitis, cytomegalovirus lymphadenitis).

Herpetic Lymphadenitis

Clinical Features

Tender enlargement of regional lymph nodes frequently accompanies cutaneous viral infections including herpes simplex type I (cervical lymph nodes), herpes simplex type II (inguinal lymph nodes), and herpes zoster. Herpes simplex lymphadenitis may also present with generalized lymphadenopathy (Tamaru et al, 1990).

Histopathology

Herpetic lymphadenitis is predominantly a paracortical process which resembles postvaccinial lymphadenitis. The paracortex is expanded and has a mottled or "moth-eaten" appearance due to immunoblastic hyperplasia (Figs. 7.3 and 7.4). Pleomorphic immunoblasts resembling Reed-Sternberg cells, foci of necrosis, and cells with typical intranuclear herpetic inclusions may be present (Tamaru et al, 1990).

Differential Diagnosis

Herpetic lymphadenitis resembles postvaccinial and other viral lymphadenitis and may mimic non-Hodgkin's lymphoma or Hodgkin's disease. The intranuclear viral inclusions of herpetic lymphadenitis may be confused with the eosinophilic inclusion-like nucleoli of Reed-Sternberg cells. Specific diagnosis rests on the demonstration of viral particles by electron microscopy or viral antigens by immunohistochemistry.

Measles Lymphadenitis

Lymphoid hyperplasia occurs during the prodromal phase of measles (rubeola). Lymph node biopsy (or tonsillectomy or appendectomy) during the prodromal phase may per-

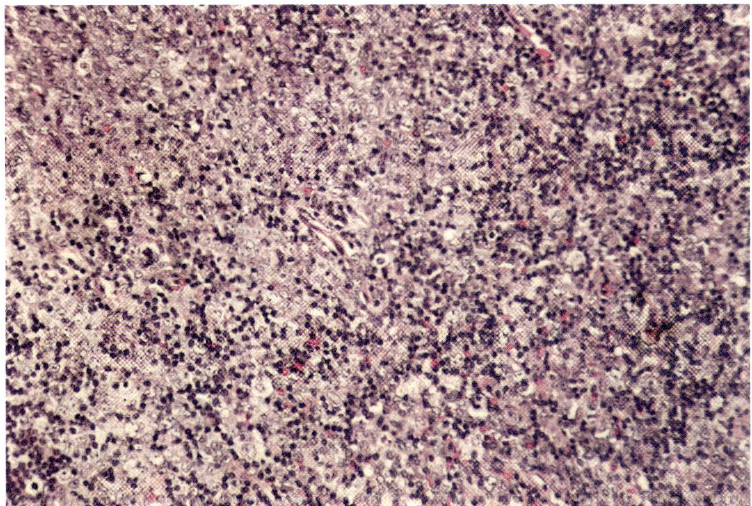

FIGURE
7.3

Herpes zoster lymphadenitis showing "mottled" or "moth-eaten" appearance of the paracortex at low magnification.

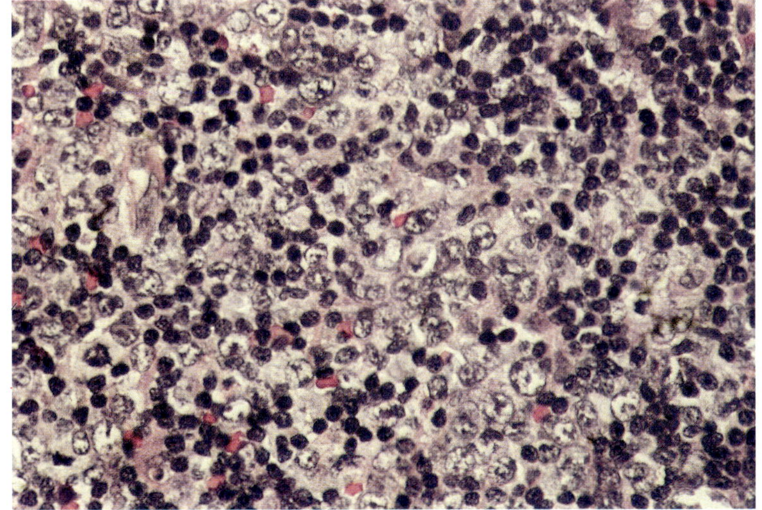

FIGURE
7.4

Herpes zoster lymphadenitis showing numerous paracortical immunoblasts.

mit the pathologist to make a diagnosis of probable measles before the appearance of the characteristic exanthem, thereby gaining great credit amongst his clinical colleagues!

Histopathology

The lymph nodes show a striking follicular lymphoid hyperplasia containing characteristic multinucleate giant cells referred to as Warthin-Finkeldey cells (Fig. 7.5). These are found within follicular centers and consist of syncytia of lymphocytes ("polykaryo-

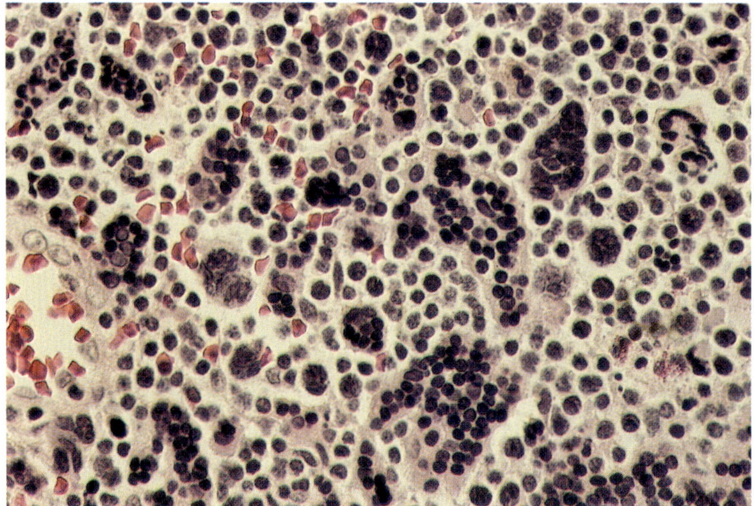

FIGURE 7.5

Warthin-Finkeldey giant cells.

cytes") with up to 100 nuclei (Strano, 1976). Intranuclear or intracytoplasmic inclusions may rarely be present. Similar changes are seen in other lymphoid tissues including the tonsils, adenoids, spleen, Peyer's patches, and appendix. The Warthin-Finkeldey cells disappear at about the time the exanthem develops.

Differential Diagnosis

Warthin-Finkeldey cells are not specific for measles and similar cells may be seen in a variety of reactive lymphoid hyperplasias, including the persistent generalized lymphadenopathy syndrome associated with HIV infection.

Cytomegalovirus Lymphadenitis

Cytomegalovirus (CMV) causes a mononucleosis-like syndrome and is one of the causes of heterophile-negative mononucleosis. Transfusion acquired CMV following cardiac surgery has been referred to as the "postpump"syndrome. CMV mononucleosis is characterized by fever, atypical lymphocytosis, and splenomegaly. Pharyngitis and cervical lymphadenopathy are less prominent than in infectious mononucleosis due to Epstein-Barr virus infection.

Histopathology

Lymph nodes in CMV lymphadenitis show changes similar to other viral lymphadenitides with paracortical immunoblastic hyperplasia and varying degrees of follicular and monocytoid B cell hyperplasia. Characteristic cytomegalic changes with intranuclear and intracytoplasmic inclusions may be found in infected T lymphocytes (Younes et al, 1991).

Differential Diagnosis

The diagnosis of CMV lymphadenitis is established by demonstration of the intranuclear and cytoplasmic inclusions characteristic of CMV histologically, demonstration of CMV antigens by immunohistochemistry, or demonstration of CMV RNA by in situ hybridization. CMV-infected cells may express CD15, causing potential confusion with Reed-Sternberg cells (Rushin et al, 1990). A morphologically similar lymphadenitis has been reported in association with human herpesvirus 6 (HHV-6) infection (Sumiyoshi et al, 1995).

Infectious Mononucleosis

Infectious mononucleosis results from primary infection with the Epstein-Barr virus and is a common cause of lymphadenopathy which may mimic malignant lymphoma.

Clinical Features

Infectious mononucleosis is an acute febrile illness resulting from primary infection with the Epstein-Barr virus (EBV). Infectious mononucleosis is principally a disease of adolescence and young adulthood and is rare past the age of 40. EBV infection in childhood likely results in nonspecific illness; by adulthood greater than 90% of individuals have antibodies to EBV indicating past infection. Infectious mononucleosis is commonly associated with the clinical triad of fever, exudative pharyngitis, and cervical lymphadenopathy. Splenomegaly and abnormal liver enzymes are a frequent feature. The hallmark of the disease, and the feature from which its name is derived, is the presence in the peripheral blood of atypical lymphocytes or Downey cells (Downey and McKinlay, 1923) (Fig. 7.6). EBV infects B cells by binding to the C3d complement receptor (CD21) and

**FIGURE
7.6**

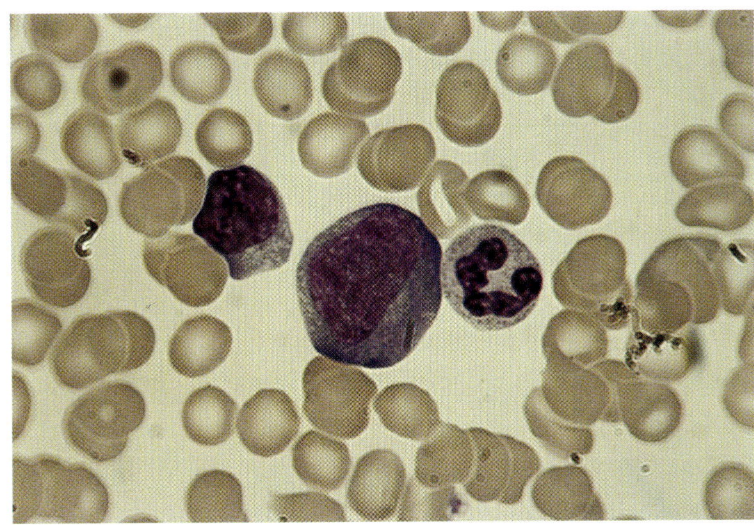

Infectious mononucleosis showing atypical lymphocytes ("Downey cells") in the peripheral blood.

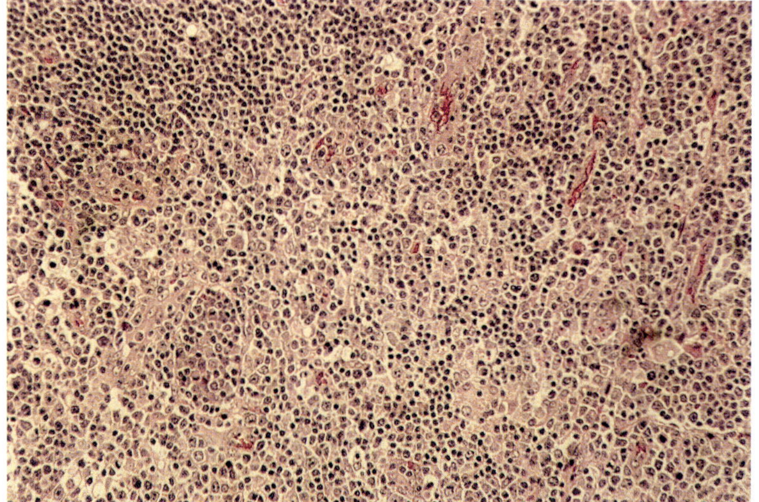

FIGURE
7.7

Infectious mononucleosis, low magnification, showing paracortical expansion by numerous immunoblasts.

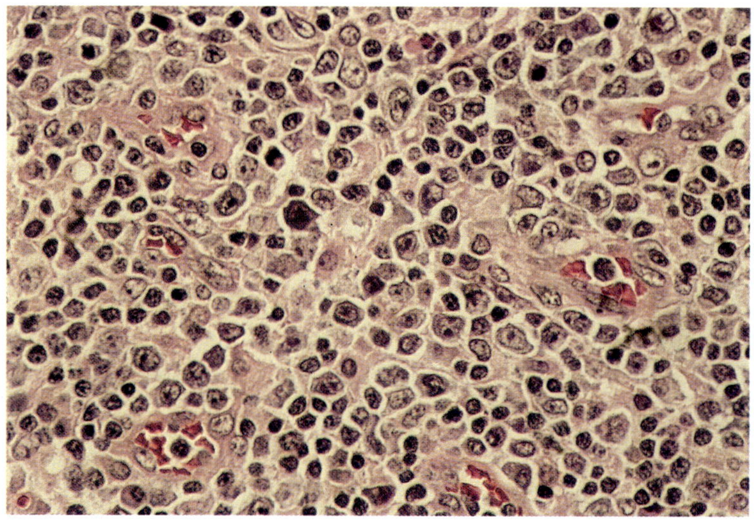

FIGURE
7.8

Infectious mononucleosis, higher magnification, showing numerous immunoblasts.

also infects oropharyngeal epithelial cells (Sixbey et al, 1984). The atypical lymphocytes in the peripheral blood are predominantly CD8 cytotoxic-suppressor T cells responding to EBV-infected B cells (DeWaele et al, 1981).

Histopathology

The lymph nodes in infectious mononucleosis exhibit a florid immunoblastic proliferation which may be confused with Hodgkin's disease or non-Hodgkin's lymphoma (Childs et al, 1987). The paracortex is expanded by proliferation of immunoblasts, pleomorphic immunoblasts, and Reed-Sternberg-like cells, frequently with foci of necrosis (Figs. 7.7,

FIGURE
7.9

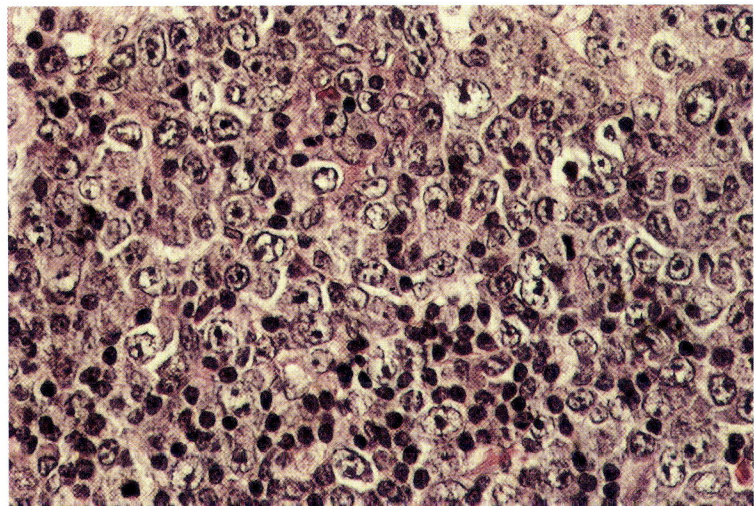

Infectious mononucleosis showing numerous immunoblasts and "mottled" appearance.

FIGURE
7.10

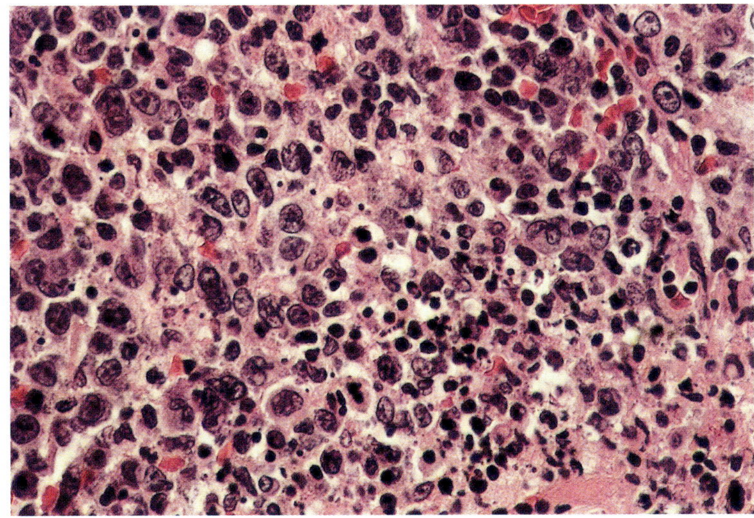

Infectious mononucleosis showing atypical cells adjacent to a focus of necrosis.

7.8, and 7.9). Reed-Sternberg-like cells and atypical cells are particularly prominent adjacent to foci of necrosis (Figs. 7.10 and 7.11). The follicles are frequently hyperplastic. The sinusoids are dilated and contain immunoblasts, plasma cells, and atypical lymphocytes, resembling those in the peripheral blood (Downey cells) (Figs. 7.12 and 7.13). The Reed-Sternberg-like cells are positive for CD30 (Abbondanzo et al, 1990).

Differential Diagnosis

Infectious mononucleosis may mimic Hodgkin's disease or non-Hodgkin's lymphoma. The presence of Reed-Sternberg-like cells (pleomorphic immunoblasts) in infectious

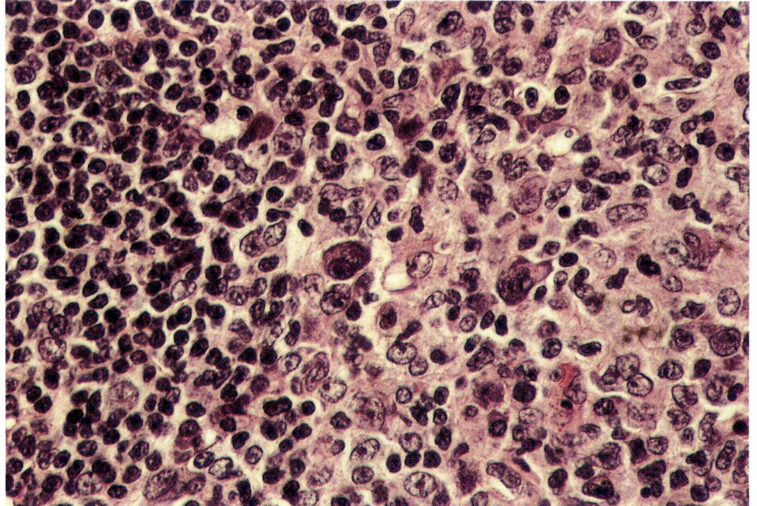

FIGURE 7.11

Infectious mononucleosis showing a Reed-Sternberg–like cell.

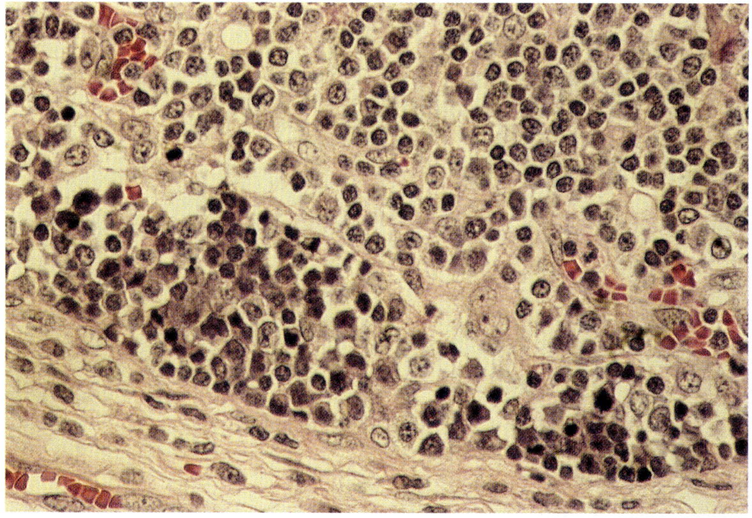

FIGURE 7.12

Infectious mononucleosis showing distention of the sinuses by atypical lymphocytes.

mononucleosis is now well recognized (Tindle et al, 1972). Pleomorphic immunoblasts may resemble Reed-Sternberg cells closely and in some cases may be indistinguishable; the nucleoli of pleomorphic immunoblasts are typically more basophilic than those of Reed-Sternberg cells and a prominent perinuclear Golgi zone may be present. The cellular background of Hodgkin's disease, however, which consists of small mature lymphocytes and admixed inflammatory cells, is distinct from that of infectious mononucleosis, which is characterized by large transformed lymphocytes and prominent immunoblasts. Immunophenotypic studies may be helpful in differential diagnosis. The Reed-Sternberg-

FIGURE
7.13

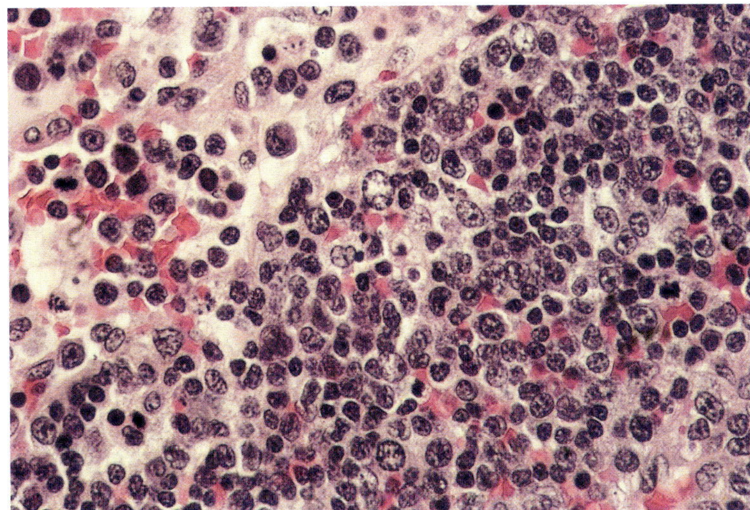

Infectious mononucleosis showing sinus involvement by atypical lymphocytes.

like cells in infectious mononucleosis are frequently positive for CD30 (Abbondanzo et al, 1990), but unlike Reed-Sternberg cells in Hodgkin's disease, they are negative for CD15 (Childs et al, 1987) and frequently express B cell antigens (CD20). Immunohistochemical staining for EBV latent membrane protein (EBV-LMP) is positive in infectious mononucleosis but may not be helpful in differential diagnosis since EBV is frequently present in Reed-Sternberg cells in Hodgkin's disease (Weiss et al, 1989). In situ hybridization for EBV, however, may reveal a characteristic pattern (Shin et al, 1991). The most useful histologic criteria for the distinction of infectious mononucleosis from Hodgkin's disease and non-Hodgkin's lymphoma are the polymorphous background of transformed lymphocytes, persistence of reactive foci, and preservation of the underlying architecture (Childs et al, 1987).

The diagnosis of infectious mononucleosis should be considered in any atypical immunoblastic proliferation, particularly in the young adult, and pursued by appropriate investigations, including examination of the peripheral blood smear for atypical lymphocytes, serum serology for heterophile antibodies (Monospot test), and serum serology for specific antibodies to Epstein-Barr virus. The presence of IgM antibodies to Epstein-Barr virus capsid antigen (VCA) indicates recent infection; IgG antibodies to VCA indicate past infection. If infectious mononucleosis is suspected clinically, laboratory confirmation of the diagnosis should be obtained, and lymph node biopsy avoided, because of the lack of diagnostic specificity and possibility of misinterpretation.

Course and Prognosis

Infectious mononucleosis is generally a benign self-limited illness. Complications include autoimmune phenomena (autoimmune hemolytic anemia and thrombocytopenia), X-linked lymphoproliferative syndrome in susceptible families (Duncan's syndrome), and, rarely, the virus-associated hemophagocytic syndrome.

REFERENCES

Abbondanzo SL, Sato N, Strauss SE, Jaffe ES. Acute infectious mononucleosis. CD30 (Ki-1) antigen expression and histologic correlations. Am J Clin Pathol 93:698–702, 1990.

Childs CC, Parham DM, Berard CW. Infectious mononucleosis. The spectrum of morphologic changes simulating lymphoma in lymph nodes and tonsils. Am J Surg Pathol 11:122–132, 1987.

DeWaele M, Thielemns C, Van Camp BKG. Characterization of immunoregulatory T cells in EBV-induced infectious mononucleosis by monoclonal antibodies. N Engl J Med 304:460, 1981.

Dorfman RF, Herweg J. Live attenuated measles virus vaccine: Inguinal lymphadenopathy complicating administration. JAMA 198:313–316, 1966.

Downey H, McKinlay CA. Acute lymphadenosis compared with acute lymphatic leukemia. Arch Intern Med 322:82, 1923.

Hartsock RJ. Postvaccinial lymphadenitis: Hyperplasia of lymphoid tissue that simulates malignant lymphoma. Cancer 21:632–649, 1968.

Rushin JM, Riordan GP, Heaton RB, Sharpe RW, Cotelingam JD, Jaffe ES. Cytomegalovirus-infected cells express Leu-M1 antigen. A potential source of diagnostic error. Am J Pathol 136:989–995, 1990.

Shin SS, Berry GJ, Weiss LM. Infectious mononucleosis. Diagnosis by in situ hybridization in two cases with atypical features. Am J Surg Pathol 15:625–631, 1991.

Sixbey JW, Nedrud JG, Raab-Traub N, Hanes RQ, Pagano JS. Epstein-Barr virus replication in oropharyngeal epithelial cells. N Engl J Med 310:1225–1230, 1984.

Strano AJ. Measles (Rubeola). In: Pathology of Tropical and Extraordinary Disease. Binford CH, Connor DH, eds. Washington, D.C., Armed Forces Institute of Pathology, pp 73–75, 1976.

Sumiyoshi Y, Kikuchi M, Ohshima K, Takeshita M, Eizuru Y, Minamishima Y. A case of human herpesvirus-6 lymphadenitis with infectious mononucleosis-like syndrome. Pathol Int 45:947–951, 1995.

Tamaru J, Atsuo M, Horie H, Itoh K, Asai T, Hondo R, Mori S. Herpes simplex lymphadenitis. Report of two cases with review of the literature. Am J Surg Pathol 14:571–577, 1990.

Tindle BH, Parker JW, Lukes RJ. "Reed-Sternberg cells" in infectious mononucleosis. Am J Clin Pathol 58:607–617, 1972.

Weiss LM, Movahed LA, Warnke RA, Sklar J. Detection of Epstein-Barr viral genomes in Reed-Sternberg cells of Hodgkin's disease. N Engl J Med 320:502–506, 1989.

Younes M, Podesta A, Helie M, Buckley P. Infection of T but not B lymphocytes by cytomegalovirus in lymph node. An immunophenotypic study. Am J Surg Pathol 15:75–80, 1991.

8

Bacterial and Mycobacterial Lymphadenitis

A variety of bacterial and mycobacterial infections produce characteristic changes in lymph nodes of diagnostic significance.

Cat Scratch Disease

Cat scratch disease (CSD) is a bacterial lymphadenitis which follows a cat scratch or other skin puncture. The etiologic agent of CSD was until quite recently unknown; for many years it was considered likely to be of chlamydial origin because of the histopathologic similarities to lymphogranuloma venereum. In 1983, Wear and his colleagues at the Armed Forces Institute of Pathology identified, for the first time, a pleomorphic Gram-negative rod in the tissue of 34 of 39 cases of CSD, using the Warthin-Starry silver impregnation technique, which they named *Afipia* (from the acronym for the Armed Forces Institute of Pathology) *felis* (Wear et al, 1983). In 1988, LeBoit and his colleagues reported on an apparently new bacterial infection in patients with AIDS, bacillary angiomatosis, which was characterized by cutaneous angiomatous lesions and contained organisms similar to CSD (LeBoit et al, 1988). These organisms were identified as members of the genus *Rochalimaea* (now *Bartonella*), principally *B. henselae* and *B. quintana* (Adal et al, 1994). Subsequently it was shown that *B. henselae* also causes cat scratch disease and is likely the more prevalent agent (Adal et al, 1994; Dolan et al, 1993).

Clinical Features

Cat scratch disease is principally a disease of children; the offending cat is usually a new kitten. The mode of inoculation is a scratch, bite, or other puncture; or it may be

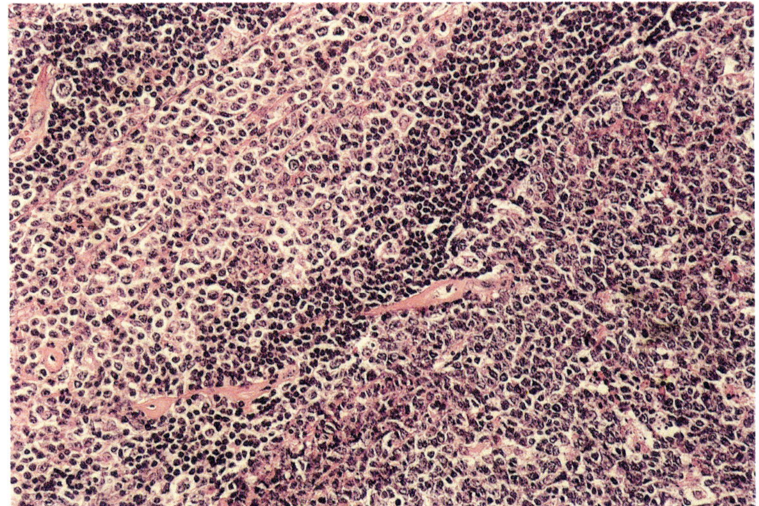

FIGURE
8.1

Cat scratch disease. Early lesion showing follicular lymphoid hyperplasia and monocytoid cells.

inapparent or mucosal (e.g., conjunctival). Several days after the scratch a papule or pustule appears at the site of inoculation, but it may be inapparent or missed. This is followed by the development, over 1–2 weeks, of tender regional lymphadenopathy, most frequently axillary or cervical, accompanied by mild systemic signs. Lymphadenopathy persists for several weeks. The oculoglandular syndrome of Parinaud refers to CSD following conjunctival inoculation with preauricular lymphadenopathy.

Histopathology

The earliest lymph node change in CSD is a nonspecific lymphoid hyperplasia; follicular lymphoid hyperplasia and monocytoid B cells may be prominent in early lesions (Fig. 8.1). Lymphoid hyperplasia is followed by the appearance of pale-staining foci of necrosis in the paracortex, surrounded by histiocytes and immunoblasts (Fig. 8.2). The characteristic well-developed lesion of CSD is the "suppurative granuloma" or "stellate microabscess." This is a confluent, ovoid-to-stellate area of necrosis bordered by a zone of palisaded histiocytes and filled with polymorphonuclear leukocytes (Figs. 8.3 and 8.4). Well-formed epithelioid granulomata or multinucleated giant cells are scarce. Dieterle or Warthin-Starry silver stains demonstrate the causative microorganisms (Fig. 8.5). These are seen as tangles of small, pleomorphic bacillary forms, which may be found in the walls of capillaries, in histiocytes, or in follicular centers (Wear et al, 1983). Paradoxically, few organisms are found in the suppurative exudate.

Differential Diagnosis

Cat scratch disease should be distinguished from other granulomatous lymphadenitides with similar morphologic changes, including fungal and mycobacterial infections, atypical mycobacteria, lymphogranuloma venereum, *Yersinia enterocolitica* and *Yersinia*

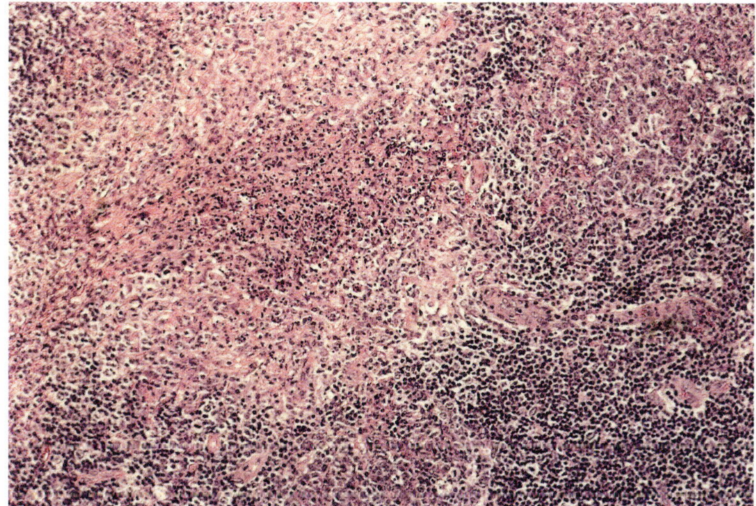

Cat scratch disease. More advanced lesion characterized by pale-staining foci of necrosis.

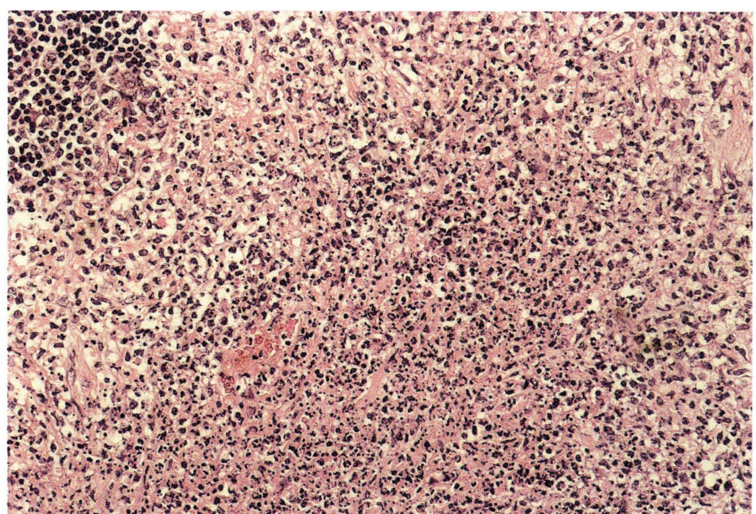

Cat scratch disease. Well-developed lesion showing suppurative granuloma or stellate microabscess surrounded by a zone of palisaded histiocytes and containing polymorphonuclear leukocytes.

pseudotuberculosis lymphadenitis, tularemia, and brucellosis. Lymphogranuloma venereum, due to venereally acquired infection with *Chlamydia trachomatis*, produces histopathologic changes virtually indistinguishable from CSD but typically involves inguinal lymph nodes. *Yersinia enterocolitica* and *Yersinia pseudotuberculosis*, also produce similar changes but are typically associated with mesenteric lymphadenitis. Hodgkin's disease may occasionally contain necrotic foci resembling the stellate microabscesses of CSD but is distinguished by the presence of diagnostic Reed-Sternberg cells.

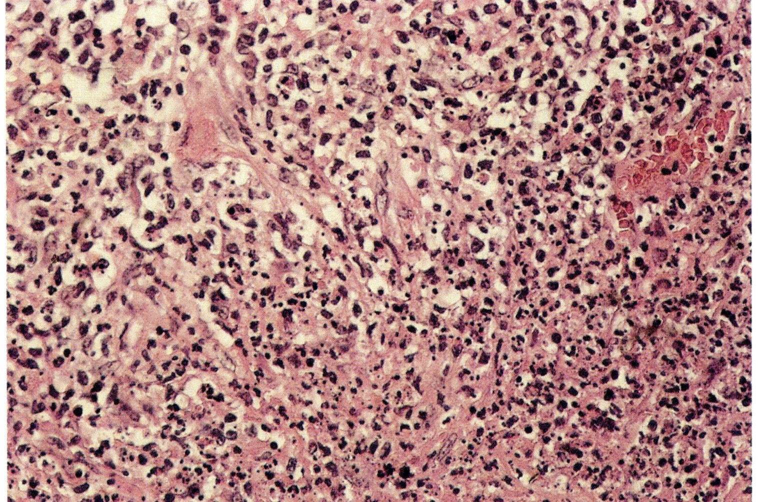

FIGURE
8.4

Cat scratch disease. Suppurative granuloma or stellate microabscess showing histiocytes and polymorphonuclear leukocytes.

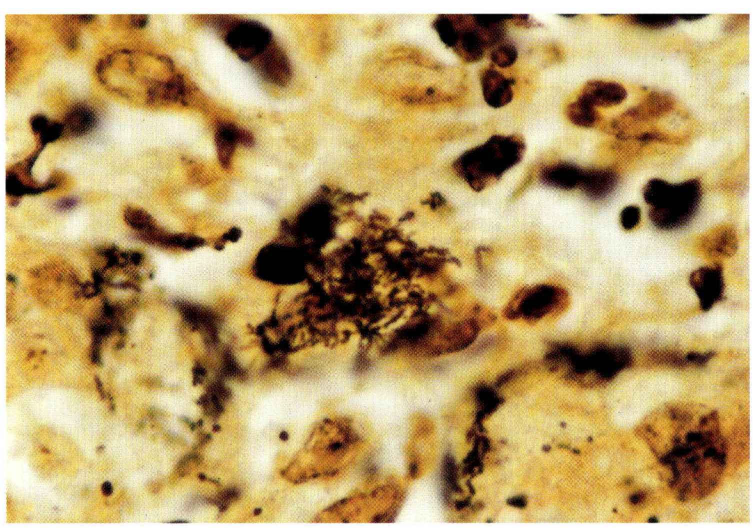

FIGURE
8.5

Cat scratch disease. Warthin-Starry silver impregnation stain showing cat scratch bacilli.

A history of exposure to cats is obtainable in 90% of patients with CSD and is helpful in diagnosis. Definitive diagnosis of CSD requires identification of the characteristic organism by Dieterle or Warthin-Starry silver stains. A skin test for CSD was formerly utilized, but the antigen, prepared from CSD lymph nodes, is no longer widely available. Serologic testing for antibodies to *B. henselae* is being increasingly utilized for diagnosis (Adal et al, 1994).

Course and Prognosis

Cat scratch disease is generally a benign self-limited illness, with spontaneous resolution of the lymphadenopathy within several weeks. Encephalitis and septic complications, principally osteomyelitis, occasionally occur. Despite the well established bacterial etiology of CSD, a beneficial effect of antibiotic therapy in uncomplicated cases has not been conclusively shown, and the role of routine antibiotic therapy of CSD is controversial (Adal et al, 1994).

Bacillary Angiomatosis

Bacillary angiomatosis was first recognized in patients with AIDS as a syndrome of multiple, cutaneous, hemangioma-like lesions caused by bacilli of the genus *Rochalimaea* (now *Bartonella*), principally *B. henselae* and *B. quintana* (Relman et al, 1990; Koehler et al, 1997). It is now recognized that visceral infection (bacillary peliosis) and lymph node involvement also occur (Chan et al, 1991; Perkocha et al, 1990).

Clinical Features

Bacillary angiomatosis occurs predominantly in patients with AIDS but has also been recognized rarely in immunocompetent individuals and transplant recipients (Tappero et al, 1993). As in cat scratch disease, a history of exposure to cats may be obtained. The skin lesions are typically multiple erythematous nodules and may be associated with constitutional symptoms of fever and weight loss (Fig. 8.6). Dissemination to extracutaneous sites, including heart, liver, spleen, lymph nodes, bone marrow, gastrointesti-

FIGURE 8.6

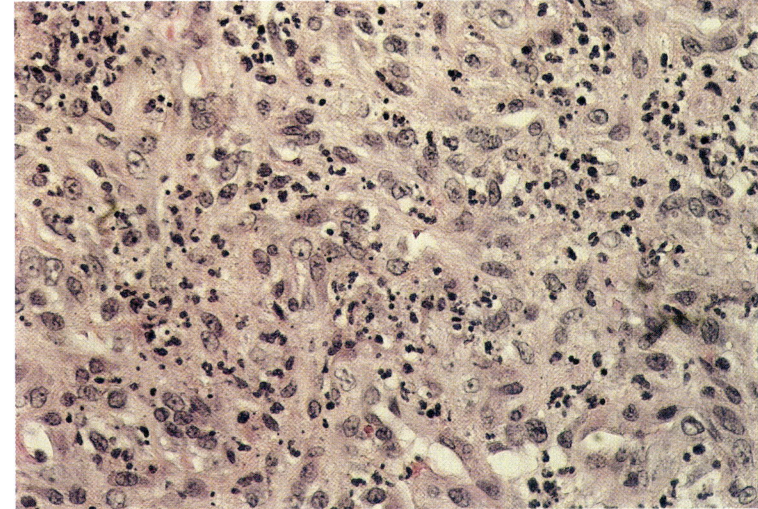

Skin lesion of bacillary angiomatosis showing epithelioid vascular proliferation and polymorphonuclear leukocytes.

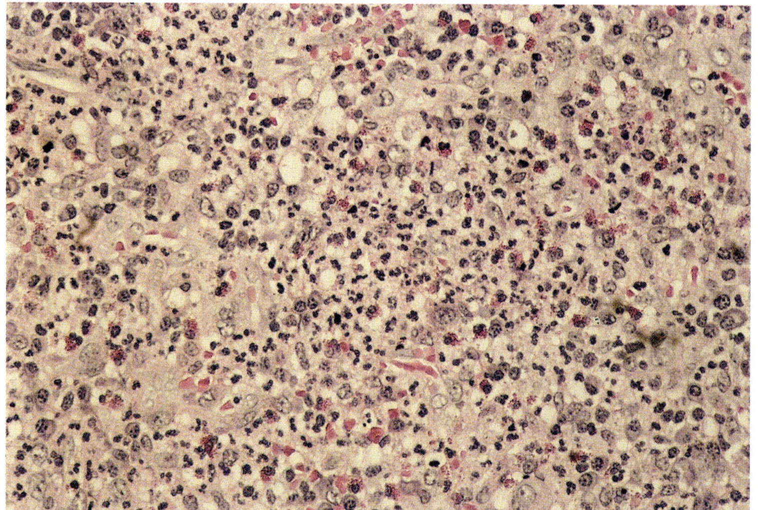

FIGURE 8.7

Lymph node involvement in bacillary angiomatosis, characterized by epithelioid vascular proliferation and polymorphonuclear leukocytes.

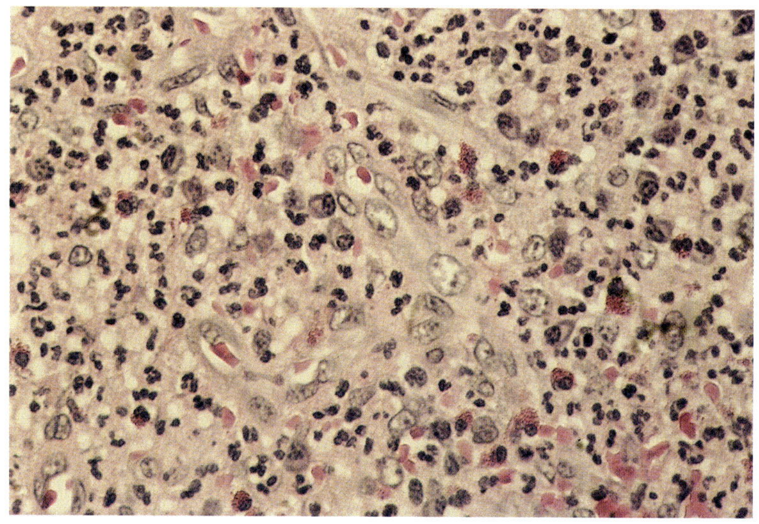

FIGURE 8.8

Lymph node involvement in bacillary angiomatosis showing atypia of proliferating endothelial cells.

nal tract, soft tissue, bone, and central nervous system occurs (Adal et al, 1994). Lymph node involvement may occur in the absence of cutaneous lesions (Chan et al, 1991).

Histopathology

The lymph node lesion of bacillary angiomatosis resembles the cutaneous lesion. The lymph node is replaced by coalescent nodules of granulation-like tissue, consisting of blood vessels lined by "plump" epithelioid endothelial cells, with mild-to-moderate nuclear atypia (Chan et al, 1991) (Figs. 8.7 and 8.8). The stroma is edematous, with varying numbers of polymorphonuclear leukocytes, and deposits of amorphous basophilic material. Warthin-Starry or Giemsa staining reveals the basophilic material to consist of masses of bacterial forms.

Differential Diagnosis

The differential diagnosis of bacillary angiomatosis in the lymph node includes other vascular proliferations, principally Kaposi's sarcoma and angiosarcoma. The distinction is critical since bacillary angiomatosis responds to antibiotic therapy. The presence of nuclear atypia and "plump" epithelioid endothelial cells may at first suggest a vascular neoplasm; however, the edematous stroma and deposits of amorphous basophilic material are characteristic of bacillary angiomatosis. The diagnosis is confirmed by Warthin-Starry or Giemsa staining, demonstrating the characteristic bacterial forms. The bacteria may also be demonstrated ultrastructurally.

Course and Prognosis

Bacillary angiomatosis responds dramatically to antibiotic therapy, with prompt resolution of the lesions and disappearance of systemic symptoms.

Lymphogranuloma Venereum

Lymphogranuloma venereum results from venereal infection with *Chlamydia trachomatis*.

Clinical Features

Lymphogranuloma venereum results from sexual transmission of *Chlamydia trachomatis*. The initial lesion is a small ulcer or papule at the site of inoculation, usually on the penis or vulva, which heals spontaneously. This is followed by the onset of tender, regional lymphadenopathy, most frequently involving inguinal lymph nodes, with fever and constitutional signs. The lymph nodes often suppurate and drain, leading to fistulae and scarring.

Histopathology

The lymph node changes of lymphogranuloma venereum are indistinguishable from cat scratch disease, with formation of "suppurative granulomas" and "stellate microabscesses." As in cat scratch disease, well-formed epithelioid granulomas and multinucleated giant cells are scarce. Warthin-Starry, Dieterle, and other stains for microorganisms are negative.

Differential Diagnosis

The primary mucosal lesion of lymphogranuloma venereum is frequently missed; however, the occurrence of suppurative inguinal lymphadenopathy in a sexually active adult should suggest the diagnosis. The diagnosis is established serologically or by isolation of *Chlamydia trachomatis.*

Course and Prognosis

Lymphogranuloma venereum is treated with antibiotics effective for *Chlamydia.* Late complications include regional scarring, lymphedema, and urethral or rectal strictures.

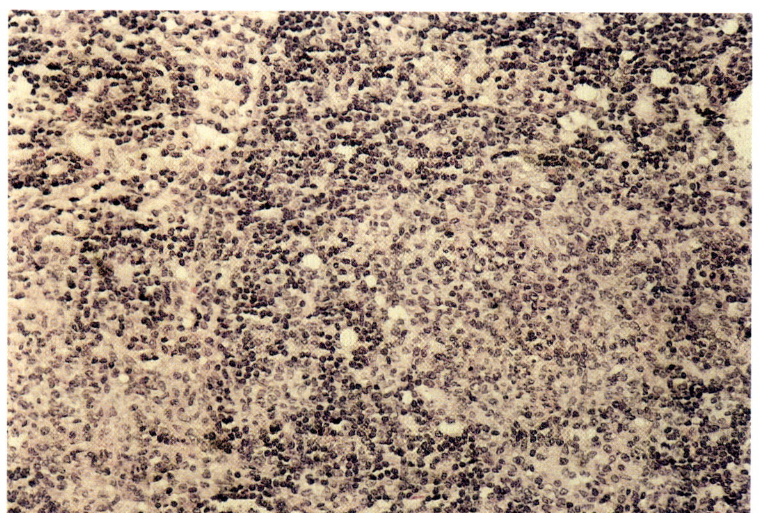

FIGURE 8.9

Mesenteric lymphadenitis due to *Yersinia* species showing early suppurative granuloma formation. Clinical findings mimic acute appendicitis.

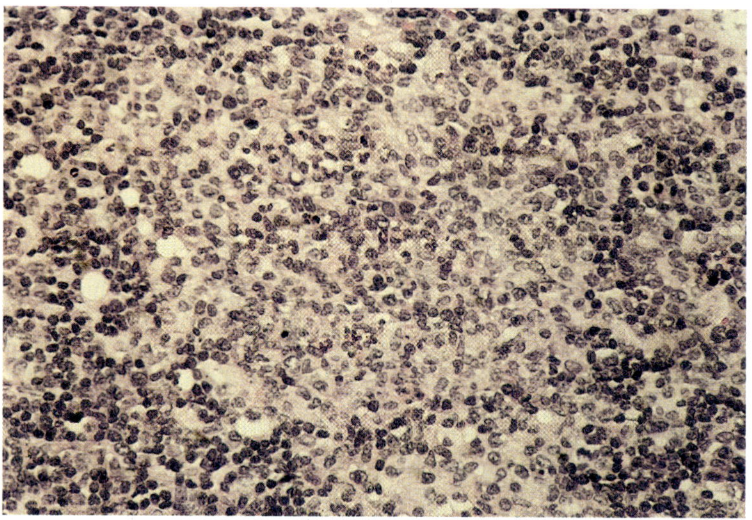

FIGURE 8.10

Mesenteric lymphadenitis due to *Yersinia* species showing early suppurative granuloma formation.

Other Causes of Suppurative Granulomas

Other causes of suppurative granulomas in lymph nodes include tularemia, due to infection with *Francisella tularensis*, acquired from rabbits; brucellosis, due to *Brucella abortus* and related *Brucella* species, acquired from cattle and other domestic animals; and *Yersinia enterocolitica* and *Yersinia pseudotuberculosis*, causes of diarrheal illness and mesenteric lymphadenitis. Mesenteric lymphadenitis due to *Yersinia enterocolitica* or *Yersinia pseudotuberculosis* is a frequent cause of enlarged mesenteric lymph nodes found at surgery for suspected acute appendicitis (Figs. 8.9 and 8.10). Specific diagnosis of suppurative granulomas in lymph nodes is based on clinical and serological findings or isolation of the organism.

Plague Lymphadenitis

Plague is epizootic in wild rodents in the western part of the United States (sylvatic plague) with occasional instances of transmission to humans. Plague is caused by a Gram-negative bacillus, *Yersinia pestis*, which is transmitted to humans from infected rodents by fleas.

Clinical Features

Plague is an acute febrile illness which occurs in bubonic, septicemic, and pneumonic forms. The bubonic form, characterized by hemorrhagic lymphadenitis, with high fever and prostration, follows the bite of an infected flea; the pneumonic form, characterized by hemorrhagic pneumonia, is acquired by inhalation. The "bubos," characteristic of the bubonic form of the disease, are greatly enlarged, tender, hemorrhagic lymph nodes. Inguinal, axillary, or cervical lymph nodes may be involved (Smith, 1976).

Histopathology

The histopathology of plague is usually only seen at autopsy. The involved lymph nodes are greatly enlarged, with massive exudation of proteinaceous fluid, hemorrhage, and necrosis. Large masses of bacteria are present, mimicking postmortem growth and eliciting little cellular response.

Differential Diagnosis

The diagnosis of plague is established bacteriologically by examination of lymph node aspirate, sputum, or blood. Blood cultures are positive in 50% of cases (Smith, 1976). In areas where plague occurs, physicians and pathologists should maintain a high index of suspicion, since early antibiotic therapy may be life saving. Necrotizing hemorrhagic lymphadenitis is also a feature of anthrax; hemorrhagic necrosis of intrathoracic lymph nodes is characteristic of inhalational anthrax (Abramova et al, 1993).

Course and Prognosis

Untreated plague has a mortality rate of 50–100%, which is reduced to 5–10% by early antibiotic therapy. Particular attention must be paid to handling infected tissue, which is highly infectious; routine prophylactic antibiotic therapy is recommended for individuals participating in a plague autopsy.

Luetic Lymphadenitis

Syphilis results from infection with the spirochete *Treponema pallidum* and is associated with lymphadenitis in the primary and secondary stages of the disease.

Clinical Features

Syphilis is usually acquired venereally. Primary syphilis is characterized by a mucosal ulcer, or chancre, at the site of inoculation and painless regional lymphadenopathy, usually involving the inguinal lymph nodes. Secondary syphilis is characterized by skin rash and generalized lymphadenopathy. Tertiary syphilis is characterized by neurologic and/or cardiovascular lesions and gummas, necrotic granuloma-like lesions.

Histopathology

Luetic lymphadenitis occurs in the primary and secondary stages of syphilis and is characterized by a florid follicular lymphoid hyperplasia with numerous interfollicular plasma cells. Scattered clusters of epithelioid histiocytes and noncaseating epithelioid granulomata are frequently present (Hartsock et al, 1970). Endarteritis, with inflammation of small vessels, is a frequent feature. Warthin-Starry silver stain reveals the presence of the characteristic spiral bacteria, which are most numerous in areas of endarteritis and granuloma formation (Hartsock et al, 1970). Immunofluorescence may also be utilized to demonstrate the spirochetes (Choi and Reiner, 1979).

Differential Diagnosis

Luetic lymphadenitis must be distinguished from other causes of florid follicular hyperplasia (rheumatoid disease, HIV infection) and from follicular lymphoma (Goffinet et al, 1970). The presence of granulomas and endarteritis may suggest the diagnosis. The diagnosis is established by demonstrating spirochetes by Warthin-Starry stain or immunofluorescence; or by serological testing with nontreponemal (VDRL or RPR) or treponemal (FTA-ABS) antigens.

Course and Prognosis

Syphilis is treated with antibiotics.

Whipple's Disease

Whipple's disease (intestinal lipodystrophy) is due to systemic infection with a previously undescribed actinomycete, *Tropheryma whippelii* (Relman et al, 1992). Whipple's disease may be a cause of mesenteric or other lymphadenopathy.

Clinical Features

Whipple's disease is a chronic disorder, characterized by arthritis, intestinal malabsorption, and central nervous system manifestations, due to accumulation of histiocytes containing characteristic periodic acid–Schiff (PAS)-positive inclusions. The PAS-positive inclusions are bacilli, now identified as *Tropheryma whippelii* (Relman et al, 1992). Mesenteric or peripheral lymphadenopathy is frequently present in Whipple's disease, and the diagnostic value of lymph node biopsy has long been recognized (Chears et al, 1959; Ereno et al, 1993).

Histopathology

The lymph nodes in Whipple's disease are characterized by PAS-positive histiocytes, as are found in other organs (Fleming et al, 1988). The sinuses are distended with histiocytes containing characteristic PAS-positive material and lipid; and epithelioid granulomas may be present. The accumulation of lipid may mimic lipogranulomata or lymphangiogram effect.

Differential Diagnosis

Whipple's disease must be distinguished from other histiocytic infiltrates involving the lymph nodes. The accumulation of histiocytes and lipid may suggest lipogranulomata or lymphangiogram effect; the presence of epithelioid granulomata may suggest sarcoidosis (Rouillon et al, 1993). The PAS stain is helpful, revealing the characteristic PAS-positive, granular, cytoplasmic inclusions of Whipple's disease. Definitive diagnosis is based on ultrastructural studies demonstrating the bacillary bodies of Whipple's disease or PCR demonstrating the presence of *Tropheryma whippelii* ribosomal RNA (Relman et al, 1992).

Course and Prognosis

Whipple's disease is treated with antibiotics. The occurrence of the BCL-2 gene rearrangement in lymphoid tissue from a patient with Whipple's disease (Fest et al, 1996) and the development of extraintestinal lymphoma have been reported (Gillen et al, 1993).

Tuberculous Lymphadenitis

Mycobacterium tuberculosis has reemerged as a major pathogen due to the effects of HIV infection and the emergence of multidrug-resistant strains. Tuberculous lymphadenitis is due to *Mycobacterium tuberculosis* infection of lymph nodes.

Clinical Features

Tuberculous lymphadenitis occurs in the course of primary infection with *Mycobacterium tuberculosis* but may also be seen in the course of reactivation tuberculosis, particularly in immunocompromised hosts. Tuberculous lymphadenitis is particularly prevalent in association with HIV infection. Involvement of mediastinal, supraclavicular, or

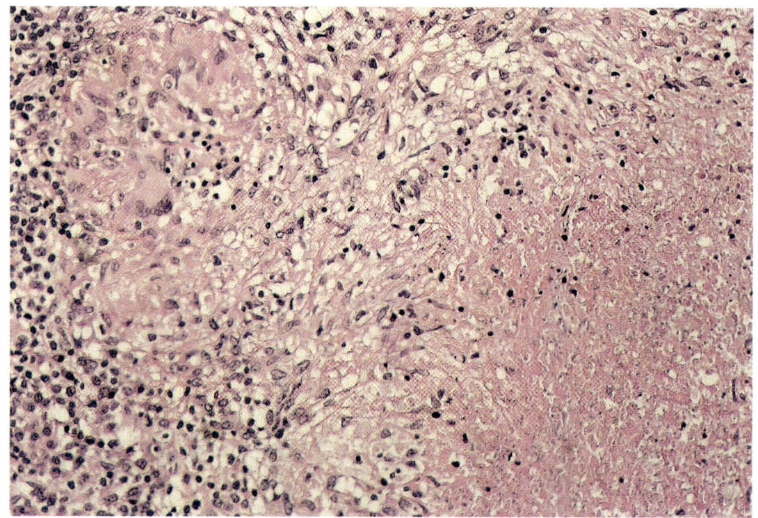

FIGURE 8.11

Tuberculous lymphadenitis showing epithelioid granulomata with caseation necrosis.

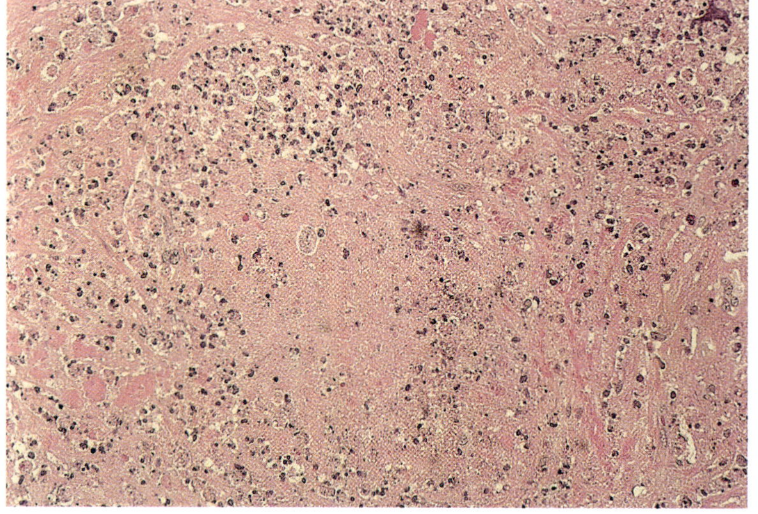

FIGURE 8.12

Tuberculous miliary necrosis. Extensive necrosis with poorly formed or absent granulomata occurs in immunosuppressed hosts and indicates a poor prognosis.

cervical lymph nodes is frequent. Concomitant pulmonary tuberculosis may or may not be present (Lee et al, 1992). Cervical lymphadenitis in children, due to tonsillar infection with *Mycobacterium bovis* acquired from milk, is now uncommon. The lymph nodes in tuberculous lymphadenitis are firm, nontender, rubbery, and may be matted.

Histopathology

Tuberculous lymphadenitis is characterized by epithelioid granulomata with caseation necrosis (Fig 8.11). Granulomata at all stages of development may be present. The earliest granulomata are noncaseating and consists of epithelioid histiocytes and multinucleated giant cells of Langhans' type. (The Langhans' cell, which is also found in sarcoidosis and other epithelioid granulomas, is characterized by a ring of nuclei arranged in a "C" configuration.) The more advanced granulomata contain well developed areas of central caseous necrosis, characterized by amorphous, eosinophilic material, which is nonsuppurative. Plasma cells and scattered neutrophils are frequently present. The late lesion consists of confluent masses of caseous material surrounded by a rim of palisaded epithelioid histiocytes and giant cells with surrounding fibrosis. Stains for acid fast bacilli (Ziehl-Neelsen, Kinyoun, or auramine-rhodamine) are frequently positive, revealing the characteristic slender, curved or "beaded," bacilli, measuring 2–8 μm in length. Bacilli may be found in the caseous material or in the cytoplasm of epithelioid histiocytes and giant cells. Bacilli may be difficult to identify in the late lesions. Tuberculous lymphadenitis in patients with HIV infection and other immunosuppressed patients is characterized by poorly formed or ill-defined granulomata and numerous acid fast bacilli (Fig. 8.12). Fulminant disseminated tuberculosis may be associated with extensive necrosis without well-formed granulomata and is associated with a poor prognosis (Medd and Hayhoe, 1955).

Differential Diagnosis

Tuberculous lymphadenitis must be distinguished from other causes of necrotizing and non-necrotizing granulomatous lymphadenitis, including atypical mycobacteria, fungi, and sarcoidosis. Definitive diagnosis of tuberculous lymphadenitis rests on identification of the organism by acid fast stains or culture. Mycobacterial cultures should be obtained on all tissues suspected of harboring *Mycobacterium tuberculosis* because of the emergence of multidrug-resistant strains and necessity of drug susceptibility testing. Newer diagnostic techniques, particularly PCR, may permit rapid diagnosis of mycobacterial infection (Sjobring et al, 1990). Fine needle aspiration biopsy may also be effectively utilized for the diagnosis of tuberculous lymphadenitis (Lee et al, 1992).

Course and Prognosis

Tuberculous lymphadenitis, like other forms of tuberculosis, is treated with combinations of antituberculous drugs. Because of the emergence of multidrug-resistant strains, initial therapy with four drugs is now recommended until drug susceptibility is confirmed by culture and susceptibility testing.

Atypical Mycobacterial Lymphadenitis

Mycobacterial lymphadenitis in childhood is frequently due to atypical mycobacteria, principally *Mycobacterium scrofulaceum* and *Mycobacterium kansasii*. Involvement of cervical lymph nodes is frequent. Histopathologic features suggestive of atypical mycobacterial infection include ill-defined and serpiginous granulomata, noncaseating or sarcoid-like granulomata, and suppurative granulomata (Pinder and Colville, 1993). Specific diagnosis requires microbiologic culture. Therapy is directed by susceptibility testing. *Mycobacterium scrofulaceum* lymphadenitis is frequently effectively managed by surgical excision of the involved lymph nodes.

Disseminated Bacillus Calmette-Guerin Lymphadenitis

Disseminated Bacillus Calmette-Guerin (BCG) infection involving lymph nodes and other organs may follow BCG inoculation in immunosuppressed hosts (Abramowsky et al, 1993) or the use of intravesical BCG for cancer immunotherapy (Ali el Dein and Nabeeh, 1996). Patients present with fever; regional or generalized lymphadenopathy may be present. The changes in involved lymph nodes range from noncaseating epithelioid granulomata, with or without acid fast bacilli, to extensive histiocytic infiltrates with numerous acid fast bacilli (Abramowsky et al, 1993). Disseminated BCG infection responds to therapy with antituberculous drugs.

Mycobacterium Avium-Intracellulare Lymphadenitis

Mycobacterium avium-intracellulare (MAI) was formerly an uncommon cause of pulmonary granulomatous disease but has now emerged as an important pathogen in patients with HIV infection.

Clinical Features

Mycobacterium avium-intracellulare occurs as a disseminated infection in patients with AIDS. MAI infection occurs principally in patients who are severely immunocompromised with CD4 counts of less than 100 per mm^3. Unlike *Mycobacterium tuberculosis*, MAI infection is environmentally acquired; person-to-person transmission is unknown. Disseminated MAI infection is characterized by fever, weight loss, and diarrhea; generalized lymphadenopathy and hepatosplenomegaly are frequently present.

Histopathology

Lymph nodes in MAI infection show a histiocytic lymphadenitis. The lymph node is infiltrated by sheets of histiocytes with abundant amphophilic cytoplasm (Figs. 8.13 and 8.14). The cytoplasm may be seen to contain delicate striations at higher magnification. Distinct granulomas or caseation necrosis are characteristically lacking. Stains for acid fast bacilli demonstrate the cytoplasm to be filled with sheaves of delicate, curved ba-

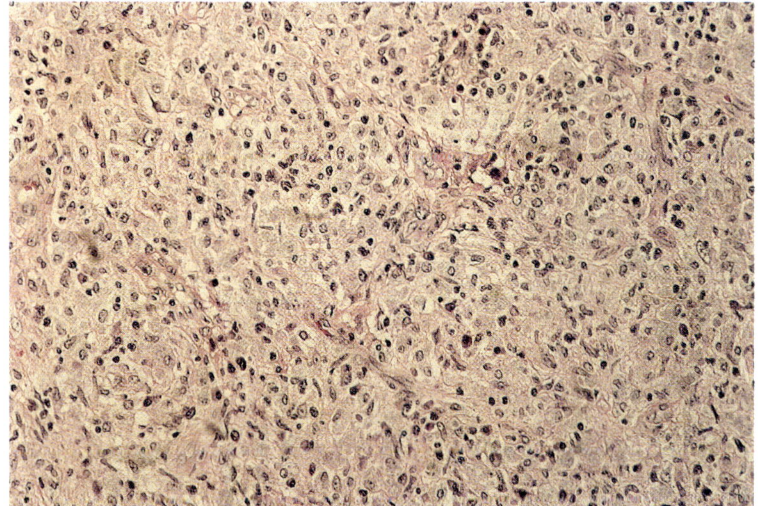

Mycobacterium avium-intracellulare lymphadenitis showing sheets of macrophage-histiocytes.

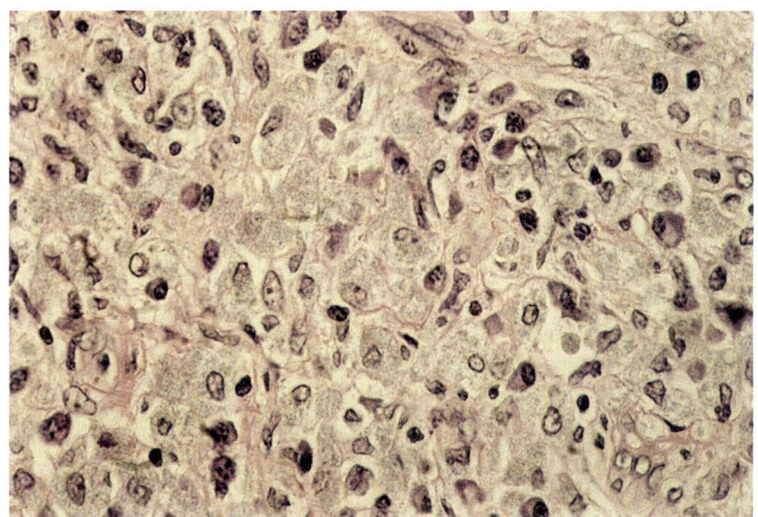

Mycobacterium avium-intracellulare lymphadenitis, higher magnification, showing histiocytes with amphophilic cytoplasm.

cilli (Fig. 8.15). The organisms are also stained by the PAS and methenamine silver techniques. Touch or imprint preparations, stained with Giemsa, demonstrate characteristic pseudo-Gaucher's cells, the nonstained intracellular organisms mimicking the cytoplasmic striations of Gaucher's disease (Solis et al, 1986). Nonstained extracellular organisms are also usually apparent. In some cases of MAI infection, the histiocytic response consists predominantly of spindled cells, which may mimic a spindle cell neoplasm (Brandwein et al, 1990; Chen, 1992) (Figs. 8.16 and 8.17).

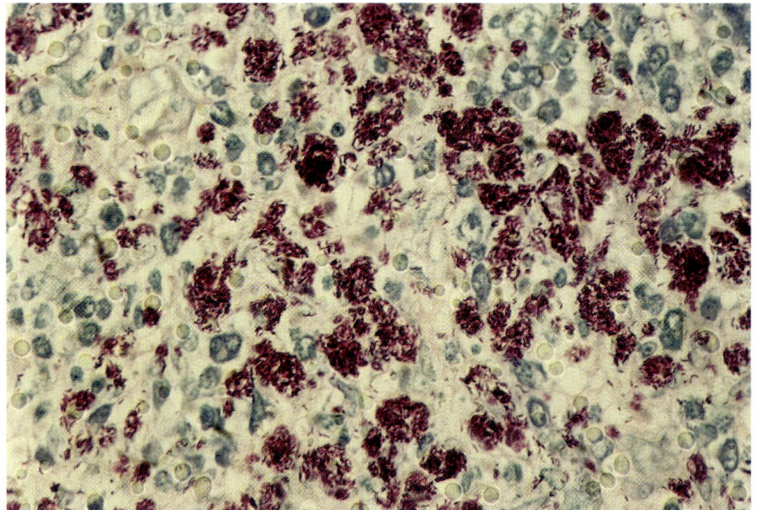

FIGURE
8.15

Mycobacterium avium-intracellulare lymphadenitis, acid fast stain, showing cytoplasm of histiocytes filled with acid bast bacilli.

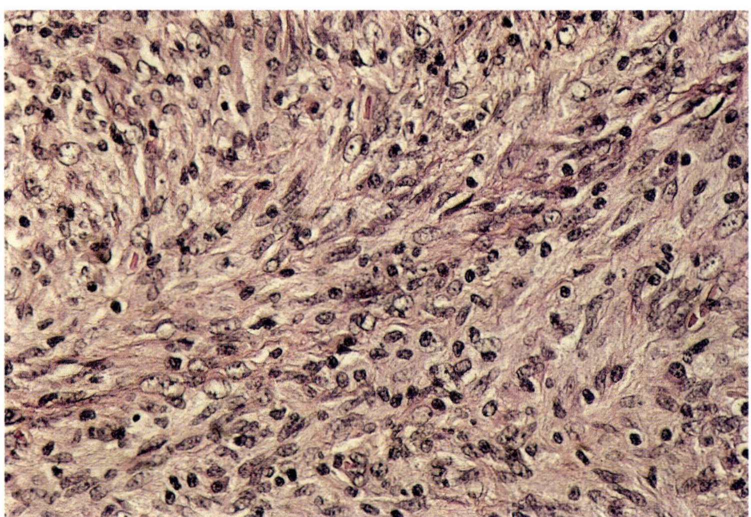

FIGURE
8.16

Pseudosarcomatous *Mycobacterium-avium intracellulare* infection with spindled histiocytes (so called "mycobacterial pseudotumor").

Differential Diagnosis

MAI lymphadenitis must be distinguished from storage disorders and from other causes of mycobacterial lymphadenitis. Although the histiocytes of disseminated MAI infection may mimic those of Gaucher's disease, stains for acid fast bacilli will be diagnostic. *Mycobacterium tuberculosis*, which also causes lymphadenitis in HIV infected patients, is distinguished by distinct granuloma formation and caseous necrosis. Bacilli of *Mycobacterium tuberculosis* are not stained by the PAS and methenamine silver techniques and are rarely as numerous as in MAI infection. *Mycobacterium leprae*, in lepromatous

**FIGURE
8.17**

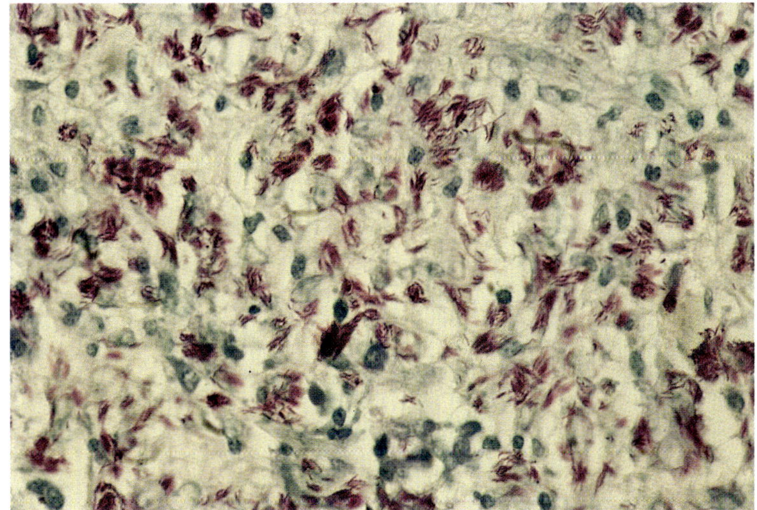

Pseudosarcomatous *Mycobacterium-avium intracellulare* infection, acid fast stain, showing numerous intracellular acid fast bacilli.

leprosy, is distinguished by the presence of "lepra cells," histiocytes containing "globi," or masses of intracellular organisms, and is only weakly acid fast and not stained by the PAS and methenamine silver techniques. MAI may also mimic Whipple's disease, particularly in biopsies from the gastrointestinal tract; the bacillus of Whipple's disease, however, *Tropheryma whippelii*, although characteristically PAS positive, is not acid fast and is not culturable (Gillin et al, 1983). MAI lymphadenitis with a predominantly spindle cell reaction ("pseudosarcomatous MAI" or "MAI pseudotumor") must be distinguished from spindle cell neoplasms involving lymph nodes, particularly Kaposi's sarcoma and fibrohistiocytic neoplasms (Brandwein et al, 1990; Chen, 1992). A similar spindle cell reaction is seen in histoid leprosy (Binford and Meyers, 1976). Stains for microorganisms will be diagnostic. Infection with an anonymous mycobacterium, with pseudo-Gaucher's cells, has been reported in a previously healthy child (Miale, 1977). The diagnosis of disseminated MAI infection may be established by endoscopic biopsy of the gastrointestinal tract, bone marrow biopsy, or lymph node biopsy. MAI is readily grown in culture and may be recovered from the peripheral blood or buffy coats.

Course and Prognosis

Disseminated MAI infection has a poor prognosis because of underlying immunodeficiency. Responses to combinations of antituberculous drugs and macrolide antibiotics occur.

Leprosy Lymphadenitis

Leprosy results from infection with *Mycobacterium leprae* and affects principally the skin and peripheral nerves. Lymph node involvement may occur, particularly in the lepromatous form of the disease.

Clinical Features

Leprosy occurs in two polar forms, tuberculoid and lepromatous, and two intermediate forms, indeterminate and borderline (Binford and Meyers, 1976). Tuberculoid leprosy is characterized by localized skin and peripheral nerve involvement, few organisms, and well-formed tuberculoid granulomas and appears to represent a strong host response to the organism. Lepromatous leprosy is characterized by disseminated involvement, numerous organisms, and poorly formed granulomas and appears to represent a poor host response to the organism. Lymph node involvement is seen predominantly in lepromatous leprosy; lymph nodes draining areas of tuberculoid leprosy may contain epithelioid granulomata (Binford and Meyers, 1976).

Histopathology

Leprosy lymphadenitis is characterized by infiltration of the lymph node sinuses and paracortex by histiocytes containing leprosy bacilli (Fig. 8.18). The histiocytes are large with abundant foamy eosinophilic cytoplasm (lepra cells). Multinucleated cells and cells containing masses of bacilli in a cytoplasmic vacuole (globi) are frequently present (Fig. 8.19). The appearance may suggest lipogranulomata. Routine acid fast stains (Ziehl-Neelsen, Kinyoun) may be negative; however, the Fite-Faraco stain demonstrates the lepra cells to be teeming with acid fast bacilli (Fig. 8.20). In tuberculoid leprosy, lymph nodes draining areas of cutaneous involvement may contain epithelioid granulomata; however, organisms are scant (Binford and Meyers, 1976).

Differential Diagnosis

Leprosy is seldom thought of in the differential diagnosis of lymphadenopathy in western countries. The characteristic skin lesions may similarly be overlooked or misinter-

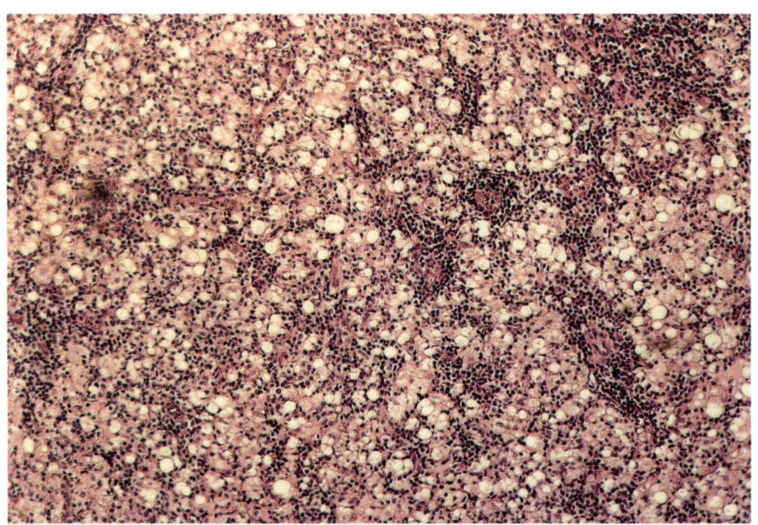

FIGURE 8.18

Leprosy lymphadenitis, low magnification, showing infiltrates of histiocytes.

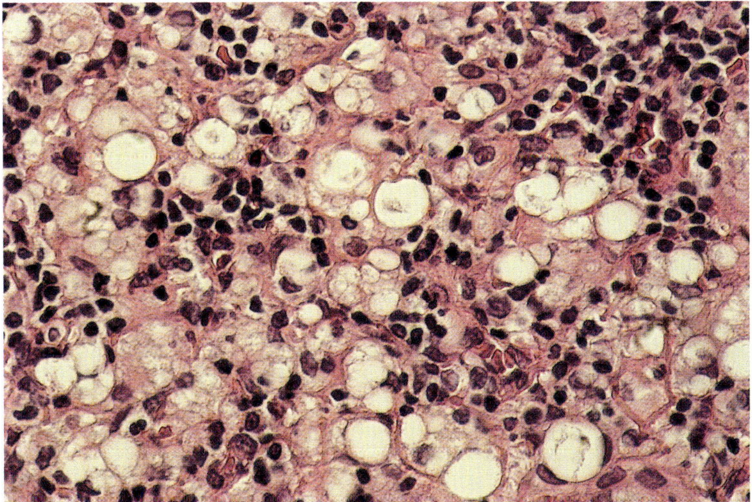

FIGURE 8.19

Leprosy lymphadenitis, higher magnification, showing characteristic "Lepra cells" and "globi," the latter consisting of masses of intracellular mycobacteria within a cytoplasmic vacuole.

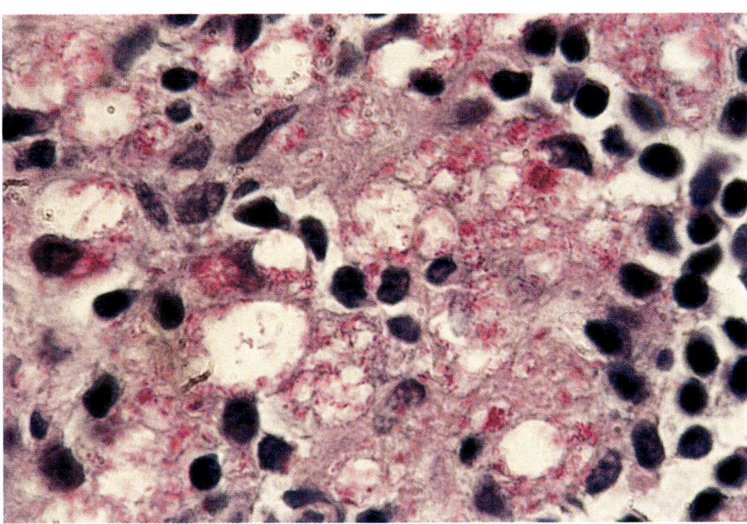

FIGURE 8.20

Leprosy lymphadenitis, Fite-Faraco stain, showing numerous intracellular acid fast bacilli.

preted. The initial histologic impression may be that of lipogranulomata or nonspecific sinus histiocytosis. The diagnostic difficulties are further compounded by the weak acid fastness of *Mycobacterium leprae*. The routine Ziehl-Neelsen and Kinyoun stains are frequently negative and the bacilli may be missed if the more sensitive Fite-Faraco stain is not performed. Leprosy lymphadenitis should be distinguished from other causes of histiocytic infiltration in lymph nodes, including MAI lymphadenitis and Whipple's disease. The presence of lepra cells and globi is characteristic. *Mycobacterium leprae*, in contrast to MAI, is not culturable.

Course and Prognosis

Leprosy is treated with combinations of antituberculous drugs and the sulfone drug dapsone.

REFERENCES

Abramova FA, Grinberg LM, Yampolaskaya OV, Walker DH. Pathology of inhalational anthrax in 42 cases from the Sverdlosvsk outbreak of 1979. Proc Natl Acad Sci USA 90:2291–2294, 1993.

Abramowsky C, Gonzalez B, Sorensen RU. Disseminated bacillus Calmette-Guerin infections in patients with primary immunodeficiencies. Am J Clin Pathol 100:52–26, 1993.

Adal KA, Cockerell CJ, Petri WA. Cat scratch disease, bacillary angiomatosis, and other infections due to Rochalemaea. N Engl J Med 330:1509–1515, 1994.

Ali el Dein B, Nabeeh A. Tuberculous iliac lymphadenitis: A rare complication of intravesical bacillus Calmette-Guerin and cause of tumor over staging. J Urol 156:1766–1767, 1996.

Binford CH, Meyers WM. Leprosy. In: Pathology of Tropical and Extraordinary Diseases. Binford CH, Connor DH, eds. Washington, D.C., Armed Forces Institute of Pathology, pp 205–225, 1976.

Brandwein M, Choi H-S H, Strauchen J, Stoler M, Jagirdar J. Spindle cell reaction to nontuberculous mycobacteriosis in AIDS mimicking a spindle cell neoplasm. Evidence for dual histiocytic and fibroblast-like characteristics of spindle cells. Virchow Arch A Pathol Anat 416:281–286, 1990.

Chan JKC, Lewin KJ, Lombard CM, Teitelbaum S, Dorfman RF. Histopathology of bacillary angiomatosis of lymph node. Am J Surg Pathol 15:430–437, 1991.

Chears WC, Smith AG, Ruffin JM. Diagnosis of Whipple's disease by peripheral lymph node biopsy: Report of a case. Am J Med 27:351–353, 1959.

Chen KTK. Mycobacterial spindle cell pseudotumor of lymph nodes. Am J Surg Pathol 16:276–281,1992.

Choi YJ, Reiner L. Syphilitic lymphadenitis: Immunofluorescent identification of spirochetes from imprints. Am J Surg Pathol 3:553–555, 1979.

Dolan MJ, Wong MT, Regnery RL, Jorgensen JH, Garcia M, Peters J, Drehner D. Syndrome of Rochalimaea henselae suggesting cat scratch disease. Ann Intern Med 118:331–336, 1993.

Ereno C, Lopez JI, Elizalde JM, Ibanez T, Fernandez-Larrinoa A, Toledo JD. A case of Whipple's disease presenting as supraclavicular lymphadenopathy. APMIS 101:865–868, 1993.

Fest T, Pron B, Lefranc MP, Pierre C, Angonin R, de Wazieres B, Soua Z, Dupond JL. Detection of a clonal BCL2 gene rearrangement in tissues from a patient with Whipple disease. Ann Intern Med 124:738–740, 1996.

Fleming JL, Wiesner RH, Shorter RG. Whipple's disease: Clinical, biochemical, and histopathologic features and assessment of treatment of 29 patients. Mayo Clin Proc 63:539–551, 1988.

Gillen CD, Coddington R, Monteith PG, Taylor RH. Extraintestinal lymphoma in association with Whipple's disease. Gut 34:1627–1629, 1993.

Gillin JS, Urmacher C, West R, Shike M. Disseminated Mycobacterium avium-intracellulare infection in acquired immunodeficiency syndrome mimicking Whipple' disease. Gastroenterology 85:1187, 1983.

Goffinet DR, Hoyt C, Eltringham JR. Secondary syphilis mis-diagnosed as lymphoma. California Med 112:22–23, 1970.

Hartsock RJ, Halling LW, King FM. Luetic lymphadenitis: A clinical and histologic study of 20 cases. Am J Clin Pathol 53:304–314, 1970.

Koehler JE, Sanchez MA, Garrido CS, Whitfeld MJ, Chen FM, Berger TG, et al. Molecular epidemiology of Bartonella infections in patients with bacillary angiomatosis-peliosis. N Engl J Med 337:1876–1883, 1997.

LeBoit PE, Berger TG, Egbert BM, Yen TSB, Stoler MH, Bonfiglio TA, Strauchen JA, English CK, Wear DJ. Epithelioid haemangioma-like vascular proliferation in AIDS: Manifestation of cat scratch disease bacillus infection? Lancet 1:960–963, 1988.

Lee KC, Tami TA, Lalwani AK, Schecter G. Contemporary management of cervical tuberculosis. Laryngoscope 102:60–64, 1992.

Medd WE, Hayhoe FGJ. Tuberculous miliary necrosis with pancytopenia. Q J Med 24:351, 1955.

Miale JB. Laboratory Medicine: Hematology, 5th ed. St Louis, CV Mosby, 1977.

Perkocha LA, Geaghan SM, Yen TSB, Nishimura SL, Chan SP, Garcia-Kennedy R, et al. Clinical and pathological features of bacillary peliosis hepatis in association with human immunodeficiency virus infection. N Engl J Med 323:1581–1586, 1990.

Pinder SE, Colville A. Mycobacterial cervical lymphadenitis in children: Can histological assessment help differentiate infections caused by nontuberculous mycobacteria from Mycobacterium tuberculosis? Histopathology 22:59–64, 1993.

Relman DA, Loutit JS, Schmidt TM, Falkow S, Tompkins LS. The agent of bacillary angiomatosis. An approach to the identification of uncultured pathogens. N Engl J Med 323:1573–1580, 1990.

Relman DA, Schmidt TM, Macdermott RP, Falkow S. Identification of the uncultured bacillus of Whipple' disease. N Engl J Med 327:293–301, 1992.

Rouillon A, Menses CJ, Gerster JC, Perez-Sawka I, Forest M. Sarcoid-like forms of Whipple's disease. Report of 2 cases. J Rheumatol 20:1070–1072, 1993.

Sjobring U, Mecklenburg M, Andersen AB, Miorner H. Polymerase chain reaction for detection of Mycobacterium tuberculosis. J Clin Microbiol 28:2200, 1990.

Smith JE. Plague. In: Pathology of Tropical and Extraordinary Disease. Binford CH, Connor DH, eds. Washington, D.C., Armed Forces Institute of Pathology, pp130–134, 1976.

Solis OG, Belmonte AH, Ramaswamy G, Tchertkoff V. Pseudo-Gaucher cells in Mycobacterium avium-intracellulare infections in acquired immunodeficiency syndrome (AIDS). Am J Clin Pathol 85:233–235, 1986.

Tappero JW, Koehler JE, Berger TG, et al. Bacillary angiomatosis and bacillary splenitis in immunocompetent adults. Ann Intern Med 118:363–365, 1993.

Wear DJ, Margileth AM, Hadfield TL, Fischer GW, Schlagel CJ, King FM. Cat scratch disease: A bacterial infection. Science 221:1403–1404, 1983.

9

Fungal, Protozoal, and Filarial Lymphadenitis and Other Lymph Node Granulomas

Fungal Lymphadenitis

Fungal lymphadenitis results from infection with several species of dimorphic fungi, including *Histoplasma capsulatum* (histoplasmosis), *Coccidioides immitis* (coccidioidomycosis), *Blastomyces dermatitidisis* (North American blastomycosis), *Paracoccidioides brasiliensis* (South American blastomycosis), and *Sporothrix schenckii* (sporotrichosis) and the yeast-like fungus *Cryptococcus neoformans* (crytococcosis). Fungal lymphadenitis in these infections is typically a manifestation of disseminated disease in the immunocompromised host.

Clinical Features

The clinical features of these fungal infections are diverse; however, they have several features in common. The primary infection is pulmonary, resulting from inhalation of contaminated dust or soil. (*Sporothrix schenckii* is an exception and is usually acquired cutaneously, by direct inoculation, while gardening.) The primary infection is frequently asymptomatic, or mildly symptomatic, and spontaneous recovery is the rule in the immunocompetent host. In the immunocompomised host, however, disseminated infection with cutaneous, visceral, or lymph node involvement occurs.

104

Histopathology

Lymph node infection with these fungi is characterized by granulomatous lymphadenitis which is frequently suppurative. *Cryptococcus neoformans* is a sometime exception, which, because of the thick, carbohydrate-rich capsule, may elicit little inflammatory response. Specific diagnosis of these fungi is based on culturing the organism or on identification of the organism in PAS- or methenamine-silver-stained sections (Woods and Gutierrez, 1993).

HISTOPLASMA CAPSULATUM *Histoplasma capsulatum* is an intracellular organism found principally in histiocytes and monocyte-macrophages. The organism is a small, ovoid, yeast-like fungus measuring 2–5 μm in diameter that frequently appears to be surrounded by a clear space or "capsule." The "capsule" is actually an artifact due to retraction of the cytoplasm. Usually, numerous organisms will be found in a single cell. African histoplasmosis is caused by a larger organism, *Histoplasma capsulatum* var. *duboisii*, which measures 12–15 μm in diameter, but is extremely rare outside of Africa. Histoplasma capsulatum must be distinguished from other intracellular organisms, principally *Leishmania donovani*, the causative protozoan of Kala-Azar (visceral leishmaniasis). The latter organism contains a nucleus and kinetoplast in a characteristic "safety pin" configuration and stains negatively with PAS and methenamine silver stains.

CRYPTOCOCCUS NEOFORMANS *Cryptococcus neoformans* is an encapsulated yeast-like fungus which measures 4–8 μm in diameter. The capsule, which stains positively with mucicarmine, appears to play an important role in pathogenicity by inhibiting phagocytosis; capsule-deficient strains may be found in individuals with AIDS. *Cryptococcus neoformans* may elicit little inflammatory response; in tissue the organisms appear to be surrounded by a clear space, corresponding to the capsule. *Cryptococcus neoformans* must be distinguished from yeast-like fungi of similar size, including *Candida* species. The mucicarmine-positive capsule is diagnostic.

COCCIDIOIDES IMMITIS *Coccidioides immitis* is the largest of this group of fungi, consisting of round spherules measuring 20–200 μm in diameter, containing smaller endospores measuring 2–5 μm in diameter. *Coccidioides immitis* is geographically restricted to areas of the southwestern United States and the San Joaquin valley of California ("valley fever").

BLASTOMYCES DERMATITIDIS *Blastomyces dermatitidis*, the causative agent of blastomycosis, is a yeast-like fungus, measuring 8–15 μm in diameter with characteristic broad-based buds. Blastomycosis is characterized by suppurative granulomatous disease involving the lungs and other organs. Blastomycosis of mucosal surfaces is frequently associated with pseudoepitheliomatous hyperplasia. The broad-based buds and suppurative tissue reaction are characteristic features.

PARACOCCIDIOIDES BRASILIENSIS *Paracoccidioides brasiliensis* is the causative agent of South American blastomycosis, a systemic mycosis prevalent in South America. Paracoccidioidomycosis is characterized by suppurative granulomatous disease involving the lungs and other organs. It is distinguished from *Blastomyces dermatitidis* by its larger size, measuring 10–40 μm in diameter, and multiple narrow-based buds.

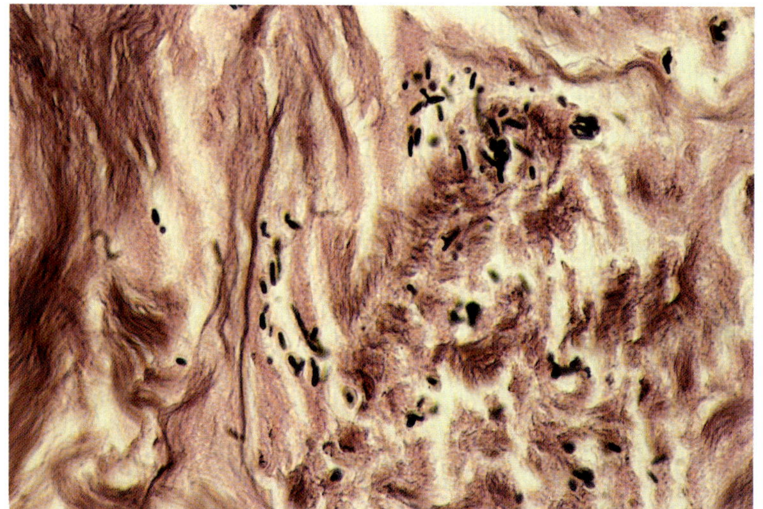

Sporotrichosis, methenamine silver stain, showing characteristic cigar-shaped organisms.

SPOROTHRIX SCHENCKII *Sporothrix schenckii* is a lymphocutaneous infection acquired from cutaneous inoculation, frequently from gardening. Osteoarticular infection may also occur; disseminated infection is rare. Sporotrichosis is characterized by suppurative granulomatous inflammation. The causative organisms are ovoid-to-cigar shaped forms, measuring 2–6 μm in diameter (Fig. 9.1). The organism are present in small numbers and may be very difficult to identify in tissue.

Differential Diagnosis

Fungal lymphadenitis must be distinguished from other causes of necrotizing or suppurative granulomatous lymphadenitis, including many of the bacterial and mycobacterial infections discussed in Chapter 8. Special stains for microorganisms, including the Ziehl-Neelsen or Kinyoun stains for acid fast bacilli, the Dieterle or Warthin-Starry stain for cat scratch and other bacilli, and the PAS and methenamine silver stains for fungi, are the appropriate starting point for differential diagnosis. The majority of fungi (*Sporothrix schenckii* is an exception) are numerous in tissue and readily identified. When special stains are negative, however, material for microbiologic culture may be necessary for diagnosis (Woods and Gutierrez, 1993).

Course and Prognosis

Disseminated fungal infections are treated with systemic antifungal drugs, principally amphotericin B and the imidazoles. Localized sporotrichosis frequently responds to oral potassium iodide.

Pneumocystis Carinii Lymphadenitis

Pneumocystis carinii is an important cause of opportunistic infection in the immuno-compromised host. *Pneumocystis carinii* was formerly classified amongst the protozo-ans; current evidence suggests it is more closely related to the fungi (Edman et al, 1988).

Clinical Features

Pneumocystis carinii is a principal cause of pneumonitis in the immunocompromised host. Patients with *Pneumocystis carinii* pneumonitis formerly included marasmic in-fants and patients with acute lymphocytic leukemia and Hodgkin's disease; most pa-tients today have AIDS. Extrapulmonary or disseminated pneumocystis infection occurs rarely and may involve lymph nodes, liver, spleen, bone marrow, or other sites (Ellison et al, 1995; Moe and Hardy, 1994). Patients with extrapulmonary pneumocystis infection frequently have concurrent or previous *Pneumocystis carinii* pneumonitis or have re-ceived prophylactic treatment with inhaled pentamidine isethionate (Moe and Hardy, 1994).

Histopathology

Pneumocystis carinii lymphadenitis is characterized by masses of foamy, eosiniphilic exudate indistinguishable from the intraalveolar exudates in the lung (Fig. 9.2). In hema-toxylin and eosin (H&E)-stained sections, the organisms (intracystic bodies) appear as tiny basophilic dots (Fig. 9.3). In methenamine-silver-stained sections, the encysted

FIGURE 9.2

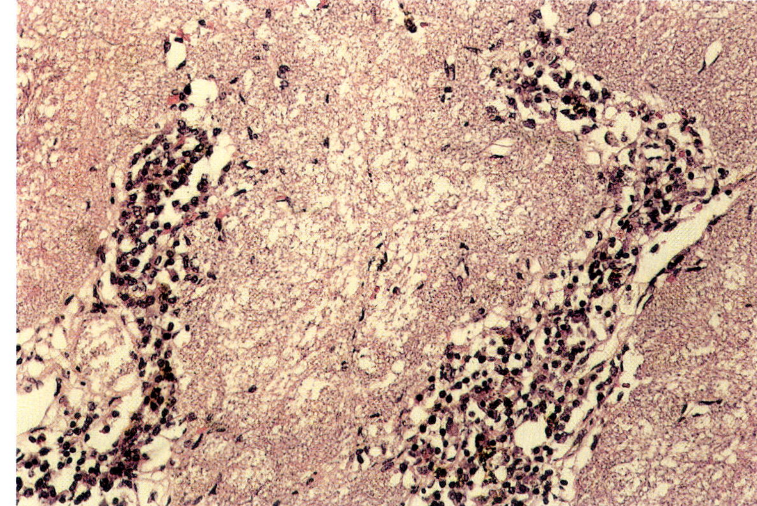

Pneumocystis carinii lymphadenitis showing masses of foamy, eosino-philic exudate identical to that seen in the lung in *pneumocystis carinii* pneumonitis.

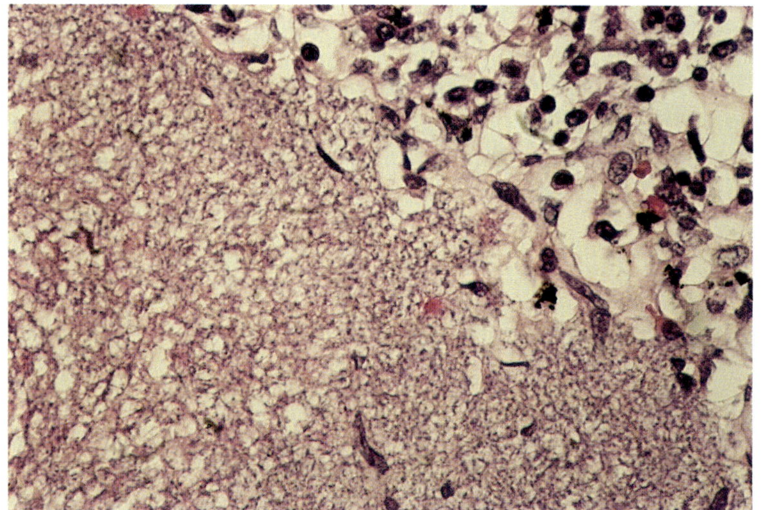

Pneumocystis carinii lymphadenitis showing basophilic intracystic bodies in the foamy exudate.

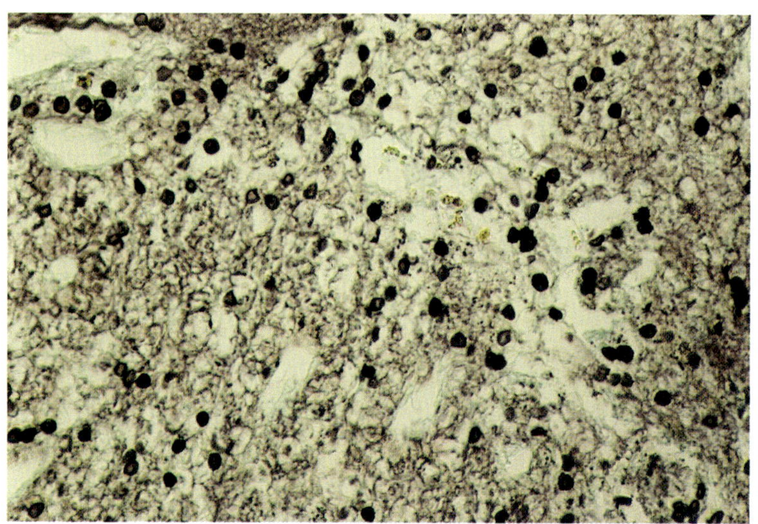

Pneumocystis carinii lymphadenitis showing encysted form of the organism, stained with methenamine silver.

forms of the organisms are visible as round to ovoid, folded or "cup-like" structures, measuring 4–6 μm in diameter (Fig. 9.4). The surrounding lymph node shows little cellular reaction to the exudate.

Differential Diagnosis

Pneumocystis carinii lymphadenitis must be distinguished from lymphadenitis due to fungal organisms, including *Histoplasma capsulatum* and *Cryptococcus neoformans.* The foamy, eosinophilic exudate in H&E-stained sections and the cup-like cysts in methenamine silver stained sections are characteristic features. *Histoplasma capsulatum* is smaller and principally intracellular; cryptococcus is slighly larger and has a characteristic mucicarmine-positive capsule. The folded, cup-like configuration of the cysts of *Pneumocystis carinii* is also helpful in distinguishing them from erythrocytes, which are sometimes stained by methenamine silver. *Pneumocystis carinii* lymphadenitis may be diagnosed by fine needle aspiration biopsy (Ellison et al, 1995).

Course and Prognosis

Pneumocystis carinii is treated with trimethoprim and sulfamethoxazole, trimethoprim and dapsone, or pentamidine isethionate. Prophylactic treatment of patients with AIDS with inhaled pentamidine isethionate may be associated with atypical presentations of *Pneumocystis carinii*, including granulomatous *Pneumocystis carinii* pneumonia (Bleiweiss et al, 1988).

Toxoplasmic Lymphadenitis

Toxoplasmic lymphadenitis occurs during primary infection with *Toxoplasma gondii*, a coccidian protozoan acquired from domestic cats. Disseminated toxoplasmosis occurs in immunocompromised hosts.

Clinical Features

Toxoplasmic lymphadenitis (acute acquired toxoplasmosis) results from infection with toxoplasma oocysts passed in the feces of domestic cats or from ingestion of cysts in undercooked meat. Toxoplasmic lymphadenitis is a mild infectious mononucleosis-like illness, characterized by posterior cervical lymphadenopathy and atypical lymphocytosis. Toxoplasmic lymphadenitis is one of the causes of the heterophile-negative mononucleosis syndrome. In immunocompetent hosts, toxoplasmic lymphadenitis is a benign, self-limited infection. In immunocompromised hosts, disseminated toxoplasmosis may develop as a result of recent or reactivated infection and is characterized by necrotizing lesions in the central nervous system, heart, and other organs.

Histopathology

Toxoplasmic lymphadenitis is characterized by the lymphadenitis of Piringer-Kuchinka, consisting of follicular lymphoid hyperplasia, clusters of epithelioid histiocytes, both within and between follicular centers, and monocytoid cells in the sinuses (Dorfman and Remington, 1973) (Figs. 9.5, 9.6, and 9.7). The last have a distinctive morphology characterized by abundant clear cytoplasm, indented or ovoid nuclei, and inconspicuous nucleoli and express B cell markers (Sheibani et al, 1984). The presence of all three histologic features correlates highly with positive serology for toxoplasmosis (Dorfman and Remington, 1973). Toxoplasma cysts are rarely identified in the lymph nodes in toxoplasmic lymphadenitis; identification may be aided by immunohistochemisty (Aisner et al, 1983). The cysts are spherical structures, measuring up to 30 μm in diameter, and contain numerous tachyzoites. Disseminated toxoplasmosis is characterized by

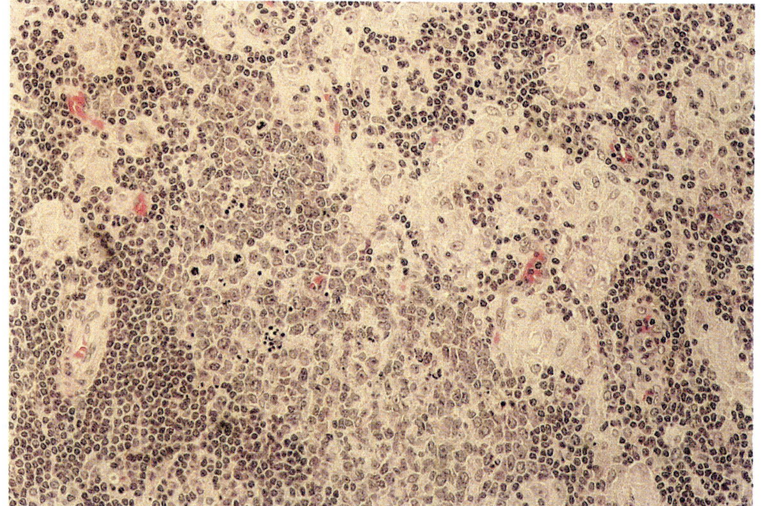

Toxoplasmic lymphadenitis showing follicular lymphoid hyperplasia and epithelioid microgranulomata.

FIGURE 9.5

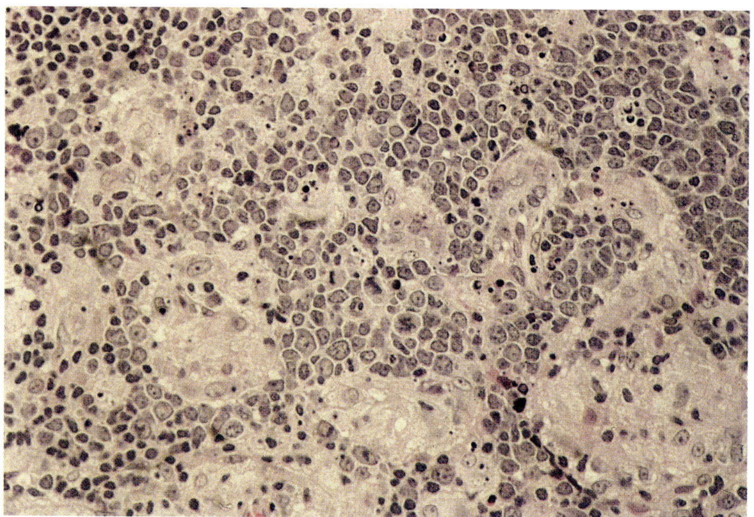

Toxoplasmic lymphadenitis showing epithelioid microgranulomata within a follicular center.

FIGURE 9.6

necrotizing lesions in the central nervous system, heart, and other organs. The areas of necrosis contain intracellular or free toxoplasma tachyzoites, ovoid or crescentic structures, measuring up to 4–6 μm in length, and toxoplasma cysts.

Differential Diagnosis

The definitive diagnosis of toxoplasmic lymphadenitis is established serologically. The presence of IgM antibodies to *Toxoplasma gondii* is indicative of recent infection. (IgG

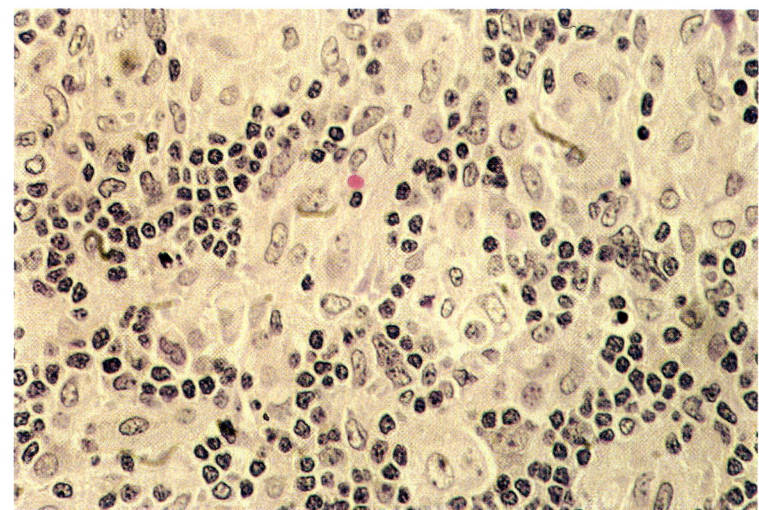

FIGURE
9.7

Toxoplasmic lymphadenitis showing clusters of epithelioid cells.

antibodies are indicative of past infection and are present in many individuals due to prior subclinical infection.) The histologic features of the lymph node are sufficiently characteristic to permit a presumptive diagnosis. The presence of the three characteristic histologic features (follicular lymphoid hyperplasia, clusters of epithelioid histiocytes, both within and between follicular centers, and monocytoid cells) correlates highly with the results of toxoplasma serology (Dorfman and Remington, 1973). Toxoplasma cysts are rarely identified in the tissue in toxoplasmic lymphadenitis and are not required for diagnosis. In contrast, the diagnosis of disseminated toxoplasmosis requires identification of toxoplasma cysts or tachyzoites in tissue.

Course and Prognosis

Toxoplasmic lymphadenitis is a benign and self-limited illness and no treatment is required. Disseminated toxoplasmosis is treated with combination of drugs including pyrimethamine, trimethoprim, and sulfadiazine. Toxoplasma infection in pregnancy may result in fetal transmission and congenital toxoplasmosis.

Leishmanial Lymphadenitis

Leishmaniasis is caused by infection with species of the flagellate protozoan *Leishmania*, and occurs in cutaneous, mucocutaneous, and visceral forms. Leishmanial lymphadenitis may accompany the visceral form of the disease (kala-azar), due to *Leishmania donovani* and related species, *Leishmania infantum* and *Leishmania chagasi*, and has been reported to accompany cutaneous leishmanias is due to *Leishmania braziliensis* (Sousa et al, 1995).

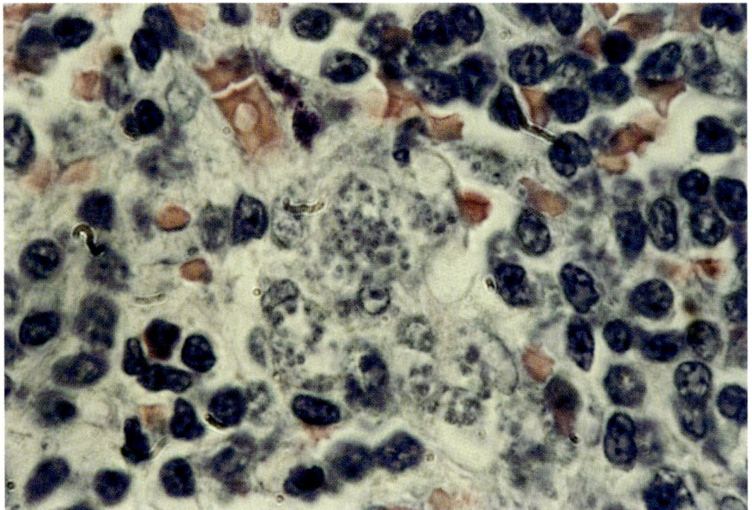

FIGURE 9.8

Kala-azar (visceral leishmaniasis) involving the spleen. Splenic macrophages are filled with amastigotes of *Leishmania donovani*.

Clinical Features

Visceral leishmaniasis (kala-azar) occurs in tropical areas, principally South America, Africa, the Mediterranean, India, and China, and is transmitted by the bites of sandflies *(Phlebotomus)*. Visceral leishmaniasis is characterized by a subacute course with fever, wasting, generalized lymphadenopathy, and hepatosplenomegaly. Pancytopenia and hypergammaglobulinemia are characteristically present; in endemic areas, the triad of splenomegaly, leukopenia, and hypergammaglobulinemia may suggest the diagnosis. An atypical form of visceral leishmaniasis has been reported in association with HIV infection (Albrecht et al, 1994).

Cutaneous leishmaniasis, prevalent in the Mediterranean and Middle East, due to *Leishmania tropica*, and in Central and South America, due to *Leishmania mexicana*, *Leishmania braziliensis*, and other leishmania species, involves the skin and occasionally regional lymph nodes (Sousa et al, 1995).

Histopathology

Visceral leishmaniasis is characterized by infiltration of the spleen, liver, lymph nodes, bone marrow, and other organs by histiocytes containing intracellular leishmanial organisms (amastigotes) (Fig. 9.8). The amastigotes are small, ovoid, intracellular structures, measuring 1.5–3 μm in size, with a well-defined nucleus and kinetoplast in a "safety pin" configuration. The morphology of the amastigotes and characteristic kinetoplast is best appreciated in imprint or touch preparations stained with Giemsa (Fig. 9.9). The number of organisms in the lymph node is variable.

Cutaneous leishmaniasis is characterized by granulomatous lesions with histiocytes containing leishmanial amastigotes. Leishmanial lymphadenitis has been reported in association with cutaneous leishmaniasis due to *Leishmania braziliensis* (Sousa et al, 1995). Localized leishmanial lymphadenitis is characterized by granulomata with varying

FIGURE
9.9

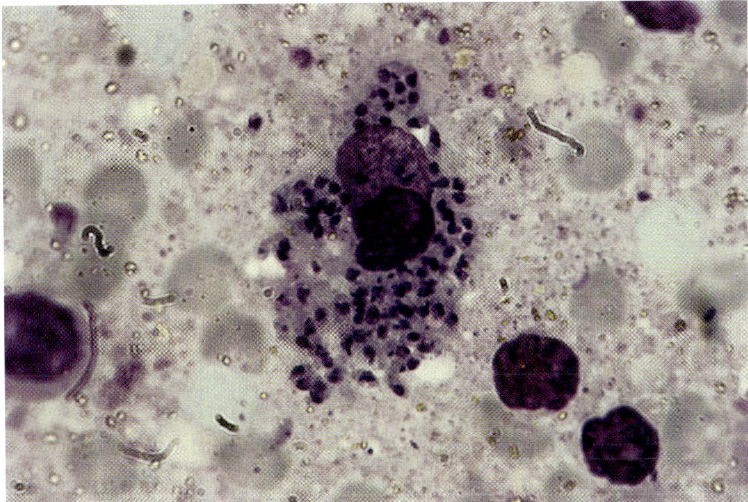

Kala-azar (visceral leishmaniasis). Splenic touch preparation stained with Giemsa showing intracellular amastigotes with characteristic kinetoplast.

FIGURE
9.10

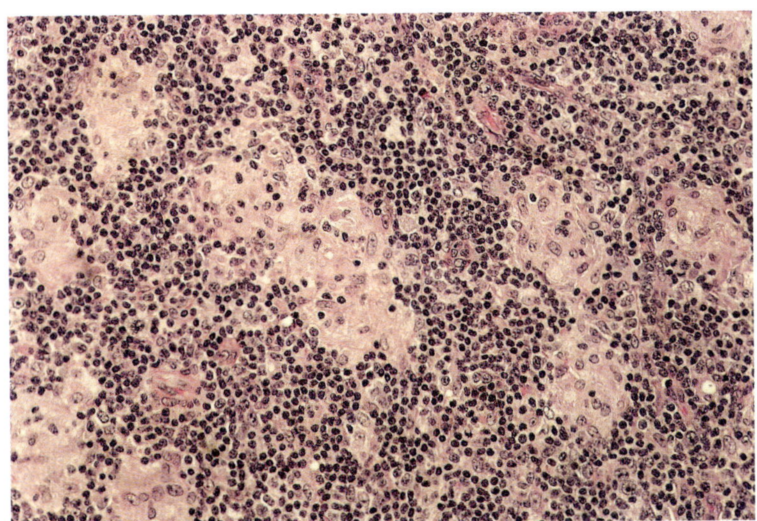

Leishmanial lymphadenitis showing clusters of epithelioid histiocytes.

degrees of necrosis, plasma cell infiltration, fibrosis, and leishmanial amastigotes (Azadeh et al, 1994). Regional lymph node involvement in cutaneous leishmaniasis may show changes resembling toxoplasmic lymphadenitis with leishmanial amastigotes present within clusters of epithelioid histiocytes (Figs. 9.10 and 9.11).

Differential Diagnosis

The diagnosis of visceral leishmaniasis is established by identification of the characteristic intracellular amastigotes in the bone marrow, liver, lymph nodes, or spleen. Leish-

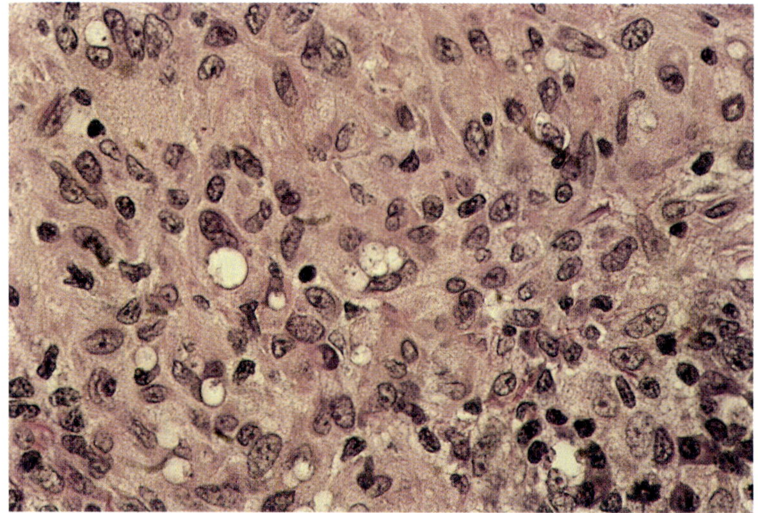

FIGURE 9.11

Leishmanial lymphadenitis showing clusters of epithelioid histiocytes containing intracellular leishmanial amastigotes.

mania must be distinguished from other intracellular organisms, in particular *Histoplasma capsulatum*, which may appear similar in tissue sections. Leishmania is distinguished by the characteristic "safety pin" configuration of the nucleus and kinetoplast, and lack of staining with methenamine silver. Leishmania may be grown in culture for definitive classification (Woods and Gutierrez, 1993).

Course and Prognosis

Visceral leishmaniasis progresses to death in the majority of untreated patients; cutaneous leishmaniasis is a chronic disorder. Leishmaniasis is treated with pentavalent antimonial compounds. Amphotericin B has also been used in refractory cases (Sundar et al, 1997). Visceral leishmaniasis may be followed by post–kala-azar dermal leishmaniasis characterized by granulomatous skin lesions containing leishmania.

Algal Lymphadenitis

Algal infections in man are caused by species of the genus *Prototheca*, an achlorophylic algae.

Clinical Features

Protothecosis typically presents as a cutaneous infection or as olecranon bursitis. *Prototheca wickerhamii* is the species most frequently isolated. Femoral lymph node involvement developed in the first reported case of cutaneous protothecosis but appears to be a rare event (Connor and Neafie, 1976). Disseminated protothecosis has also been rarely reported (Iacoviello et al, 1992).

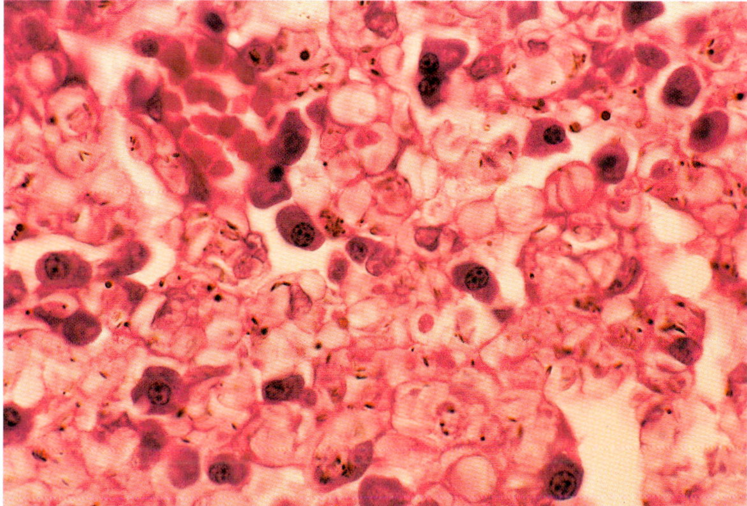

Protothecosis showing thick-walled structures with characteristic endoseptations.

Histopathology

Protothecosis is characterized by suppurative granulomatous inflammation. The organisms of protothecosis are readily demonstrated in PAS- or methenamine-silver-stained sections and consist of round-to-ovoid thick-walled structures, measuring 5–15 μm in diameter, with characteristic endoseptations (Fig. 9.12).

Differential Diagnosis

Protothecosis must be distinguished from fungal infections, which it may resemble. The endoseptations (as opposed to the budding of fungi) are characteristic. The organisms can also be grown in culture.

Course and Prognosis

Protothecosis has been treated by surgical excision and systemic therapy with amphotericin B (Iacoviello et al, 1992). Olecranon bursitis due to protothecosis is frequently cured by surgical excision alone.

Filarial Lymphadenitis

Lymphatic filariasis is caused by infection with filarial nematode worms, principally *Wucheria bancrofti*, prevalent in Africa, Asia, Central and South America, and *Brugia malayi*, prevalent in Southeast Asia. Zoonotic filarial infections have also been reported in the United States (Eberhard et al, 1993).

Clinical Features

The adult filarial worms inhabit the lymphatics and lymph node sinuses of the lower extremities and inguinal region, resulting in recurrent episodes of lymphangitis and lymphadenitis, eventually progressing to fibrosis and lymphedema. Elephantiasis of the scrotum or lower extremity may result. The progeny of the adult worms are microfilaria, measuring 200–300 μm in length and 5–10 μm in diameter, which are released into the lymph and enter the blood (Fig. 9.13). Microfilaria circulate with nocturnal periodicity, with a peak between 10:00 PM and 2:00 AM (Woods and Gutierrez, 1993). Eosinophilia is frequently present.

Histopathology

The adult filaria are found in dilated lymph node sinuses or perinodal lymphatics. In tissue sections, the adult worms, which measure 5–10 cm in length, are seen in cross section and consist of rounded structures, measuring 100–200 μm in diameter, with an outer cuticle and complex internal structure. There is little tissue reaction to the living worms. When the worms die, there is an intense inflammatory response, with numerous eosinophils and granulomatous reaction, followed by fibrosis and calcification (Jungmann et al, 1992).

Differential Diagnosis

The diagnosis of filariasis is usually established by identification of microfilaria in the peripheral blood. Microfilaria measure 200–300 μm in length and 5–10 μm in diameter and circulate at night. Speciation of the filaria is based on the morphology of the microfilaria, or of the adult worms, but is beyond the scope of the discussion here (Meyers et al, 1976).

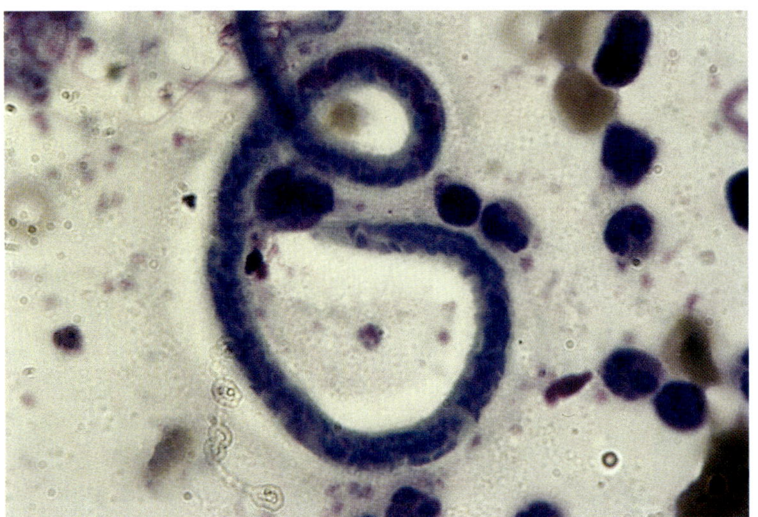

FIGURE
9.13

Filariasis showing microfilaria in peripheral blood buffy coat.

Course and Prognosis

Lymphatic filariasis is treated with diethylcarbamazine, which eliminates the adult worms. The fibrosis and lymphedema are not reversed, however.

Sarcoid Lymphadenopathy

Sarcoidosis is an idiopathic granulomatous disorder which is characterized by noncaseating epithelioid granulomata in the lungs, lymph nodes, and other organs and by progression to fibrosis.

Clinical Features

The etiology of sarcoidosis is unknown; reaction to an environmental antigen (pine pollens) or infectious agent (mycobacterial L-forms) has been considered (Newman et al, 1997). Sarcoidosis is most prevalent among young black women, but no age or ethnic group is immune. Involvement of the lungs and hilar lymph nodes is most frequent; however, almost any organ may be involved. Peripheral lymphadenopathy (particularly epitrochlear lymph nodes), skin or ocular involvement, splenomegaly, and bone marrow involvement are not infrequent. Bronchial lavage in patients with active pulmonary sarcoidosis demonstrates increased activated CD4 T cells, suggesting an immune response to an unknown antigen; paradoxically, there is frequently cutaneous anergy to delayed hypersensitivity skin tests. The T lymphocytes in affected organs are predominantly of the T helper 1 phenotype (TH1), as in other granulomatous disorders (Newman et al, 1997). Serum angiotensin converting enzyme levels are increased.

Histopathology

Sarcoid lymphadenopathy is characterized by multiple noncaseating epithelioid granulomata replacing all or part of the lymph node (Figs. 9.14 and 9.15). The granulomata are composed of epithelioid histiocytes with abundant eosinophilic cytoplasm and multinucleate giant cells of Langhans' and foreign-body type. The latter may contain a variety of intracytoplasmic inclusions including asteroid bodies (stellate or "spiked" inclusions) and Schaumann bodies (round or ovoid, laminated inclusions); none is specific to sarcoidosis. The granulomata in sarcoidosis are small and well circumscribed and frequently surrounded by a delicate rim of collagen. Surrounding inflammatory cells are characteristically scant ("naked" granulomas). Although the granulomas are noncaseating, foci of central necrosis of a fibrinoid type are not uncommon and should not dissuade one from making the diagnosis (Fig. 9.15). The granulomas heal by fibrosis and in late cases may be surrounded by dense collagen.

Differential Diagnosis

Sarcoid lymphadenopathy must be distinguished from infectious causes of granulomatous lymphadenitis and from reactive sarcoid-like granulomata seen in a variety of conditions (see below). Stains for acid fast bacilli and fungi should be routinely performed

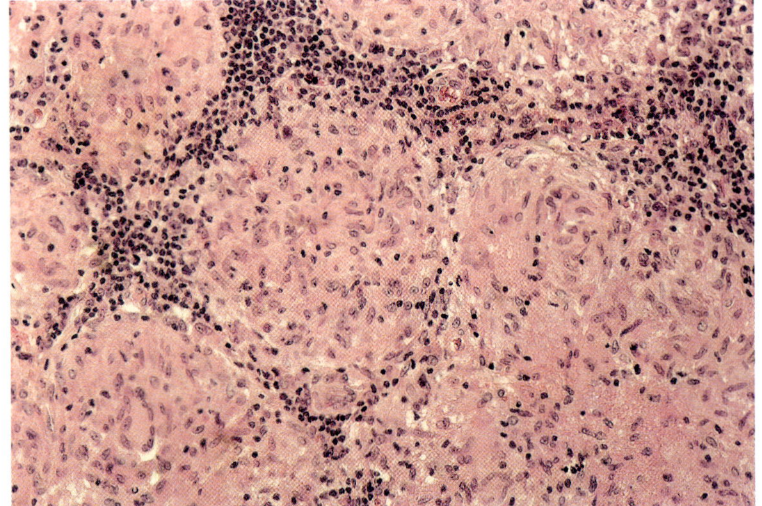

FIGURE 9.14

Sarcoid lymphadenopathy showing multiple, noncaseating epithelioid granulomata.

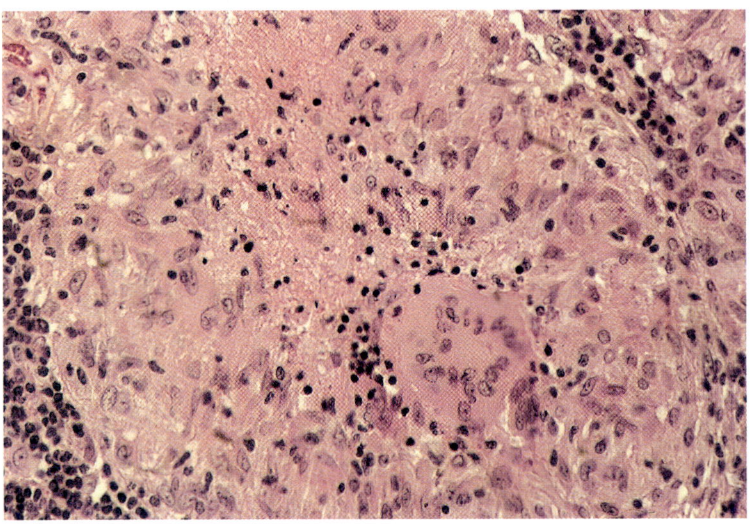

FIGURE 9.15

Sarcoid lymphadenopathy showing epithelioid granulomata with central fibrinoid necrosis and Langhans' giant cell.

in cases of suspected sarcoid lymphadenopathy, which is a diagnosis of exclusion. The Kveim test, based on the appearance of a granulomatous reaction at the site of injection of an antigen derived from sarcoid tissue, has been used in the diagnosis of sarcoidosis at some centers, but the antigen is not widely available.

Course and Prognosis

The course of sarcoidosis is highly variable, with some patients progressing to pulmonary fibrosis and others remaining asymptomatic. In most patients the course is benign. Active sarcoidosis is treated with corticosteroids.

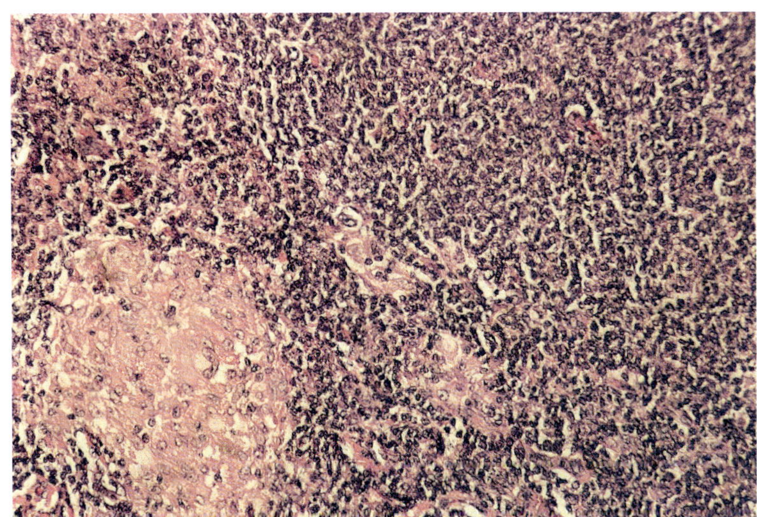

FIGURE
9.16

Sarcoid-like granulomata in non-Hodgkin's lymphoma.

Sarcoid-like Granulomata

Noncaseating epithelioid granulomata, morphologically indistinguishable from those of sarcoidosis, may be seen in lymph nodes in a variety of reactive conditions. These include berylliosis, immunodeficiency disorders (Mechanic et al, 1997), and lymph nodes draining the sites of various malignant tumors, including carcinoma of the lung and germ cell tumors (Brincker, 1986), and lymph nodes in patients with Hodgkin's disease (Sacks et al, 1978). The presence of granulomata does not indicate lymph node involvement; sarcoid-like granulomata in patients with Hodgkin's disease have been associated with an improved prognosis (Sacks et al, 1978). Malignant lymphoma may be obscured by a marked granulomatous reaction (Hollingsworth et al, 1993) (Fig. 9.16).

REFERENCES

Aisner SC, Aisner J, Moravec C, Arnett EN. Acquired toxoplasmic lymphadenitis with demonstration of the cyst form. Am J Clin Pathol 79:125–127, 1983.

Albrecht H, Stellbrink HJ, Gross G, Gerg B, Helmchen U, Mensing H. Treatment of atypical leishmaniasis with interferon gamma resulting in progression of Kaposi's sarcoma in an AIDS patient. Clin Investig 72:1041–1047, 1994.

Azadeh B, Sells PG, Ejeckam GC, Rampling D. Localized leishmania lymphadenitis. Immunohistochemical studies. Am J Clin Pathol 102:11–15, 1994.

Bleiweiss I, Jagirdar JS, Klein MJ, Siegel JL, Krellenstein DJ, Gribetz AR, Strauchen JA. Granulomatous pneumocystis carinii pneumonia in patients with the acquired immunodeficiency syndrome. Chest 94:580–583, 1988.

Brincker H. Sarcoid reactions in malignant tumors. Cancer Treat Rev 13:147–156, 1986.

Connor DH, Neafie RC. Protothecosis. In: Pathology of Tropical and Extraordinary Disease. Binford CH, Connor DH, eds. Washington, D.C., Armed Forces Institute of Pathology, pp 684–689, 1976.

Dorfman RF, Remington JF. Value of lymph node biopsy in the diagnosis of acute acquired toxoplasmosis. N Engl J Med 289:878–881, 1973.

Eberhard ML, DeMeester LJ, Martin DW, Lammie PJ. Zoonotic Brugia infection in western Michigan. Am J Surg Pathol 17:1058–1061, 1993.

Edman JC, Kordes JA, Masur H, et al. Ribosomal RNA sequence shows Pneumocystis carinii to be a member of the fungi. Nature 334:519, 1988.

Ellison E, Yuen SY, Lawson L, Chan NH. Fine-needle aspiration diagnosis of extrapulmonary pneumocystis carinii lymphadenitis in a human immunodeficiency virus positive patient. Diagn Cytopathol 12:251–253, 1995.

Hollingsworth HC, Longo DL, Jaffe ES. Small non-cleaved cell lymphoma associated with florid epithelioid granulomatous response. A clinicopathologic study of seven patients. Am J Surg Pathol 17:51–59, 1993.

Iacoviello VR, DeGirolami PC, Lucarini J, Sutker K, Williams ME, Wanke CA. Protothecosis complicating prolonged endotracheal intubation: case report and literature review. Clin Infect Dis 15:959–967, 1992.

Jungmann P, Figueredo-Silva J, Dreyer G. Bancroftian lymphangitis in northeastern Brazil: A histopathological study of 17 cases. J Trop Med Hyg 95:113–118, 1992.

Mechanic LJ, Dikman S, Cunningham-Rundles C. Granulomatous disease in common variable immunodeficiency. Ann Intern Med 127:613–617, 1997.

Meyers WM, Neafie RC, Connor DH. Bancroftian and Malayan filariasis. In: Pathology of Tropical and Extraordinary Diseases. Binford CH, Connor DH, eds. Washington, D.C., Armed Forces Institute of Pathology, pp 340–355, 1976.

Moe AA, Hardy WD. Pneumocystis carinii infection in the HIV-seropositive patient. Infect Dis Clin North Am 8:331–364, 1994.

Newman LS, Rose CS, Maier LA. Sarcoidosis. N Engl J Med 336:1224–1234, 1997.

Sacks EL, Donaldson SS, Gordon J, Dorfman RF. Epithelioid granulomas associated with Hodgkin's disease—Clinical correlations in 55 previously untreated patients. Cancer 41:562–567, 1978.

Sheibani K, Fritz RM, Winberg CD, Burke JS, Rappaport H. "Monocytoid" cells in reactive follicular hyperplasia with and without multifocal histocytic reactions: An immunohistochemical study of 21 cases including suspected cases of toxoplasmic lymphadenitis. Am J Clin Pathol 81:453–458, 1984.

Sousa A de Q, Parise MER, Pompeu MM, Coehlo-Filho JM, Vasconcelos IA, Lima JW, et al. Bubonic leishmaniasis: A common manifestation of Leishmania (Viannia) braziliensis infection in Ceara, Brazil. Am J Trop Med Hyg 53:380–385, 1995.

Sundar S, Agrawal NK, Sinha PR, Horwith G, Murray HW. Short-course, low-dose amphotericin B lipid complex therapy for visceral leishmaniasis unresponsive to antimony. Ann Intern Med 127:133–137, 1997.

Woods GK, Gutierrez Y. Diagnostic Pathology of Infectious Diseases. Philadelphia, Lea & Febiger, 1993.

10

Autoimmune Lymphadenopathy and Lymph Node Infarction

Morphologically distinctive lymph node changes accompany several autoimmune disorders, including rheumatoid arthritis, Sjögren's syndrome, and lupus erythematosus, which are considered in this chapter. Lymph node infarction, characterized by coagulative lymph node necrosis, is also considered in this chapter.

Rheumatoid Lymphadenopathy

Rheumatoid arthritis is a systemic disease characterized by polyarthritis, serum antibodies to IgG (rheumatoid factor) and extraarticular manifestations including localized or generalized lymphadenopathy.

Clinical Features

Lymphadenopathy is a frequent accompaniment of rheumatoid arthritis. Lymphadenopathy may be localized, affecting lymph nodes draining affected joints, or generalized. The lymphadenopathy exhibits no special clinical features. Generalized lymphadenopathy is frequent in cases of juvenile rheumatoid arthritis and may precede the appearance of joint involvement. Lymphadenopathy may also be present in Felty's syndrome (rheumatoid arthritis, splenomegaly, and leukopenia).

Histopathology

Lymph node involvement in rheumatoid arthritis is characterized by florid follicular lymphoid hyperplasia and marked interfollicular plasmacytosis (Nosanchuk and Schnit-

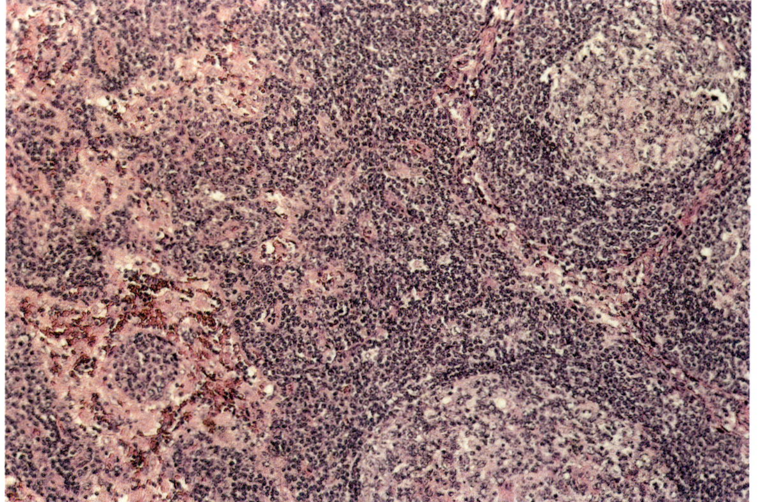

FIGURE 10.1

Rheumatoid lymphadenopathy showing follicular lymphoid hyperplasia.

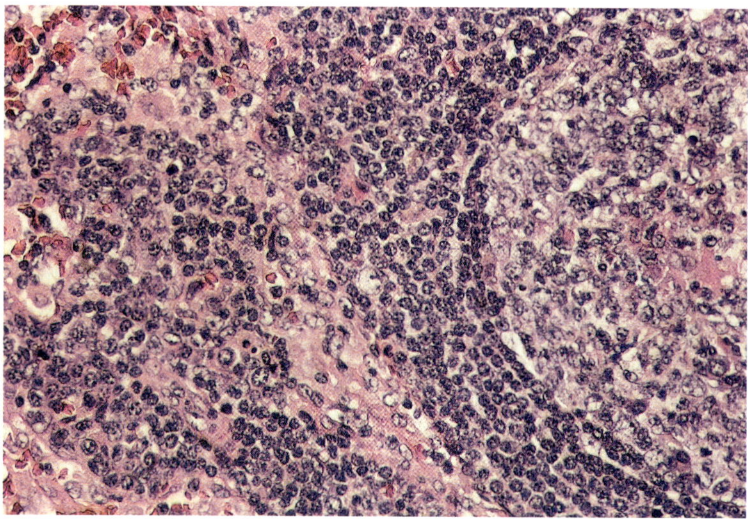

FIGURE 10.2

Rheumatoid lymphadenopathy showing follicular lymphoid hyperplasia
and plasmacytosis.

izer, 1969) (Figs. 10.1 and 10.2). The follicles are increased in number and size with
prominent follicular centers, attenuated mantle zones, and compressed paracortex, containing numerous plasma cells (Fig.10.3). Plasma cells containing Russell bodies, globular intracytoplasmic immunoglobulin inclusions, are frequently present. The plasma
cells are polyclonal by immunoglobulin light chain staining.

Differential Diagnosis

Rheumatoid lymphadenopathy should be distinguished from other causes of florid follicular lymphoid hyperplasia, including luetic lymphadenitis, persistent generalized lymph-

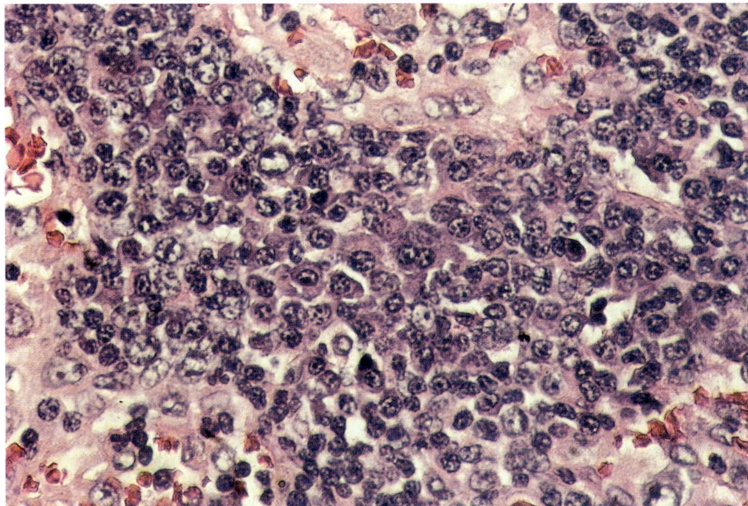

Rheumatoid lymphadenopathy showing marked plasmacytosis.

adenopathy associated with HIV infection, and nonspecific follicular lymphoid hyperplasia.

Course and Prognosis

There is no specific therapy for rheumatoid lymphadenopathy.

Sjögren's Syndrome

Sjögren's syndrome is a systemic disorder characterized by lymphocytic infiltration and atrophy of the salivary and lacrimal glands resulting in the "sicca" syndrome with xerostomia and keratoconjunctivitis. Patients with Sjögren's syndrome have an increased incidence of nodal and extranodal lymphoid proliferations, including lymphoid hyperplasias and non-Hodgkin's lymphomas.

Clinical Features

Patients with Sjögren's syndrome are predominantly women presenting with xerostomia and keratoconjunctivitis sicca; an underlying autoimmune disorder, principally rheumatoid arthritis, but occasionally systemic lupus erythematosus, scleroderma, or mixed connective tissue disease may be evident. Salivary gland enlargement due to lymphoid hyperplasia (benign lymphoepithelial lesion, myoepithelial sialadenitis) is frequent, and nodal or extranodal lymphoid hyperplasia (pseudolymphoma) may be present. The incidence of B cell non-Hodgkin's lymphoma is increased, including mucosa-associated lymphoid tissue (MALT) and monocytoid B cell lymphomas (Royer et al, 1997; Sheibani et al, 1988) and B cell large cell lymphomas. Dysglobulinemias, including γ heavy chain disease, may also be associated with Sjögren's syndrome (Fermand et al, 1989).

Histopathology

The characteristic extranodal salivary lesion of Sjögren's syndrome is the benign lymphoepithelial lesion (myoepithelial sialadenitis). The salivary gland contains a polymorphous infiltrate of small and large lymphocytes and plasma cells, frequently with formation of follicular centers. The salivary acini are atrophic; however, epimyoepithelial
islands, focal proliferations of ductal epithelial and myoepithelial cells, are characteristically present. Epimyoepithelial islands are frequently surrounded by a pale zone of
larger transformed lymphoid cells. Although characteristic of benign lymphepithelial lesions, epimyoepithelial islands are not specific and are also found in non-Hodgkin's
lymphoma involving the salivary glands, particularly of MALT or monocytoid B cell type.
Benign lymphoepithelial lesions of the salivary gland may occur in the absence of clinical evidence of Sjögren's syndrome. Lymphoid hyperplasias, analogous to benign lymphepithelial lesions of the salivary glands, also occur in the lung in Sjögren's syndrome
(pulmonary pseudolymphoma) and are characterized by polymorphous lymphoid infiltrates. The lymph nodes in Sjögren's syndrome may show lymphoid hyperplasia, which
resembles rheumatoid lymphadenopathy (Talal and Schnitizer, 1977) or diffuse atypical
lymphoid hyperplasia with prominent immunoblasts ("pseudolymphoma") (Figs. 10.4
and 10.5).

Differential Diagnosis

Benign lymphoepithelial lesions and pseudolymphomas in Sjögren's syndrome must be
distinguished from nodal and extranodal non-Hodgkin's lymphoma, which occur with
increased incidence. Mucosa associated lymphoid tissue (MALT) and monocytoid B cell
lymphomas frequently coexist with benign lymphepithelial lesions in Sjögren's syndrome; recognition is aided by infiltration of the epimyoepithelial islands by monomorphic monocytoid B cells (Sheibani et al, 1988); however, immunohistochemical studies

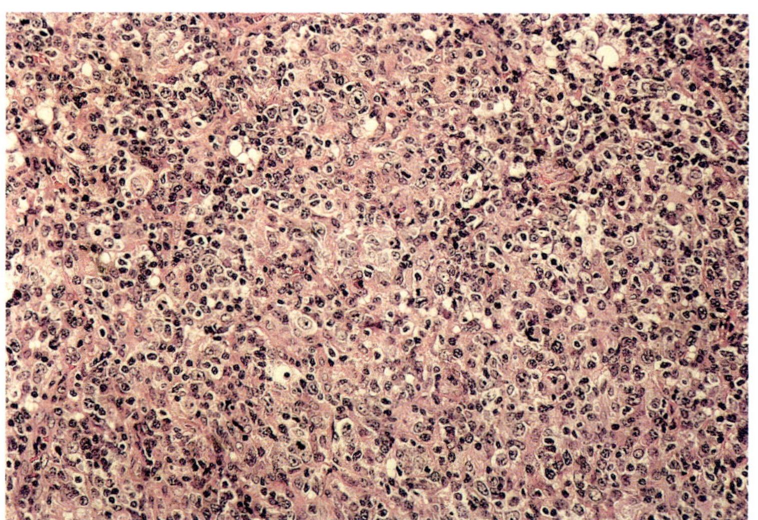

**FIGURE
10.4**

Sjögren's syndrome with diffuse atypical lymphoid hyperplasia in a
lymph node.

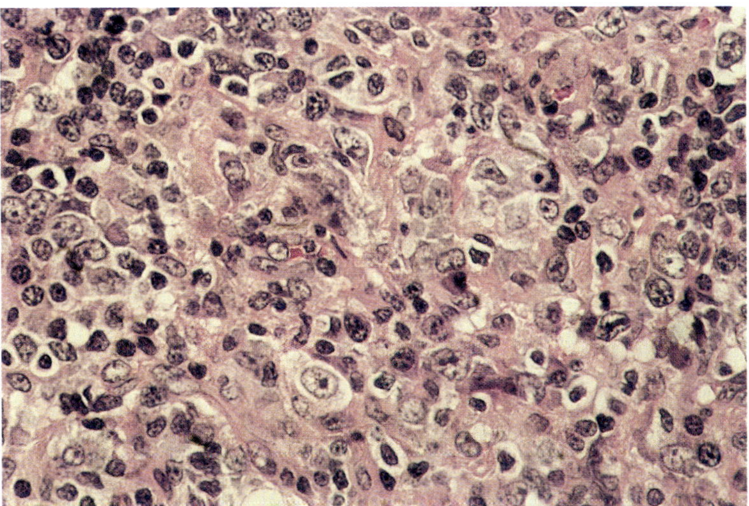

FIGURE
10.5

Sjögren's syndrome with diffuse atypical lymphoid hyperplasia in a lymph node, higher magnification, showing pleomorphic immunoblasts. Gene rearrangement studies revealed a germline configuration and patient was alive without evidence of lymphoma 2 years later.

showing immunoglobulin light chain restriction are frequently necessary for diagnosis (Falzon and Isaacson, 1991). Molecular studies show a high incidence of clonal immunoglobulin gene rearrangements in benign lymphepithelial lesions, even in the absence of complicating non-Hodgkin's lymphoma (Fishleder et al, 1987). Diffuse lymphoid hyperplasias involving nodal and extranodal sites (pseudolymphoma) in Sjögren's syndrome may be difficult to distinguish from non-Hodgkin's lymphoma. Attention to the polymorphous cell population and immunophenotypic studies may be helpful.

Lymphoid hyperplasias in juxtaparotid lymph nodes and parotid lymphoid tissue in HIV infection may also be associated with epimyoepithelial islands and epithelial cysts and closely resemble the benign lymphoepithelial lesion of Sjögren's syndrome (Ioachim et al, 1988). The sicca syndrome, however, is not observed.

Course and Prognosis

Therapy for Sjögren's syndrome is symptomatic. Corticosteroids and cytotoxic drugs have been used in the management of pulmonary pseudolymphoma. The increased incidence of both low- and high-grade B cell non-Hodgkin's lymphoma has been noted. The MALT and monocytoid B cell lymphomas of the salivary glands have an indolent natural history; however, transformation to diffuse large B cell lymphoma may occur (Sheibani et al, 1988).

Lupus Lymphadenitis

Lupus lymphadenitis occurs in systemic lupus erythematosus (SLE), occasionally in lymph nodes draining areas of discoid lupus erythematosus (DLE), and in mixed connective tissue disease (Shiokawa et al, 1993).

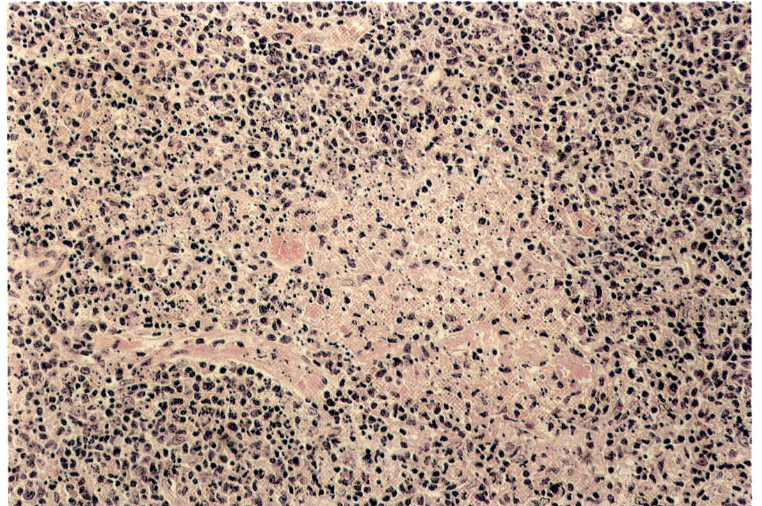

FIGURE
10.6

Lupus lymphadenitis showing foci of necrosis.

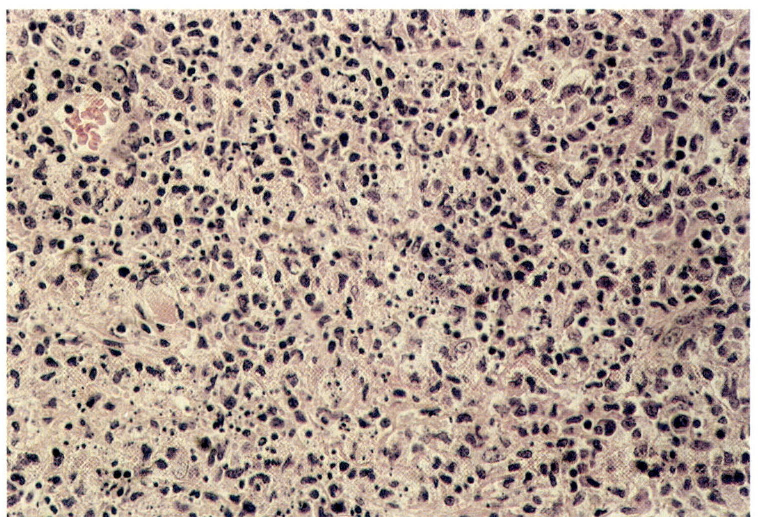

FIGURE
10.7

Lupus lymphadenitis showing necrosis with karyorrhectic debris.

Clinical Features

Systemic lupus erythematosus (SLE) is an autoimmune disorder characterized by the occurrence of antinuclear and anti-double stranded DNA antibodies, with cutaneous, rheumatologic, renal and other manifestations. Most patients with SLE are young women. Lymphadenopathy, cervical or generalized, is present frequently during the course of the disease. Lymph nodes in SLE may show only nonspecific follicular lymphoid hyperplasia or characteristic features of lupus lymphadenitis.

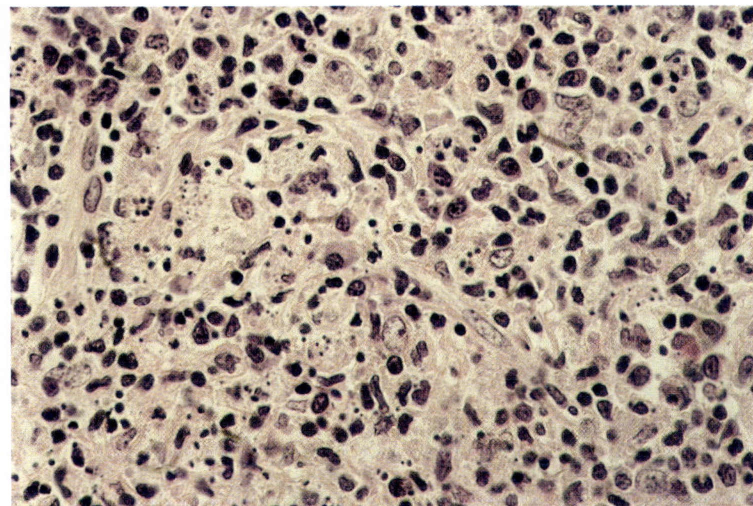

Lupus lymphadenitis showing necrosis and plasma cells. The presence of plasma cells is helpful in distinguishing lupus lymphadenitis from Kikuchi's disease.

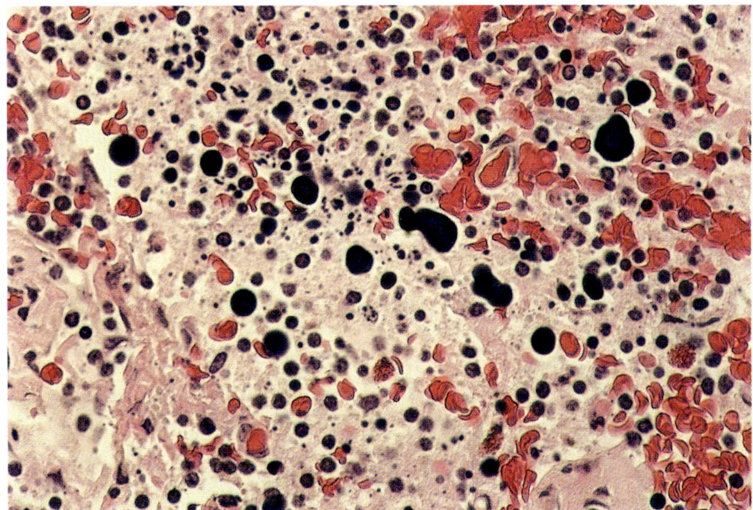

Hematoxylin bodies, consisting of amorphous, basophilic masses of DNA, are a specific finding in lupus lymphadenitis.

Histopathology

Lupus lymphadenitis is characterized by follicular lymphoid hyperplasia with paracortical foci of necrosis (Medeiros et al, 1989) (Figs. 10.6, 10.7 and 10.8). The necrosis may be minor or major in extent, is characteristically coagulative, with abundant eosinophilic cell "ghosts" and nuclear karyorrhexis, and may be associated with formation of "hematoxylin bodies," amorphous masses of homogenous basophilic material found in the sinuses and around blood vessels (Fig. 10.9). The "hematoxylin bodies" are Feulgen-positive masses of altered DNA, analogous to the material phagocytosed in the LE cell phenomenon, and are specific to lupus lymphadenitis. Polymorphonuclear leukocytes are characteristically absent in lupus lymphadenitis; however, immunoblasts and plasma cells may be prominent (Fig. 10.8).

Differential Diagnosis

Necrotizing lymphadenitis, nearly indistinguishable from lupus lymphadenitis, occurs in Kickuchi's disease, an idiopathic form of lymphadenopathy in young women (Turner et al, 1983; Unger et al, 1987; Kuo, 1995). The similarities have raised the suspicion that Kikuchi's disease is a "forme fruste" of lupus lymphadenitis; nevertheless, plasma cells, frequently prominent in lupus lymphadenitis, are usually absent in Kikuchi's lymphadenitis, and the development of SLE in patients with Kikuchi's disease is exceptional (Kuo, 1995).

Course and Prognosis

Lupus lymphadenitis is present during active SLE and frequently disappears during remission induced by corticosteroids or other therapy.

Lymph Node Infarction

Lymph node infarction refers to spontaneous coagulative necrosis of lymph nodes, a phenomenon which may be associated with the subsequent development of malignant lymphoma (Cleary et al, 1982; Maurer et al, 1986).

Clinical Features

Lymph node infarction occurs predominantly in middle-aged or older adults. Cervical lymph nodes are most frequently involved; affected lymph nodes may be painful or nontender and firm. The etiology of lymph node infarction is obscure; evidence of vascular disease has been present in some patients (Maurer et al, 1986); however, lymph node infarction frequently precedes the development of malignant lymphoma.

Histopathology

The hallmark of lymph node infarction is coagulative necrosis of all or of a portion of the lymph node, with residual eosinophilic cell "ghosts" (Fig. 10.10). The latter are homogeneously stained eosinophilic bodies devoid of nuclear or cytoplasmic detail. The infarcted area is surrounded by a peripheral zone of granulation tissue; macrophages and foamy macrophages may be present at the periphery of the infarcted area. The lymph node capsule is intact and frequently fibrotic.

Differential Diagnosis

Lymph node infarction must be distinguished from other causes of lymph node necrosis, including necrotizing granulomatous lymphadenitis, lupus lymphadenitis, Kikuchi's dis-

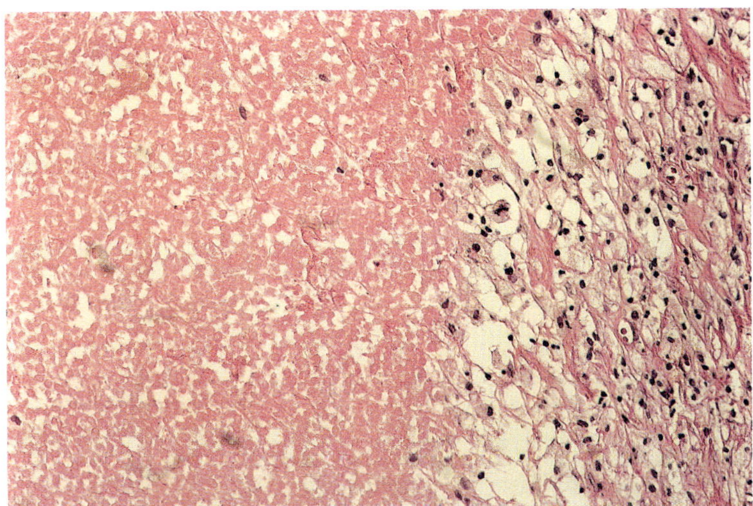

Lymph node infarction. Eosinophilic cell ghosts and peripheral zone of granulation tissue are characteristic features.

ease, and malignant lymphoma with extensive necrosis. Necrotizing granulomatous lymphadenitis is classically characterized by caseous, rather than coagulative, necrosis; cell "ghosts" are typically absent and the periphery consists of epithelioid histiocytes and multinucleate giant cells rather than granulation tissue. Nevertheless, it is prudent to obtain stains for AFB and fungi in cases of apparent lymph node infarction. Lupus lymphadenitis or Kikuchi's disease, when lymph node necrosis is extensive, may mimic lymph node infarction; however, islands of viable lymph node tissue with extensive nuclear karyorrhexis remain to suggest the correct diagnosis. Malignant lymphoma with extensive necrosis is the most difficult and significant differential diagnosis. Malignant lymphoma with extensive necrosis is frequently of diffuse large cell or other high-grade type. Careful examination of the extensively necrotic lymph node may reveal residual viable foci of lymphoma, usually surrounding blood vessels. The diagnosis of malignant lymphoma with extensive necrosis can be made only by identifying areas of viable lymphoma; the diagnosis cannot be made on eosinophilic cell "ghosts" alone. Immuno-phenotypic studies on necrotic tissue are often uninterpretable because of nonspecific staining of necrotic cells.

Course and Prognosis

Patients with lymph node infarction are at increased risk of malignant lymphoma. Malignant lymphoma may be present at the time of initial biopsy or develop later. Cleary and colleagues reported malignant lymphoma in 16 of 18 patients with lymph node infarction diagnosed within 2–6 months of the initial biopsy (Cleary et al, 1982). Maurer and colleagues, in a review of their own cases and cases gathered from the literature, reported malignant lymphoma in 26 of 81 patients, diagnosed within 2 years of the initial biopsy (Maurer et al, 1986). Our own experience is closer to that of Maurer and colleagues. Biopsy of recurrent or persistent lymphadenopathy is, therefore, always recommended when the diagnosis of lymph node infarction is made. The lymphomas following lymph node infarction have been predominantly of diffuse large cell type; however, other lymphomas, including Hodgkin's disease, may occur (Cleary et al, 1982; Maurer et al, 1986).

REFERENCES

Cleary KR, Osborne BM, Butler JJ. Lymph node infarction foreshadowing malignant lymphoma. Am J Surg Pathol 6:435–442, 1982.

Falzon M, Isaacson PG. The natural history of benign lymphoepithelial lesions of the salivary gland in which there is a monoclonal population of B cells. A report of two cases. Am J Surg Pathol 15:59–65, 1991.

Fermand J-P, Brouet J-C, Danon F, Seligmann M. Gamma heavy chain "disease": Heterogeneity of the clinicopathologic features. Report of 16 cases and review of the literature. Medicine (Baltimore) 68:321–333, 1989.

Fishleder A, Tubbs R, Hesse B, Levine H. Uniform detection of immunoglobulin-gene rearrangment in benign lymphoepithelial lesions. N Engl J Med 316:1118–1121, 1987.

Ioachim HL, Ryan JR, Blaugrund SM. Salivary gland lymph nodes. The site of lymphadenopathies and lymphomas associated with human immunodeficiency virus infection. Arch Pathol Lab Med 112:1224–1228, 1988.

Kuo TT. Kikuchi's disease (histiocytic necrotizing lymphadenitis). A clinicopathologic study of 79 cases with an analysis of histologic subtypes, immunohistology, and ploidy. Am J Surg Pathol 19:798–809, 1995.

Maurer R, Schmid U, Davie JD, Mahy J, Stansfield AG, Lukes RJ. Lymph node infarction and malignant lymphoma: A multicentre survey of European, English, and American cases. Histopathol 10:571–588, 1986.

Medeiros LJ, Raynor B, Harris NL. Lupus lymphadenitis: Report of a case with immunohistochemical studies on frozen sections. Hum Pathol 20:295–299, 1989.

Nosanchuk JS, Schnitizer B. Follicular hyperplasia in lymph nodes from patients with rheumatoid arthritis. Cancer 24:343–354, 1969.

Royer B, Cazals-Hatem D, Sibilia J, Agbalika F, Cayuela J-M, Soussi T, et al. Lymphomas in patients with Sjögren's syndrome are marginal zone B-cell neoplasms, arise in diverse extranodal and nodal sites, and are not associated with viruses. Blood 90:766–775, 1997.

Sheibani K, Burke JS, Swartz MS, Nademanee A, Winberg CD. Monocytoid B cell lymphoma. Clinicopathologic study of 21 cases of a unique type of low-grade lymphoma. Cancer 62:1531–1538, 1988.

Shiokawa S, Yasuda M, Kikuchi M, Yoshikawa Y, Nobunga M. Mixed connective tissue disease associated with lupus lymphadenitis. J Rheumatol 20:147–150, 1993.

Talal N, Schnitizer B. Lymphadenopathy and Sjogren's syndrome. Clin Rheum Dis 3:421–432, 1977.

Turner RR, Martin J, Dorfman RF. Necrotizing lymphadenitis: A study of 30 cases. Am J Surg Pathol 7:115–124, 1983.

Unger PD, Rappaport K, Strauchen JA. Necrotizing lymphadenitis (Kikuchi's disease). Report of four cases of an unusual pseudolymphomatous lesion and immunologic marker studies. Arch Pathol Lab Med 111:1031–1034, 1987.

Kikuchi's Disease, Kawasaki's Disease, and Kimura's Disease

Kikuchi's disease, Kawasaki's disease, and Kimura's disease are causes of lymphadenopathy which are seen most frequently in the Far East, but they are also seen in Europe and North America. All are peculiar reactive lymphadenopathies of unknown etiology.

Kikuchi's Disease

Kikuchi's disease (Kikuchi-Fujimoto disease, histiocytic necrotizing lymphadenitis) is an idiopathic lymphadenopathy which was first recognized in Japan, from which the majority of cases continue to originate, but it has a worldwide distribution (Kikuchi, 1972; Kickuchi et al, 1977; Dorfman and Berry, 1988).

Clinical Features

The majority of patients with Kikuchi's disease are young women presenting with persistent tender or nontender cervical lymphadenopathy (Turner et al, 1983; Unger et al, 1987). Fever and a viral-like prodrome are frequently present; mild leukopenia may be present. Cervical lymph nodes are most frequently involved; however, involvement of virtually any lymph node group has been described, including mesenteric and mediastinal lymph nodes. Patients with inconspicuous or inapparent lymphadenopathy may present as fever of unknown origin (Norris et al, 1996; Pearl and Strauchen, 1989). We have seen one case of mesenteric Kikuchi's disease mimicking acute appendicitis. Extranodal cutaneous involvement is rare, but has also been reported (Kuo, 1995). The etiology of Kikuchi's disease is obscure. A possible relation to lupus lymphadenitis is

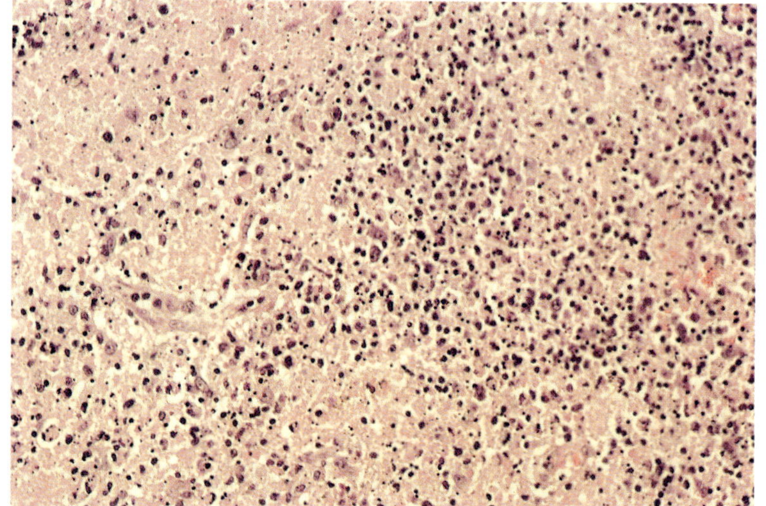

FIGURE 11.1

Kikuchi's disease showing a focus of necrosis.

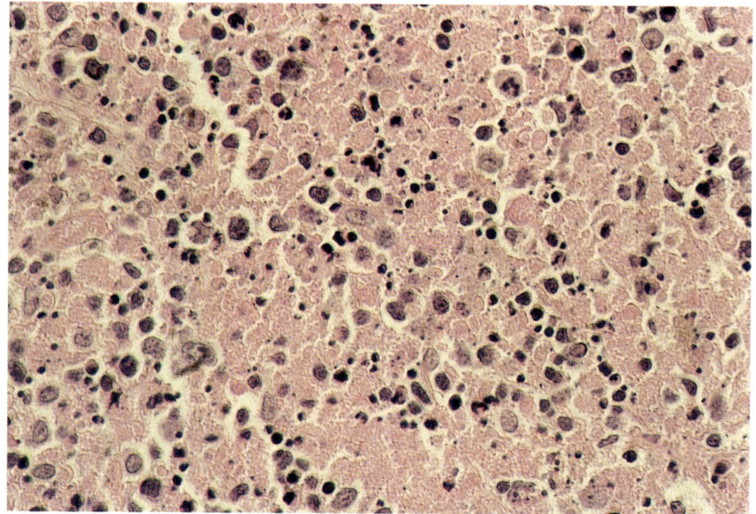

FIGURE 11.2

Kikuchi's disease showing necrosis and karyorrhectic debris.

suggested by the histopathologic similarities; however, the development of systemic lupus erythematosus (SLE) in patients with Kikuchi's disease is exceptional. Despite the viral-like prodrome in some patients, no virus, including Epstein-Barr virus and human herpesvirus 6, has been consistently demonstrated (Hollingsworth et al, 1994).

Histopathology

The lymph node in Kikuchi's disease is characterized by paracortical foci of necrosis with abundant karyorrhectic debris (Turner et al, 1983) (Figs.11.1 and 11.2). The foci of

FIGURE
11.3

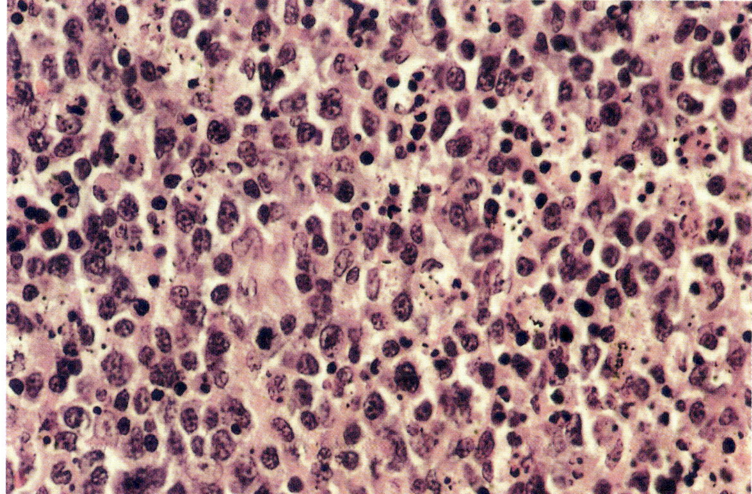

Kikuchi's disease showing numerous immunoblasts at the periphery of a focus of necrosis.

FIGURE
11.4

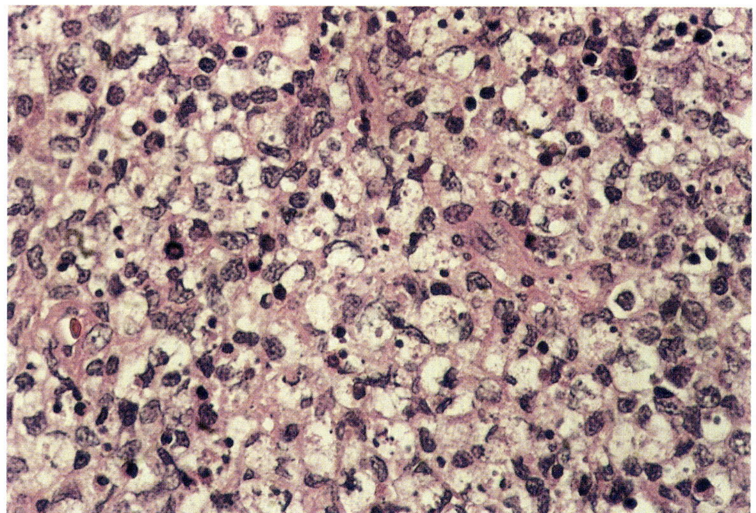

Kikuchi's disease showing numerous macrophages with "C-shaped" nuclei or "crescentic histiocytes."

necrosis may be minimal, or confluent and extensive, and are characteristically well circumscribed and surrounded by a zone of immunoblasts and macrophages (Fig.11.3). Macrophages with distinctive C-shaped nuclei ("crescentic histiocytes") and plasmacytoid monocytes are prominent (Hansmann et al, 1992; Kuo, 1995) (Fig.11.4). Polymorphonuclear leukocytes and plasma cells are characteristically scant; xanthoma cells may be prominent in late lesions (Kuo, 1995). Three histopathologic subtypes of Kikuchi's disease have been identified: proliferative, necrotizing, and xanthomatous; these may represent stages in development of the lesion (Kuo, 1995). Immunohistochemical stud-

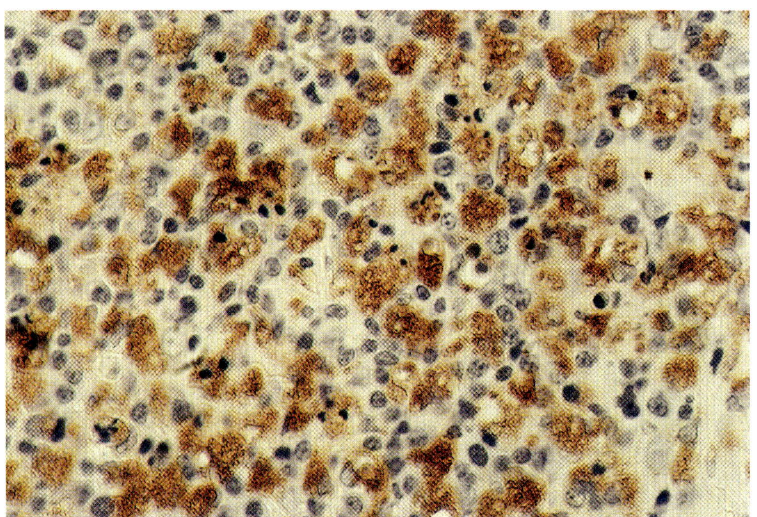

FIGURE
11.5

Kikuchi's disease showing numerous macrophages stained with monoclonal antibody to CD68.

ies in Kikuchi's disease demonstrate a preponderance of CD8 T cells and macrophages
in the necrotic zones (Kuo, 1995; Turner et al, 1983; Unger et al, 1987) (Fig.11.5).

Differential Diagnosis

Kikuchi's disease must be distinguished from other causes of necrotizing lymphadenopathy including necrotizing granulomatous lymphadenitis, lupus lymphadenitis, lymph
node infarction, and malignant lymphoma with extensive necrosis. The absence of granulomata and polymorphonuclear leukocytes, and abundance of karyorrhectic debris and
"crescentic histiocytes" are features distinguishing Kikuchi's disease from the usual infectious causes of necrotizing lymphadenitis. Lupus lymphadenitis may appear indistinguishable in some cases (Kuo, 1995); however, the prominence of plasma cells in lupus
lymphadenitis will usually permit distinction (Dorfman and Berry, 1988). In equivocal
cases, serology for antinuclear antibodies (ANA) may be helpful. Distinction from malignant lymphoma is usually not difficult once the pathologist is familiar with the histopathologic features of Kikuchi's disease. The abundance of karyorrhectic debris, focal
pattern of involvement, and "crescentic histiocytes" are distinctive.

Course and Prognosis

Kikuchi's disease is, in almost all cases, a benign, self-limited process with spontaneous
resolution of the lymphadenopathy without treatment, usually within 6 months. Recurrence is uncommon, but has been reported. Kuo observed two cases of recurrence in
his series of 79 cases, occurring 4 and 7 years after diagnosis (Kuo, 1995). We have seen
one case with multiple recurrences over a several year period; she is now alive and well
without specific therapy. There is one fatal case of Kikuchi's disease recorded in the
literature, with death attributed to myocarditis (Chan et al, 1989).

Kawasaki's Disease

Kawasaki's disease (mucocutaneous lymph node syndrome) is an acute febrile illness of childhood, characterized by skin rash, cervical lymphadenopathy, and systemic vasculitis with coronary artery involvement and coronary artery aneurysms. Most cases originate in the Far East and Japan, where the entity was first described (Kawasaki, 1967); however, the distribution is worldwide.

Clinical Features

Kawasaki's disease is a disorder of infancy and childhood with most cases under the age of 6 years; rare cases have been reported in young adults (Schlossberg et al, 1979). Affected children present with fever, cervical lymphadenopathy, and mucocutaneous manifestations, including erythema of the conjunctiva, lips, and oral mucosa, and desquamation of the skin of the palms, soles, and fingertips. Coronary artery vasculitis with coronary artery aneurysms is the principal complication and typically develops in the third to fourth week of illness. The etiology of Kawasaki's disease is unknown; the occurrence in outbreaks has suggested an infectious or postinfectious etiology (Bell et al, 1981). There is evidence of abnormal T cell and macrophage activation, leading to systemic vasculitis (Abe et al, 1993).

Histopathology

The histopathology of the skin and mucosa is nonspecific with perivascular lymphocytes and macrophages. The lymph nodes are infrequently biopsied. The changes observed in the lymph nodes include fibrin thrombi in small vessels and multiple irregular foci of necrosis involving the paracortex and follicles (Giesker et al, 1982; Marsh et al, 1980) (Figs.11.6, 11.7, and 11.8).

FIGURE 11.6

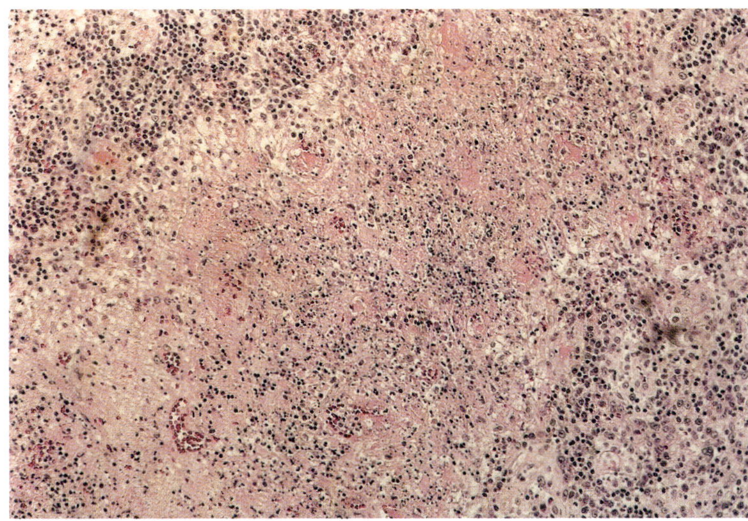

Kawasaki's disease showing focus of lymph node necrosis.

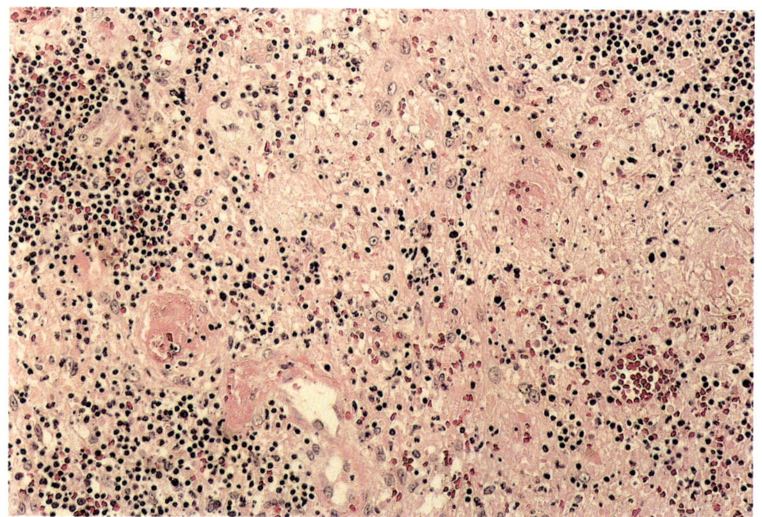

FIGURE 11.7

Kawasaki's disease showing lymph node necrosis and fibrin thrombi.

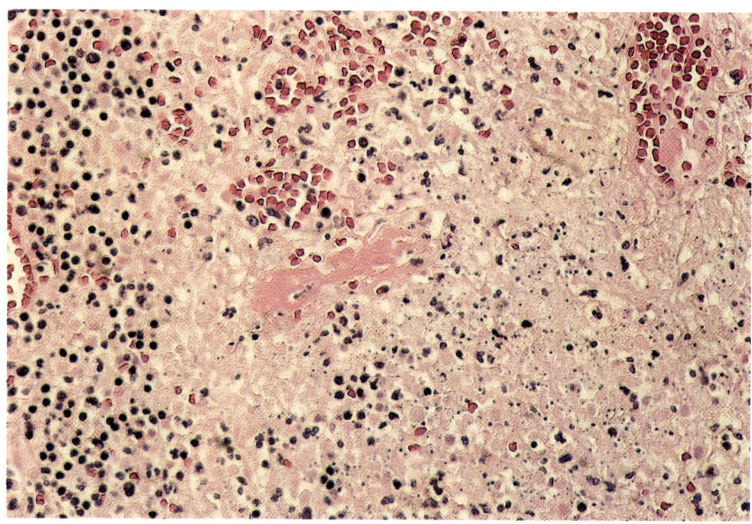

FIGURE 11.8

Kawasaki's disease showing fibrin thrombi.

Differential Diagnosis

Kawasaki's disease is principally diagnosed clinically. Lymph node biopsy has been advocated for early diagnosis (Giesker et al, 1982). The foci of lymph node necrosis may resemble those in Kikuchi's disease and lupus lymphadenitis. Fibrin thrombi, however, are not seen in the latter two conditions.

Course and Prognosis

Kawasaki's disease is associated with the development of coronary artery aneurysms in up to 25% of patients, with a 1–3% mortality rate. Kawasaki's disease is treated with high doses of intravenous immunoglobulin, which reduces the rate of cardiac complications

(Newberger et al, 1991). Intravenous immunoglobulin is likely active by binding to the Fc receptors of macrophages, inhibiting their activity.

Kimura's Disease

Kimura's disease is an unusual angiolymphoid proliferation which involves the subcutaneous tissues, salivary glands, and regional lymph nodes of the neck (Kuo et al, 1988). Kimura's disease was originally reported from Japan (Kimura et al, 1948); and cases continue to occur almost exclusively in individuals from the Far East. Kimura's disease is frequently confused with angiolymphoid hyperplasia with eosinophilia (ALHE), a distinct disorder, which occurs in western countries.

Clinical Features

Patients with Kimura's disease are typically young men presenting with soft tissue swelling, involving the preauricular or submandibular regions, and regional lymph node enlargement. Isolated cervical lymphadenopathy may also occur (Hui et al, 1989). Peripheral blood eosinophilia and elevation of serum IgE are characteristically present. The nephrotic syndrome has been reported in association with Kimura's disease (Quinibi et al, 1988). The etiology of Kimura's disease is obscure.

Histopathology

Kimura's disease involves the subcutaneous tissue of the neck, parotid and submandibular salivary glands, and cervical lymph nodes. The histopathologic changes consist of follicular lymphoid hyperplasia with interfollicular eosinophils and proliferation of thin-walled blood vessels (Kuo et al, 1988) (Figs. 11.9 and 11.10). Warthin-Finkeldey–like giant cells, formation of eosinophilic microabscesses, and infiltration of follicular cen-

FIGURE 11.9

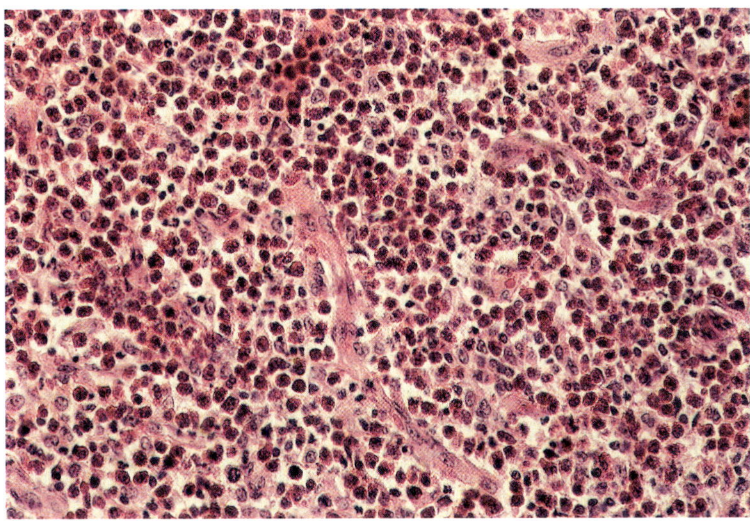

Kimura's disease showing proliferation of thin-walled blood vessels and numerous eosinophils.

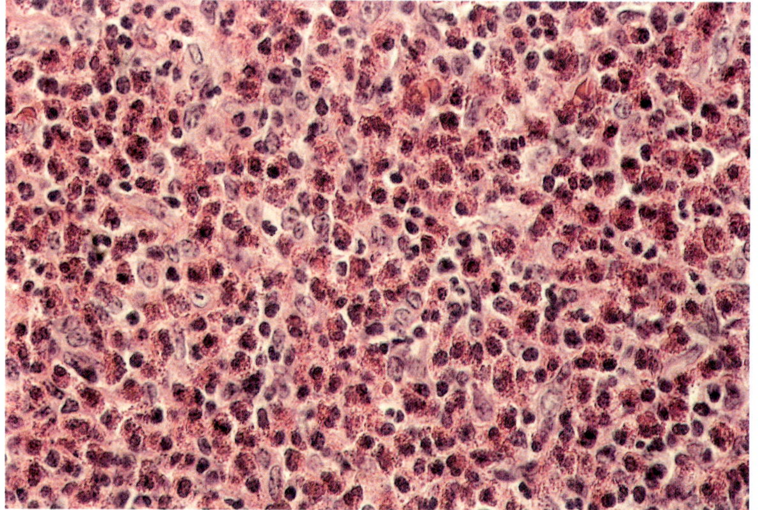

FIGURE
11.10

Kimura's disease showing marked eosinophilic infiltration of the para-cortex.

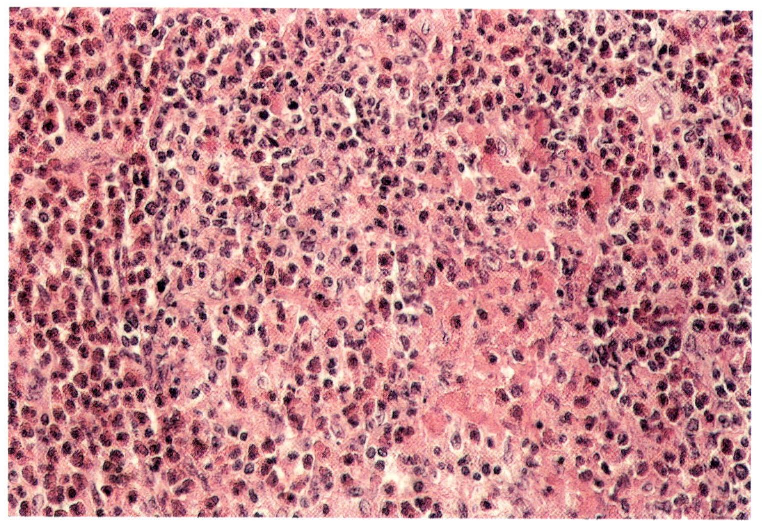

FIGURE
11.11

Kimura's disease showing infiltration of a follicular center by eosino-phils (eosinophilic folliculolysis) and deposition of hyaline material.

ters by eosinophils (eosinophilic folliculolysis) are frequently present (Hui et al, 1989) (Fig. 11.11). Deposition of hyaline material in follicular centers and foci of sclerosis may be present (Hui et al, 1989); Charcot-Leyden crystals may also be present (Kuo et al, 1988). Immunophenotypic studies demonstrate a preponderance of B cells and deposition of IgE in follicular centers (Kuo et al, 1988).

Differential Diagnosis

Kimura's disease should be distinguished from angiolymphoid hyperplasia with eosinophilia (ALHE), with which it has been confused in the past (Kuo et al, 1988). ALHE, in contrast to Kimura's disease, occurs frequently in western countries, affects women more often than men, and most frequently presents as superficial cutaneous lesions on the head and neck. ALHE is characterized by proliferation of histiocytoid or epithelioid endothelial cells and is considered by most authors to be an epithelioid hemangioma (Rosai et al, 1979; Urabe et al, 1987) (Figs. 11.12 and 11.13). Peripheral eosinophilia and elevated serum IgE are absent in patients with ALHE.

Kimura's disease should also be distinguished from other causes of reactive lymphoid

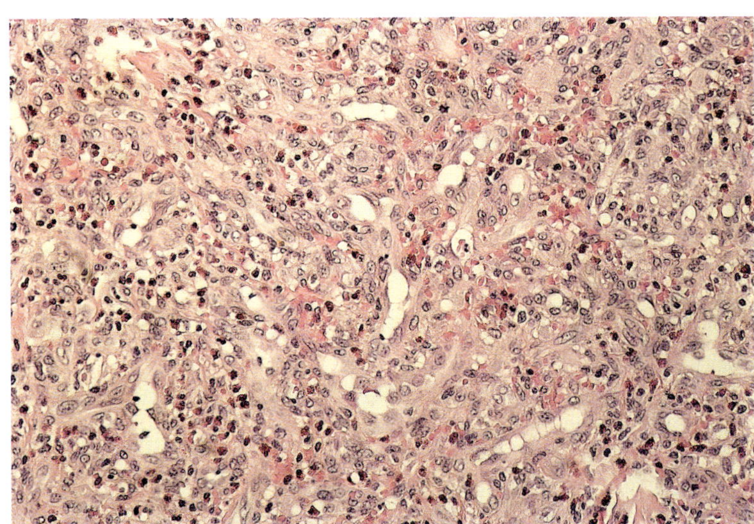

FIGURE 11.12

Angiolymphoid hyperplasia with eosinophilia is characterized by proliferation of blood vessels lined by plump, epithelioid or histiocytoid endothelial cells, in contrast to the thin-walled blood vessels in Kimura's disease.

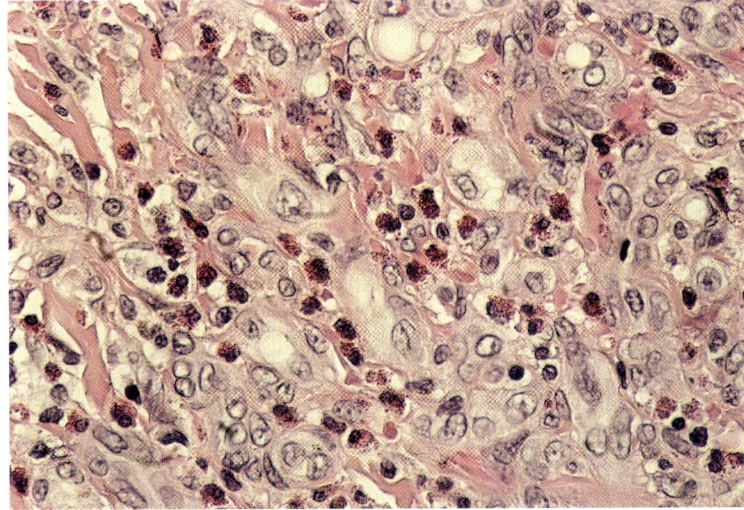

FIGURE 11.13

Angiolymphoid hyperplasia with eosinophilia showing epithelioid endothelial cells and eosinophils.

hyperplasia with eosinophilia including drug reactions and parasitic disease. The florid follicular hyperplasia and eosinophilic folliculolysis are characteristic features of Kimura's disease. Immunohistochemical staining for IgE, demonstrating characteristic follicular center deposits, will be helpful in equivocal cases. Eosinophilic microabscesses may be seen in other conditions, including filariasis, Hodgkin's disease, and eosinophilic granuloma (Langerhans' cell histiocytosis). Fragments of adult worm are regularly found in the eosinophilic microabscesses of filariasis, which usually involves inguinal lymph nodes; Hodgkin's disease and eosinophilic granuloma are distinguished by the presence of Reed-Sternberg cells and Langerhans' cells, respectively.

Course and Prognosis

Kimura's disease is treated by surgical excision. Recurrence is frequent.

REFERENCES

Abe J, Kotzin EL, Meissner C, Melish ME, Takahashi M, Fulton D, Romagne F, Malissen B, Leung DT. Characterization of T cell repertoire changes in acute Kawasaki disease. J Exp Med 177:791–196, 1993.

Bell DM, Brink EW, Nitzkin JL, Hall EB, Wulff H, Berkowitz ID, et al. Kawasaki syndrome: Description of two outbreaks in the U.S. N Engl J Med 304:1568–1575, 1981.

Chan JKC, Wong K-C, Ng C-S. A fatal case of multicentric Kikuchi's histiocytic necrotizing lymphadenitis. Cancer 63:1856–1862, 1989.

Dorfman RF, Berry GJ. Kikuchi's histiocytic necrotizing lymphadenitis: An analysis of 108 cases with emphasis on differential diagnosis. Semin Diagn Pathol 5:329–345, 1988.

Giesker DW, Pastuszak WT, Forouhar FA, Krause PJ, Hine P. Lymph node biopsy for early diagnosis in Kawasaki disease. Am J Surg Pathol 6:493–501, 1982.

Hansmann ML, Kikuchi M, Wacker HH, Radzun HJ, Nathwani BN, Hesse K, Parwaresch MR. Immunohistochemical monitoring of plasmacytoid cells in lymph node sections of Kikuchi-Fujimoto disease by a new pan-macrophage antibody Ki-M1P. Hum Pathol 23:676–680, 1992.

Hollingsworth HC, Peiper SC, Weiss LM, Raffeld M, Jaffe ES. An investigation of the viral pathogenesis of Kikuchi-Fujimoto disease. Lack of evidence for Epstein-Barr virus or human herpesvirus 6 as the causative agents. Arch Pathol Lab Med 118:134–140, 1994.

Hui PK, Chan JKC, Ng CS, Kung ITM, Gwi E. Lymphadenopathy of Kimura's disease. Am J Surg Pathol 13:177–186, 1989.

Kawasaki T. Acute febrile mucocutaneous syndrome with lymphoid involvement with specific desquamation of fingers and toes in children. Jpn J Allerg 16:178–222, 1967.

Kikuchi M. Lymphadenitis showing focal reticulum cell hyperplasia with nuclear debris and phagocytes. Acta Hematol Jpn 35:379–380, 1972.

Kikuchi M, Yoshizumi T, Nakamura H. Necrotizing lymphadenitis: Possible acute toxoplasmic infection. Virchows Arch A 376:247–253, 1977.

Kimura T, Yoshimura S, Ishikawa E. On the unusual granulation combined with hyperplastic changes of lymphatic tissues. Trans Soc Pathol Jpn 37:179–180, 1948.

Kuo T-T. Kikuchi's disease (histiocytic necrotizing lymphadenitis). A clinicopathologic study of 79 cases with an analysis of histologic subtypes, immunohistology, and DNA ploidy. Am J Surg Pathol 19:798–809, 1995.

Kuo T-T, Shih L-Y, Chan H-L. Kimura's disease. Involvement of regional lymph nodes and distinction from angiolymphoid hyperplasia with eosinophilia. Am J Surg Pathol 12:843–854, 1988.

Marsh WL, Bishop JW, Koenig HM. Bone marrow and lymph node findings in a fatal case of Kawasaki's disease. Arch Pathol Lab Med 14:563–567, 1980.

Newberger JW, Takahashi M, Beiser AS, Burns JC, Bastian J, Chung KJ, et al. A single intravenous infusion of gamma globulin as compared with four infusions in the treatment of acute Kawasaki disease. N Engl J Med 324:1633–1643, 1991.

Norris AH, Krasinskas AM, Salhany KE, Gluckman SJ. Kikuchi-Fujimoto disease: A benign cause of fever and lymphadenopathy. Am J Med 101:401–405, 1996.

Pearl D, Strauchen JA. Kikuchi's disease as a cause of fever of unknown origin. N Engl J Med 320:1147–1148, 1989.

Quinibi WY, Al-Sibai MB, Akhar M. Mesangioproliferative glomerulonephritis associated with Kimura's disease. Clin Nephrol 30:111, 1988.

Rosai J, Gold J, Landy R. The histiocytoid hemangiomas: a unifying concept embracing several previously described entities of the skin, soft tissue, large vessel, bone, and heart. Hum Pathol 10:707, 1979.

Schlossberg D, Kandra J, Kreiser J. Possible Kawasaki disease in a 20 year old woman. Arch Dermatol 115:1435–1436, 1979.

Turner RD, Martin J, Dorfman RF. Necrotizing lymphadenitis. A study of 30 cases. Am J Surg Pathol 7:115–123, 1983.

Unger PD, Rappaport KM, Strauchen JA. Necrotizing lymphadenitis (Kikuchi's disease). Report of four cases of an unusual pseudolymphomatous lesion and immunologic marker studies. Arch Pathol Lab Med 111:1031–1034, 1987.

Urabe A, Tsuneyoshi M, Enjoji M. Epithelioid hemangioma versus Kimura's disease: A comparative clinicopathologic study. Am J Surg Pathol 11:758, 1987.

Castleman's Disease and Progressive Transformation of Germinal Centers

Castleman's disease (CD) and progressive transformation of germinal centers (PTGC) are abnormal follicular proliferations which are non-neoplastic and of uncertain pathogenesis.

Castleman's Disease

Castleman's disease (angiofollicular lymph node hyperplasia, "giant" lymph node hyperplasia) is an abnormal follicular lymphoid proliferation of uncertain pathogenesis which occurs in two major histologic forms, hyaline-vascular and plasma cell, and two clinical forms, localized and multicentric. Multicentric Castleman's disease is associated with infection with the Kaposi's sarcoma–associated herpesvirus (KSHV) (Soulier et al, 1995a).

Clinical Features

Patients with Castleman's disease of the hyaline-vascular type are usually asymptomatic and present with disease localized to mediastinal lymph nodes (Castleman et al, 1956). Patients with Castleman's disease of the plasma cell type are often symptomatic and present with a localized mass with systemic symptoms, including fever, anemia, and hyperglobulinemia, which remit on resection of the mass (Keller et al, 1972), or with multicentric Castleman's disease (Frizzera et al, 1983). Multicentric Castleman's disease is a systemic lymphoproliferative disorder characterized by fever, generalized lymphade-

FIGURE 12.1

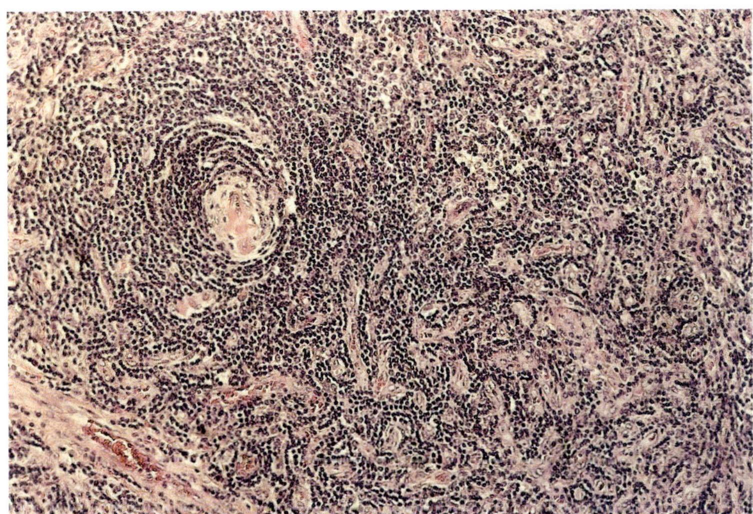

Hyaline-vascular Castleman's disease showing atrophic follicular center, onionskin arrangement of mantle zone lymphocytes, and interfollicular vascular proliferation.

nopathy, splenomegaly, hyperglobulinemia, abnormal liver function tests, and an increased incidence of infections and malignant neoplasms, particularly Kaposi's sarcoma and malignant lymphoma (Frizzera et al, 1985). The POEMS syndrome (polyneuropathy, organomegaly, endocrinopathy, monoclonal gammopathy, and skin abnormalities) may be associated (Bitter et al, 1985; Miralles et al, 1992). Lymph node changes indistinguishable from multicentric Castleman's disease occur in association with HIV infection (Oksenhendler et al, 1996) and Kaposi's sarcoma (Chen, 1984). The etiology of Castleman's disease is unknown. Multicentric Castleman's disease in both HIV-infected and non–HIV-infected patients is associated with infection with KSHV (Soulier et al, 1995a). Clonal immunoglobulin gene rearrangements have been detected in some cases of multicentric Castleman's disease (Hanson et al, 1988; Soulier et al, 1995b). Monoclonal antibody to interleukin-6 was reported to induce remission in the systemic manifestations of Castleman's disease, suggesting a role of the cytokine in the pathogenesis of the disorder (Beck et al, 1994).

Histopathology

HYALINE-VASCULAR CASTLEMAN'S DISEASE   The mass in the hyaline-vascular form of Castleman's disease usually consists of a single greatly enlarged lymph node. The characteristic histopathologic feature is the presence, throughout the affected lymph node, of abnormal follicles, consisting of atrophic, hyalinized follicular centers, with a broad mantle zone of small lymphocytes in a concentric or onionskin arrangement and one or more penetrating blood vessels (Fig. 12.1). The low-magnification appearance of the abnormal follicle and penetrating blood vessel has been likened to a "lollipop on a stick" (Fig 12.2). The abnormal follicular center is depleted of follicular center cells and consists of a concentric whorl of "naked" follicular dendritic cells, resembling the Hassall's corpuscle of the thymus. Multiple atrophic follicular centers may be present in a single

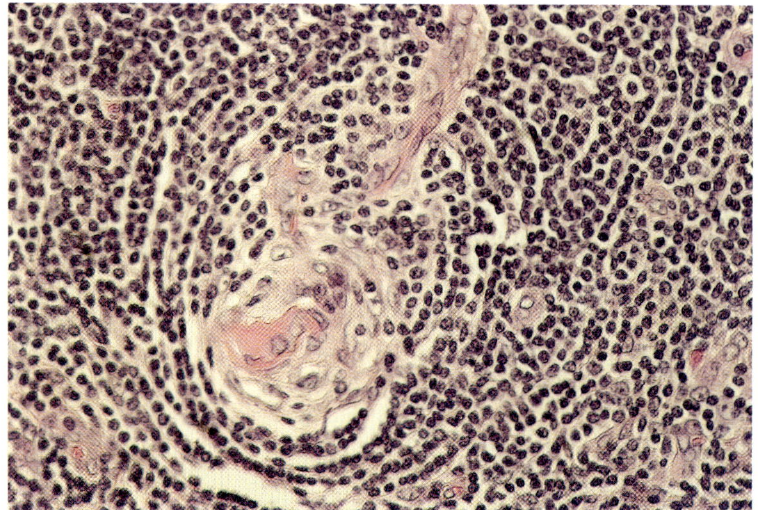

FIGURE
12.2

Hyaline-vascular Castleman's disease showing "lollipop on a stick" appearance of follicular center and concentric onionskin arrangement of mantle zone lymphocytes.

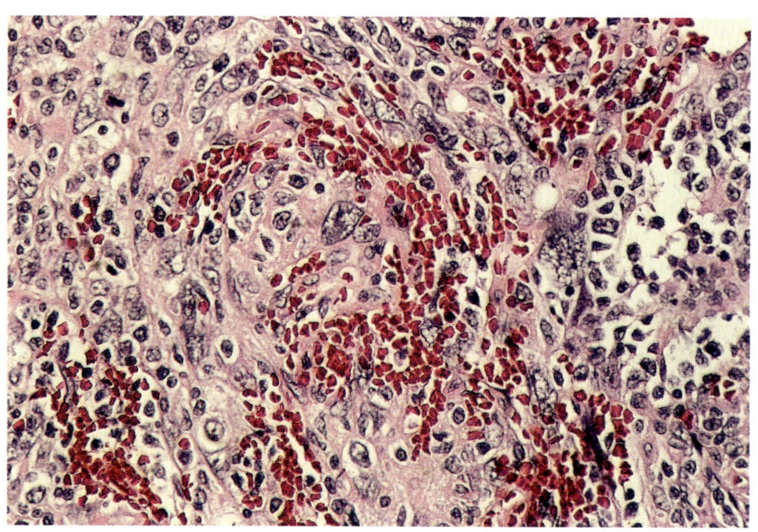

FIGURE
12.3

Hyaline-vascular Castleman's disease showing nuclear atypia of follicular dendritic cells ("dendritic cell dysplasia").

abnormal follicle. The interfollicular zone is hypervascular with a dense meshwork of proliferating blood vessels, foci of fibrosis, and scattered small lymphocytes, plasma cells, and immunoblasts. The sinuses are effaced. Follicular, classic, and stroma-rich histopathological variants of hyaline-vascular Castleman's disease have been recognized, with varying proportion of follicles and interfollicular stromal cells (Danon et al, 1993). Striking atypia of stromal cells, considered to represent dendritic cell dysplasia (Fig. 12.3), nodules of proliferating follicular dendritic cells and vascular cells (Fig. 12.4), and development of follicular dendritic cell and vascular neoplasms (Fig 12.5), may be seen (Chan et al, 1994; Lin and Frizzera, 1997).

FIGURE
12.4

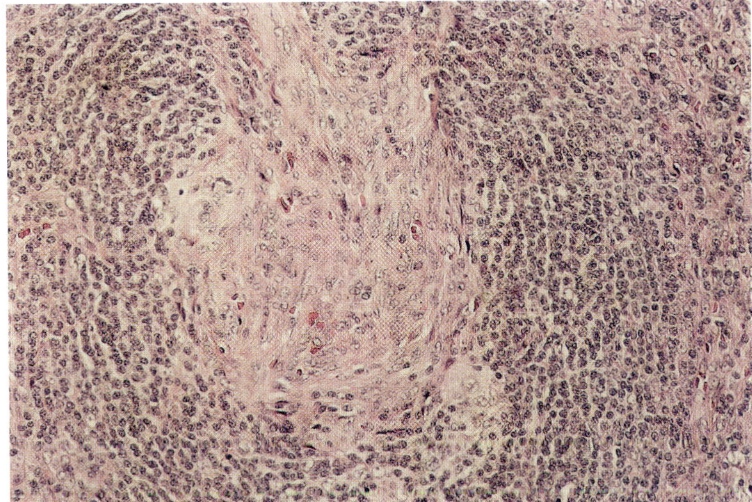

Hyaline-vascular Castleman's disease showing spindle cell proliferation.

FIGURE
12.5

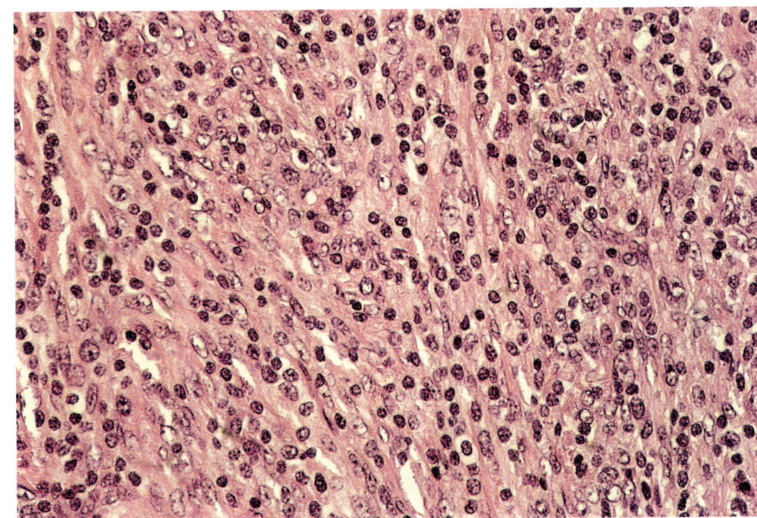

Follicular dendritic cell tumor developing in hyaline-vascular Castleman's disease.

Immunohistochemical studies in hyaline-vascular Castleman's disease demonstrate abnormal, enlarged follicular dendritic cells, decreased follicular center proliferation, and an aberrant population of mantle zone lymphocytes (Menke et al, 1996). Plasmacytoid monocytes and fibroblastic reticulum cells are also prominent (Danon et al, 1993).

PLASMA CELL CASTLEMAN'S DISEASE   The mass in the plasma cell form of Castleman's disease usually consists of a group of enlarged lymph nodes. The characteristic histopathologic feature is the presence, in the interfollicular areas, of solid, confluent sheets of plasma cells (Figs. 12.6 and 12.7). The follicular centers are usually enlarged and

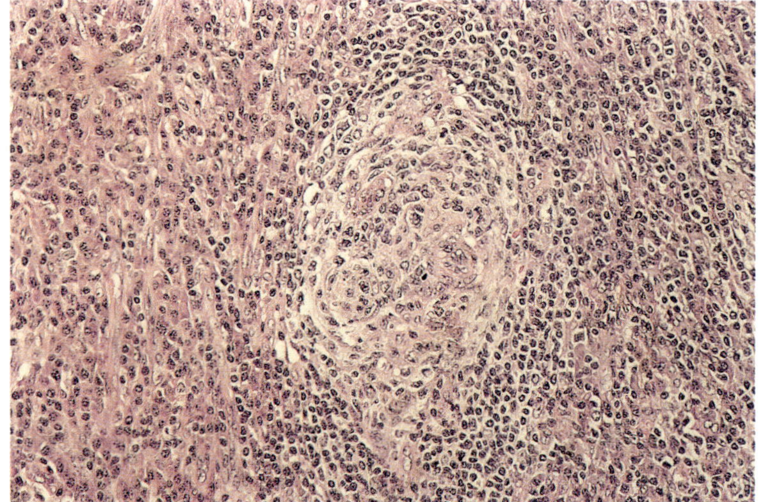

FIGURE 12.6

Plasma cell Castleman's disease showing hyperplastic follicular center and interfollicular plasma cells.

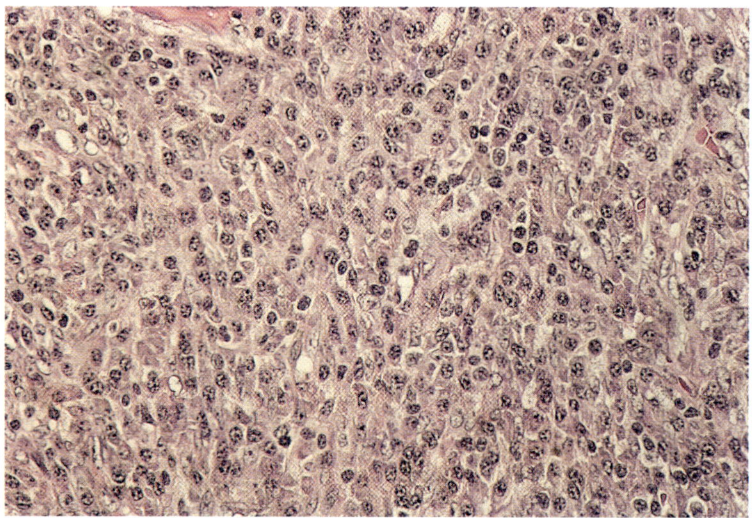

FIGURE 12.7

Plasma cell Castleman's disease showing sheets of interfollicular plasma cells.

hyperplastic, in contrast to the atrophic follicular centers of hyaline-vascular Castleman's disease; paracortical hypervascularity and onionskin mantle zones are typically absent.

Immunohistochemical studies in plasma cell Castleman's disease demonstrate changes similar to those observed in hyaline-vascular Castleman's disease, with abnormal follicular dendritic cells, decreased follicular center cell proliferation, and aberrant mantle zone lymphocytes (Menke et al, 1996); plasmacytoid monocytes were, however, less frequent. The plasma cells in plasma cell Castleman's disease are usually polyclonal by immunoglobulin light chain staining; however, monoclonal plasma cells may be found in some cases (Radaszkiewicz et al, 1989; Menke et al, 1996). The development of plasmacytoma in lymph nodes with plasma cell Castleman's disease has been reported (Schlosnagle et al, 1982).

MIXED AND TRANSITIONAL FORMS OF CASTLEMEN'S DISEASE Castleman's disease with features of both the hyaline-vascular and plasma cell variants is occasionally encountered and is referred to as the mixed or transitional form of Castleman's disease. These cases are heterogeneous and include cases clinicopathologically resembling the hyaline-vascular form of Castleman's disease, but with the presence of plasmacytosis, and other cases clinicopathologically resembling the plasma cell form of Castleman's disease, but with the presence of hyalinized follicular centers. Multicentric Castleman's disease accounts for a disproportionate number of the latter cases.

MULTICENTRIC CASTLEMAN'S DISEASE Multicentric Castleman's disease affects multiple groups of enlarged lymph nodes and shows a spectrum of lymph node changes which may resemble the plasma cell, hyaline-vascular, or mixed forms of Castleman's disease. Most cases are of the plasma cell or mixed type, with diffuse plasmacytosis, hyperplastic or involuted follicular centers, variable admixture of immunoblasts, and partial preservation of lymph node architecture (Frizzera et al, 1983; Weisenberger et al, 1985) (Figs. 12.8 and 12.9).

CASTLEMAN'S DISEASE-LIKE CHANGES IN HIV INFECTION AND KAPOSI'S SARCOMA Lymph nodes from patients with HIV infection (Oksenhendler et al, 1996) and from patients with Kaposi's sarcoma (Chen, 1984) may show changes indistinguishable from the multicentric form of Castleman's disease. Kaposi's sarcoma–associated herpesvirus (KSHV) may play an etiologic role (Soulier et al, 1995a).

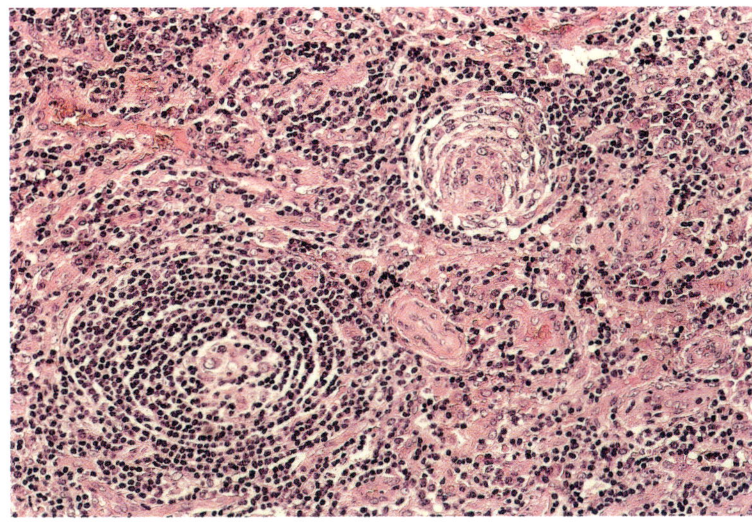

FIGURE 12.8

Multicentric Castleman's disease in a patient presenting with the POEMS syndrome showing hyaline-vascular changes with atrophy of follicular centers and marked vascular proliferation.

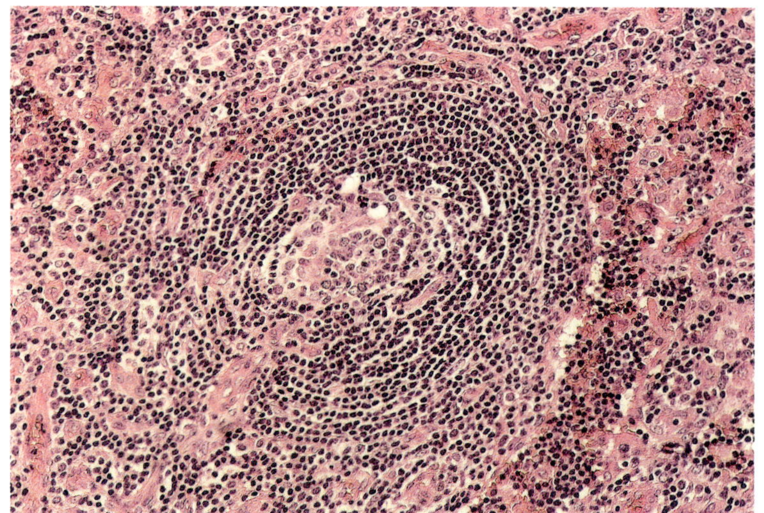

Multicentric Castleman's disease in a patient presenting with the POEMS
syndrome showing hyaline-vascular changes with a "lollipop" follicle.

Differential Diagnosis

The hyaline-vascular form of Castleman's disease must be distinguished from other
forms of reactive follicular lymphoid hyperplasia. The diagnosis of hyaline-vascular Castleman's disease should be made only when abnormal follicles are present throughout
the lymph node in association with interfollicular hypervascularity and effacement of
the sinus architecture. The presence of a few involuted or hyalinized follicles is not
specific to Castleman's disease and is frequently seen in nonspecific reactive follicular
lymphoid hyperplasias. The plasma cell form of Castleman's disease must be distinguished from other causes of lymph node plasmacytosis, including rheumatoid lymphadenopathy and luetic lymphadenitis.

Castleman's disease is usually readily distinguished from malignant lymphoma. Hodgkin's disease occasionally is found to coexist in lymph nodes with Castleman's disease
(Abdel-Reheim et al, 1996) and a relation between follicular dendritic cells and Reed-
Sternberg cells has been proposed (Delsol et al, 1993). Rarely, follicular lymphoma, or
mantle cell lymphoma with a pronounced mantle-zone pattern, may mimic the abnormal
follicles of Castleman's disease. Immunohistochemical staining for immunoglobulin light
chain restriction and BCL-2 oncoprotein (in follicular lymphoma) or BCL-1 oncoprotein
(in mantle-cell lymphoma) will resolve the diagnostic difficulty.

Course and Prognosis

The localized forms of Castleman's disease are treated by surgical resection; systemic
symptoms, when present, remit with resection and recurrence is infrequent. The multicentric forms of Castleman's disease are difficult to treat; some cases respond to cytotoxic chemotherapy (Frizzera et al, 1985; Oksenhendler, 1996). Multicentric Castleman's
disease is associated with an increased incidence of neoplasms, including Kaposi's sarcoma and malignant lymphoma (Frizzera et al, 1985). The development of other neo-

plasms in association with Castleman's disease has been rarely reported, including vascular neoplasms (Gerald et al, 1990), follicular dendritic cell neoplasms (Chan et al, 1994), osteoblastic myeloma and POEMS syndrome (Bitter et al, 1985), and plasmacytoma of lymph node (Schlosnagle et al, 1982) and bone (Gould et al, 1990).

Progressive Transformation of Germinal Centers

PTGC is a peculiar form of follicular lymphoid hyperplasia which occurs in children and young adults (Ferry et al, 1992; Osborne et al, 1992) and is also associated with nodular lymphocyte predominance Hodgkin's disease (Burns et al, 1984; Poppema et al, 1979).

Clinical Features

PTGC occurs predominantly in male children and young adults (Ferry et al, 1992; Osborne et al, 1992). Lymphadenopathy is usually solitary and asymptomatic (Osborne and Butler, 1984) but may be tender or involve more than one lymph node group (Ferry et al, 1992). PTGC occurring in association with nodular lymphocyte predominance Hodgkin's disease may occur prior to the diagnosis of Hodgkin's disease, in the same lymph node biopsy as Hodgkin's disease, or following Hodgkin's disease (Osborne and Butler, 1984).

Histopathology

Progressive transformation of germinal centers occurs in association with reactive follicular lymphoid hyperplasia. The hyperplastic follicular centers become progressively infiltrated with small lymphocytes and enlarged (Figs. 12.10 and 12.11). The fully transformed germinal center is several times the size of the surrounding hyperplastic follicles and consists predominantly of small lymphocytes, with loss of the boundary between the follicular center and the mantle zone (Fig. 12.10). Scattered clusters of residual follicular center cells are usually present amongst the small lymphocytes (Fig. 12.11). Adjacent follicles may show folliculolysis; noncaseating epithelioid granulomata may be present (Ferry et al, 1992; Osborne et al, 1992). Immunohistochemistry demonstrates the small lymphocytes in progressively transformed germinal centers to consist of mantle zone B lymphocytes and CD4 T cells (Ferry et al, 1992).

Differential Diagnosis

Progressive transformation of germinal centers must be distinguished from nodular lymphocyte predominance Hodgkin's disease and from follicular lymphomas. PTGC may closely resemble nodular lymphocyte predominance Hodgkin's disease and may frequently coexist in the same lymph node (Burns et al, 1984). Distinction is based on the identification of the characteristic L&H Reed-Sternberg–variant cells in the latter. L&H cells must be carefully distinguished from residual follicular center cells, which are frequently present in the nodules of PTGC. Immunohistochemical studies are less useful than morphology in making this distinction, since both L&H cells and residual follicular center cells express B cell antigens; however, EMA positivity and a ring of surrounding

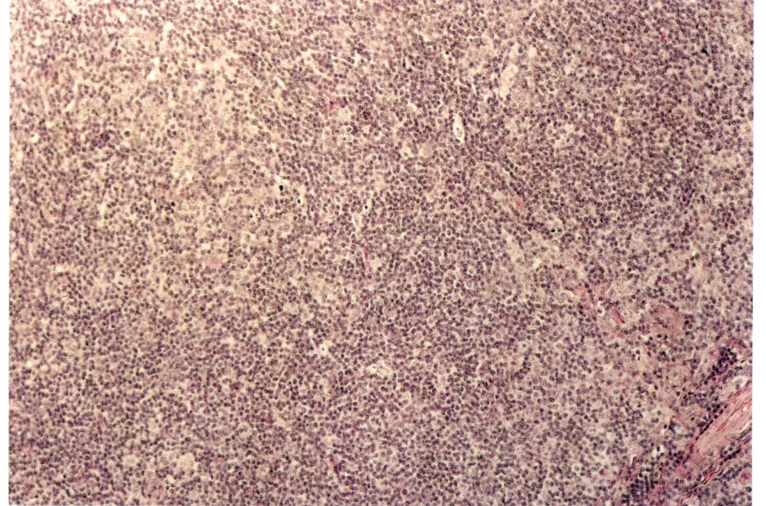

FIGURE
12.10

Progressive transformation of germinal centers showing greatly expanded follicular center infiltrated by mantle-zone lymphocytes.

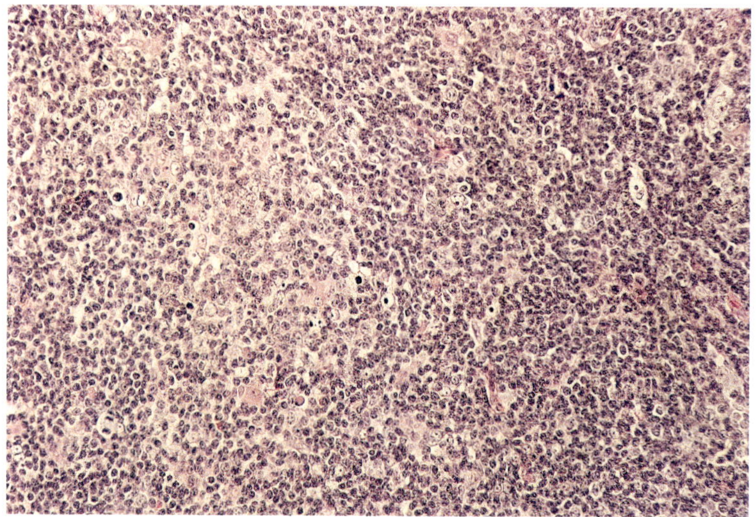

FIGURE
12.11

Progressive transformation of germinal centers, higher magnification, showing scattered residual follicular center cells amongst the mantle-zone lymphocytes.

CD57+ T cells are features supporting a diagnosis of nodular lymphocyte predominance Hodgkin's disease.

Follicular lymphoma may rarely mimic the appearance of progressively transformed germinal centers (Osborne and Butler, 1987). The "floral variant" of follicular lymphoma is characterized by neoplastic follicles which are surrounded and irregularly infiltrated by mantle-zone lymphocytes, imparting a flower-like appearance (Goates et al, 1994). The neoplastic follicles may closely simulate the appearance of progressively transformed germinal centers. Distinction from PTGC is aided by recognition of the crowding and cytologic monomorphism of the neoplastic follicles. In difficult cases, immunohisto-chemical demonstration of immunoglobulin light chain restriction or BCL-2 oncoprotein expression may be helpful (Goates et al, 1994).

Course and Prognosis

Progressive transformation of germinal centers is a benign process. The lymphadenopathy may persist or recur—in some cases, over several years (Ferry et al, 1992). The risk of development of Hodgkin's disease appears to be quite small in recent series (Ferry et al, 1992; Osborne and Butler, 1984; Osborne et al; 1992). In patients with prior nodular lymphocyte predominance Hodgkin's disease, the development of PTGC is not related to recurrence of Hodgkin's disease (Osborne and Butler, 1984).

REFERENCES

Abdel-Reheim FA, Koss W, Rappaport ES, Arber DA. Coexistence of Hodgkin's disease and giant lymph node hyperplasia of the plasma cell type (Castleman's disease). Arch Pathol Lab Med 120:91–96, 1996.

Beck JT, Hsu S-M, Wijdenes J, Bataille R, Klein B, Vesole D, Hayden K, Jagannath S, Barlogie B. Brief report: Alleviation of systemic manifestations of Castleman's disease by monoclonal anti-interleukin-6 antibody. N Engl J Med 330:602–605, 1994.

Bitter MA, Komaiko W, Franklyn WA. Giant lymph node hyperplasia with osteoblastic bone lesions and the POEMS (Takatsuki's) syndrome. Cancer 56:188–194, 1985.

Burns BF, Colby TV, Dorfman RF. Differential diagnostic features of nodular L&H Hodgkin's disease, including progressive transformation of germinal centers. Am J Surg Pathol 8:253–261, 1984.

Castleman B, Iverson I, Menendez VP. Localized mediastinal lymph node hyperplasia resembling thymoma. Cancer 9:822–830, 1956.

Chan JKC, Tsang WYW, Ng CS. Follicular dendritic cell tumor and vascular neoplasm complicating hyaline-vascular Castleman's disease. Am J Surg Pathol 18:517–525, 1994.

Chen KTK. Multicentric Castleman's disease and Kaposi's sarcoma. Am J Surg Pathol 8:287–293, 1984.

Danon AD, Krishnan J, Frizzera G. Morpho-immunophenotypic diversity of Castleman's disease, hyaline-vascular type: With emphasis on a stroma-rich variant and a new pathogenetic hypothesis. Virchows Arch A Pathol Anat Histopathol 423:369–382, 1993.

Delsol G, Meggetto F, Brousset P, Cohen-Knafo E, al Saati T, Rochaix P, Gorguet B, et al. Relation of follicular dendritic cells to Reed-Sternberg cells of Hodgkin's disease with emphasis on the expression of CD21 antigen. Am J Pathol 142:1729–1738, 1993.

Ferry JA, Zukerberg LR, Harris NL. Florid progressive transformation of germinal centers. A syndrome affecting young men without early progression to nodular lymphocyte predominance Hodgkin's disease. Am J Clin Pathol 16:252–258, 1992.

Frizzera G, Massarelli G, Banks PM, Rosai J. A systemic lymphoproliferative disorder with morphologic features of Castleman's disease: Pathological findings in 15 patients. Am J Surg Pathol 7:211–231, 1983.

Frizzera G, Peterson BA, Bayrd ED, Goldman A. A systemic lymphoproliferative disorder with morphologic features of Castleman's disease: Clinical findings and clinicopathologic correlations in 15 patients. J Clin Oncol 3:1202–1216, 1985.

Gerald W, Kostianovsky M, Rosai J. Development of vascular neoplasia in Castleman's disease. Report of seven cases. Am J Surg Pathol 14:603–614, 1990.

Goates JJ, Kamel OW, LeBrun DP, Benharroch D, Dorfman RF. Floral variant of follicular lymphoma. Immunological and molecular studies support a neoplastic process. Am J Surg Pathol 18:37–47, 1994.

Gould JS, Diss T, Isaacson PG. Multicentric Castleman's disease in association with a solitary plasmacytoma: A case report. Histopathol 17:135–140, 1990.

Hanson CA, Frizzera G, Patton DF, Peterson BA, McClain KL, Gajl-Peczalska KJ, Kersey JH. Clonal rearrangements for immunoglobulin and T-cell receptor genes in systemic Castleman's disease. Association with Epstein-Barr virus. Am J Pathol 131:84–91, 1988.

Keller AF, Hochholzer L, Castleman B. Hyaline-vascular and plasma-cell types of giant lymph node hyperplasia of the mediastinum and other locations. Cancer 29:670–683, 1972.

Lin O, Frizzera G. Angiomyoid and follicular dendritic cell proliferative lesions in Castleman's disease of hyaline-vascular type: A study of 10 cases. Am J Surg Pathol 21:1295–1306, 1997.

Menke DM, Tiemann M, Camoriano JK, Chang SF, Madan A, Chow M, Haberman TM, Parwaresch R. Diagnosis of Castleman's disease by identification of an immunophenotypically aberrant population of mantle zone B lymphocytes in paraffin-embedded lymph node biopsies. Am J Clin Pathol 105:268–276, 1996.

Miralles GD, O'Fallon JR, Talley NJ. Plasma cell dyscrasia with polyneuropathy: The spectrum of POEMS syndrome. N Engl J Med 327:1919–1927, 1992.

Oksenhendler E, Duarte M, Soulier J, Cacoub P, Welker Y, Cadranel J, Cazals-Hatem D, et al. Multicentric Castleman's disease in HIV infection: A clinical and pathological study of 20 patients. AIDS 10:61–67, 1996.

Osborne BM, Butler JJ. Clinical implications of progressive transformation of germinal centers. Am J Surg Pathol 8:725–733, 1984.

Osborne BM, Butler JJ. Follicular lymphoma mimicking progressive transformation of germinal centers. Am J Clin Pathol 88:264–269, 1987.

Osborne BM, Butler JJ, Gresik MV. Progressive transformation of germinal centers: comparison of 23 pediatric patients to the adult population. Mod Pathol 5:135–140, 1992.

Poppema S, Kaiserling E, Lennert K. Hodgkin's disease with lymphocytic predominance nodular type (nodular paragranuloma) and progressively transformed germinal centers. A cytohistological study. Histopathol 3:285–308, 1979.

Radaszkiewicz T, Hansmann ML, Lennert K. Monoclonality and polyclonality of plasma cells in Castleman's disease of the plasma cell variant. Histopathology 14:11–24, 1989.

Schlosnagle DC, Chan WC, Hargreaves HK, Nolting SF, Bryne RK. Plasmacytoma arising in giant lymph node hyperplasia. Am J Clin Pathol 78:541–544, 1982.

Soulier J, Grollet L, Oksenhendler E, Cacoub P, Cazals-Hatem D, Babinet P, et al. Kaposi's sarcoma-associated herpesvirus-like DNA sequences in multicentric Castleman's disease. Blood 86:1276–1280, 1995a.

Soulier J, Grollet L, Oksenhendler E, Miclea JM, Cacoub P, Baruchel A, et al. Molecular analysis of clonality in Castleman's disease. Blood 86:1131–1138, 1995b.

Weisenberger DD, Nathwani BN, Winberg CD, Rappaport H. Multicentric angiofollicular lymph node hyperplasia: A clinicopathologic study of 16 cases. Hum Pathol 16:162–172, 1985.

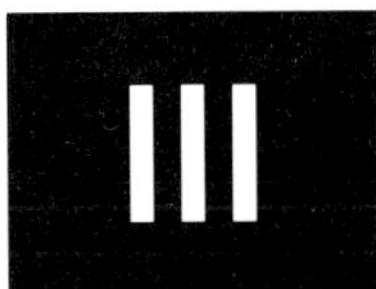

Lymphoproliferative Disorders

13

Classification of the Non-Hodgkin's Lymphomas

The classification of the non-Hodgkin's lymphomas has been a major area of controversy and confusion, in no small amount due to the clinical, biological, and immunological heterogeneity of these neoplasms (Kay, 1974). The recognition of the non-Hodgkin's lymphomas as neoplasms of specific elements of the immune system suggests a rational approach to classification by analogy with normal stages of lymphoid differentiation and development (Lukes and Collins, 1974). The classification of the non-Hodgkin's lymphomas has evolved from a purely morphologic descriptive approach to a multidisciplinary approach incorporating immunophenotypic, cytogenetic, and molecular data (Harris et al, 1994). In this same period, the advances in the clinical management of these neoplasms have demanded increasingly precise classification. A classification of the non-Hodgkin's lymphomas would, ideally, be simple, reproducible, biologically precise, and clinically relevant. Unfortunately, no ideal classification currently exists.

Historical Perspectives

Widely used classifications of the non-Hodgkin's lymphomas were introduced by Rappaport (Rappaport, 1966) and Lukes and Collins (Lukes and Collins, 1974) in North America and by the Kiel group (Lennert et al, 1975) in Europe. To address the need for consistent classification in clinical trials, the National Cancer Institute sponsored a study of the classifications of non-Hodgkin's lymphomas, which, in 1982, culminated in the publication of a Working Formulation for Clinical Usage (Non-Hodgkin's Lymphoma Pathologic Classification Project, 1982) based on a review of 1,175 cases of non-Hodgkin's lymphoma and six systems of classification then in use. The Working Formulation (WF), based on morphology in routine H&E-stained sections, was originally intended as a means of translating among the classifications then in use but was itself widely accepted as a classification, and it has remained, until recently, the major classification of the non-Hodgkin's lymphomas in use by pathologists and clinicians in North America. Since the publication of the WF, however, the development of new immunophenotypic and molecular techniques, the widespread application of immunophenotypic studies on paraffin-embedded tissue, and the description of several new lymphoma entities have made it apparent that the classification of the non-Hodgkin's lymphomas should not remain static. In 1994, the International Lymphoma Study group, consisting of 19 eminent North American and European hematopathologists, proposed a comprehensive classification termed the Revised European-American Classification of Lymphoid Neoplasms (Harris et al, 1994) to incorporate these advances. The Revised European-American Classification of Lymphoid Neoplasms (REAL) is a list of 23 immunophenotypically distinct B and T cell neoplasms. Since, at the present time, both the WF and REAL classifications are in use in North America, these two classifications will be discussed in further detail.

Working Formulation

The WF (Table 13.1) is based on descriptive morphology in routine H&E-stained sections. The diagnostic categories are based on Rappaport's classification, with updated, descriptive terms (e.g., small lymphocytic, small cleaved cell, and large cell replace well-differentiated lymphocytic, poorly differentiated lymphocytic, and histiocytic). The term "follicular" was selected to replace "nodular" to emphasize the relatedness of the follicular lymphomas to follicular center cells. The diffuse large cell lymphomas are divided into two morphologic categories: (1) malignant lymphoma, diffuse, large cell, cleaved and noncleaved, and (2) malignant lymphoma, large cell, immunoblastic. No distinction is made between B and T cell lymphomas; immunophenotypic studies are not applied to classification. Some WF categories are immunologically homogeneous (e.g., malignant lymphoma, follicular); others are immunologically heterogenous and include B and T cell lymphomas of diverse origin (e.g., malignant lymphoma, diffuse, mixed small and large cell). A unique feature of the WF is the division of the non-Hodgkin's lymphomas into clinical grades. The clinical grades are based on median survival of 1,175 patients treated at four university medical centers from 1971 to 1975 and define groups of lymphomas with differing natural histories and responses to therapy. The low-grade lymphomas (malignant lymphoma, small lymphocytic; malignant lymphoma, follicular, predominantly small cleaved cell; and malignant lymphoma, follicular, mixed small cleaved and large cell) are indolent systemic disorders characterized by advanced stage at presentation, lack of durable responses to therapy, and prolonged median survival (5–7 years). The high-grade lymphomas (malignant lymphoma, large cell, immunoblastic; malignant lymphoma, small noncleaved cell; and malignant lymphoma, lymphoblastic) in contrast, are rapidly progressive disorders with brief median survival (1–2 years) but durable responses to therapy. The intermediate grade includes lymphomas with features in common with both the low-grade lymphomas (malignant lymphoma follicular, predominantly large cell; malignant lymphoma, diffuse, small cleaved cell) and the high-grade lymphomas (malignant lymphoma, diffuse, mixed small and large cell; malignant lymphoma, diffuse, large cell).

Table 13.1 Working Formulation of Non-Hodgkin's Lymphomas for Clinical Usage

Low Grade
A. Malignant lymphoma
 Small lymphocytic
  consistent with chronic lymphocytic leukemia
  plasmacytoid
B. Malignant lymphoma, follicular
 Predominantly small cleaved cell
  diffuse areas
  sclerosis
C. Malignant lymphoma, follicular
 Mixed, small cleaved and large cell
  diffuse areas
  sclerosis

Intermediate grade
D. Malignant lymphoma, follicular
 Predominantly large cell
  diffuse areas
  sclerosis
E. Malignant lymphoma, diffuse
 Small cleaved cell
  sclerosis
F. Malignant lymphoma, diffuse
 Mixed, small and large cell
  sclerosis
  epithelioid cell component
G. Malignant lymphoma, diffuse
 Large cell
  cleaved cell
  noncleaved cell
  sclerosis

High Grade
H. Malignant lymphoma
 Large cell, immunoblastic
  plasmacytoid
  clear cell
  polymorphous
  epithelioid cell component
I. Malignant lymphoma
 Lymphoblastic
  convoluted cell
  nonconvoluted cell
J. Malignant lymphoma
 Small noncleaved cell
  Burkitt's
  follicular areas
 Miscellaneous
  Composite
  Mycosis fungoides
  Histiocytic
  Extramedullary plasmacytoma
  Unclassifiable
  Other

Revised European-American Classification

The Revised European-American Classification (Table 13.2) is based on immunophenotypically defined entities. The diagnostic categories are based, with some exceptions, on those of the updated Kiel classification (Stansfield et al, 1988). The REAL classification permits the recognition of several lymphoma types not separately distinguished in the WF, including mantle cell lymphoma, marginal-zone B cell lymphoma, and anaplastic large cell lymphoma. The distinction between immunoblastic and other types of large cell lymphoma found in the WF and Kiel classifications is not made because of the lack of objective immunophenotypic differences and high interobserver variability (Harris et al, 1994). Clinical grading is also abandoned. Although many of the REAL categories can be recognized in routine H&E-stained sections, immunophenotypic studies are necessary for recognition of some categories. In a study of 670 cases of non-Hodgkin's

Table 13.2 Revised European-American Classification of Lymphoid Neoplasms

B Cell Neoplasms
  I. Precursor B cell neoplasm: Precursor B lymphoblastic leukemia/lymphoma
 II. Peripheral B cell neoplasms
     1. B cell chronic lymphocytic leukemia/prolymphocytic leukemia/small lymphocytic lymphoma
     2. Lymphoplasmacytoid lymphoma/immunocytoma
     3. Mantle cell lymphoma
     4. Follicle center lymphoma, follicular
        Provisional cytologic grades: I (small cell), II (mixed small and large cell), III (large cell)
        Provisional subtype: diffuse, predominantly small cell type
     5. Marginal zone B cell lymphoma
        Extranodal (MALT-type $\pm$ monocytoid B cells)
        Provisional subtype: nodal ($\pm$ monocytoid B cells)
     6. Provisional entity: splenic marginal zone lymphoma ($\pm$ villous lymphocytes)
     7. Hairy cell leukemia
     8. Plasmacytoma/plasma cell myeloma
     9. Diffuse large B cell lymphoma
        Subtype: primary mediastinal (thymic) B cell lymphoma
    10. Burkitt's lymphoma
    11. Provisional entity: high-grade B cell lymphoma, Burkitt-like

T Cell and Putative NK Cell Neoplasms
  I. Precursor T cell neoplasm: Precursor T lymphoblastic lymphoma/leukemia
 II. Peripheral T cell and NK cell neoplasms
     1. T cell chronic lymphocytic leukemia/prolymphocytic leukemia
     2. Large granular lymphocyte leukemia (LGL)
        T cell type
        NK cell type
     3. Mycosis fungoides/Sezary's syndrome
     4. Peripheral T cell lymphomas, unspecified
        Provisional cytologic categories: medium-sized cell, mixed medium and large cell, large cell, lympho-
          epithelioid cell
        Provisional subtype: hepatosplenic γ-δ T cell lymphoma
        Provisional subtype: subcutaneous panniculitic T cell lymphoma
     5. Angioimmunoblastic T cell lymphoma (AILD)
     6. Angiocentric lymphoma
     7. Intestinal T cell lymphoma ($\pm$ enteropathy associated)
     8. Adult T cell lymphoma/leukemia (ATL/L)
     9. Anaplastic large cell lymphoma (ALCL), CD30+, T and null cell types
    10. Provisional entity: anaplastic large cell lymphoma, Hodgkin's-like

lymphomas, 77% of the cases could be categorized in the REAL classification from H&E-stained sections alone; immunophenotypic studies were necessary principally for recognition of T cell and anaplastic large cell lymphoma categories (Pittaluga et al, 1996). The ability to recognize lymphoma entities with distinctive natural histories, which are not distinguished in the WF, is the principal advantage of the REAL classification (Fisher et al, 1995; Pittaluga et al, 1996). The practicability and clinical relevance of the REAL classification has recently been validated in two large series (Melnyk et al, 1997; Non-Hodgkin's Lymphoma Classification Project, 1997). The REAL classification will also serve as the basis of a new World Health Organization (WHO) classification being developed (Jaffe, 1997).

Current Approaches to Classification

Both the WF and REAL classifications are in clinical use in North America. The WF has the advantage of simplicity and immediate clinical relevance. The REAL classification is biologically and immunologically more precise than the WF and permits the recognition of lymphomas not distinguished in the WF. The REAL classification is, however, significantly more complex than the WF, with 23 major categories, compared to 10 in the WF. Clinicians and pathologists (as well organizers of clinical trials and their statistician colleagues) may find the REAL classification daunting; however, many of the major and most common lymphoma entities (small lymphocytic lymphoma, follicular lymphomas, and most diffuse large cell lymphomas) are classified similarly in the REAL and WF. In the following discussion we will follow the recommendations of the International Lymphoma Study Group for the classification of the non-Hodgkin's lymphomas, using the REAL classification, and also providing the equivalent WF terminology. For non-Hodgkin's lymphomas in the REAL classification occurring in more than one WF category, the most frequent WF category will be given.

REFERENCES

Fisher RI, Dahlberg S, Nathwani BN, Banks PM, Miller TP, Grogan TM. A clinical analysis of two indolent lymphoma entities: Mantle cell lymphoma and marginal zone lymphoma (including the mucosa-associated lymphoid tissue and monocytoid B-cell categories): A Southwest Oncology Group Study. Blood 85:1075–1082, 1995.

Harris NL, Jaffe ES, Stein H, Banks PM, Chan JKC, Cleary ML, Delsol G, De Wolf-Peeters C, Falini B, Gatter KC, Grogan TM, Isaacson PG, Knowles DM, Mason DY, Muller-Hermelink H-K, Pileri SA, Piris MA, Ralfkiaer E, Warnke RA. A revised European-American classification of lymphoid neoplasms: A proposal from the international lymphoma study group. Blood 84:1361–1392, 1994.

Jaffe ES. Introduction to the WHO classification. Society for Hematopathology. Am J Surg Pathol 21:114–115, 1997.

Kay HEM. Classification of the non-Hodgkin's lymphomas (letter). Lancet 2:586, 1974.

Lennert K, Mohri N, Stein H, Kaiserling E. The histopathology of malignant lymphoma. Br J Haematol (suppl) 31:193–203, 1975.

Lukes RJ, Collins RD. Immunological characterization of human malignant lymphomas. Cancer 34:1488–1503, 1974.

Melnyk A, Rodriguez A, Pugh WC, Cabannillas F. Evaluation of the Revised European-American Lymphoma Classification confirms the clinical relevance of immunophenotype in 560 cases of aggressive non-Hodgkins lymphoma. Blood 89:4514–4520, 1997.

Non-Hodgkin's Lymphoma Classification Project. A clinical evaluation of the International Lymphoma Study Group classification of non-Hodgkin's lymphoma. Blood 89:3909–3918, 1997.

Non-Hodgkin's Lymphoma Pathologic Classification Project. National Cancer Institute-sponsored study of classifications of non-Hodgkin's lymphomas: Summary and description of a working formulation for clinical usage. Cancer 49:2112–2135, 1982.

Pittaluga S, Bijnens L, Teodorovic I, Hagenbeek A, Meerwaldt JH, Somers R, Thomas J, Noordijk EM, De Wolf-Peeters C. Clinical analysis of 670 cases in two trials of the European Organization for the Reseach and Treatment of Cancer Lymphoma Cooperative Group subtyped according to the re-vised European-American Classification of Lymphoid Neoplasms: A comparison with the Working Formulation. Blood 87:4358–4367, 1996.

Rappaport H. Tumors of the hematopoietic system. In: Atlas of Tumor Pathology, Section 3, Fascicle 8. Washington, D.C., Armed Forces Institute of Pathology, 1966.

Stansfield A, Diebold J, Kapanci Y, Kelenyi G, Lennert K, Mioduszewska O, Noel H, Rike F, Sundstrom C, van Unnik J, Wright D. Updated Kiel classification for lymphomas. Lancet 1:292, 1988.

14

Precursor B and T Cell Neoplasms

Precursor B and T cell neoplasms include precursor B lymphoblastic leukemia/lymphoma and precursor T lymphoblastic lymphoma/leukemia in the REAL classification and lymphoblastic lymphoma in the WF. The terms leukemia/lymphoma for precursor B cell neoplasms and lymphoma/leukemia for precursor T cell neoplasms reflect the more frequent leukemic presentation of precursor B cell neoplasms and lymphomatous presentation of precursor T cell neoplasms. The precursor B and T cell neoplasms are characterized by an immature, terminal deoxynucleotidyl transferase (TdT)-positive lymphoid phenotype and lymphoblastic morphology.

Precursor B Lymphoblastic Leukemia/Lymphoma

Classification

REAL: Precursor B lymphoblastic leukemia/lymphoma.
WF: Malignant lymphoma, lymphoblastic.

Immunophenotype

TdT+, CD10+, HLA-DR+, CD19+, cytoplasmic CD22+, SIg$-$, cytoplasmic μ+ in pre-B types.

Clinical Features

Precursor B lymphoblastic leukemia/lymphoma accounts for most cases of acute lymphoblastic leukemia of childhood and adults; lymphomatous presentations are infrequent (Copelan and McGuire, 1995; Pui et al, 1993). Precursor B lymphoblastic leukemia/lymphoma presents as French-American-British (FAB) classification FAB L1 and L2 acute lymphoblastic leukemia with an early pre–B cell or pre–B cell phenotype. (Cases of acute lymphoblastic leukemia of FAB L3 type with a mature B cell phenotype are considered the leukemic phase of Burkitt's lymphoma.) Lymphomatous presentations of precursor B lymphoblastic leukemia/lymphoma are infrequent (Sheibani et al, 1987). The distinction between acute lymphoblastic leukemia and lymphoblastic lymphoma is based on the extent of bone marrow involvement at presentation. Patients with precursor B lymphoblastic leukemia/lymphoma diagnosed at an extramedullary site and less than 25% bone marrow involvement are classified as lymphoblastic lymphoma (lymphomatous presentation); patients with greater than 25% bone marrow involvement are classified as acute lymphoblastic leukemia (leukemic presentation). Patients with lymphomatous presentations of precursor B cell lymphoblastic leukemia/lymphoma have an aggressive clinical course with high incidence of lymph node and bone marrow involvement (Cheng et al, 1994). Extranodal involvement is not infrequent. Extranodal cutaneous involvement was reported in two cases reported by Sheibani and colleagues (Sheibani et al, 1987) and we have seen two cases in adults presenting with extranodal involvement of the ovaries and endometrium. In contrast to precursor T lymphoblastic lymphoma/leukemia, mediastinal involvement is rare (Sander et al, 1992).

Histopathology

Lymph node involvement in precursor B lymphoblastic leukemia/lymphoma is morphologically indistinguishable from the more frequent involvement in T lymphoblastic lymphoma/leukemia, discussed in detail below. Lymphoblasts are small to medium-sized cells with characteristically scant cytoplasm, finely dispersed chromatin, inconspicuous nucleoli, and numerous mitoses (Fig. 14.1). A "starry sky" pattern with admixture of benign phagocytic macrophages may be present. In imprint or touch preparations stained with Giemsa, the cells are indistinguishable from the cells of acute lymphoblastic leukemia (Fig. 14.2).

Differential Diagnosis

Precursor B lymphoblastic leukemia/lymphoma must be distinguished from other high grade B cell neoplasms, principally Burkitt's lymphoma and Burkitt-like lymphoma. The cells of Burkitt's lymphoma are characteristically larger than lymphoblasts, approximately the size of a macrophage nucleus, in contrast to lymphoblasts, which are smaller, have coarse chromatin, two to five distinct, basophilic nucleoli, and a rim of basophilic cytoplasm. The distinction is particularly evident in Giemsa-stained imprint or touch preparations; the cells of Burkitt's lymphoma have coarsely reticular chromatin and deeply basophilic cytoplasm with neutral fat vacuoles, in contrast to the fine chromatin and scant, pale blue cytoplasm of lymphoblasts. Immunophenotypic studies are also helpful in distinction. Burkitt's lymphoma characteristically expresses a mature B cell phenotype (TdT-negative, surface immunoglobulin positive) in contrast to the early pre–B cell or pre–B cell phenotype of precursor B lymphoblastic leukemia/lymphoma (TdT-positive, surface immunoglobulin negative). Both Burkitt's lymphoma and precursor B lymphoblastic leukemia/lymphoma, however, are frequently positive for the common acute lymphocytic leukemia antigen (CALLA) or CD10. As noted previously, the FAB L3

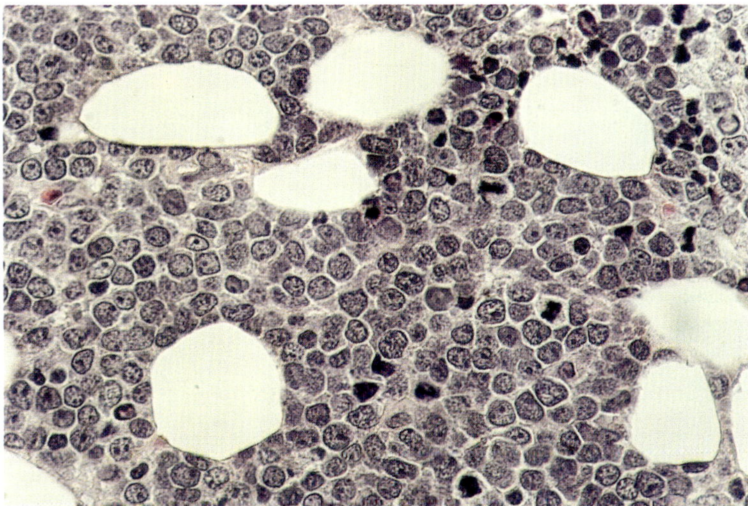

Precursor B lymphoblastic leukemia/lymphoma showing perinodal infiltration by lymphoblasts with finely dispersed chromatin, inconspicuous nucleoli, and numerous mitoses.

FIGURE
14.1

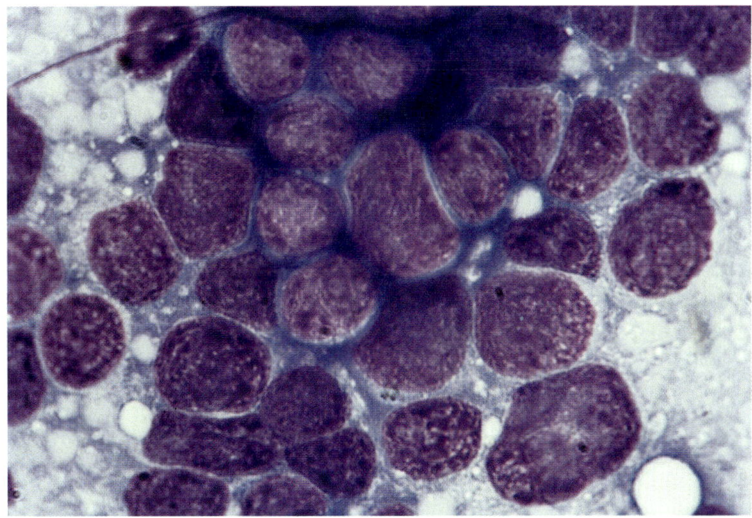

Precursor B lymphoblastic leukemia/lymphoma, touch preparation stained with Giemsa, showing cells indistinguishable from the blasts of acute lymphoblastic leukemia.

FIGURE
14.2

form of acute lymphoblastic leukemia is distinct from precursor B lymphoblastic leukemia/lymphoma in that it demonstrates a mature B cell phenotype, indistinguishable from that of Burkitt's lymphoma, of which it is considered the leukemic phase (Pui et al, 1993).

Precursor B lymphoblastic leukemia/lymphoma must also be distinguished from an uncommon "blastic" variant of mantle cell lymphoma which it may resemble closely (Lardelli et al, 1990). The "blastic" variant of mantle cell lymphoma is characterized by cells closely resembling lymphoblasts with finely dispersed chromatin, inconspicuous nucleoli, and scant cytoplasm. The cells, however, retain the characteristic CD5-positive mature B cell phenotype of mantle cell lymphoma and are negative for TdT (Cheng et al, 1994).

Course and Prognosis

Precursor B lymphoblastic leukemia/lymphoma is an aggressive neoplasm. Therapy for lymphomatous presentations is similar to that for acute lymphoblastic leukemia, with intensive remission induction, consolidation, and central nervous system prophylaxis (Copelan and McGuire, 1995). Responses to therapy are frequently durable. The prognosis in adults is less favorable than in children.

Precursor T Lymphoblastic Lymphoma/Leukemia

Classification

REAL: Precursor T lymphoblastic lymphoma/leukemia.
WF: Malignant lymphoma, lymphoblastic.

Immunophenotype

TdT+, CD7+, cytoplasmic CD3+, CD10 may be +, CD1, CD4, CD8 may be coexpressed.

Clinical Features

Precursor T lymphoblastic lymphoma/leukemia is predominantly a disease of male adolescents presenting with mediastinal mass; in contrast to precursor B lymphoblastic leukemia/lymphoma, lymphomatous presentations are frequent. The distinction between T lymphoblastic lymphoma and T acute lymphoblastic leukemia is based on the extent of marrow involvement at presentation: Cases of precursor T lymphoblastic lymphoma/leukemia with less than 25% marrow involvement are classified as T lymphoblastic lymphoma (lymphomatous presentation); cases with greater than 25% marrow involvement are classified as T cell acute lymphoblastic leukemia (leukemic presentation). Leukemic presentations are characterized by more immature T cell phenotypes (Pui et al, 1993; Weiss et al, 1986). Leukemic lymphoblasts may be of either FAB L1 or L2 type. Involvement of peripheral lymph nodes and extranodal sites, including the central nervous system, is frequent.

Histopathology

Lymph node involvement in precursor T lymphoblastic lymphoma/leukemia is characterized by infiltration with lymphoblasts (Figs. 14.3 and 14.4). Lymphoblasts are small to medium-sized cells with scant cytoplasm, finely dispersed chromatin with a characteristic "dusty" or delicately stippled appearance, inconspicuous nucleoli, and numerous mitoses. A variant with larger cells with more prominent nucleoli also occurs (Griffith

FIGURE 14.3

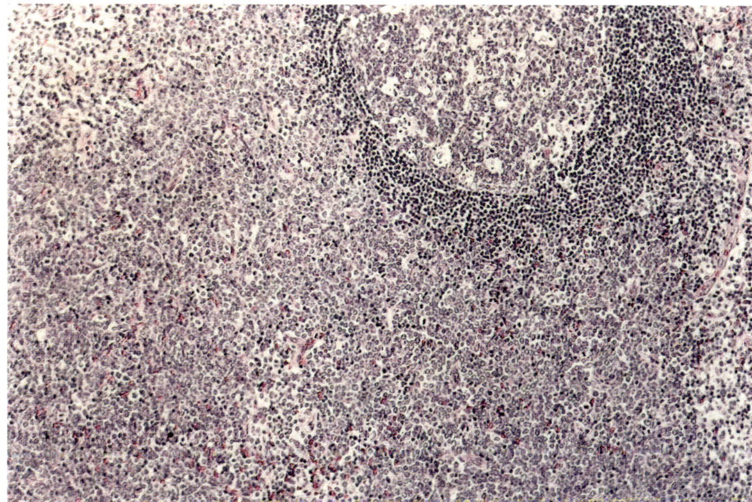

Precursor T lymphoblastic lymphoma/leukemia showing a paracortical pattern of infiltration with sparing of the lymph node follicles.

FIGURE 14.4

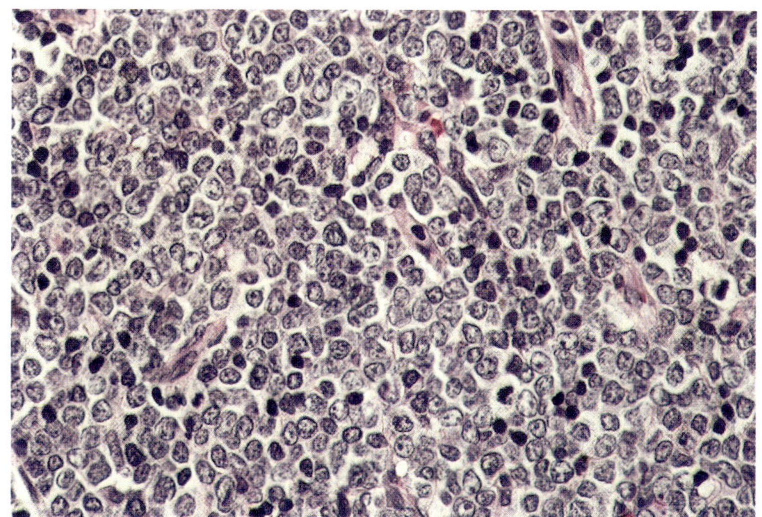

Precursor T lymphoblastic lymphoma/leukemia showing lymphoblasts with finely dispersed chromatin, inconspicuous nucleoli, and numerous mitoses.

et al, 1987). Cells with complexly folded and indented nuclei are present in some cases; these characterize the "convoluted cell" type in the WF. However, there is no clinical or immunophenotypic significance to the presence of convoluted or nonconvoluted cells (Figs. 14.5 and 14.6). A starry-sky pattern with admixture of benign phagocytic macrophages may be present. Lymph node involvement is usually diffuse with effacement of lymph node architecture and involvement of perinodal soft tissue, which may be extensive. In some cases, a leukemic pattern of infiltration is evident, with paracortical infiltration and sparing of the follicles (Fig. 14.3). In other cases, a striking pseudonodular

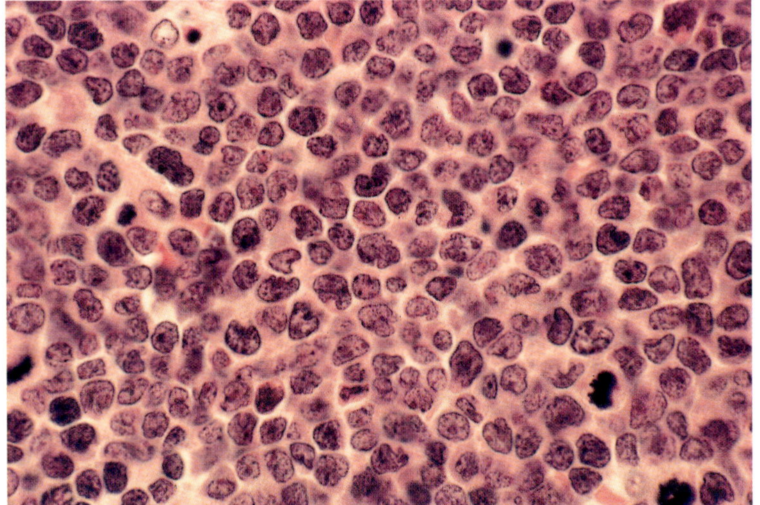

FIGURE 14.5

Precursor T lymphoblastic lymphoma/leukemia showing convoluted cells.

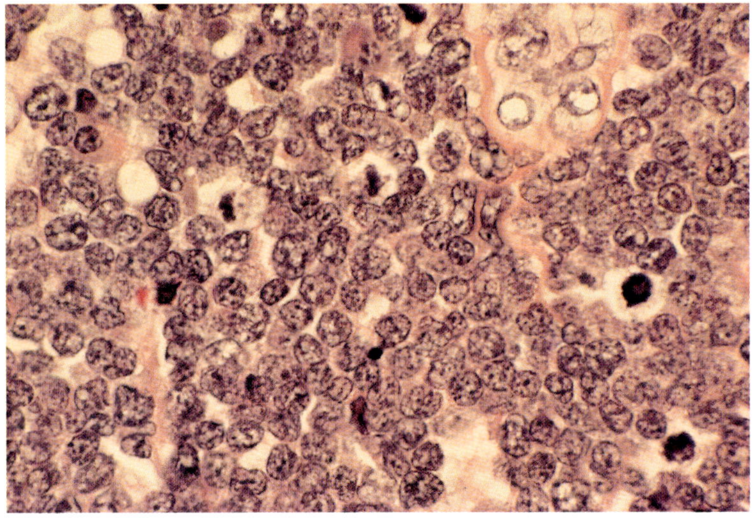

FIGURE 14.6

Precursor T lymphoblastic lymphoma/leukemia showing nonconvoluted cells.

or lobular pattern of infiltration is evident. Soft tissue infiltration is frequently characterized by single cells in an "Indian file" arrangement. "Streaming" of the nuclear chromatin and crush artifact may be prominent, especially in small biopsies. In imprint or touch preparations stained with Giemsa, the cells are indistinguishable from the cells of acute lymphoblastic leukemia.

Variants

LYMPHOBLASTIC LYMPHOMA/LEUKEMIA WITH NK CELL ANTIGENS Some cases of precursor lymphoblastic lymphoma/leukemia express NK cell antigens (CD16, CD56,

CD57) suggesting possible precursor NK cell neoplasms (Koita et al, 1997). These neoplasms are morphologically indistinguishable from other lymphoblastic lymphomas. The expression of NK cell antigens has been associated with an aggressive clinical course (Sheibani et al, 1987).

T LYMPHOBLASTIC LYMPHOMA/LEUKEMIA WITH EOSINOPHILIA   Some cases of T lymphoblastic lymphoma have been associated with striking eosinophilia and subsequent development of myeloid neoplasms, suggesting lineage infidelity (Abruzzo et al, 1992). Hypereosinophilia has also been associated with cases of acute lymphoblastic leukemia (Catovsky et al, 1980; Hogan et al, 1987). Biphenotypic lymphoblastic lymphoma with precursor T lymphoblastic phenotype and granulocytic differentiation has been reported (Childs et al, 1986) (Figs. 14.7 and 14.8).

Differential Diagnosis

Precursor T lymphoblastic lymphoma/leukemia must be distinguished from other high grade non-Hodgkin's lymphomas and from other tumors involving mediastinum. Lymphomatous presentations of precursor B lymphoblastic leukemia/lymphoma are less frequent and seldom involve the mediastinum (Sander et al, 1992). Distinction from Burkitt's lymphoma and the "blastic" variant of mantle cell lymphoma has been considered in the differential diagnosis of B lymphoblastic leukemia/lymphoma. Immunophenotypic studies are helpful in difficult cases. The frequent mediastinal presentation of precursor T lymphoblastic lymphoma/leukemia raises specific issues in differential diagnosis. Mediastinal biopsies are frequently small and distorted by crush artifact; patients may have received prior glucocorticosteroids for respiratory distress or the superior vena cava syndrome with resultant tumor necrosis. Precursor T lymphoblastic lymphoma/leukemia must be distinguished from other neoplasms occurring in the mediastinum, including thymomas and small cell neuroendocrine neoplasms. Thymomas are thymic epithelial neoplasms which are frequently obscured by a non-neoplastic lymphocytic component which may appear morphologically immature. Immunohistochemical studies may cause further confusion, since the lymphocytic component of thymomas expresses an immature thymic T cell phenotype which is TdT positive and mimics that of precursor T lymphoblastic lymphoma/leukemias (Mokhtar et al, 1984). The diagnosis of thymoma is established by the presence of fibrous bands, characteristic of thymoma, and the identification of neoplastic thymic epithelial cells. Identification of the latter is aided by immunohistochemical staining for cytokeratin. Small cell neuroendocrine carcinomas frequently also involve the mediastinum. Small cell neuroendocrine carcinomas may arise in the mediastinum or, more frequently, they are metastatic from the lung. Distinction from lymphoblastic lymphoma is usually not a problem because of the larger size and organoid arrangement of the carcinoma cells, but it may be a problem in small biopsies distorted by crush artifact. In difficult cases, immunohistochemical staining for cytokeratin will resolve the issue. Primitive neuroectodermal tumors (PNET) and Ewing's sarcoma also enter into the differential diagnosis. The p30/32MIC2 glycoprotein recognized by the monoclonal antibody 013 and characteristically expressed on the cells of PNET and Ewing's sarcoma is also frequently expressed on the cells of lymphoblastic lymphoma (Weidner and Tjoe, 1994). Uncritical interpretation of 013 staining, and the tendency of lymphoblastic lymphomas to stain inconsistently for CD45 in paraffin-embedded tissue may lead to misinterpretation (Parham, 1995).

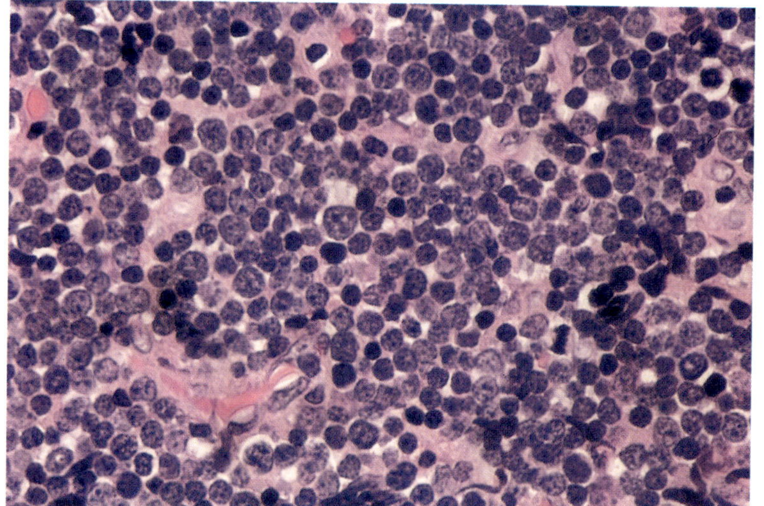

FIGURE 14.7

Biphenotypic lymphoblastic lymphoma/leukemia showing lymphoblast-like cells which expressed T cell markers and granulocytic differentiation.

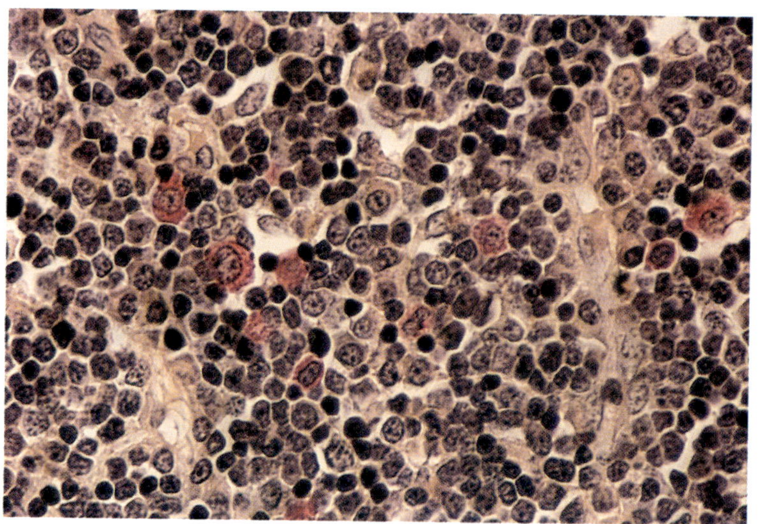

FIGURE 14.8

Biphenotypic lymphoblastic lymphoma/leukemia showing chloroacetate-esterase-positive immature granulocytes.

Course and Prognosis

Precursor T lymphoblastic lymphoma/leukemia is an aggressive neoplasm. Therapy for lymphomatous presentations is similar to that for acute lymphoblastic leukemia (Copelan and McGuire, 1995). Responses to therapy are frequently durable. The prognosis of T lymphoblastic lymphoma/leukemia is less favorable than for B lymphoblastic leukemia/lymphoma in most series (Pui et al, 1993).

REFERENCES

Abruzzo LV, Jaffe ES, Cotelingam JD, Whang-Peng J, Del Duca V, Medeiros LJ. T cell lymphoblastic lymphoma with eosinophilia associated with subsequent myeloid malignancy. Am J Surg Pathol 16:236–245, 1992.

Catovsky D, Bernasconi C, Verdonck PJ, Postma A, Hows J, van der Does-van den Berg A, Rees JKH, Castelli G, Morra E, Galton DAG. The association of eosinophilia with lymphoblastic leukemia or lymphoma: A study.of seven patients. Br J Haematol 45:523–534, 1980.

Cheng A-L, Su I-J, Tien H-F, Wang C-C, Chen Y-C, Wang C-H. Characteristic clinicopathologic features of adult B cell lymphoblastic lymphoma with special emphasis on differential diagnosis with an atypical form of probably blastic lymphocytic lymphoma of intermediate differentiation origin. Cancer 73:706–710, 1994.

Childs CC, Chrystal GC, Strauchen JA. Biphenotypic lymphoblastic lymphoma: An unusual tumor with lymphocytic and granulocytic differentiation. Cancer 57:1019–1023, 1986.

Copelan EA, McGuire EA. The biology and treatment of acute lymphoblastic leukemia in adults. 85:1151–1168, 1995.

Griffith RC, Kelly DR, Nathwani BN, Shuster JJ, Murphy SB, Hvizdala E, Sullivan MP, Berard CW. A morphologic study of childhood lymphoma of lymphoblastic type. The Pediatric Oncology Group experience. Cancer 59:1126–1131, 1987.

Hogan TF, Koss W, Murgo AJ, Amato RS, Fontana JA, VanScoy FL. Acute lymphoblastic leukemia with chromosomal 5;14 translocation and hypereosinophila. Case report and literature review. J Clin Oncol 5:382–390, 1987.

Koita H, Suzumiya J, Ohshima K, Takeshita M, Kimura N, Kikuchi M, Koono M. Lymphoblastic lymphoma expressing natural killer cell phenotype with involvement of the mediastinum and nasal cavity. Am J Surg Pathol 21:242–248, 1997.

Lardelli P, Bookman MA, Sundeen J, Longo DL, Jaffe ES. Lymphocytic lymphoma of intermediate differentiation: Morphologic and immunophenotypic spectrum and clinical correlation. Am J Surg Pathol 14:752–763, 1990.

Mokhtar N, Hsu S-M, Lad RP, Haynes BF, Jaffe ES. Thymoma: Lymphoid and epithelial components mirror the phenotype of normal thymus. Hum Pathol 15:378–384, 1984.

Parham DM. Anti-CD45 (letter). Am J Surg Pathol 19:732–733, 1995.

Pui C-H, Behm FG, Crist WM. Clinical and biologic relevance of immunologic marker studies in childhood acute lymphoblastic leukemia. Blood 82:343–362, 1993.

Sander CA, Jaffe ES, Gebhart FC, Yano T, Medeiros LJ. Mediastinal lymphoblastic lymphoma with an immature B cell immunophenotype. Am J Surg Pathol 16:300–305, 1992.

Sheibani K, Nathwani BN, Winberg CD, Burke JS, Swartz WG, Blayney D, van de Velde S, Hill LR, Rappaport H. Antigenically defined subgroups of lymphoblastic lymphoma. Relationship to clinical presentation and biologic behavior. Cancer 60:183–190, 1987.

Weidner N, Tjoe K. Immunohistochemical profile of monoclonal antibody 013: an antibody that recognizes glycoprotein p30/32MIC2 and is useful in diagnosing Ewing's sarcoma and peripheral neuroepithelioma. Am J Surg Pathol 18:486–494, 1994.

Weiss LM, Bindl J, Picozzi VJ, Link MP, Warnke RA. Lymphoblastic lymphoma: An immunophenotypic study of 26 cases with comparison to T cell acute lymphocytic leukemia. Blood 67:474–478, 1986.

15

Peripheral B Cell Neoplasms: I. B Cell Chronic Lymphocytic Leukemia, Small Lymphocytic Lymphoma, and Lymphoplasmacytoid Lymphoma

B cell chronic lymphocytic leukemia, small lymphocytic lymphoma, and lymphoplasmacytoid lymphoma are small lymphocytic proliferations characterized by advanced age at presentation and indolent natural history. This group of lymphoid neoplasms in the REAL classification corresponds to the category of small lymphocytic lymphoma in the WF.

B Cell Chronic Lymphocytic Leukemia and Small Lymphocytic Lymphoma

Classification

REAL: B cell chronic lymphocytic leukemia/prolymphocytic leukemia/small lymphocytic lymphoma.

WF: Malignant lymphoma, small lymphocytic, consistent with chronic lymphocytic leukemia

Immunophenotype.

CD5+, CD10−, CD19+, CD20+, CD22 dim+, CD23+, SIg dim+.

Clinical Features

B cell chronic lymphocytic leukemia (CLL) and small lymphocytic lymphomas (SLL) are indolent systemic proliferations of mature CD5-positive B lymphocytes which occur in adults principally past the age of 40. The CLL phenotype corresponds to a normal CD5-positive subset of circulating B lymphocytes which is expanded in autoimmune diseases and is hypothesized to play a role in autoantibody formation (Mayer et al, 1990). CD5 negative cases of CLL also occur and in some cases demonstrate expression of myelomonocytic antigens (CD13) and more aggressive clinical course (Ikematsu et al, 1994). Chronic lymphocytic leukemia is distinguished from small lymphocytic lymphoma principally by the presence of peripheral lymphocytosis (greater than 5,000 lymphocytes per mm^3) (Fig. 15.1). Lymphadenopathy, hepatosplenomegaly, and bone marrow involvement are frequent in both. A monoclonal gammopathy is present in some cases. B CLL is associated with trisomy 12 in 30% of cases.

Histopathology

Lymph node involvement in B cell chronic lymphocytic leukemia is indistinguishable from small lymphocytic lymphoma. The pattern of infiltration may be diffuse, with complete effacement of lymph node architecture (Figs. 15.2 and 15.3), or involvement may be partial, with an interfollicular or mantle zone pattern of involvement (Figs. 15.4 and 15.5), or preservation of the lymph node sinuses. The cells of CLL and SLL are monotonous, small, mature, round to ovoid lymphocytes with coarsely clumped chromatin and inconspicuous nucleoli. Pseudofollicular proliferation centers, consisting of aggregates of larger, nucleolated cells (called prolymphocytes or paraimmunoblasts) are frequently

FIGURE 15.1

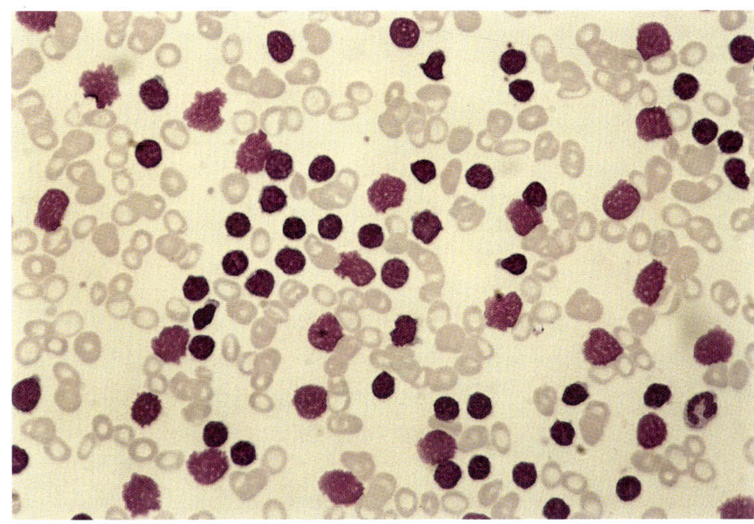

B cell chronic lymphocytic leukemia showing peripheral lymphocytosis.

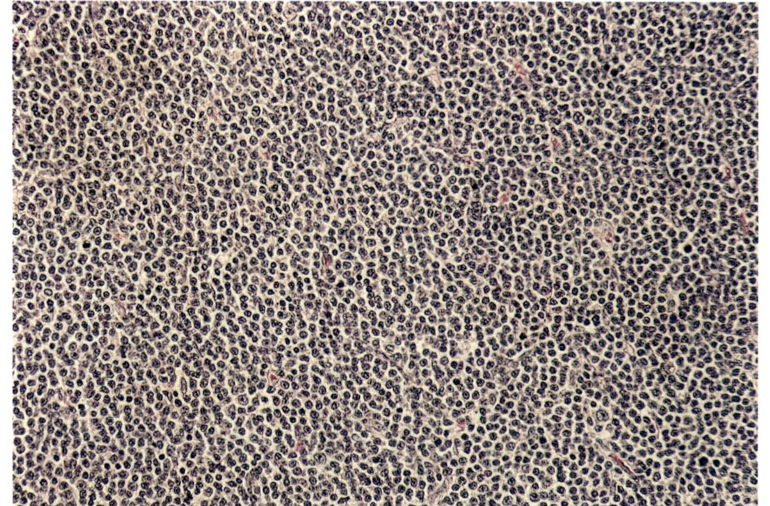

FIGURE 15.2

Small lymphocytic lymphoma showing diffuse effacement by small mature lymphocytes.

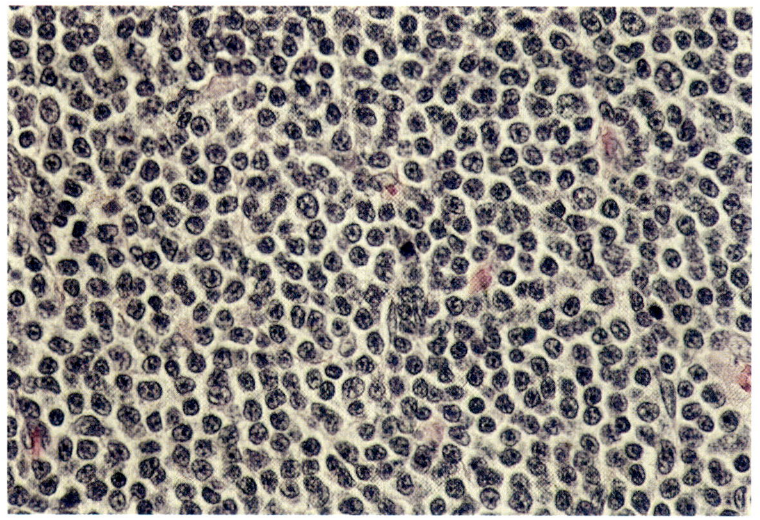

FIGURE 15.3

Small lymphocytic lymphoma showing small mature lymphocytes with coarsely clumped chromatin and small nucleoli.

present, and they are an important diagnostic feature (Fig. 15.6). At low magnification, pseudofollicular proliferation centers appear as characteristic "pale" areas that may impart a pseudonodular appearance. Mitoses are frequently present in the pseudofollicular proliferation centers. Occasional plasmacytoid cells are present in some cases of CLL and SLL.

Variants

CLL OR SLL WITH CLEAVED CELLS In some cases of CLL or SLL, the lymphocytes depart from the typical appearance described above and show nuclear irregularities and

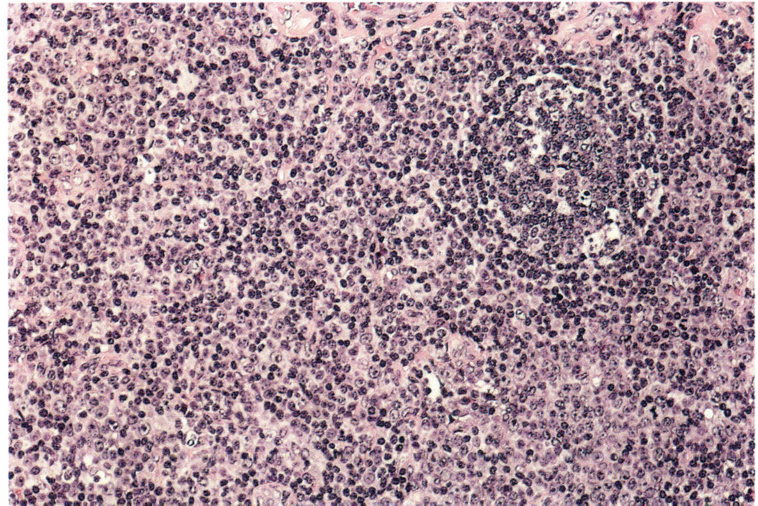

Small lymphocytic lymphoma showing interfollicular pattern of involvement.

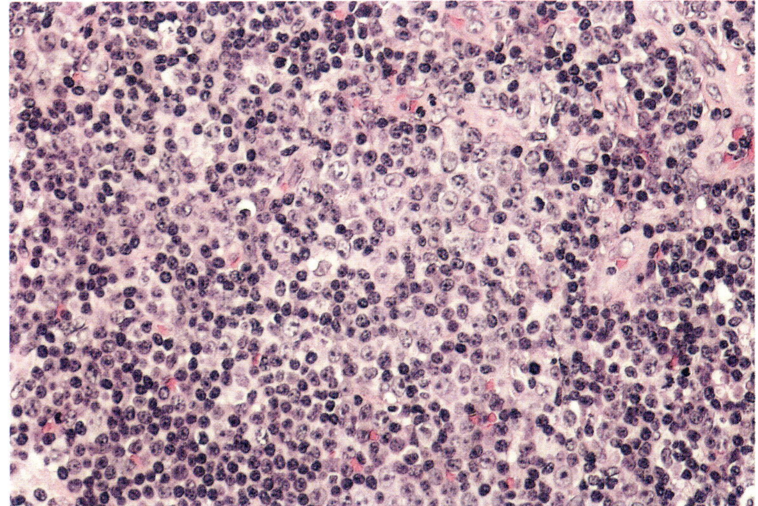

Small lymphocytic lymphoma with interfollicular pattern of involvement and pseudofollicular proliferation center.

clefts reminiscent of the cells of small cleaved cell lymphoma or mantle cell lymphoma (Bonato et al, 1998) (Fig. 15.7). In the presence of characteristic pseudofollicular proliferation centers, however, the natural history appears to be indistinguishable from that of typical CLL or SLL (Perry et al, 1990).

LARGE CELL–RICH CLL OR SLL   Some cases of CLL or SLL are characterized by numerous larger, nucleolated cells, distributed diffusely, rather than in pseudofollicular proliferation centers (Fig. 15.8). These have frequent mitoses and obscure the small lymphocytic proliferation. These cases have been termed "large-cell–rich immunocytoma" (Berger et al, 1994) or "paraimmunoblastic variant of small lymphocytic lymphoma/leu-

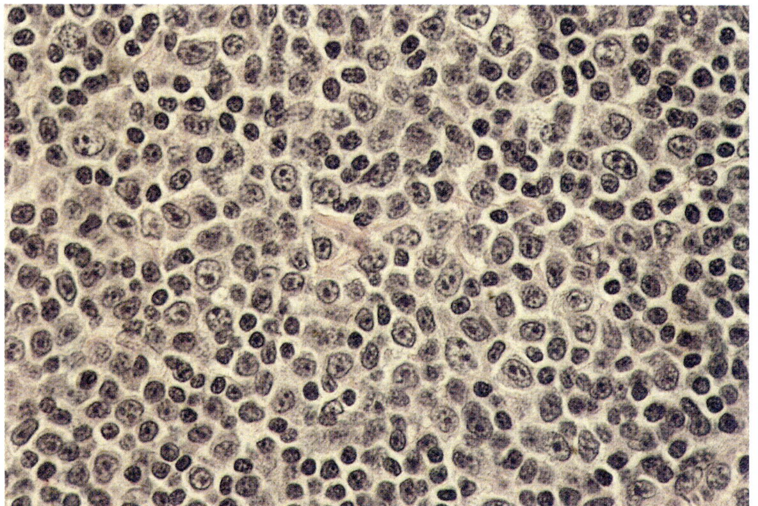

FIGURE 15.6

Small lymphocytic lymphoma showing pseudofollicular proliferation center composed of larger, nucleolated cells.

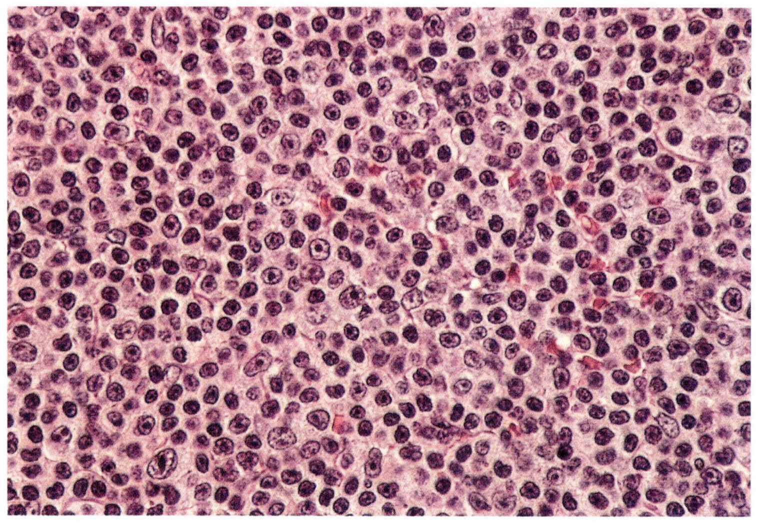

FIGURE 15.7

Small lymphocytic lymphoma composed of irregular lymphocytes with pseudofollicular proliferation centers.

kemia" (Pugh et al, 1988); they have a more aggressive course with shorter survival than typical CLL or SLL.

B CELL PROLYMPHOCYTIC LEUKEMIA   B cell prolymphocytic leukemia is classified with B cell chronic lymphocytic leukemia and small lymphocytic lymphoma in the REAL classification but is clinically and immunophenotypically a distinct disorder (Batata and Shen, 1992). Patients with B cell prolymphocytic leukemia (PLL) are adults presenting with marked peripheral lymphocytosis (frequently 200,000 per mm^3 or greater), greater than 55% nucleolated prolymphocytes in the peripheral blood, and marked splenomegaly. In contrast to CLL and SLL, lymphadenopathy is usually inconspicuous. The prolym-

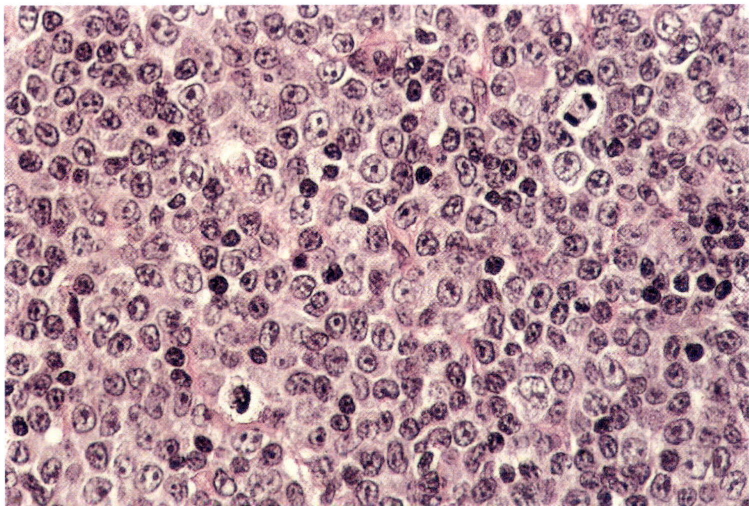

Small lymphocytic lymphoma with numerous larger, nucleolated cells, referred to as the paraimmunoblastic variant of small lymphocytic lymphoma.

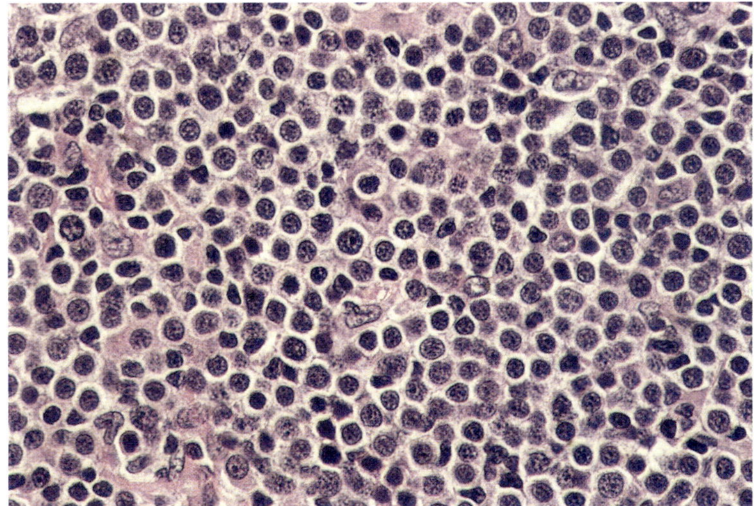

Small lymphocytic lymphoma showing features of B cell prolymphocytic leukemia.

phocytes are CD5-negative and demonstrate bright surface immunoglobulin staining (Batata and Shen, 1992). Lymph nodes in cases with peripheral lymphadenopathy show diffuse infiltration by prolymphocytes with prominent central nucleoli (Owens et al, 1984) or pseudonodularity (Bearman et al, 1978) (Fig. 15.9). Prolymphocytic leukemia is an aggressive disorder which is refractory to therapy.

Transformations of Chronic Lymphocytic Leukemia

PROLYMPHOCYTOID TRANSFORMATION B cell chronic lymphocytic leukemia may enter a refractory phase characterized by progressive anemia, thrombocytopenia, lymph-

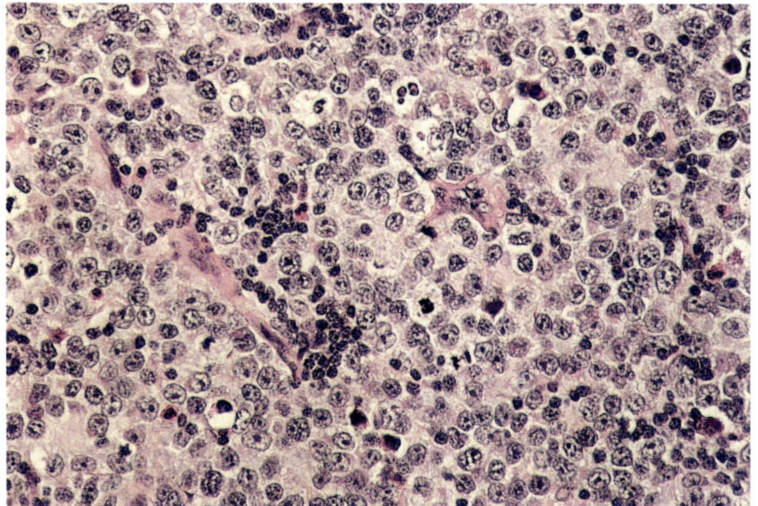

FIGURE
15.10

Richter's syndrome showing transformation of chronic lymphocytic leukemia to diffuse large B cell lymphoma.

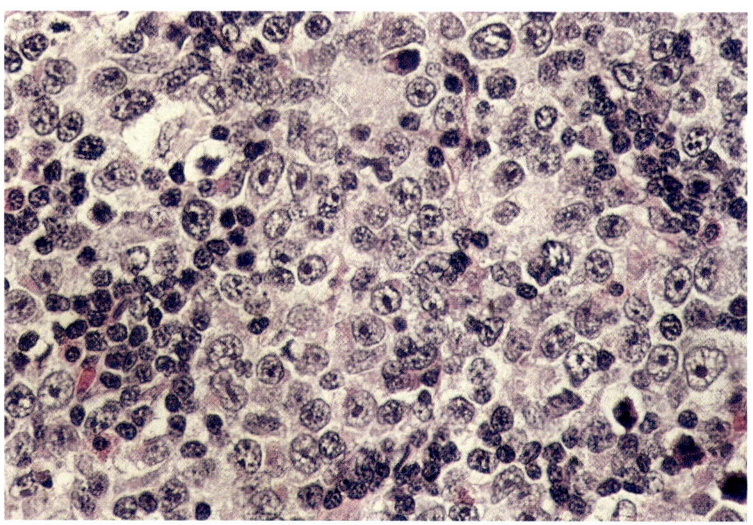

FIGURE
15.11

Richter's syndrome, higher magnification, showing immunoblastic features of the transformed cells.

adenopathy, and hepatosplenomegaly, with increasing numbers of larger nucleolated lymphocytes ("prolymphocytes") in the peripheral blood, a phenomenon which is referred to as "prolymphocytoid" transformation of chronic lymphocytic leukemia (Enno et al, 1979). Lymph nodes in prolymphocytoid transformation show increased numbers of larger nucleolated cells, either in pseudofollicular proliferation centers or diffusely (Kjeldsberg and Marty, 1981). In contrast to de novo prolymphocytic leukemia, the cells in prolymphocytoid transformation usually retain the typical B CLL phenotype and are CD5-positive with dim staining for surface immunoglobulin (Foon et al, 1993).

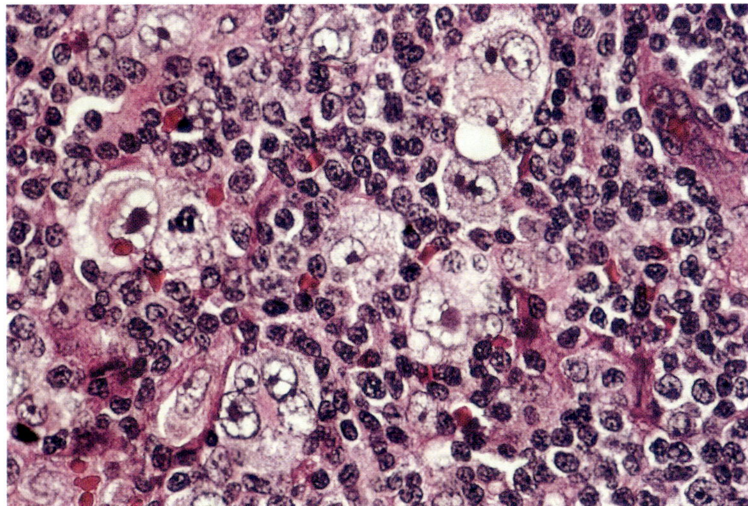

FIGURE
15.12

Hodgkin's disease variant of Richter's syndrome, showing pleomorphic Reed-Sternberg–like cells.

RICHTER'S SYNDROME   Richter's syndrome refers to the development of diffuse large B cell lymphoma in patients with chronic lymphocytic leukemia (Richter, 1928). The large cell lymphoma typically develops in the setting of advanced CLL or SLL, with the onset of fever, weight loss, and progressive lymphadenopathy; but occasionally it is the presenting feature of CLL or SLL (Strauchen et al, 1987). The lymphomas are diffuse large B cell lymphomas, which are frequently pleomorphic, with large immunoblastic cells with prominent central nucleoli, classified as large cell immunoblastic lymphoma in the WF (Figs. 15.10 and 15.11). Pleomorphic Reed-Sternberg–like cells may be prominent in some cases (Fig. 15.12) (see Hodgkin's disease variant of Richter's syndrome, below). In approximately 50% of cases, the large cell lymphoma and the CLL contain identical immunoglobulin gene rearrangements, indicating clonal transformation of the CLL (Foon et al, 1993). In the remaining cases, the large cell lymphoma appears genetically unrelated to the CLL and may represent a second neoplasm.

HODGKIN'S DISEASE VARIANT OF RICHTER'S SYNDROME   Some patients with B cell chronic lymphocytic leukemia develop a malignant lymphoma morphologically indistinguishable from Hodgkin's disease, a phenomenon which has been termed the "Hodgkin's disease variant of Richter's syndrome" (Brecher and Banks, 1990). The Hodgkin's disease may be of any of the usual histologic types, including nodular sclerosis and mixed cellularity. Cases of coexistent Hodgkin's disease and CLL or SLL in the same lymph node have also been reported (Momose et al, 1992; Williams et al, 1991). The Reed-Sternberg–like cells in these cases express the Hodgkin's disease marker CD15, and in some cases the B cell marker CD20, suggesting derivation of Reed-Sternberg cells from neoplastic B cells (Momose et al, 1992; Williams et al, 1991). Epstein-Barr virus is detected in the Reed-Sternberg–like cells and may play a role in transformation (Momose et al, 1992).

OTHER TRANSFORMATIONS OF CHRONIC LYMPHOCYTIC LEUKEMIA   Transformation of B cell chronic lymphocytic leukemia to acute lymphoblastic leukemia and to plasma cell myeloma has been reported rarely (Foon et al, 1993).

Differential Diagnosis

B cell chronic lymphocytic leukemia and small lymphocytic lymphoma must be distinguished form other low-grade B cell lymphomas composed of small lymphoid cells, including lymphoplasmacytoid lymphoma, mantle cell lymphoma, and marginal-zone lymphomas of nodal (monocytoid B cell lymphoma) and extranodal (mucosa associated lymphoid tissue) types. The recognition of pseudofollicular proliferation centers is a useful diagnostic feature, since these are not found in other lymphomas (Ellison et al, 1989). In difficult cases, immunophenotypic studies are helpful. B cell CLL and SLL are typically CD5- and CD23-positive. Lymphoplasmacytoid lymphoma and marginal-zone lymphomas are usually CD5-negative; mantle cell lymphoma is CD5-positive but is distinguished by lack of expression of CD23.

The "large-cell–rich" variants of B cell CLL and SLL should be distinguished from malignant lymphoma, diffuse, mixed small and large cell in the WF. The distinction is based principally on the lack of atypia of the small lymphocytes in B cell CLL and SLL. B cell CLL and SLL with prominent pseudofollicular proliferation centers should also be distinguished from follicular lymphoma. The distinction is based on the cytology of the pseudofollicular proliferation centers, which are characterized by pale, medium sized cells with prominent central nucleoli (prolymphocytes or paraimmunoblasts), in contrast to the small cleaved cells and large noncleaved cells of follicular lymphomas. The phenotype of CLL and SLL (CD5-positive, CD10-negative, dim SIg staining) is also distinct from the phenotype of follicular lymphoma (CD5-negative, CD10-positive, bright SIg staining).

Course and Prognosis

CLL and SLL are indolent systemic lymphoproliferative disorders. Treatment has conventionally consisted of alkylating-agent–based chemotherapy, usually with the orally administered alkylating agent chlorambucil. Responses to therapy are not durable. The newer purine analogues, fludarabine and 2-chlorodeoxyadenosine, have major activity in CLL and SLL (Rozman and Montserrat, 1995). Transformations of CLL and SLL, including Richter's syndrome and prolymphocytoid transformation of chronic lymphocytic leukemia, have a poor prognosis. The Hodgkin's disease variant of Richter's syndrome may have a better prognosis than usual Richter's syndrome (Brecher and Banks, 1990).

Lymphoplasmacytoid Lymphoma

Classification

REAL: Lymphoplasmacytoid lymphoma/immunocytoma.
WF: Malignant lymphoma, small lymphocytic, plasmacytoid.

Immunophenotype

CD5−, CD10−, CD19+, CD20+, CD22+, CD23−, SIg+, cytoplasmic Ig+.

Molecular Pathology

PAX-5 rearrangement with t(9;14) translocation in 50%

Clinical Features

Lymphoplasmacytoid lymphoma is a systemic indolent lymphoproliferative disorder characterized by proliferation of plasmacytoid lymphocytes in the lymph nodes, spleen, and bone marrow, with frequent IgM or other paraproteinemia. Patients may present with the clinical syndrome of Waldenström's macroglobulinemia and symptoms related to hyperviscosity, or with other dysglobulinemia. Hepatitis C virus has been detected in lymph nodes from patients with lymphoproliferative disorders associated with chronic hepatitis C and mixed cryoglobulinemia, suggesting a possible role in lymphomagenesis (Sansonno et al, 1996; Silvestri et al, 1996). Lymphoplasmacytoid lymphoma is associated with the t(9;14) chromosome translocation and rearrangement of the PAX-5 oncogene in 50% of cases (Lida et al, 1996).

Histopathology

Lymph node involvement in lymphoplasmacytoid lymphoma is characterized by infiltration with lymphocytes, plasma cells, and plasmacytoid lymphocytes (Figs. 15.13, 15.14 and 15.15). The latter are cells with cytologic features intermediate between those of a lymphocyte and a plasma cell; typically, the nucleus resembles that of a lymphocyte,

FIGURE 15.13

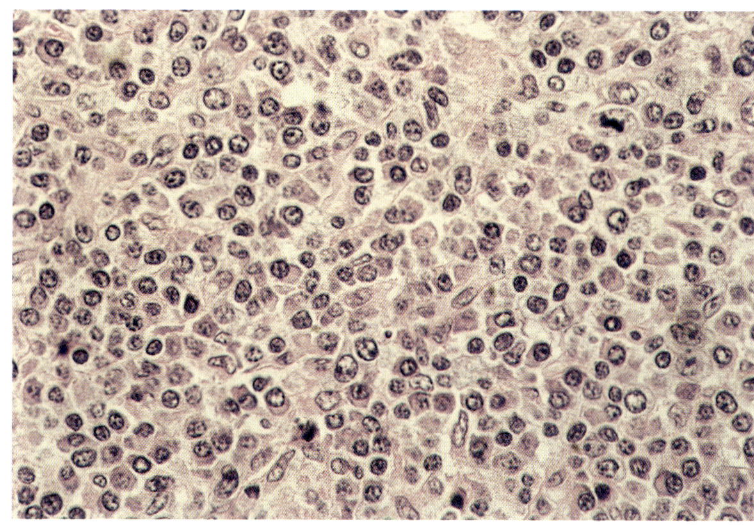

Lymphoplasmacytoid lymphoma showing lymphocytes, plasmacytoid lymphocytes, and plasma cells.

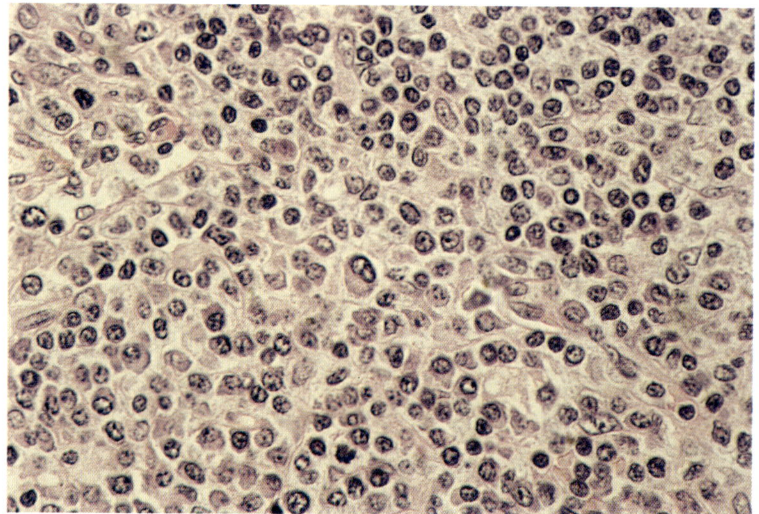

FIGURE
15.14

Lymphoplasmacytoid lymphoma showing lymphocytes, plasmacytoid lymphocytes, and plasma cells.

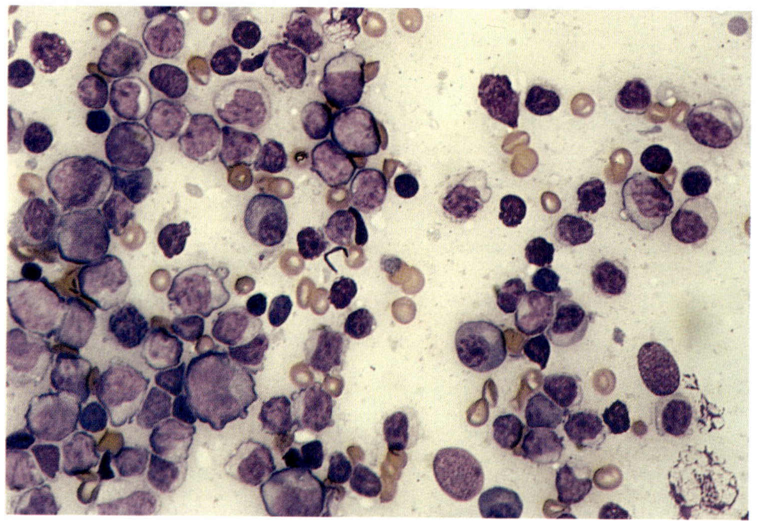

FIGURE
15.15

Lymphoplasmacytoid lymphoma, touch preparation stained with Giemsa, showing population of lymphocytes, plasmacytoid lymphocytes, and plasma cells.

with an eccentric rim of moderate to abundant amphophilic or basophilic cytoplasm resembling that of a plasma cell. Nuclear inclusions of dilated cytoplasmic Golgi cisternae (Dutcher bodies) are frequently present and a variety of cytoplasmic immunoglobulin inclusions may be present, including large eosinophilic globular inclusions (Russell bodies) (Figs. 15.16 and 15.17) and crystalline immunoglobulin inclusions (Figs. 15.18 and 15.19). The latter may accumulate in macrophages, mimicking the histologic appearance of rhabdomyoma (Friedman et al, 1996). The nuclear and cytoplasmic inclusions are frequently PAS-positive due to the high carbohydrate content of IgM (Fig. 15.17).

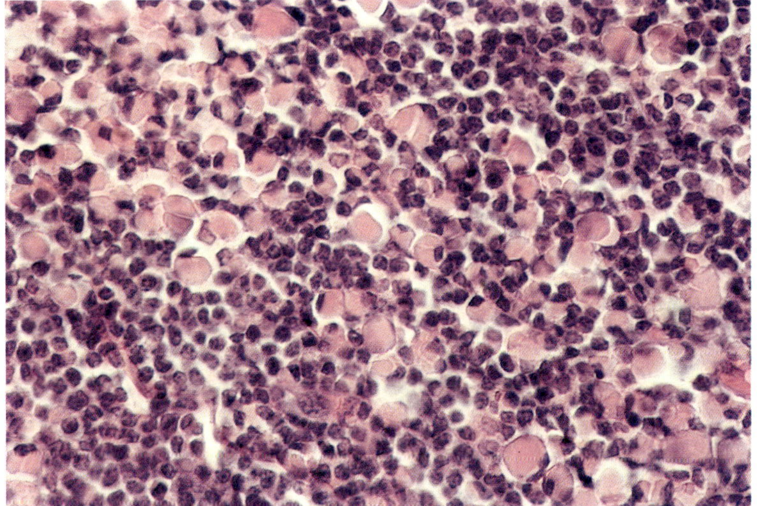

Lymphoplasmacytoid lymphoma showing numerous Russell bodies.

FIGURE
15.16

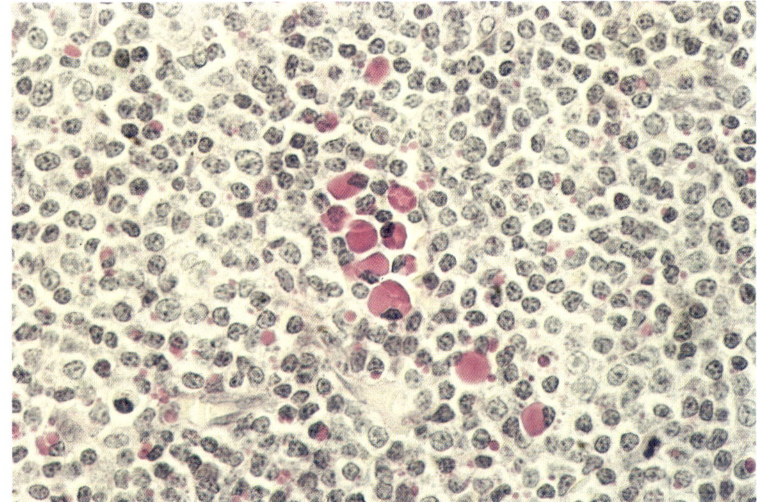

Lymphoplasmacytoid lymphoma showing Russell bodies stained with PAS.

FIGURE
15.17

Mature plasma cells are frequently present and may be distributed diffusely or in discrete aggregates. The relative proportion of lymphocytes, plasma cells, and plasmacytoid cells varies from case to case. Deposition of hemosiderin is frequent in cases associated with autoimmune hemolysis. The lymph node architecture may be completely effaced, or lymph node involvement may be partial, with preservation of the sinuses. A polymorphic variant of lymphoplasmacytoid lymphoma is occasionally encountered which is characterized by admixture of larger cells, including immunoblasts, Reed-Sternberg–like cells, and epithelioid histiocytes (Patsouris et al, 1990) (Fig. 15.20). Cases

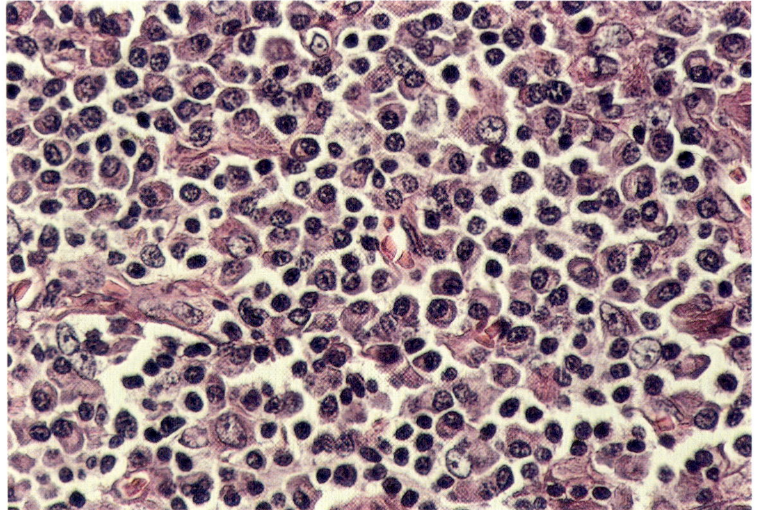

**FIGURE
15.18**

Lymphoplasmacytoid lymphoma associated with deposition of crystalline immunoglobulin inclusions (same case as Fig 15.19).

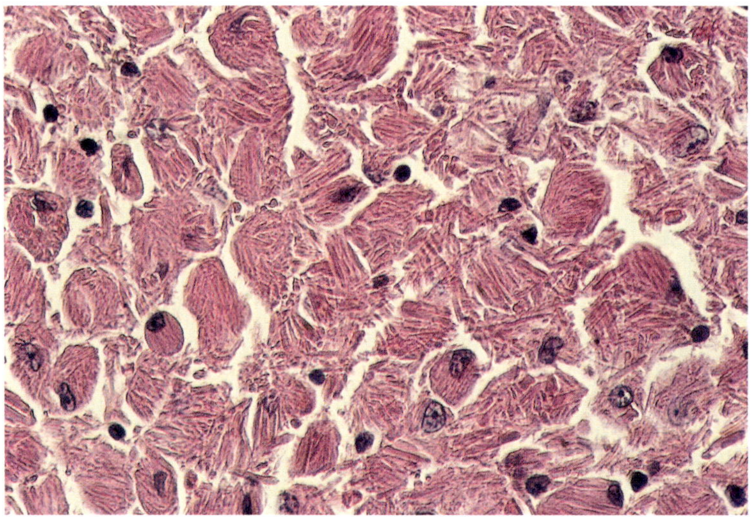

**FIGURE
15.19**

Crystalline immunoglobulin inclusions in a case of lymphoplasmacytoid
lymphoma (same case as Fig 15.18).

with this histology are classified as malignant lymphoma, diffuse, mixed small and large
cell in the WF.

Other Lymphoplasmacytoid Proliferations with Paraproteinemia

GAMMA HEAVY CHAIN DISEASE Gamma heavy chain disease (Franklin's disease) is a
lymphoplasmacytoid proliferation involving the lymph nodes, spleen, and bone marrow,
associated with the presence in the serum and urine of fragments consisting of the Fc

**FIGURE
15.20**

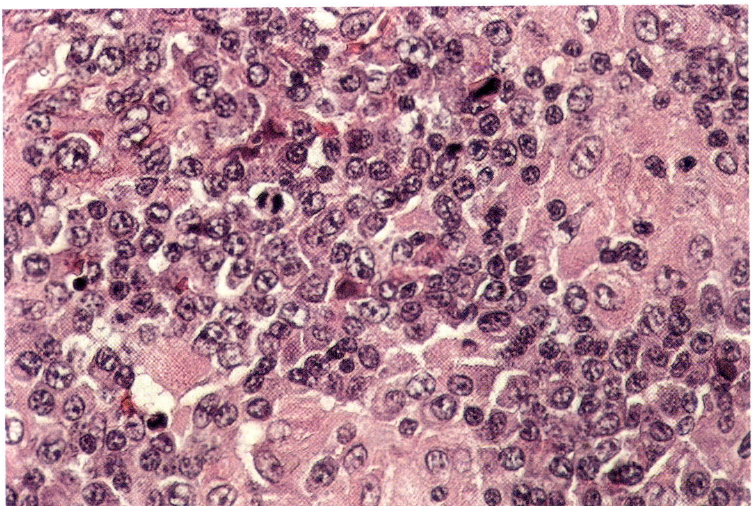

Polymorphic variant of lymphoplasmacytoid lymphoma showing admixture of larger cells and epithelioid histiocytes.

portion of the γ heavy chain (Franklin, 1964). Involvement of Waldeyer's ring has been frequent in some series. The underlying lymphoproliferation may be a lymphoplasmacytoid lymphoma of usual appearance; a polymorphous lymphoplasmacytoid proliferation with lymphocytes, plasma cells, immunoblasts, epithelioid cells, and eosinophils; or rarely, another type of non-Hodgkin's lymphoma (Fermand et al, 1989). Diagnosis is established by demonstration of the abnormal immunoglobulin, which consists of a fragment of the Fc portion of the γ heavy chain, in the serum or urine. The abnormal immunoglobulin is frequently missed on routine electrophoresis but is detected on immunoelectrophoresis by characteristic reaction with antibodies to the gamma heavy chain with no corresponding reaction to kappa or lambda light chain (Fermand et al, 1989).

MU HEAVY CHAIN DISEASE Mu heavy chain disease is variant of chronic lymphocytic leukemia, associated with the presence of μ heavy chains in the serum and free light chains in the urine (Forte et al, 1970). Lymphadenopathy is an infrequent occurrence; the bone marrow frequently contains abnormal vacuolated plasma cells in addition to small lymphocytes.

ALPHA HEAVY CHAIN DISEASE Alpha heavy chain disease (Mediterranean lymphoma, immunoproliferative small-bowel disease) is a lymphoplasmacytoid proliferation involving the small bowel which occurs most frequently in the Middle East and is associated with a syndrome of chronic diarrhea, weight loss, malabsorption, and the presence in the serum of α heavy chain fragments (Price, 1990). The early intestinal lesion is characterized by dense mucosal plasma cell infiltration, which may be reversible with antibiotic treatment. The advanced lesion is characterized by transformation to diffuse large B cell lymphoma, which is frequently pleomorphic with large immunoblastic and Reed-Sternberg–like cells, classified as large cell immunoblastic lymphoma in the WF.

Differential Diagnosis

Plasmacytoid differentiation is not specific to lymphoplasmacytoid lymphoma and may be observed in low-grade B cell non-Hodgkin's lymphoma of a variety of other types, including chronic lymphocytic leukemia, marginal-zone lymphomas of nodal (monocytoid B cell) and extranodal (mucosa associated lymphoid tissue) types, and some cases of follicular lymphoma. IgM or IgG paraproteins may also occur in the course of these lymphomas, but the level of paraproteinemia is not symptomatic. The distinguishing feature of lymphoplasmacytoid lymphoma is the presence of plasmacytoid differentiation in the absence of specific features of other lymphomas. Lymphomas with plasmacytoid differentiation at extranodal sites (e.g., gastrointestinal tract and lung) are most frequently found to be of extranodal marginal-zone (MALT) type. Gamma heavy chain disease may be associated with unusual polymorphous lymphoplasmacytoid infiltrates in lymph nodes or extranodal sites (Fermand et al, 1989).

Course and Prognosis

Lymphoplasmacytoid lymphoma is an indolent disorder which is treated with alkylating agent based chemotherapy. Responses to therapy are not durable. Hyperviscosity symptoms in Waldenström's macroglobulinemia are treated with plasmapheresis. Large cell transformation of lymphoplasmacytoid lymphoma may occur.

REFERENCES

Batata A, Shen B. Immunophenotyping of subtypes of B chronic (mature) lymphoid leukemia: Study of 242 cases. Cancer 70:2436–2443, 1992.

Bearman RM, Pangalis G, Rappaport H. Prolymphocytic leukemia. Clinical, histopathological, and cytochemical observations. Cancer 42:2360–2372, 1978.

Berger F, Felman P, Sonet A, Salles G, Bastion Y, Byron PA, Coiffier B. Nonfollicular small B cell lymphomas: A heterogeneous group of patients with distinct clinical features and outcome. Blood 63:2829–2835, 1994.

Bonato M, Pittaluga S, Tierens A, Criel A, Verhoef G, Wlodarska I, et al. Lymph node histology in typical and atypical chronic lymphocytic leukemia. Am J Surg Pathol 22:49–56, 1998.

Brecher M, Banks PM. Hodgkin's disease variant of Richter's syndrome. Report of eight cases. Am J Clin Pathol 93:333–339, 1990.

Ellison DJ, Nathwani BN, Cho SY, Martin SE. Interfollicular small lymphocytic lymphoma. The diagnostic significance of pseudofollicles. Hum Pathol 20:1108, 1989.

Enno A, Catovsky D, O'Brien M, Cherchi M, Kumaran TO, Galton DAG. "Prolymphocytoid" transformation of chronic lymphocytic leukemia. Br J Haematol 41:9–18, 1979.

Fermand J-P, Brouet J-C, Danon F, Seligmann M. Gamma heavy chain "disease": Heterogeneity of the clinicopathologic features. Report of 16 cases and review of the literature. Medicine (Baltimore) 68:321–333, 1989.

Foon KA, Thiruvengadam R, Saven A, Bernstein ZP, Gale RP. Genetic relatednes of lymphoid malignancies. Transformation of chronic lymphocytic leukemia as a model. Ann Intern Med 119:63–73, 1993.

Forte FA, Prelli F, Yount WJ, Jerry LM, Kochwa S, Franklin EC, Kunkel HI. Heavy chain disease of the mu (μM) type: Report of the first case. Blood 36:137–144, 1970.

Franklin EC, Lowenstein J, Bigelow B, Meltzer M. Heavy chain disease—a new disorder of serum gamma-globulins. Report of the first case. Am J Med 37:332–350, 1964.

Friedman MT, Mohlo L, Valderrama E, Kahn LB. Crystal-storing histiocytosis associated with a lymphoplasmacytic neoplasm mimicking adult rhabdomyoma: A case report and review of the literature. Arch Pathol Lab Med 120:1133–1136, 1996.

Ikematsu W, Ikematsu H, Okamura S, Otsuka T, Harada M, Niho Y. Surface phenotype and Ig heavy-chain gene usage in chronic B cell leukemia: Expression of myelomonocytic surface markers in CD5− chronic B cell leukemia. Blood 83:2602–2610, 1994.

Kjeldsberg CR, Marty J. Prolymphocytic transformation of chronic lymphocytic leukemia. Cancer 48:2447–2457, 1981.

Lida S, Rao PH, Nallasivam P, Hibshoosh H, Butler M, Louie DC, Dyomin V, Ohno H, Chaganti RSK, Dalla-Favera R. The t(19;14)(p13;q32) chromosomal translocation associated with lymphoplasmacytoid lymphoma involves the PAX-5 gene. Blood 88:4110–4117, 1996.

Mayer R, Logtenberg T, Strauchen J, Dimitriu-Bona A, Mayer L, Mechanic S, Chiorazzi N, Borche L, Dighiero G, Mannheimer-Lory A, Diamond B, Alt F, Bona C. CD5 and immunoglobulin V gene expression in B cell lymphomas and chronic lymphocytic leukemia. Blood 75:1518–1524, 1990.

Momose H, Jaffe ES, Shin SS, Chen Y-Y, Weiss LM. Chronic lymphocytic leukemia/small lymphocytic lymphoma with Reed-Sternberg-like cells and possible transformation to Hodgkin's disease. Mediation by Epstein-Barr virus. Am J Surg Pathol 15:859–867, 1992.

Owens MR, Strauchen JA, Rowe JM, Bennett JM. Prolymphocytic leukemia: Histologic findings in atypical cases. Hematol Oncol 2:249–257, 1984.

Patsouris E, Noel H, Lennert K. Lymphoplasmacytic/lymphoplasmacytoid immunocytoma with a high content of epithelioid cells. Histologic and immunohistologic findings. Am J Surg Pathol 14:660–670, 1990.

Perry DA, Bast MA, Armitage JO, Weisenberger DD. Diffuse intermediate lymphocytic lymphoma. A clinicopathologic study with comparison to small lymphocytic lymphoma and diffuse small cleaved cell lymphoma. Cancer 66:1995–2000, 1990.

Price SK. Immunoproliferative small intestinal disease: A study of 13 cases with alpha heavy-chain disease. Histopathology 17:7–17, 1990.

Pugh W, Manning JT, Butler JJ. Paraimmunoblastic variant of small lymphocytic lymphoma/leukemia. Am J Surg Pathol 12:907–917, 1988.

Richter MN. Generalized reticular cell sarcoma of lymph nodes associated with lymphatic leukemia. Am J Pathol 4:285–292, 1928.

Rozman C, Montserrat E. Current concepts. Chronic lymphocytic leukemia. N Engl J Med 333:1052–1057, 1995.

Sansonno D, De Vita S, Cornacchiulo V, Carbone A, Boiocchi M, Dammacco F. Detection and distribution of hepatitis C virus-related proteins in lymph nodes of patients with type II mixed cryoglobulinemia and neoplastic or non-neoplastic lymphoproliferation. Blood 88:4638–4645, 1996.

Silvestri F, Pipan C, Barillari G, Zaja F, Fanin R, Infanti L, et al. Prevalence of hepatitis C virus infection in patients with lymphoproliferative disorders. Blood 87:4296–4301, 1996.

Strauchen JA, May MM, Crown J. Large cell transformation of subclinical small lymphocytic leukemia/lymphoma: A variant of Richter's syndrome. Hematol Oncol 5:167–174, 1987.

Williams J, Schned A, Cotelingam JD, Jaffe ES. Chronic lymphocytic leukemia with coexistent Hodgkin's disease. Implications for the origin of the Reed-Sternberg cell. Am J Surg Pathol 15:33–42, 1991.

16

Peripheral B Cell Neoplasms: II. Mantle Cell Lymphoma and Follicle Center Lymphoma

Mantle cell lymphoma and follicle center lymphomas are lymphoid neoplasms related to the lymphoid follicle. Mantle cell lymphoma arises from B cells of the mantle zone, the residual portion of the primary lymphoid follicle, which surrounds the follicular center in secondary follicles. Mantle cell lymphoma may be derived from a subset of CD5-positive, CD23-negative inner mantle B lymphocytes (Inghirami et al, 1991). Follicle center lymphomas are derived from follicular center B cells.

Mantle Cell Lymphoma

Classification

REAL: Mantle cell lymphoma.
WF: Malignant lymphoma, diffuse, small cleaved cell.

Immunophenotype

CD5+, CD10–, CD19+, CD20+, CD22+, CD23–, CD43+, SIg+, $\lambda > \kappa$.

Molecular Pathology

BCL-1 (PRAD1/CYCLIN D1) rearrangement with t(11;14) chromosome translocation in 50–70%

186

**FIGURE
16.1**

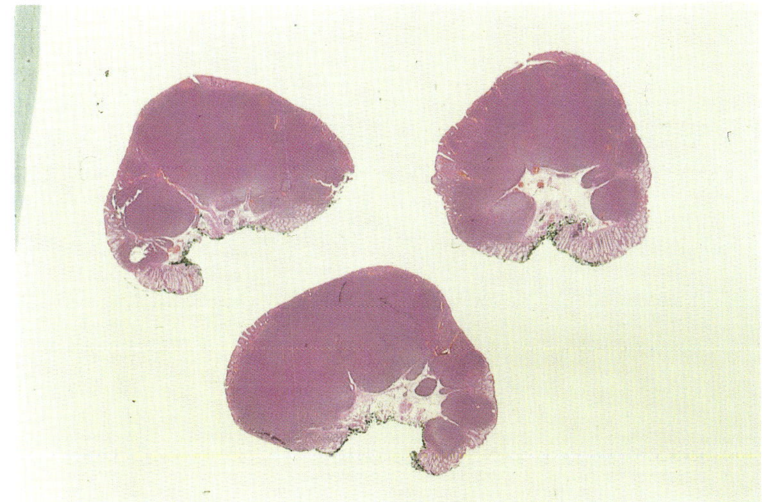

Mantle cell lymphoma showing multiple lymphomatous polyposis (whole mount).

Clinical Features

Mantle cell lymphoma is the presently accepted term for lymphomas formerly considered lymphocytic lymphoma of intermediate differentiation, intermediate lymphocytic lymphoma, mantle zone lymphoma, and centrocytic lymphoma (in the Kiel classification) (Banks et al, 1992; Weisenberger and Armitage, 1996). Mantle cell lymphoma is a relatively infrequent systemic lymphoproliferative disorder affecting predominantly male patients over the age of 40. Generalized lymphadenopathy, splenomegaly, and bone marrow involvement are frequently present at diagnosis. Extranodal involvement is also frequent. Gastrointestinal involvement is present in 20% and takes the form of multiple lymphomatous polyposis, consisting of multiple mucosal and submucosal polypoid lymphoid masses involving the stomach, small bowel, and colon (O'Briain et al, 1988) (Fig. 16.1). Multiple lymphomatous polyposis is a specific feature of mantle cell lymphoma and rarely of follicle center lymphoma, involving the gastrointestinal tract (Moynihan et al, 1996). Leukemic transformation of mantle cell lymphoma occurs and may mimic chronic lymphocytic leukemia, or lymphosarcoma cell leukemia with circulating cleaved cells (Vadlamudi et al, 1996).

Mantle cell lymphoma is characterized by a t(11;14) chromosomal translocation and rearrangement of the PRAD1/CYCLIN D1 (BCL-1) oncogene in 50–70% of cases (de Boer et al, 1995). Overexpression of cyclin D1 protein can be detected immunohistochemically in nearly all cases (Yatabe et al, 1996). Cyclin D1 is a cell cycle regulatory protein and dysregulation of cyclin D1 likely plays a role in lymphomagenesis.

Histopathology

Mantle cell lymphoma is characterized by monotonous proliferation of round to irregular or cleaved small lymphocytes (Fig. 16.2). Pseudofollicular proliferation centers, transformed cells, and large noncleaved cells are characteristically absent (Figs. 16.3,

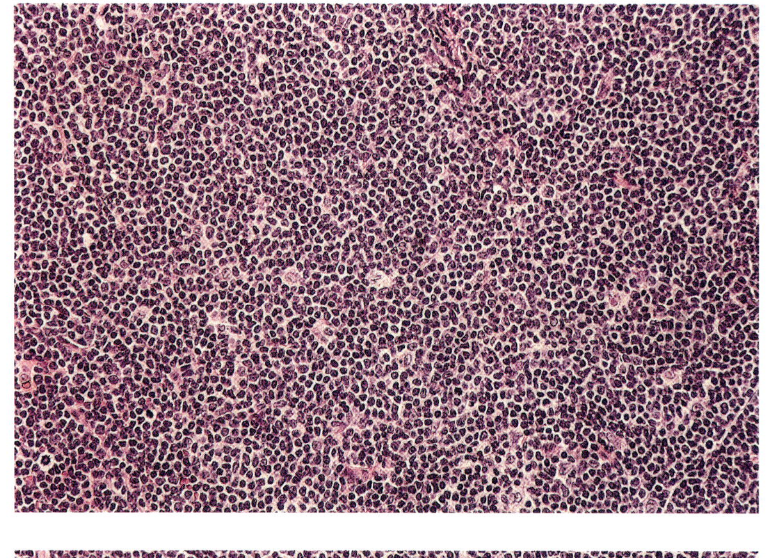

A

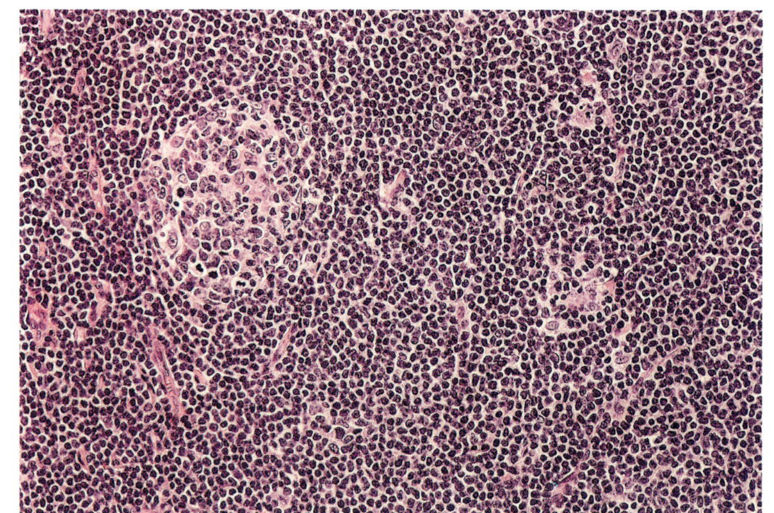

B

Mantle cell lymphoma showing diffuse proliferation of small irregular lymphocytes (A) and residual "naked" follicular center (B).

16.4, and 16.5). Residual follicular centers are frequently present and appear as "naked" follicular centers, surrounded by lymphoma cells (Fig. 16.2). The pattern of infiltration may be diffuse or vaguely nodular; in some cases a pronounced mantle-zone pattern of involvement is evident, with proliferation of neoplastic cells in broad zones around reactive follicular centers (Duggan et al, 1990) (Fig. 16.6). Scattered benign histiocytes with abundant eosinophilic granular cytoplasm ("pink histiocytes") are a frequent feature of mantle cell lymphomas (Figs. 16.3 and 16.4). The "pink histiocytes" are infrequently found in other low-grade B cell lymphomas and are a helpful clue to the diagnosis. A variable number of mitoses are present.

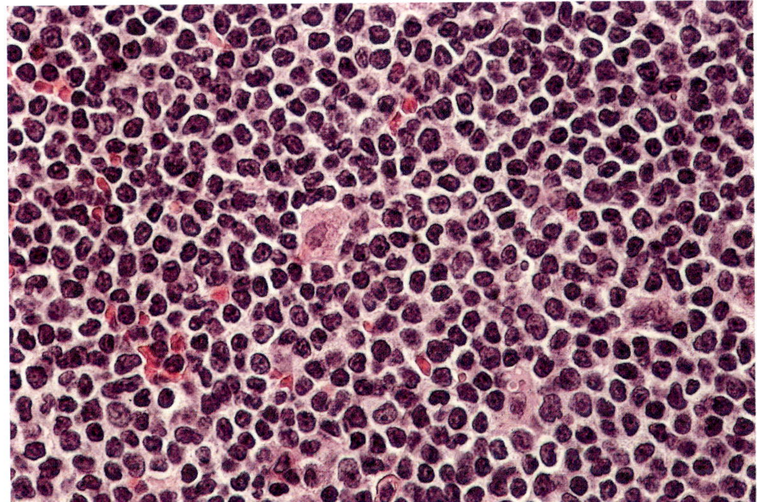

Mantle cell lymphoma showing round to irregular lymphocytes and scattered granular, eosinophilic histiocytes.

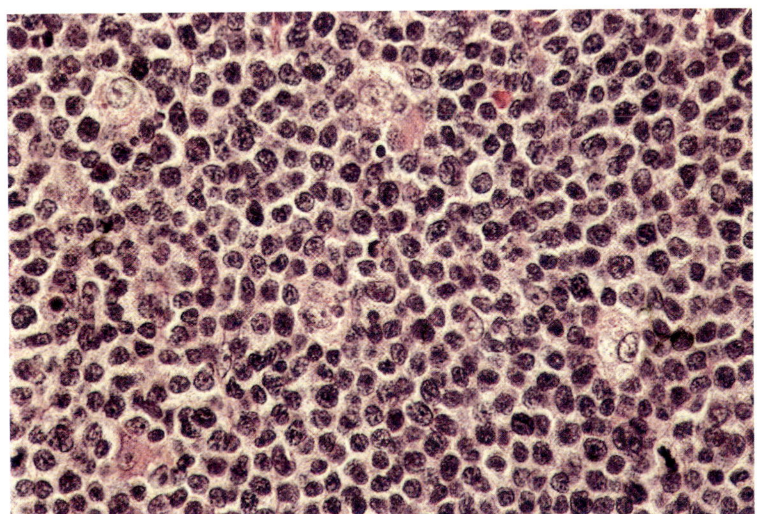

Mantle cell lymphoma showing round to irregular lymphocytes and scattered granular, eosinophilic histiocytes.

Variants

NODULAR OR MANTLE-ZONE MANTLE CELL LYMPHOMA   In approximately 30% of mantle cell lymphomas, a pronounced nodular or mantle-zone pattern is present at diagnosis and may represent an earlier stage in the development of the lymphoma (Weisenberger and Armitage, 1996) (Fig. 16.6). Subclassification of mantle cell lymphoma into diffuse, nodular, and mantle-zone categories may be clinically relevant, with lymphomas with a

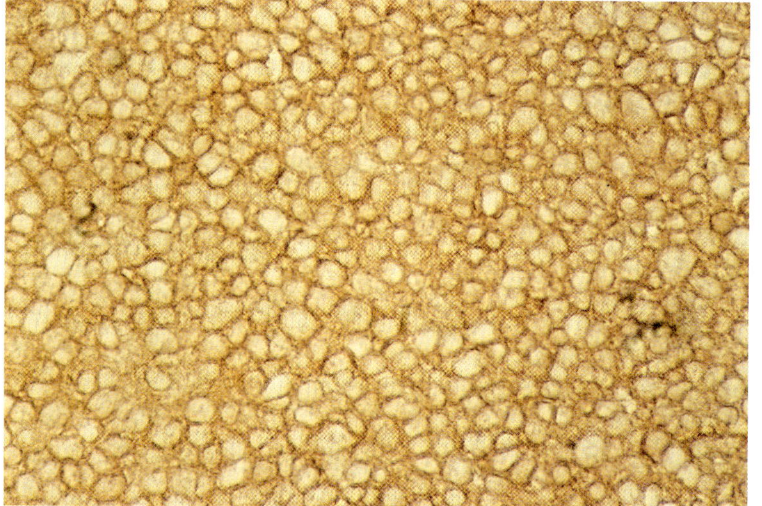

FIGURE 16.5

Mantle cell lymphoma showing diffuse positivity for CD5 in frozen tissue.

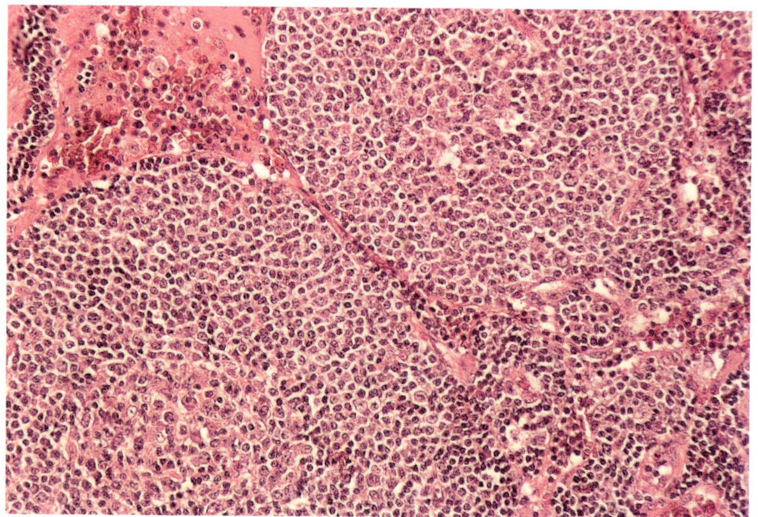

FIGURE 16.6

Mantle cell lymphoma showing mantle-zone pattern of involvement.

mantle-zone pattern demonstrating improved survival in some (Majlis et al, 1997) but not all series (Argatoff et al, 1997).

BLASTIC MANTLE CELL LYMPHOMA In some cases of mantle cell lymphoma, the cells depart from the classic appearance and are larger and blastic in appearance, with finely dispersed chromatin, inconspicuous nucleoli, and numerous mitoses (Lardelli et al, 1990) (Figs. 16.7 and 16.8). Mantle cell lymphomas with this appearance closely resemble lymphoblastic lymphoma morphologically, but are TdT negative and retain the CD5-positive B cell phenotype of typical mantle cell lymphoma (Cheng et al, 1994). Blastic

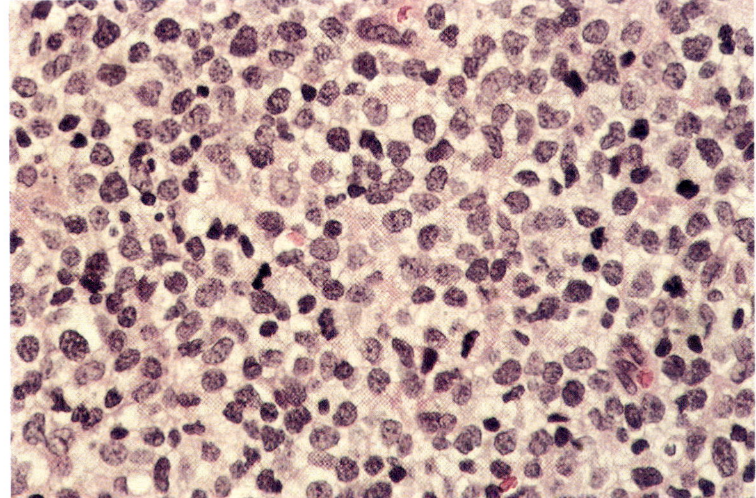

Mantle cell lymphoma, blastic variant, with frequent mitoses.

FIGURE 16.7

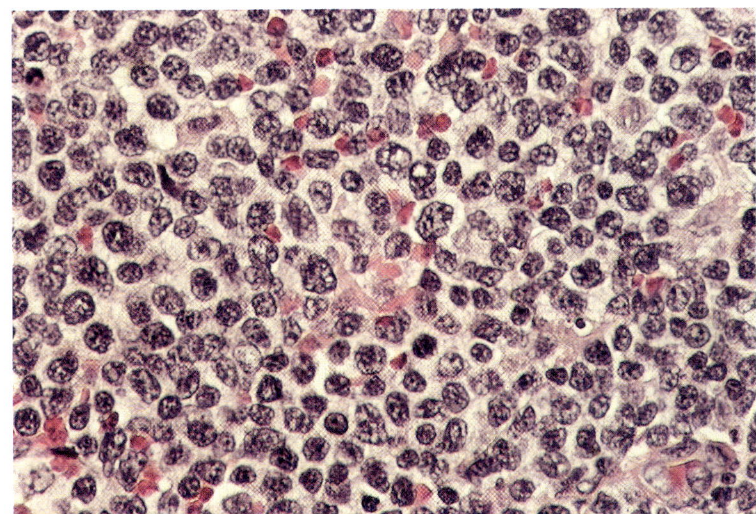

Mantle cell lymphoma, blastic variant.

FIGURE 16.8

mantle cell lymphomas have a poor prognosis (Lardelli et al, 1990). A large cell variant of mantle cell lymphoma has also been described (Zoldan et al, 1996).

Differential Diagnosis

Mantle cell lymphoma must be distinguished from other low-grade B cell lymphomas composed of small lymphoid cells, including chronic lymphocytic leukemia and small lymphocytic lymphoma, marginal-zone lymphomas of nodal (monocytoid B cell lymphoma) and extranodal (MALT) type, and follicle center lymphomas. The mantle-zone pattern is not specific to mantle cell lymphoma and is found occasionally in other low-grade B cell lymphomas including small lymphocytic lymphoma and marginal-zone lymphomas. Chronic lymphocytic leukemia and small lymphocytic lymphoma are distinguished from mantle cell lymphoma by the presence of pseudofollicular proliferation centers and by phenotype. CLL and SLL are CD5- and CD23-positive; mantle cell lymphomas are CD5-positive, but CD23-negative. Marginal-zone lymphomas are distinguished morphologically by the presence of cells with more abundant cytoplasm (monocytoid B cells and centrocyte-like cells), plasmacytoid differentiation, and admixture of larger transformed cells. Residual follicular centers are frequently present in both; however, in marginal-zone lymphoma, the follicular centers are separated from the lymphoma cells by an attenuated zone of residual non-neoplastic mantle cells, in contrast to the "naked" follicular centers in mantle cell lymphoma. In difficult cases, immunophenotypic studies are helpful, since marginal-zone lymphomas are CD5-negative in most cases. Mantle cell lymphomas with a pronounced mantle-zone or nodular pattern may mimic follicle center lymphomas. Immunophenotypic studies are helpful in distinction, since follicle center lymphomas are CD5-negative and CD10-positive.

Mantle cell lymphoma must be distinguished from widened mantle zones in benign conditions. Widened mantle zones are encountered in the hyaline-vascular form of Castleman's disease and in occasional cases of reactive lymphoid hyperplasia (mantle-zone hyperplasia). Distinction from mantle cell lymphoma is based on the presence of typical morphologic features of Castleman's disease (hyaline-vascular follicular centers, paracortical hypervascularity) or reactive lymphoid hyperplasia and is aided by immunophenotypic studies. The mantle cells in Castleman's disease and mantle-zone hyperplasia are polyclonal by immunoglobulin light chain restriction and CD5- and CD43-negative; the cells of mantle cell lymphoma, in contrast, are monoclonal by immunoglobulin light chain restriction and CD5- and CD43-positive.

Immunohistochemical staining for cyclin D1 protein has been shown to be helpful in the differential diagnosis of mantle cell lymphoma (de Boer et al, 1995; Yatabe et al, 1996). Characteristic nuclear staining for cyclin D1 can be demonstrated in frozen or deparaffinized sections in most cases. Mantle cell lymphomas are positive for BCL-2 oncoprotein, as are normal mantle cells (Pezzella et al, 1990).

Course and Prognosis

Mantle cell lymphoma is an aggressive disorder with poorer survival than other low grade B cell lymphomas (Fisher et al, 1995). Responses to therapy are not durable. Mantle cell lymphomas with a mantle-zone pattern may have improved survival (Duggan et al, 1990; Majlis et al, 1997; Weisenberger and Armitage, 1996).

Follicle Center Lymphoma, Follicular

Classification

REAL: Follicle center lymphoma, follicular; provisional cytologic grades: I (predominantly small cell), II (mixed small and large cell), III (predominantly large cell).
WF: Malignant lymphoma, follicular, predominantly small cleaved cell; malignant

lymphoma, follicular, mixed small cleaved and large cell; malignant lymphoma, follicular, predominantly large cell.

Immunophenotype

CD5−, CD10+, CD19+, CD20+, CD22+, CD43−, SIg+

Molecular Pathology

BCL-2 oncogene rearrangement with t(14;18) chromosome translocation in 90%

Clinical Features

Follicle center lymphoma, follicular (follicular lymphoma, FL) occurs predominantly in adults over the age of 40 but is seen occasionally in younger patients and even in children (Pinto et al, 1990). Patients usually present with advanced disease (Ann Arbor stages III and IV); occasional patients present with localized disease (Ann Arbor stages I and II). Lymphadenopathy is the most frequent presenting sign; bone marrow involvement is frequent and is characteristically paratrabecular. Leukemic transformation may occur and is characterized by circulating small cleaved cells (lymphosarcoma cell leukemia) of follicle center lymphoma cell phenotype.

FL are characterized by the t(14;18) chromosome translocation and rearrangement of the BCL-2 oncogene (Weiss et al, 1987). BCL-2 oncoprotein is a mitochondrial protein which inhibits apoptosis (programmed cell death); dysregulation of BCL-2 expression results in "immortalization" of follicular center B cells. Small numbers of B cells with the t(14;18) translocation are detected in the blood of normal individuals (Limpens et al, 1995). FL have extensively mutated immunoglobulin V region genes, indicating derivation from antigenically stimulated B cells (Stewart and Schwartz, 1994).

Histopathology

Follicle center lymphoma, follicular is characterized by proliferation of abnormal follicles throughout the lymph node (Fig. 16.9). The abnormal follicles are rounded or polygonal with relatively little variation in size and shape; are characteristically crowded, with a "back-to-back" or "touching" arrangement with little or no intervening lymphoid tissue; and have absent or attenuated mantle zones (Nathwani et al, 1981). In occasional cases, there is greater variation in follicle size and shape and the follicles may be more loosely arranged with partial preservation of the mantle zones. The "cracking" phenomenon, characterized by separation of the follicles by an artifactual cleft or space, was previously considered a feature of FL but is now recognized as an artifact which occurs as frequently in follicular hyperplasia as in follicular lymphoma, and it is not of diagnostic value (Nathwani et al, 1981). At higher magnification, the abnormal follicles of FL are cytologically monotonous, with a paucity or absence of tingible body macrophages and mitoses (Figs. 16.10, 16.11, and 16.12). Phagocytic macrophages (starry-sky cells) and mitoses, however, may be seen in high-grade FL. The follicles in FL are frequently poorly demarcated, blending imperceptibly into the surrounding lymphoid tissue, with

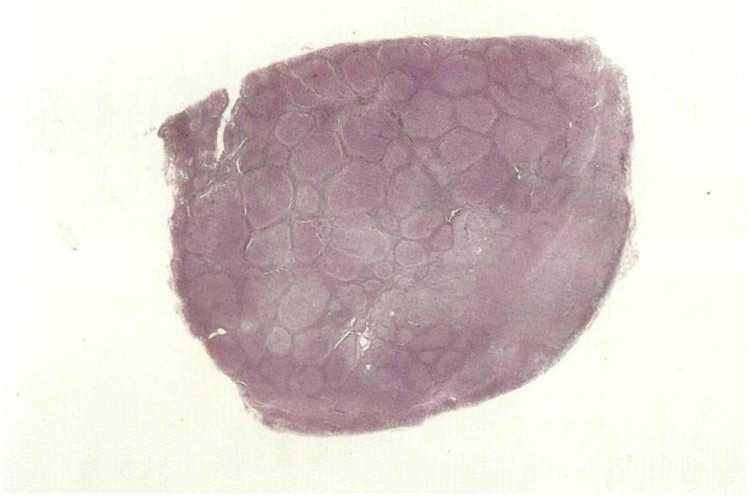

FIGURE 16.9

Follicular lymphoma, whole mount, showing crowding of abnormal, "back-to-back" follicles.

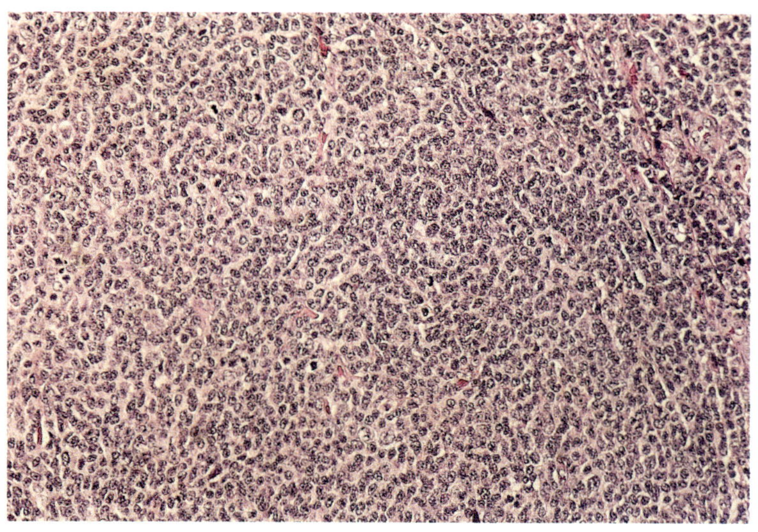

FIGURE 16.10

Follicular lymphoma, predominantly small cleaved cell (provisional cytologic grade I). Cytologically monotonous small cleaved cells with absence of tingible body macrophages.

follicle center cells present outside the follicles. Polarity of follicles, a characteristic feature of follicular hyperplasia, is absent in FL.

Subclassification of Follicle Center Lymphoma, Follicular

Follicular lymphomas have traditionally been subclassified according to the relative proportion of small cleaved cells (centrocytes) and large noncleaved cells (centroblasts)

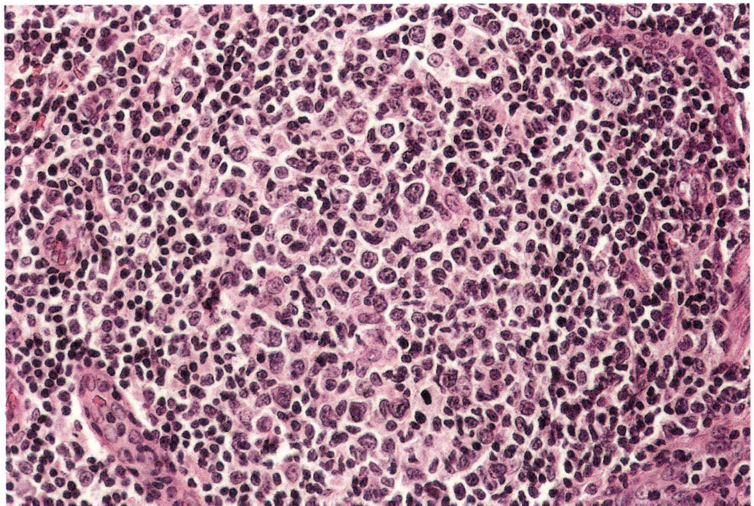

FIGURE 16.11

Follicular lymphoma, mixed small cleaved and large cell (provisional cytologic grade II). Admixture of small cleaved and large cells with absence of tingible body macrophages.

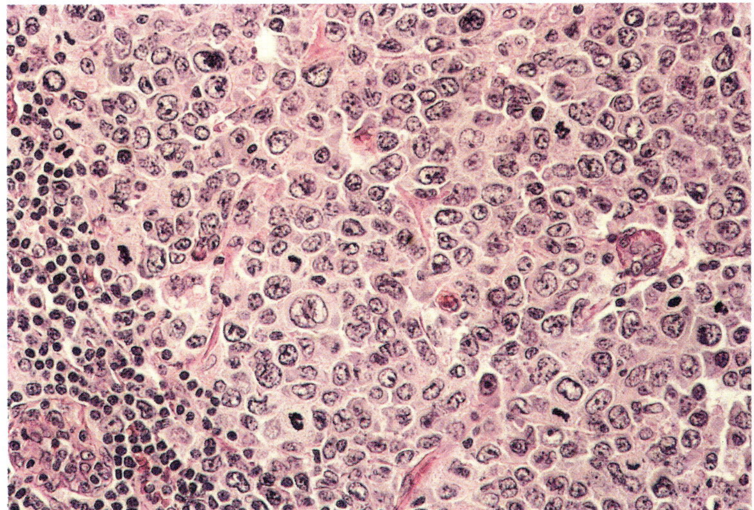

FIGURE 16.12

Follicular lymphoma, predominantly large cell (provisional cytologic grade III). Large cells with frequent mitoses and absence of tingible body macrophages.

present. The distribution of these cell types, however, represents a continuum, rather than distinct entities. In the WF, the FL are divided into three categories: predominantly small cleaved cell, mixed small cleaved and large cell, and predominantly large cell (Figs. 16.10, 16.11, and 16.12). In the REAL classification, these categories are reflected in three provisional cytologic grades: I (predominantly small cell), II (mixed small and large cell), III (predominantly large cell). The WHO has proposed a two grade scheme: I (centroblasts <50% of the follicle area) and II (centroblasts>50% of the follicle area)

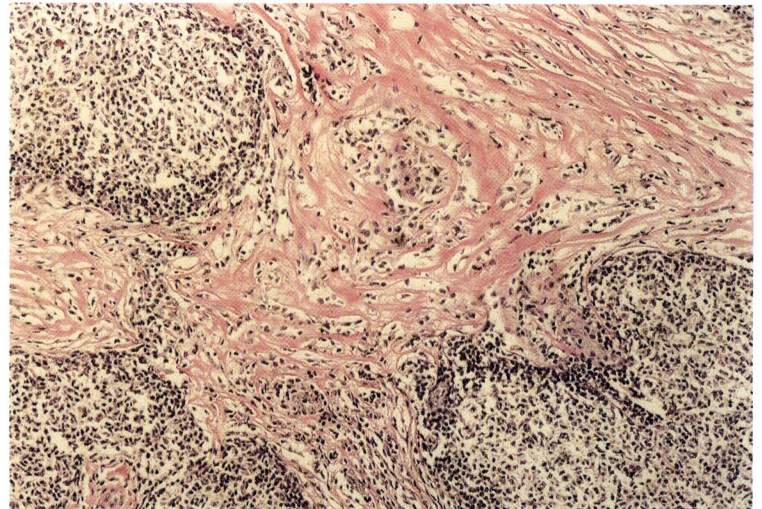

FIGURE 16.13

Follicular lymphoma with sclerosis.

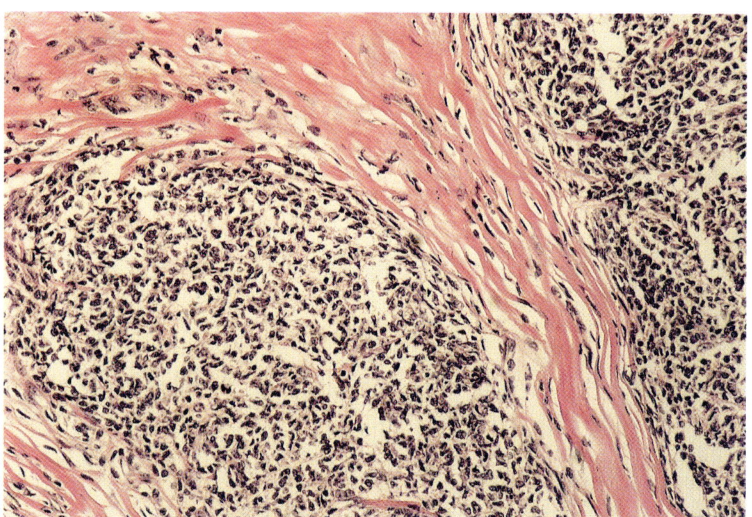

FIGURE 16.14

Follicular lymphoma with sclerosis showing broad fibrous bands.

(Harris, 1997). There is no unanimity of opinion on the specific criteria for distinguishing categories (or grades) of follicular lymphoma. The criteria proposed by Mann and Berard, which are based on the number of large noncleaved cells within the follicles per high-power ($40\times$ objective) field (hpf), have been widely used (Mann and Berard, 1983): <5 large noncleaved cells per hpf (predominantly small cleaved cell), 5 or >, but <15 large noncleaved cells per hpf (mixed small cleaved and large cell), and 15 or > large noncleaved cells per hpf (predominantly large cell). Subclassification (or grading) of FL by these criteria appears to be clinically relevant and to identify subgroups of FL with prolonged and possibly durable responses to therapy (Longo et al, 1984; Martin et

**FIGURE
16.15**

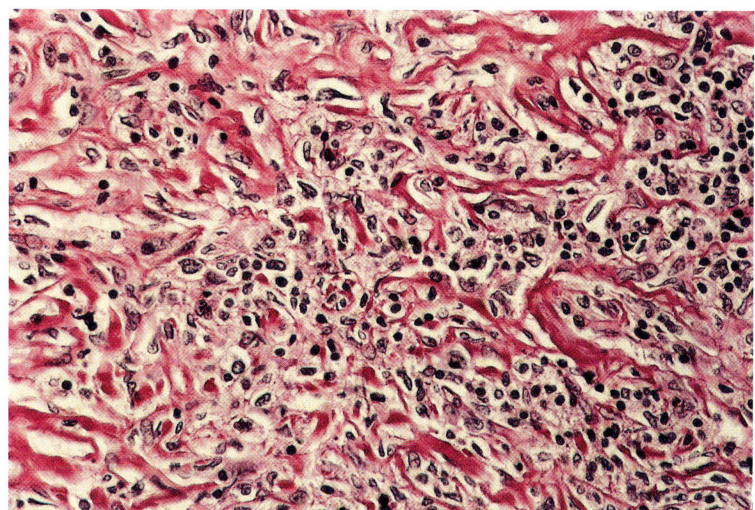

Follicular lymphoma with diffuse sclerosis.

al, 1995). The clinical and therapeutic significance of distinctions between subcategories of FL, however, continues to be debated.

Variants of Follicle Center Lymphoma, Follicular

FOLLICULAR LYMPHOMA WITH DIFFUSE AREAS   Follicular lymphomas are defined by the presence of a follicular component of any extent. Diffuse areas are frequently present in follicular lymphomas; the effect on prognosis is contradictory in different studies, but is likely adverse for an extensive diffuse component. In general, lymphomas with follicular and diffuse components behave as follicular lymphoma when of predominantly small cleaved cell or mixed small cleaved and large cell type, and as diffuse lymphoma when of predominantly large cell type (Warnke et al, 1977; Bartlett et al, 1994).

FOLLICULAR LYMPHOMA WITH SCLEROSIS   Sclerosis is a frequent feature of follicular lymphoma. Sclerosis may be present in the form of a delicate compartmentalizing sclerosis surrounding single or small groups of cells, broad fibrous bands, or both (Figs. 16.13 and 16.14). Sclerosis may extend into the perinodal soft tissue and may obscure the follicular architecture (Fig. 16.15). Follicular lymphoma with sclerosis has been reported as both prognostically favorable and prognostically unfavorable. Sclerosis in follicular lymphomas appears to have no independent effect on prognosis (Warnke et al, 1995).

FLORAL VARIANT OF FOLLICULAR LYMPHOMA   Rare cases of follicular lymphoma are characterized by neoplastic follicles which are surrounded and irregularly infiltrated by an expanded mantle zone, imparting a "floral" appearance (Goates et al, 1994) (Figs. 16.16 and 16.17). The abnormal follicles may mimic those of progressive transformation of germinal centers (Osborne and Butler, 1987). Diagnosis is aided by recognition of the

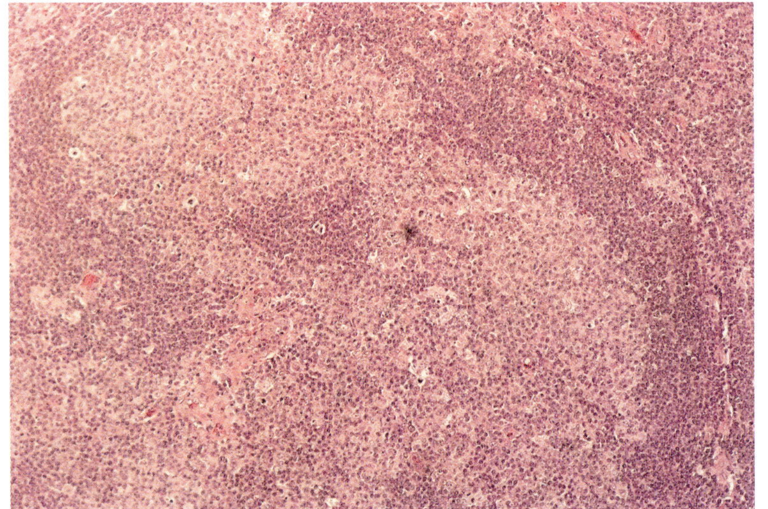

FIGURE 16.16

Floral variant of follicular lymphoma showing a neoplastic follicle surrounded and irregularly infiltrated by mantle zone lymphocytes.

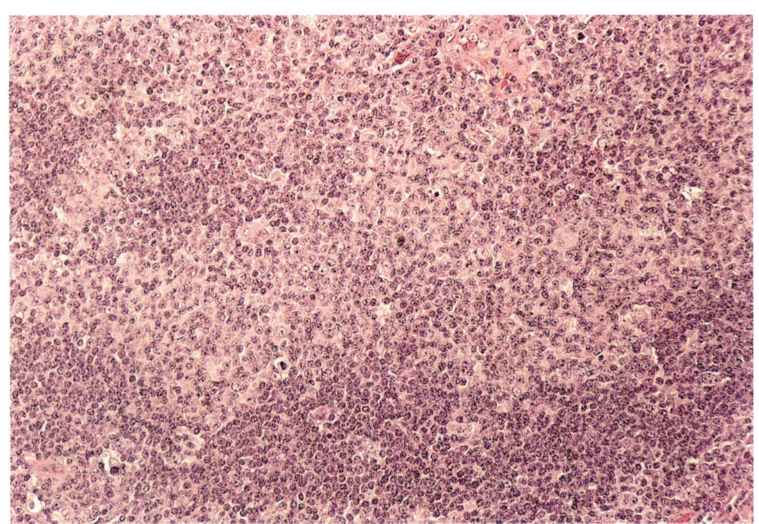

FIGURE 16.17

Floral variant of follicular lymphoma, higher magnification, showing intermingling of neoplastic follicular center cells and mantle zone lymphocytes.

crowding of the abnormal follicles and monomorphic cytology. Immunophenotypic studies for immunoglobulin light chain restriction and BCL-2 oncoprotein are diagnostic (Goates et al, 1994). The clinical behavior is similar to other FL.

SIGNET RING CELL LYMPHOMA Rare cases of follicular lymphoma are characterized by "signet ring" cells in which the nucleus is displaced by a clear cytoplasmic vacuole (Figs. 16.18 and 16.19) or PAS-positive eosinophilic cytoplasmic inclusion (Russell-like body) (Figs. 16.20 and 16.21). The cytoplasmic inclusions result from abnormal intracellular accumulation of immunoglobulin. The clear vacuoles are dilated Golgi cisternae or

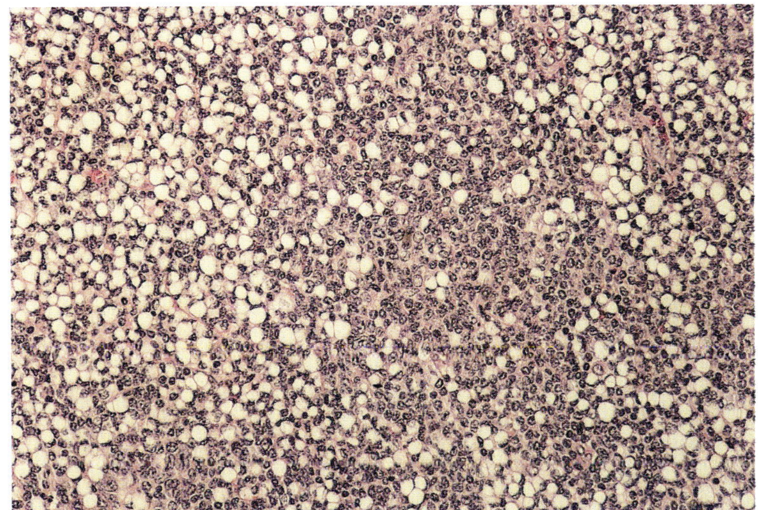

Signet ring cell lymphoma showing numerous signet ring cells.

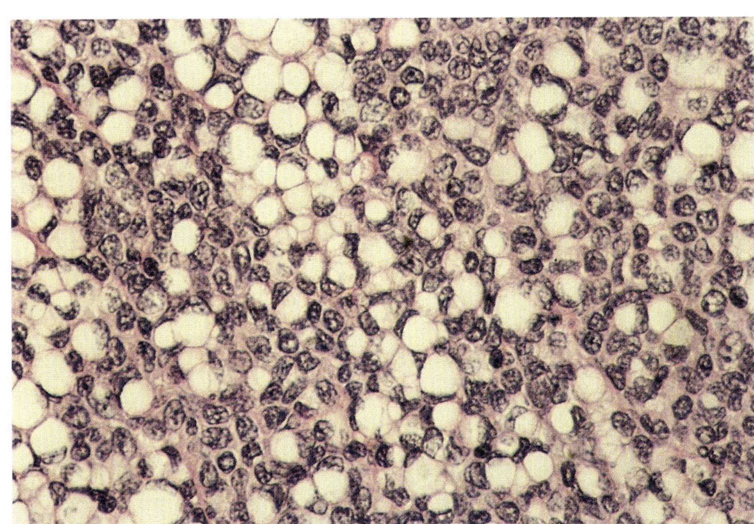

Signet ring cell lymphoma, higher magnification, showing displacement of the nucleus by a clear cytoplasmic vacuole. Vacuoles are dilated Golgi cisternae or endocytic vesicles containing IgG.

endocytic vesicles containing IgG; the eosinophilic inclusion consists of IgM (Warnke et al, 1995). Signet ring lymphoma cells must be distinguished from the more common signet ring cells associated with gastric and other adenocarcinomas. The latter stain positive for mucin. Signet ring cell lymphomas behave similarly to other follicular lymphomas.

FOLLICULAR LYMPHOMA WITH EXTRACELLULAR EOSINOPHILIC DEPOSITS   Rare cases of follicular lymphoma are characterized by extracellular deposits of eosinophilic, PAS positive, hyaline material in the neoplastic follicles (Figs. 16.22 and 16.23). The material

FIGURE
16.18

FIGURE
16.19

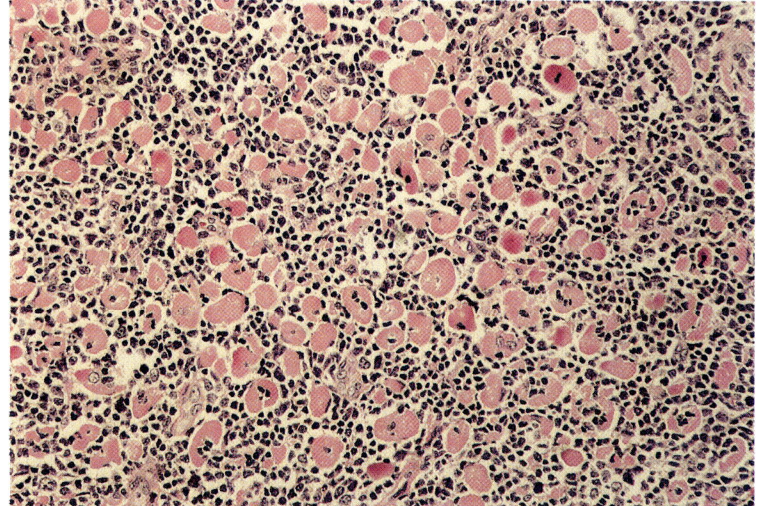

FIGURE 16.20

Follicular lymphoma with eosinophilic cytoplasmic inclusions (Russell-like bodies).

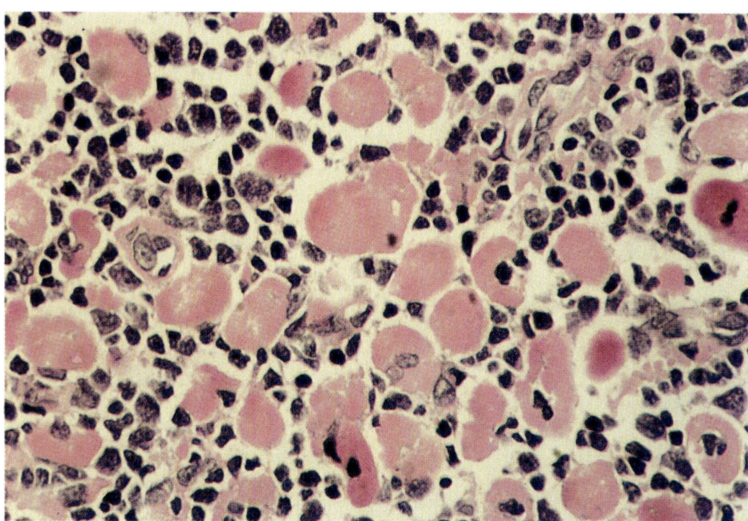

FIGURE 16.21

Follicular lymphoma with eosinophilic cytoplasmic inclusions (Russell-like bodies). The eosinophilc material consists of intracellular accumulation of IgM.

consists of extracellular accumulation of cell membrane and membrane bound vesicles bearing immunoglobulin (Chittal et al, 1987). Follicular lymphomas with extracellular eosinophilic deposits behave similarly to other follicular lymphomas.

OTHER VARIANTS OF FOLLICULAR LYMPHOMA Follicular lymphomas with Homer-Wright rosette-like structures, hyaline-vascular Castleman's disease-like follicles, plasmacytosis, monocytoid B cell differentiation, cerebriform or multilobated nuclei, a "reverse" variant with darkly staining follicles surrounded by transformed cells, and a variant consisting predominantly of small round lymphocytes have been reported rarely

FIGURE
16.22

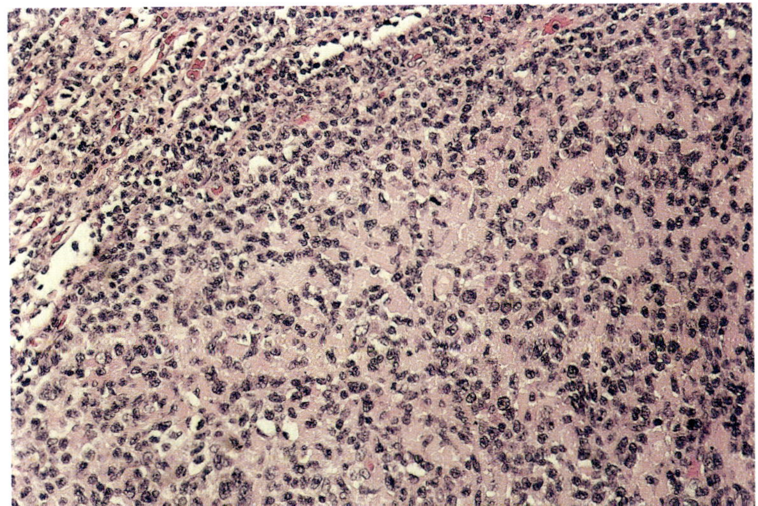

Follicular lymphoma with extracellular eosinophilic deposits.

FIGURE
16.23

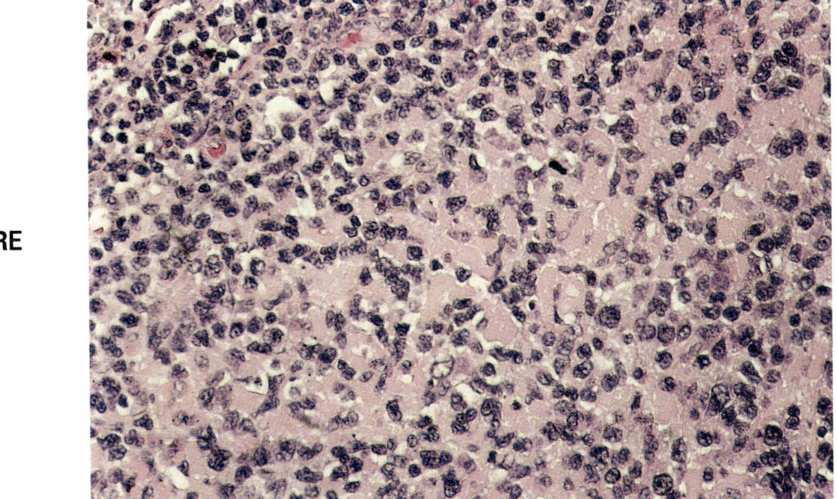

Follicular lymphoma with extracellular eosinophilic deposits. The extracellular material consists of cell membrane and membrane-bound vesicles associated with immunoglobulin.

(Warnke et al, 1995). A blastic variant of follicular lymphoma associated with leukemic
transformation has been reported (Come et al, 1980) but would now be interpreted as
the blastic variant of mantle cell lymphoma (Lardelli et al, 1990).

Transformation of Follicular Lymphoma

Follicular lymphomas may undergo transformation to more aggressive histologic types.
Transformation is characterized by an increasing diffuse component and an increased

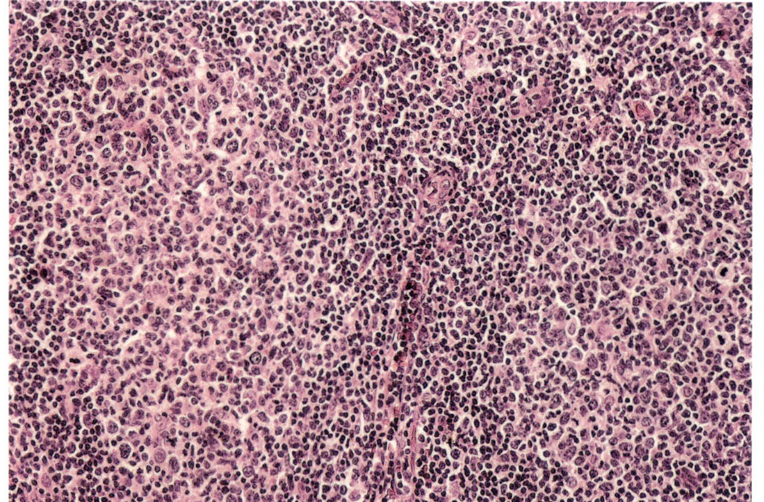

Follicular lymphoma with transformation to large cell anaplastic lymphoma showing follicular lymphoma at initial diagnosis.

FIGURE 16.24

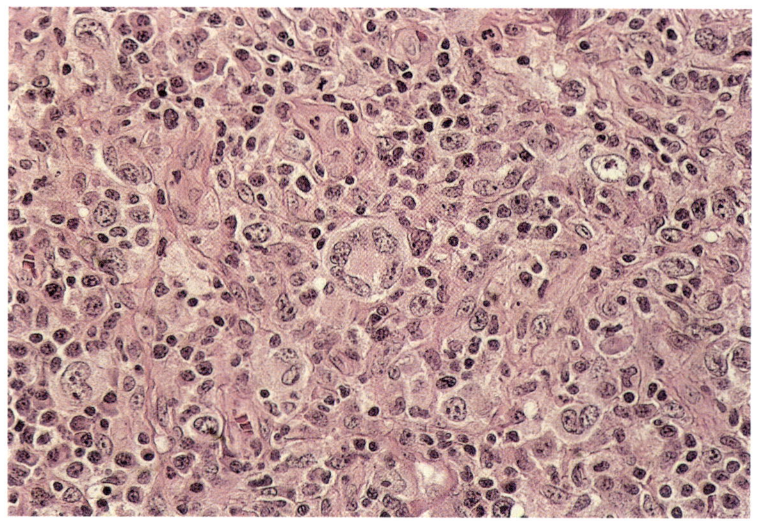

Follicular lymphoma with transformation to large cell anaplastic lymphoma showing CD30 positive large cell anaplastic lymphoma developing 5 years after diagnosis.

FIGURE 16.25

number of large cells. Therefore, malignant lymphoma, follicular, predominantly small cleaved cell (follicle center lymphoma, follicular, small cell type) may eventually transform to diffuse large B cell lymphoma. The risk factors for transformation are unknown. The risk of transformation was 19% in initially untreated patients, and 23% in treated patients, at 8 years of follow-up (Horning and Rosenberg, 1984). Transformation is characterized by additional oncogene mutations in particular mutations of the p53 gene (Lo Coco et al, 1993). Transformation of follicular lymphoma to CD30-positive B cell ana-

**FIGURE
16.26**

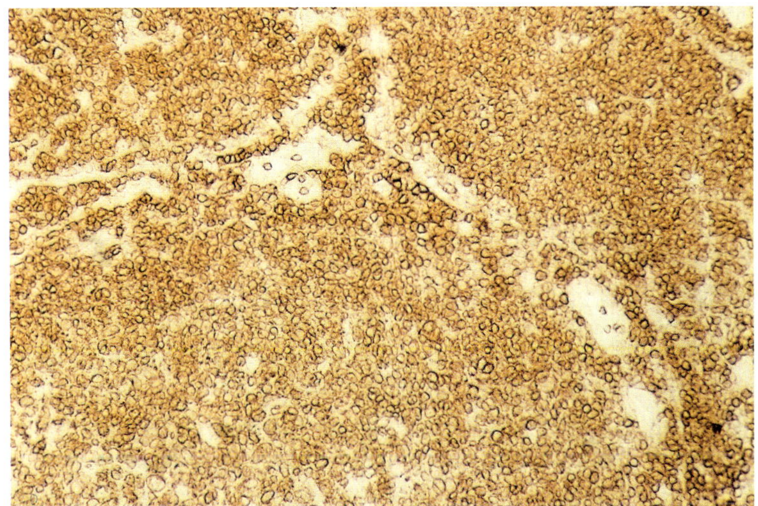

Follicular lymphoma showing positive staining for BCL-2 oncoprotein.

plastic large cell lymphoma has also been recognized (Alsabeh et al, 1997) (Figs. 16.24 and 16.25).

Differential Diagnosis

Follicle center lymphoma, follicular must be distinguished from other lymphomas which may have a nodular or pseudonodular pattern and from reactive follicular lymphoid hyperplasia. The morphological criteria for the recognition of follicular lymphomas and distinction from reactive follicular lymphoid hyperplasia are those enumerated by Nathwani and colleagues (Nathwani et al, 1981). The single most useful criterion identified was the presence throughout the lymph node of abnormally crowded follicles with little or no intervening lymphoid tissue (Nathwani et al, 1981). This pattern was observed in 85% of FL but in no case of reactive follicular lymphoid hyperplasia. Other important criteria were cytologic monotony of the follicles, absence of tingible body macrophages, and presence of follicular center cells outside of follicles. Immunophenotypic and immunohistochemical studies are an important adjunct in the diagnosis of follicular lymphomas. The demonstration of follicular B cell monoclonality by immunoglobulin light chain restriction or the demonstration of follicular BCL-2 oncoprotein overexpression is diagnostic (Ngan et al, 1988). BCL-2 is not expressed in normal or hyperplastic follicular centers but is characteristically expressed in follicle center lymphomas associated with the t(14;18) chromosome translocation (Fig. 16.26). Care must be taken in interpretation, however, since normal mantle cells and a variety of lymphomas unassociated with the t(14;18) translocation (including small lymphocytic lymphomas, mantle cell lymphomas, marginal-zone lymphomas, and peripheral T cell lymphomas) may express BCL-2 oncoprotein (Pezzella et al, 1990). The presence of normal mantle cells staining positively for BCL-2 is a useful internal positive control for immunohistochemical studies. BCL-2 oncoprotein expression may be detected in frozen or deparaffinized tissue (Utz and Swerdlow, 1993). Immunohistochemical studies are also helpful in distinguishing follicular lymphomas from other follicular lymphoid proliferations including Castleman's disease and progressive transformation of germinal centers (Goates et al, 1994).

A variety of other low-grade B cells lymphomas may present a nodular or pseudonodular appearance in the lymph node, including small lymphocytic lymphoma and chronic lymphocytic leukemia with prominent pseudofollicular proliferation centers, mantle cell lymphoma with a nodular or mantle-zone pattern, and marginal-zone lymphomas with colonization of residual follicular centers. Nodular lymphocyte predominance Hodgkin's disease and, rarely, peripheral T cell lymphomas may also present a nodular appearance (Macon et al, 1995). Follicle center lymphoma, follicular is distinguished by the presence of cleaved cells; the cells of mantle cell lymphoma and marginal-zone lymphoma are frequently irregular but are seldom as angular and irregular as the cleaved cells of FL. Immunophenotypic studies are also helpful. Follicular lymphomas are negative for CD5, in contrast to small lymphocytic lymphoma and mantle cell lymphoma, which are CD5 positive. Follicular lymphomas are positive for CD10 (CALLA), in contrast to small lymphocytic, mantle cell, and marginal-zone lymphomas, which are CD10-negative. CD43 is a useful marker in paraffin-embedded tissue. Follicular lymphomas are negative for CD43, in contrast to small lymphocytic lymphoma, mantle cell lymphoma, and marginal-zone lymphoma, which are frequently positive. Follicular lymphomas contain abundant follicular dendritic cells which are recognized by immunohistochemical staining for CD21 and CD35; follicular dendritic cells, however, may also be present in mantle cell and marginal-zone lymphomas and are prominent in nodular lymphocyte predominance Hodgkin's disease. BCL-2 oncoprotein expression is useful in distinguishing follicular lymphoma from follicular lymphoid hyperplasia but is not useful in lymphoma classification, since BCL-2 is frequently expressed in lymphomas unrelated to the t(14;18) translocation (Pezzella et al, 1990).

Course and Prognosis

Follicle center lymphoma, follicular, grade I (small cell) and grade II (mixed small and large cell) are indolent neoplasms with prolonged survival. Therapeutic approaches for patients who present with advanced disease (the great majority are Ann Arbor stage III or IV) range from observation without initial therapy to combination chemotherapy with alkylating-agent– or adriamycin-based regimens (Longo et al, 1984). Observation is a reasonable option for asymptomatic patients. In patients managed without initial therapy, the median time until therapy was required was 3 years, and 20–30% of the patients experienced spontaneous regressions (Horning and Rosenberg, 1984). Responses to conventional chemotherapy in patients with follicle center lymphoma, follicular, grade I (small cell) and II (mixed small and large cell) are generally not durable. In some but not all series, follicle center lymphoma, follicular, grade II (mixed small and large cell) was associated with prolonged initial remission following alkylating based chemotherapy (Longo et al, 1984). Follicle center lymphoma, follicular, grade III (large cell) is an aggressive neoplasm (Bartlett et al, 1994); the long-term natural history is uncertain; however, some responses to therapy may be durable (Martin et al, 1995; Wendum et al, 1997). The possibility that follicle center lymphoma, follicular can be eliminated by high dose chemotherapy with autologous stem cell rescue or bone marrow transplantation is being investigated. Occasional patients presenting with localized involvement with follicle center lymphoma, follicular (Ann Arbor stage I and II) are effectively managed with involved field radiotherapy; approximately 50% remain disease free (Paryani et al, 1983).

Follicle Center Lymphoma, Diffuse

Classification

REAL: Provisional subtype: follicle center lymphoma, diffuse, predominantly small cell type.
WF: Malignant lymphoma, diffuse, small cleaved cell.

Immunophenotype

CD5−, CD10+, CD19+, CD20+, CD22+, CD43−, SIg+.

Molecular Pathology

BCL-2 oncogene rearrangement and t(14;18) chromosomal translocation as in follicle center lymphoma, follicular

Clinical Features

Follicle center lymphoma, diffuse, predominantly small cell type is infrequent. The majority of malignant lymphomas, diffuse, small cleaved cell in the WF are mantle cell lymphomas. Nevertheless, diffuse small cleaved cell lymphomas of follicular center cell origin occur. The clinical features are not well characterized and are probably similar to other follicle center lymphomas.

Histopathology

Follicle center lymphoma, diffuse, predominantly small cell type, is characterized by diffuse infiltration of the lymph node by small cleaved cells, identical to those of follicle center lymphoma, follicular, but lacking a follicular pattern (Figs. 16.27 and 16.28). The small cleaved cells are irregular with angular nuclei. Small numbers of large noncleaved cells are admixed; some cases may be classified as malignant lymphoma, diffuse, mixed small and large cell in the WF.

Differential Diagnosis

Follicle center lymphoma, diffuse, predominantly small cell type, should be distinguished from other low-grade forms of diffuse B cell lymphomas. The lack of follicles may be due to sampling, and in some cases additional sections will show typical follicular lymphoma. Distinction from the occasional small lymphocytic lymphoma with cleaved or irregular cells is based on the absence of pseudofollicular proliferation centers; distinction from mantle cell lymphoma is based on the presence of admixed large

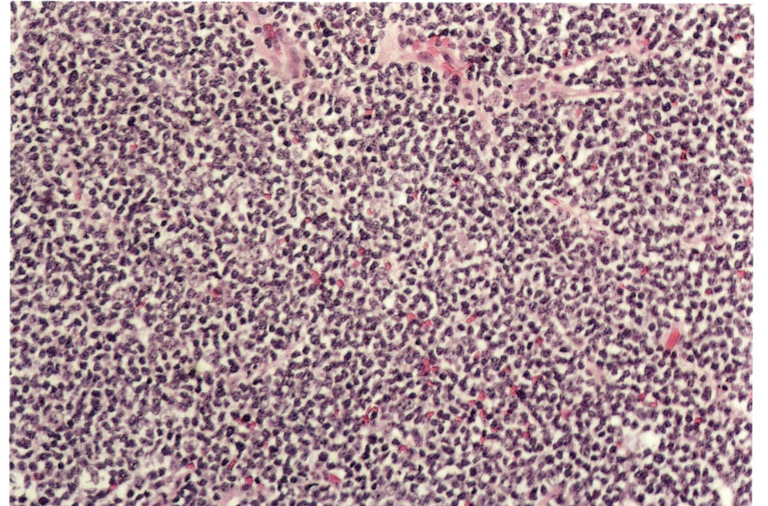

FIGURE 16.27

Follicle center lymphoma, diffuse, predominantly small cell is the diffuse counterpart of follicular small cleaved cell lymphoma.

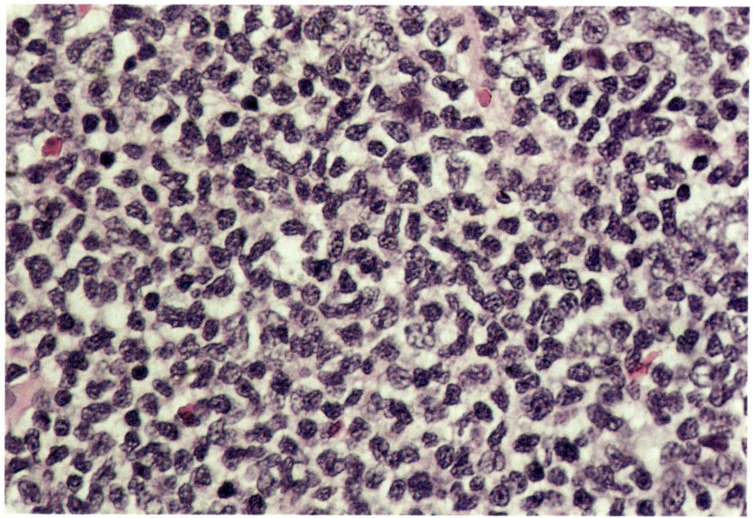

FIGURE 16.28

Follicle center lymphoma, diffuse, predominantly small cell consists of small irregular lymphocytes which are more angular and cleaved than the cells of mantle cell lymphoma or small lymphocytic lymphoma. A small number of large noncleaved cells are usually admixed.

noncleaved cells. Follicle center lymphoma, diffuse, predominantly small cell type shares the typical phenotype of follicular lymphoma (CD5−, CD10+, CD43−), which distinguishes it from other diffuse low grade B cell lymphomas, including small lymphocytic and mantle cell lymphoma (CD5+, CD10−, CD43+) and marginal zone lymphoma (CD5−, CD10−, CD43+).

Course and Prognosis

The natural history of follicle center lymphoma, diffuse, predominantly small cell type is not well characterized but probably differs little from that of other follicle center lymphomas. Responses to therapy are not durable.

REFERENCES

Alsabeh R, Medeiros LJ, Glackin C, Weiss LM. Transformation of follicular lymphoma into CD30–large cell lymphoma with anaplastic cytologic features. Am J Surg Pathol 21:528–536, 1997.

Argatoff LH, Connors JM, Klasa RJ, Horsman DE, Gascoyne RD. Mantle cell lymphoma: A clinicopathologic study of 80 cases. Blood 89:2067–2078, 1997.

Banks PM, Chan J, Cleary ML, Delsol G, De Wolf-Peeters C, Gatter K, et al. Mantle cell lymphoma: A proposal for unification of morphologic, immunologic, and molecular data. Am J Surg Pathol 16:636–640, 1992.

Bartlett NL, Rizeq M, Dorfman RF, Halpern J, Horning SJ. Follicular large cell lymphoma: Intermediate or low grade? J Clin Oncol 12:1349–1357, 1994.

Cheng A-L, Su I-J, Tien H-F, Wang C-C, Chen Y-C, Wang C-H. Characteristic clinicopathologic features of adult B cell lymphoblastic lymphoma with special emphasis on differential diagnosis with an atypical form probably of blastic lymphocytic lymphoma of intermediate differentiation origin. Cancer 73:706–710, 1994.

Chittal SM, Careriviere P, Voight JJ, Dumont J, Benevent B, Raure P, Bordessoule GD, Delsol G. Follicular lymphoma with abundant PAS positive extracellular material. Immunohistochemical and ultrastructural observations. Am J Surg Pathol 11:618–624, 1987.

Come SE, Jaffe ES, Andersen JC et al. Non-Hodgkin's lymphoma in leukemic phase: Clinicopathologic correlations. Am J Med 69:667–674, 1980.

de Boer CJ, Schuuring E, Dreef E, Peters G, Bartek J, Kluin PM, van Krieken JHJM. Cyclin D1 protein analysis in the diagnosis of mantle cell lymphoma. Blood 86:2715–2723, 1995.

Duggan MJ, Weisenberger DD, Ye JL, Bast MA, Pierson JL, Linder J, Armitage JO. Mantle zone lymphoma: A clinicopathologic study of 22 cases. Cancer 66:522–529, 1990.

Fisher RI, Dahlberg S, Nathwani BN, Banks PM, Miller TP, Grogan TM. A clinical analysis of two indolent lymphoma entities: Mantle cell lymphoma and marginal zone lymphoma (including mucosa associated lymphoid tissue and monocytoid B cell subcategories): A southwest oncology group study. Blood 85:1075–1082, 1995.

Goates JJ, Kamel O, LeBrun DP, Benharroch D, Dorfman RF. Floral variant of follicular lymphoma. Immunological and molecular studies support a neoplastic process. Am J Surg Pathol 18:37–47, 1994.

Harris NL. Peripheral B cell neoplasms. In: Society for Hematopathology Program (abstracts). Am J Surg Pathol 21:114–121, 1997.

Horning SJ, Rosenberg SA. The natural history of initially untreated low grade non-Hodgkin's lymphomas. N Engl J Med 311:1471–1475, 1984.

Inghirami G, Foitl D, Sabichi A, Zhu B, Knowles D. Autoantibody-associated cross-reactive idiotype bearing human B lymphocytes: Distribution and characterization, including IgVH gene and CD5 antigen expression. Blood 78:1503, 1991.

Lardelli P, Bookman MA, Sundeen J, Longo DL, Jaffe ES. Lymphocytic lymphoma of intermediate differentiation: Morphologic and immunophenotypic spectrum and clinical correlations. Am J Surg Pathol 14:752–763, 1990.

Limpens J, Stad R, Vos C, de Vlaam C, de Jong D, van Ommen G-Jb, Schuuring E, Kluin PM. Lymphoma-associated tranlocation t(14;18) in blood B cells of normal individuals. Blood 85:2528–2536, 1995.

Lo Coco F, Gaidano G, Louie DC, Offit K, Chaganti RSK, Dalla-Favera R. p53 mutations are associated with histologic transformation of follicular lymphoma. Blood 82:2289–2295, 1993.

Longo DL, Young RC, Hubbard SM, Wesley M, Fisher RI, Jaffe E, Berard C, DeVita VT. Prolonged initial remission in patients with nodular mixed lymphoma. Ann Intern Med 100:651–656, 1984.

Macon WR, Williams ME, Greer JP, Cousar JB. Paracortical nodular T cell lymphoma. Identification of an unusual variant of peripheral T cell lymphoma. Am J Surg Pathol 19:297–303, 1995.

Majlis A, Pugh WC, Rodriguez MA, Benedict WF, Cabanillas F. Mantle cell lymphoma: Correlation of clinical outcome and biologic features with three histologic variants. J Clin Oncol 15:1664–1671, 1997.

Mann RB, Berard CW. Criteria for the cytologic subclassification of follicular lymphomas: A proposed alternative method. Hematol Oncol 1:187–192, 1983.

Martin AR, Weisenberger DD, Chan WC, Ruby EI, Andersen JR, Vose JM, Bierman PJ, Bast MA, Daley DT, Armitage JO. Prognostic value of cellular proliferation and histologic grade in follicular lymphoma. Blood 85:3671–3678, 1995.

Moynihan MJ, Bast MA, Chan WC, Delabie J, Wickert RS, Guanquing W, Weisenberger DD. Lymphomatous polyposis: A neoplasm of either follicular mantle or germinal center cell origin. Am J Surg Pathol 20:442–452, 1996.

Nathwani BN, Winberg C, Diamond LW, Bearman RM, Kim H. Morphologic criteria for the differentiation of follicular lymphoma from florid reactive follicular hyperplasia: A study of 80 cases. Cancer 48:1794–1806, 1981.

Ngan B-Y, Chen-Levy Z, Weiss LM, Warnke RA, Cleary ML. Expression in non-Hodgkin's lymphoma of the bcl-2 protein associated with the t(14;18) chromosomal translocation. N Engl J Med 318:1638–1644, 1988.

O'Briain DS, Kennedy MJ, Daly PA, O'Brien AAJ, Tanner WA, Rogers P, Lawlor E. Multiple lymphomatous polyposis of the gastrointestinal tract: A clinicopathologically distinctive form of non-Hodgkin's lymphoma of B cell centrocytic type. Am J Surg Pathol 13:691–699, 1989.

Osborne BM, Butler JJ. Follicular lymphoma mimicking progressive transformation of germinal centers. Am J Clin Pathol 88:264–269, 1987.

Paryani SB, Hoppe RT, Cox RS, Colby TV, Rosenberg SA, Kaplan HS. Analysis of non-Hodgkin's lymphomas with nodular and favorable histologies, Stage I and II. Cancer 52:2300–2307, 1983.

Pezzella F, Tse AG, Cordell JL, Pulford KA, Gatter DC, Mason DY. Expression of bcl-2 oncoprotein is not specific for the t(14;18) chromosome translocation. Am J Pathol 137:225–232, 1990.

Pinto A, Hutchinson RE, Grant LH, Trevenen CL, Berard CW. Follicular lymphomas in pediatric patients. Mod Pathol 3:308–313, 1990.

Stewart AK, Schwartz RS. Immunoglobulin V regions and the B cell. Blood 83:1717–1730, 1994.

Utz GL, Swerdlow SH. Distinction of follicular hyperplasia from follicular lymphoma in B5 fixed tissue: Comparison of MT2 and bcl-2 antibodies. Hum Pathol 24:1155–1158, 1993.

Vadlamudi G, Lionetti KA, Greenberg S, Mehta K. Leukemic phase of mantle cell lymphoma. Two case reports and review of the literature. Arch Pathol Lab Med 120:35–40, 1996.

Warnke RA, Kim H, Fuks Z, Dorfman RF. The coexistence of nodular and diffuse patterns in nodular non-Hodgkin's lymphomas: Significance and clinicopathologic correlation. Cancer 40:1229–1233, 1977.

Warnke RA, Weiss LM, Chan JKC, Cleary ML, Dorfman RF. Tumors of the lymph nodes and spleen. In: Atlas of Tumor Pathology, Third series, Fascicle 14. Rosai J, Sobin LH, eds. Washington, D.C.: Armed Forces Institute of Pathology, 1995.

Weisenberger DD, Armitage JO. Mantle cell lymphoma—an entity comes of age. Blood 87:4483–4494, 1996.

Weiss LM, Warnke RA, Sklar J, Cleary ML. Molecular analysis of the t(14;18) chromosome translocation in malignant lymphomas. N Engl J Med 317:1185–1189, 1987.

Wendum D, Sebban C, Gaulard P, Coiffier B, Tilly H, Cazals D, et al. Follicular large-cell lymphoma treated with intensive chemotherapy: An analysis of 89 cases included in the LNH87 trial and comparison with the outcome of diffuse large B-cell lymphoma. J Clin Oncol 15:1654–1663, 1997.

Yatabe Y, Nakamura S, Seto M, Kuroda H, Kagami Y, Suzuki R et al. Clinicopathologic study of PRAD1/Cyclin D1 overexpressing lymphoma with special reference to mantle cell lymphoma. A distinct molecular pathologic entity. Am J Surg Pathol 20:1110–1122, 1996.

Zoldan MC, Inghirami G, Masuda Y, Vanderkerckhove F, Raphael B, Amorosi E, Hymes K, Frizzera G. Large-cell variants of mantle cell lymphoma: Cytologic characteristics and p53 anomalies may predict poor outcome. Br J Haematol 93:475–486, 1996.

17

Peripheral B Cell Neoplasms: III. Marginal-Zone B Cell Lymphoma, Hairy Cell Leukemia, and Plasmacytoma/Plasma Cell Myeloma

Marginal-zone B cell lymphoma, splenic marginal-zone lymphoma, hairy cell leukemia, and plasmacytoma/plasma cell myeloma are B cell neoplasms which are frequently extranodal and exhibit plasmacytoid differentiation.

Marginal-Zone B Cell Lymphoma

Classification

REAL: Marginal zone B cell lymphoma, extranodal (MALT type +/- monocytoid B cells); provisional subtype: nodal (+/- monocytoid B cells).
WF: Malignant lymphoma, small lymphocytic.

Immunophenotype

CD5−, CD10−, CD11c+, CD19+, CD20+, CD22+, CD23−, CD43+ or −, SIg+, CIg may be +.

Clinical Features

Marginal-zone B cell lymphoma (MZBL) includes extranodal low-grade B cell lymphoma of mucosa-associated lymphoid tissue (MALT) type and nodal monocytoid B cell lymphoma (Sheibani et al, 1988). Evidence suggests the two are related; lymph node involvement in cases of extranodal low-grade B cell lymphoma of MALT type may be indistinguishable from monocytoid B cell lymphoma; trisomy 3 or trisomy 18 is frequently present in both (Dierlamm et al, 1996).

MZBL of extranodal (MALT) type is a low-grade lymphoma which occurs in the salivary glands, orbit, lung, stomach and gastrointestinal tract, thymus, and other sites, including the dura and skin (Bailey et al, 1996; Kumar et al, 1997). MZBL accounts for the great majority of low-grade B cell lymphomas of extranodal sites. Prior to the advent of immunophenotypic studies these lesions were often considered "pseudolymphomas" because of the frequent presence of plasma cells and reactive lymphoid follicles and the indolent natural history following surgical resection. MZBL of extranodal (MALT) type of the stomach is uniquely associated with infection with *Helicobacter pylori;* the lymphoma frequently regresses following eradication of the infection (Roggero et al, 1995; Wotherspoon et al, 1993). MZBL of extranodal (MALT) type usually presents as localized extranodal disease (Ann Arbor stage I or IIE); systemic dissemination may occur and frequently involves other extranodal MALT sites. Lymph node involvement may be indistinguishable from MZBL of nodal (monocytoid B cell) type. The natural history of systemic MZBL of extranodal (MALT) type is similar to that of other systemic low-grade B cell lymphomas (Fisher et al, 1995). Transformation to diffuse large B cell lymphoma may occur; transformation of underlying MZBL of extranodal (MALT) type accounts for the development of some diffuse large B cell lymphomas of extranodal sites (Hsi et al, 1998).

MZBL of nodal type (monocytoid B cell lymphoma, parafollicular B cell lymphoma) occurs in lymph nodes with involvement of extranodal sites and salivary glands (Cousar et al, 1987; Sheibani et al, 1988). Extranodal involvement is indistinguishable from MZBL of extranodal (MALT) type. Monocytoid B cell lymphoma is frequently associated with Sjögren's syndrome (Sheibani et al, 1988). MZBL of nodal (monocytoid B cell) type most frequently presents as localized lymphadenopathy (Ann Arbor stage I or II); systemic dissemination and bone marrow involvement may occur, but is less frequent than in other low-grade B cell lymphomas (Sheibani et al, 1988). The natural history of systemic MZBL of nodal (monocytoid B cell) type is indolent (Fisher et al, 1995). Transformation to diffuse large B cell lymphoma may occur.

Histopathology

MARGINAL-ZONE B CELL LYMPHOMA, EXTRANODAL (MALT) TYPE   MZBL of extranodal (MALT) type is characterized by proliferation of small lymphocytes with admixture of monocytoid B cells, centrocyte-like cells, plasma cells, and admixed large cells (Figs. 17.1 and 17.2). Reactive follicular centers are frequently present and may become colonized with neoplastic cells. Lymphoepithelial lesions, characterized by infiltration of epithelial structures by neoplastic B cells, are an important diagnostic feature (Figs. 17.3 and 17.4). Lymph node involvement in MZBL of extranodal (MALT) type may be indistinguishable from MZBL of nodal (monocytoid B cell) type (Figs. 17.5 and 17.6).

FIGURE
17.1

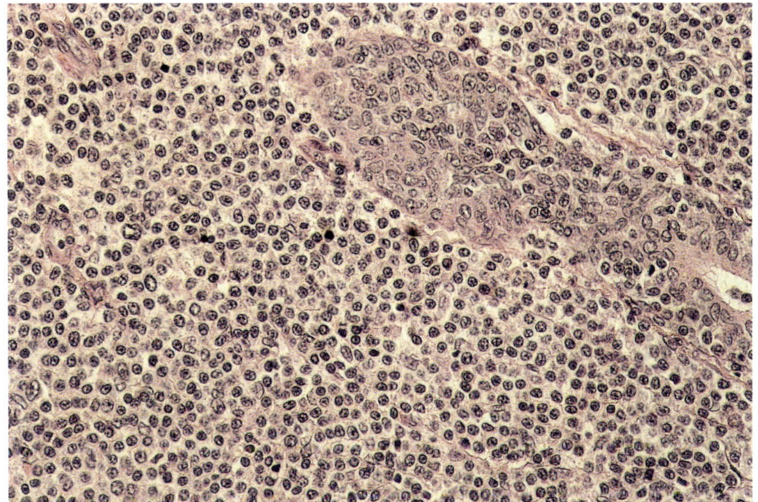

Marginal-zone B cell lymphoma, extranodal (MALT) type, involving parotid salivary gland, showing monocytoid lymphocytes and epimyoepithelial island.

FIGURE
17.2

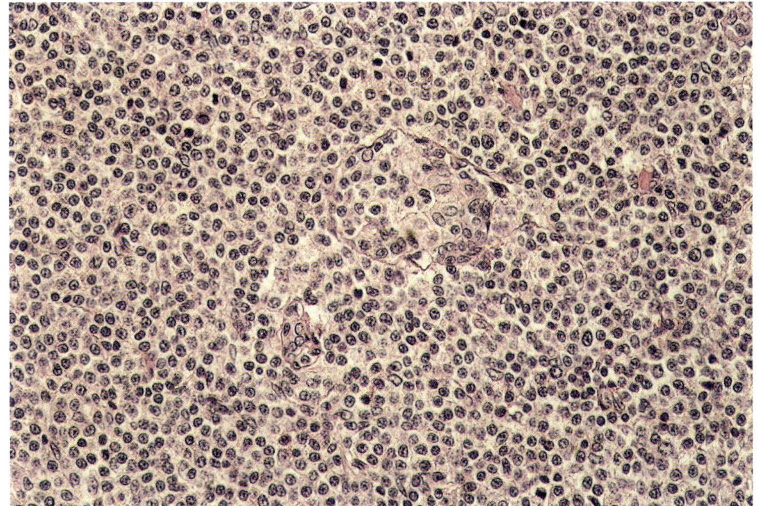

Marginal-zone B cell lymphoma, extranodal (MALT) type, involving parotid salivary gland, showing infiltration of an epimyoepithelial island (at center).

MARGINAL-ZONE B CELL LYMPHOMA, NODAL TYPE   MZBL of nodal type is characterized by proliferation of monocytoid B cells in the sinuses, paracortex, and parafollicular areas of the lymph node (Figs. 17.7, 17.8, and 17.9). The monocytoid B cells, which resemble the reactive monocytoid B cells of toxoplasmic lymphadenitis, are characterized by bland, round to ovoid nuclei, inconspicuous nucleoli, and abundant clear to faintly eosinophilic cytoplasm (Sheibani et al, 1988). Polymorphonuclear leukcoytes and large lymphoid cells may be admixed. Plasmacytoid differentiation is frequent and may

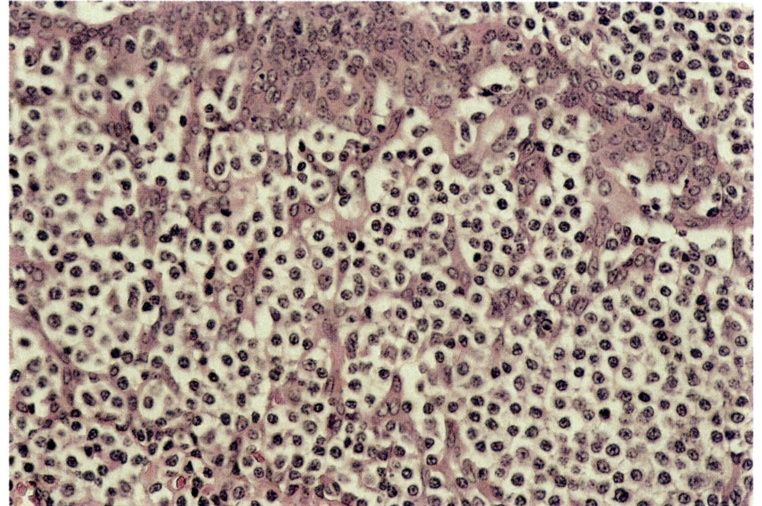

FIGURE 17.3

Marginal-zone B cell lymphoma, extranodal (MALT) type, involving parotid salivary gland, showing infiltration of an epimyoepithelial island, forming a "lymphoepithelial lesion."

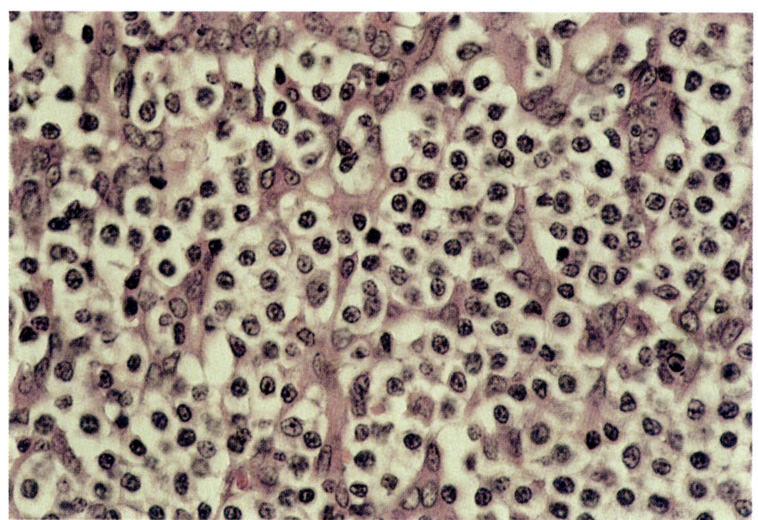

FIGURE 17.4

Marginal-zone B cell lymphoma, extranodal (MALT) type, involving parotid salivary gland, higher magnification of a lymphoepithelial lesion showing infiltration by monocytoid cells.

be focal with aggregates of mature plasma cells (Fig. 17.10). Mitoses are scant. In some cases, proliferation of monocytoid B cells is confined to the lymph node sinuses, a pattern which has been referred to as "localized" or "in situ" monocytoid B cell lymphoma (Sheibani et al, 1988).

Differential Diagnosis

MZBL of extranodal (MALT) type must be distinguished from extranodal lymphoid hyperplasia and from other types of low-grade B cell lymphoma. Distinction from extra-

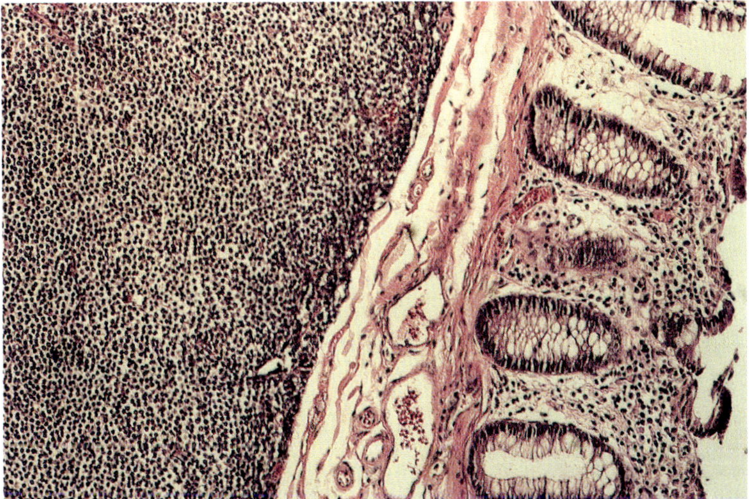

Marginal-zone B cell lymphoma, extranodal (MALT) type, involving the colon.

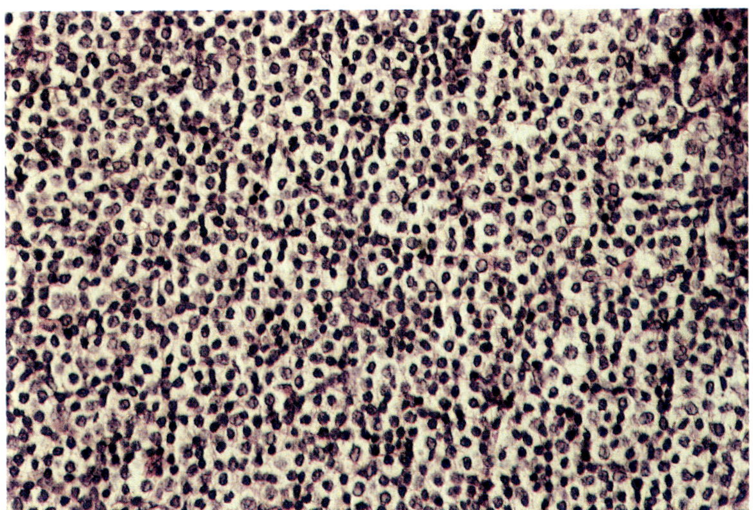

Marginal-zone B cell lymphoma, extranodal (MALT) type of colon, show-ing involvement of a regional lymph node. The histopathologic findings are indistinguishable from marginal-zone B cell lymphoma of nodal (monocytoid B cell) type.

nodal lymphoid hyperplasia may be difficult on morphological grounds alone because of the polymorphous cell population and reactive follicular centers encountered in MALT lymphomas. Irregular centrocyte-like cells, intranuclear Dutcher bodies, and lymphoepi-thelial lesions are features favoring MALT lymphoma. In difficult cases, determination of B cell clonality by immunoglobulin light chain restriction is frequently diagnostic. Immunohistochemical studies for CD43 on deparaffinized sections may also be helpful; CD43 expression on B cells favors lymphoma; however, plasma cells may normally ex-press CD43.

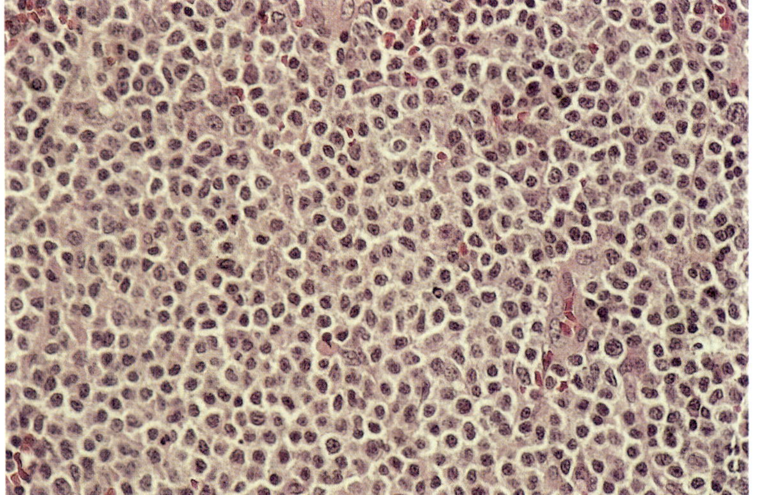

FIGURE 17.7

Marginal-zone B cell lymphoma, nodal (monocytoid B cell) type.

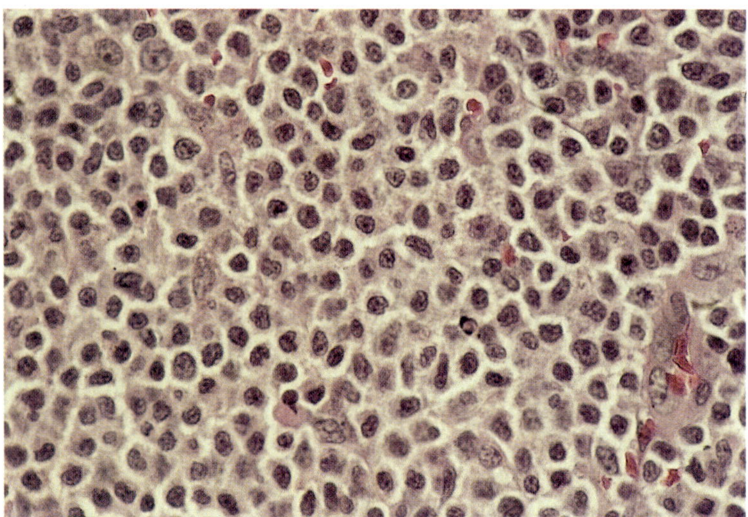

FIGURE 17.8

Marginal-zone B cell lymphoma, nodal (monocytoid B cell) type, higher magnification, showing cells resembling the monocytoid cells seen in toxoplasmic lymphadenitis and other reactive lymphadenopathies.

MZBL of extranodal (MALT) type should also be distinguished from extranodal involvement with other forms of low-grade B cell lymphoma, including CLL and SLL, mantle cell lymphoma, and follicle center cell lymphoma. CLL and SLL are distinguished by pseudofollicular proliferation centers and CD5-positive phenotype; rare CD5-positive extranodal marginal-zone lymphomas have been reported (Ferry et al, 1996). Mantle cell lymphoma is distinguished by more monotonous cytology, paucity of admixed plasma cells and large lymphoid cells, paucity of lymphoepithelial lesions, and CD5-positive phenotype. The residual follicular centers in MZBL are frequently surrounded by an attenuated mantle zone, in contrast to the naked follicular centers of mantle cell lymphoma. MZBL of extranodal (MALT) type may be associated with colonization of

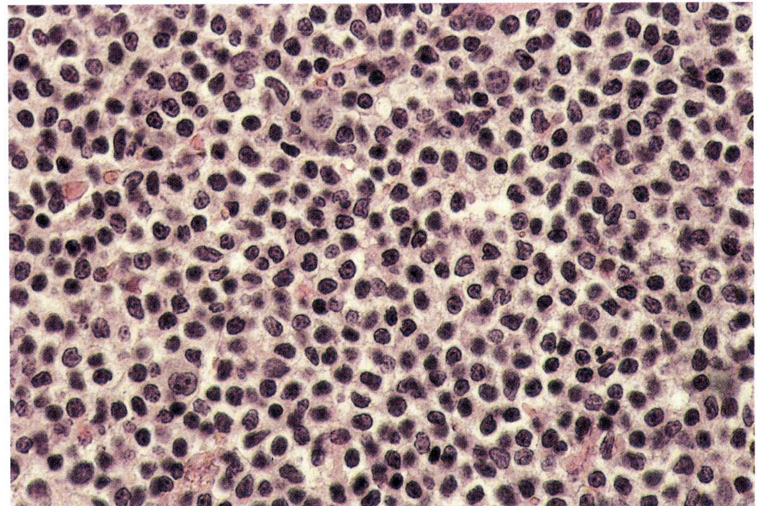

Marginal-zone B cell lymphoma, nodal (monocytoid B cell) type.

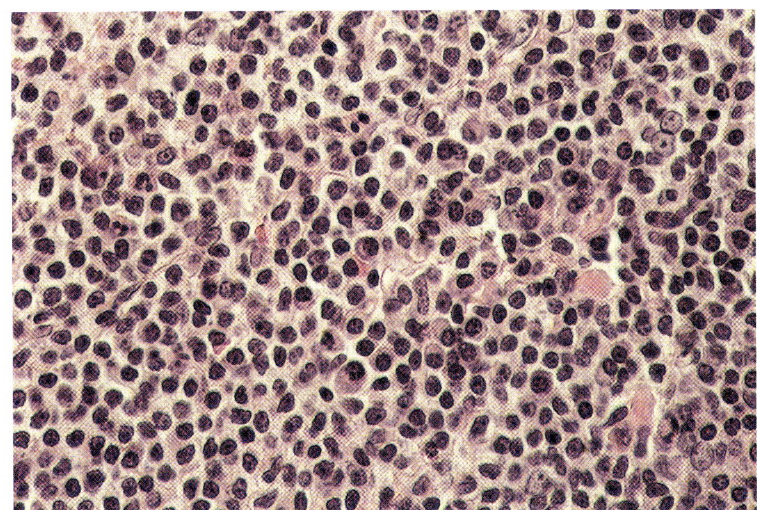

Marginal-zone B cell lymphoma, nodal (monocytoid B cell) type, showing plasmacytoid differentiation.

residual follicular centers by marginal-zone lymphoma cells, mimicking follicle center lymphoma. Distinction is based on the presence of other features of marginal-zone lymphoma and immunophenotypic studies.

MZBL of nodal (monocytoid B cell) type must be distinguished from monocytoid B cell hyperplasia, which frequently accompanies follicular lymphoid hyperplasia, including toxoplasmic lymphadenitis and persistent generalized lymphadenopathy associated with HIV infection. In cases of MZBL confined to the lymph node sinuses (the localized or in situ form of monocytoid B cell lymphoma), demonstration of B cell clonality by immunoglobulin light chain restriction may be necessary for diagnosis (Sheibani et al, 1988).

MZBL of nodal (monocytoid B cell) type should be distinguished from other low-grade forms of nodal B cell lymphoma, including CLL and SLL, and mantle cell lymphoma. CLL and SLL are distinguished by small lymphocytes with scant cytoplasm, presence of pseudofollicular proliferation centers, and CD5-positive phenotype. Mantle cell lymphoma is distinguished by cells with irregular or cleaved nuclei, presence of mitoses, and CD5-positive phenotype. The residual follicular centers in MZBL are separated from the monocytoid B cells by an intact mantle zone; the residual follicular centers in mantle cell lymphoma are naked. Unlike other low-grade B cell lymphomas, MZBL is frequently positive for CD11c (Sheibani et al, 1988). MZBL of nodal (monocytoid B cell) type may be indistinguishable from lymph node involvement in cases of MZBL of extranodal (MALT) type (Dierlamm et al, 1996). Monocytoid B cell lymphoma may closely resemble extramedullary involvement in hairy cell leukemia (Sheibani et al, 1988).

Course and Prognosis

MZBL of extranodal (MALT) type is frequently localized and cured by surgical resection. MZBL of the stomach frequently regresses following eradication of *Helicobacter pylori* infection with antibiotic therapy. Complete regression occurs in up to 60% of patients but may be delayed for up to 6 or more months (Roggero et al, 1995). The natural history of disseminated MZBL of extranodal (MALT) type appears similar to that of other systemic low-grade forms of B cell lymphoma with lack of durable responses to therapy (Fisher et al, 1996). The natural history of MZBL of nodal (monocytoid B cell) type is indolent (Sheibani et al, 1988); survival appears to be better than in other low-grade forms of B cell lymphoma (Fisher et al, 1996). Transformation to diffuse large B cell lymphoma may occur.

Splenic Marginal-Zone Lymphoma

Classification

REAL: Provisional entity: splenic marginal zone lymphoma (+/- villous lymphocytes).
WF: Malignant lymphoma, small lymphocytic.

Immunophenotype

CD5 −, CD10 −, CD11c + or −, CD19 +, CD20 +, CD22 +, CD23 −, CD25 − or +, SIg +.

Clinical Features

Splenic marginal-zone lymphoma (SMZL) and splenic lymphoma with villous lymphocytes (SLVL) are closely related entities which are clinicopathologically distinct from MZBL of extranodal (MALT) and nodal (monocytoid B cell) types. Patients with SMZL and SLVL are adults presenting with splenomegaly and anemia; peripheral lymphadenopathy is infrequent. Patients with SLVL have, in addition, moderate lymphocytosis, characterized by circulating atypical lymphocytes with scant basophilic cytoplasm and

FIGURE
17.11

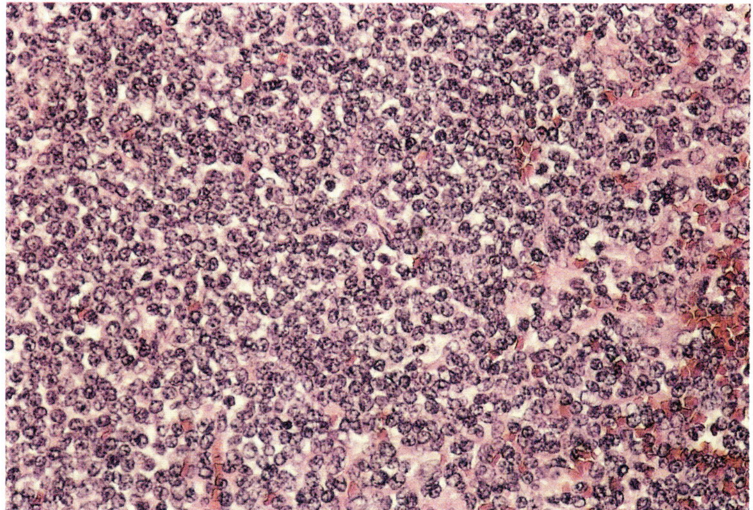

Splenic marginal-zone lymphoma showing involvement of the red and white pulp of the spleen.

FIGURE
17.12

Splenic marginal-zone lymphoma, higher magnification, showing splenic infiltrates composed of medium-sized lymphocytes with round to ovoid nuclei.

irregular cytoplasmic projections (Matutes et al, 1994). The circulating cells may mimic those of hairy cell leukemia or chronic lymphocytic leukemia. An IgM monoclonal paraprotein is frequently present.

Histopathology

The histopathology of SMZL and SLVL is virtually identical (Hammer et al, 1996; Isaacson et al, 1994). Splenic involvement is characterized by infiltration of the red and white

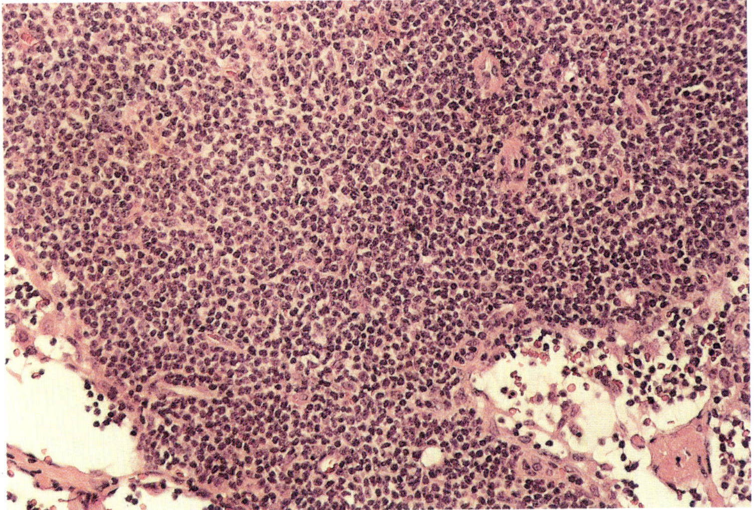

FIGURE 17.13

Splenic marginal-zone lymphoma showing involvement of splenic hilar lymph node with infiltration of the marginal zone and preservation of the sinuses.

pulp by small to medium-sized lymphocytes with round to ovoid nuclei and moderately abundant cytoplasm and admixed larger lymphoid cells (Figs. 17.11 and 17.12). The marginal and mantle zones of the splenic white pulp are expanded; residual follicular centers are frequently present and may be involuted or hyperplastic. Splenic hilar lymph nodes are frequently involved; the marginal and mantle zones are expanded with preservation of the sinuses (Fig. 17.13); residual follicular centers may be present (Mollejo et al, 1997).

Differential Diagnosis

SMZL is distinguished from SLVL principally by the absence of lymphocytes with villous projections (Hammer et al, 1996). SMZL may be difficult to distinguish histologically from other low-grade B cell lymphomas involving the spleen, including CLL and SLL, lymphoplasmacytoid lymphoma, mantle cell lymphoma, MZBL of nodal (monocytoid B cell) or extranodal (MALT) type, and follicle center lymphoma. Differential diagnosis is aided by the clinicopathologic and immunophenotypic features (Isaacson et al, 1994). SLVL may mimic hairy cell leukemia or chronic lymphocytic leukemia. The immunophenotype of SLVL is heterogeneous (Matutes et al, 1994). SLVL lacks the characteristic histopathologic features of hairy cell leukemia in the bone marrow and spleen and is tartrate-resistant acid phosphatase negative; a sinusoidal pattern of bone marrow involvement may be evident (Labouyrie et al, 1997).

Course and Prognosis

SMZL and SLVL are indolent disorders. Clinical improvement frequently follows splenectomy.

Hairy Cell Leukemia

Classification

REAL: Hairy cell leukemia.
WF: Unclassified.

Immunophenotype

CD5 −, CD10 −, CD11c +, CD19 +, CD20 +, CD22 +, CD25 +, SIg +.

Clinical Features

Hairy cell leukemia (HCL, formerly leukemic reticuloendotheliosis) is a chronic lympho-proliferative disorder of adults characterized by the presence in the spleen, bone marrow, and peripheral blood of lymphoid cells with characteristic "hairy" cytoplasmic projections (Catovsky et al, 1974). The hairy cells are characterized by ovoid to bilobed nuclei, abundant clear cytoplasm, and delicate cytoplasmic projections best seen by phase contrast or electron microscopy; in conventionally stained smears or touch imprints the projections appear as a "fuzzy" cell border; in routine histologic sections they are not appreciated at all. Hairy cells exhibit a distinct phenotype characterized by bright positivity for CD11c, CD22, and CD25 (Robbins et al, 1993). The presence of tartrate-resistant acid phosphatase (TRAP) is characteristic. Hairy cells correspond to a late stage in B cell development with pre-plasma cell differentiation (Anderson et al, 1985). A variant of hairy cell leukemia presents with immature blastic-appearing cells (Diez Martin et al, 1987).

Patients with hairy cell leukemia are usually elderly men with pancytopenia and splenomegaly; lymphadenopathy is infrequent. The white blood cell count is most often low and few hairy cells are present in the peripheral blood smear; rarely, overt leukemia with numerous circulating hairy cells is present. The bone marrow is frequently inaspirable due to reticulin fibrosis.

Histopathology

Splenic involvement in hairy cell leukemia is characterized by red pulp infiltration with hairy cells, with small to medium-sized, round to ovoid nuclei, and abundant clear to eosinophilic cytoplasm (Fig. 17.14). The individual cells frequently have a distinctive "fried egg" appearance. The infiltrate is characteristically loosely arranged, with admixed red blood cells, and formation of blood filled spaces lined by hairy cells (pseudosinuses) (Fig. 17.15). The white pulp is atrophic. The bone marrow in hairy cell leukemia is characterized by "loose" infiltrates of hairy cells with reticulin fibrosis. Plasma cells are frequently admixed. Lymph node involvement is infrequent in hairy cell leukemia and is characterized by patchy, subcapsular, interfollicular, or diffuse infiltrates of hairy cells, with frequent preservation of the follicles (Figs. 17.16, 17.17, and 17.18).

Differential Diagnosis

Hairy cell leukemia should be distinguished from other low-grade B cell lymphoproliferative disorders with circulating abnormal lymphocytes and splenomegaly, including

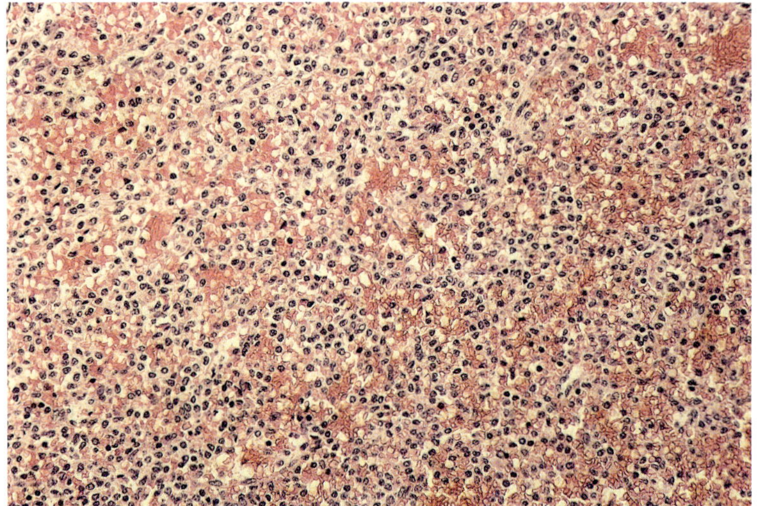

FIGURE
17.14

Hairy cell leukemia showing splenic involvement with infiltration of the red pulp by cytologically bland cells with clear to eosinophilic cytoplasm.

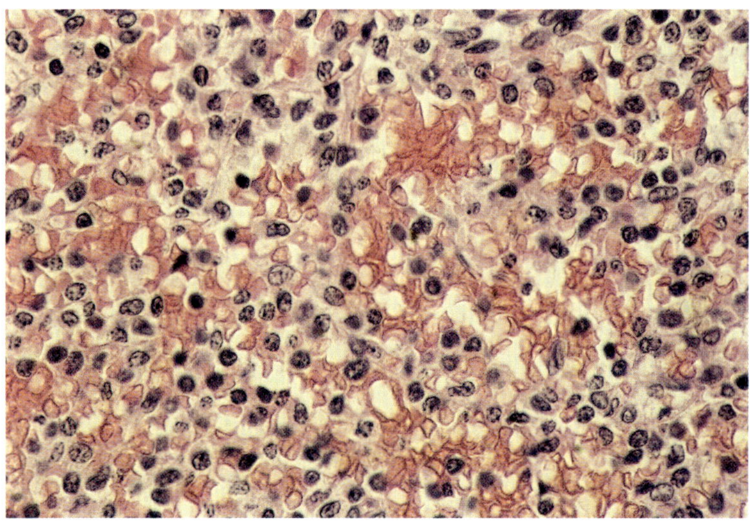

FIGURE
17.15

Hairy cell leukemia, higher magnification, showing splenic red pulp infiltration with formation of blood filled spaces lined by hairy cells ("pseudosinuses").

chronic lymphocytic leukemia, prolymphocytic leukemia, leukemic phase of mantle cell or follicle center lymphoma (lymphosarcoma cell leukemia), and splenic lymphoma with villous lymphocytes. The immunophenotype of hairy cell leukemia, with strong staining for CD11c, CD22, and CD25, is characteristic and usually permits distinction (Robbins et al, 1993). Splenic lymphoma with villous lymphocytes, however, may express CD11c and CD25 (Matutes et al, 1994). Tartrate-resistant acid phosphatase is positive in almost all cases of hairy cell leukemia but is occasionally also positive in other

FIGURE
17.16

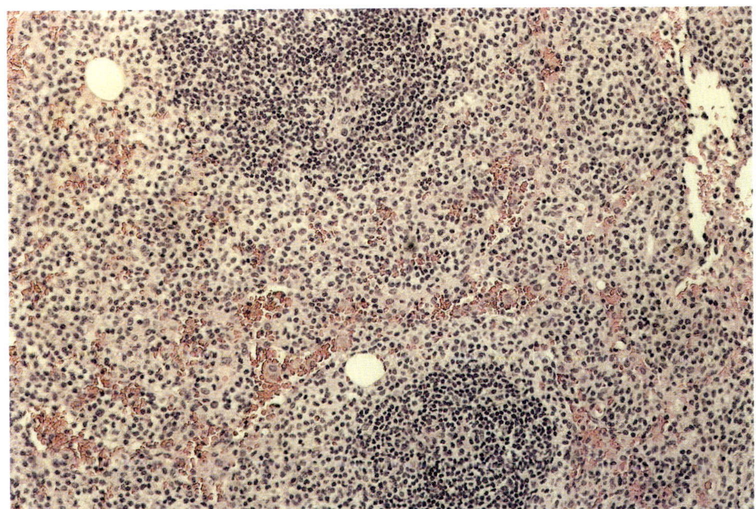

Hairy cell leukemia, lymph node involvement, showing interfollicular pattern of infiltration with preservation of the follicles.

FIGURE
17.17

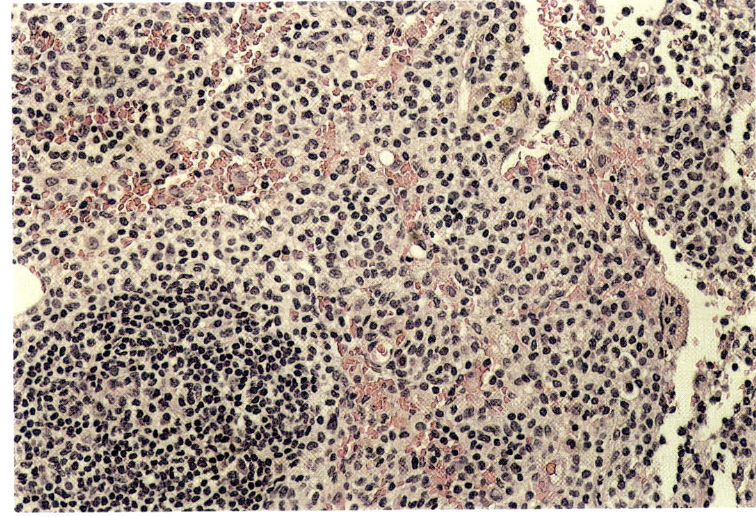

Hairy cell leukemia, lymph node involvement, showing infiltration of the marginal zone.

low-grade B cell lymphoproliferative disorders. The histopathological findings in the bone marrow in hairy cell leukemia are characteristic.

Lymph node involvement or extramedullary infiltrates in hairy cell leukemia may closely resemble marginal-zone B cell lymphoma of nodal (monocytoid B cell) type (Fig 17.19). Hairy cells bear a striking resemblance to monocytoid B cells morphologically, may have a similar pattern of lymph node involvement, and express CD11c (Sheibani et al, 1988). MZBL of nodal (monocytoid B cell) type, however, typically presents as local-

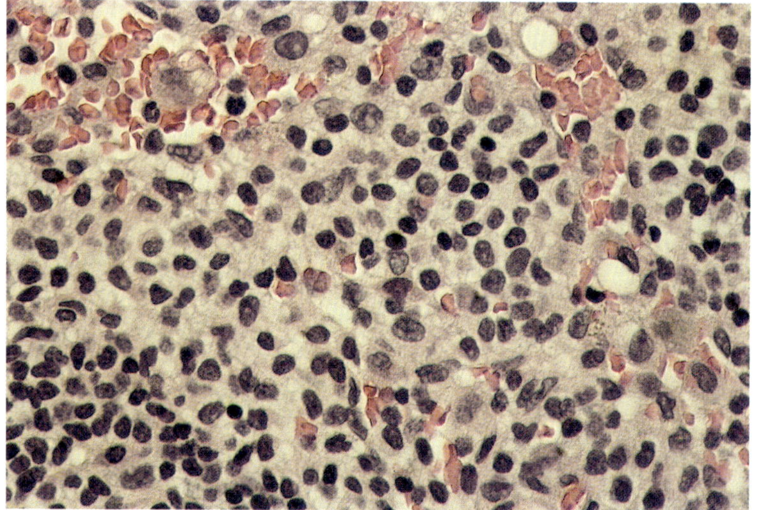

FIGURE 17.18

Hairy cell leukemia, lymph node involvement, higher magnification, showing characteristic hairy cells.

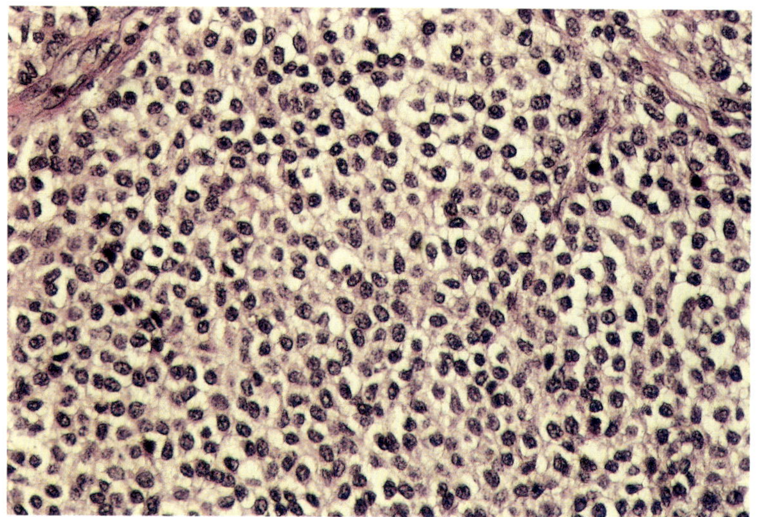

FIGURE 17.19

Hairy cell leukemia, extramedullary infiltrates, mimicking marginal-zone B cell lymphoma of nodal (monocytoid B cell) type.

ized lymph node involvement (Ann Arbor stage I or II); peripheral blood and bone marrow findings characteristic of hairy cell leukemia, TRAP, and bright CD25 positivity are absent.

Course and Prognosis

Hairy cell leukemia is an indolent disorder which, until recently, was usually treated with splenectomy or interferon-α. Introduction of the purine analogue, 2-chlorodeoxyadenosine, has revolutionized the treatment of hairy cell leukemia, with durable complete responses in up to 90% of cases, following a single 7-day infusion (Piro et al, 1990).

The availability of specific therapy for hairy cell leukemia makes accurate recognition and diagnosis critical.

Plasmacytoma/Plasma Cell Myeloma

Classification

REAL: Plasmacytoma/plasma cell myeloma.
WF: Extramedullary plasmacytoma.

Immunophenotype

CD5 , CD10   or I , CD19 −, CD20 −, CD22 −, CD38 +, CD45 − or +, EMA +, SIg −, CIg +.

Clinical Features

Plasmacytoma/plasma cell myeloma is a neoplasm of differentiated plasma cells, usually associated with disseminated skeletal involvement and monoclonal serum immunoglobulin. Solitary plasmacytomas of bone and extramedullary plasmacytomas of the upper respiratory tract and other locations also occur. Plasmacytomas of lymph nodes are infrequent and may be a manifestation of disseminated plasma cell myeloma, metastasis of extramedullary plasmacytoma (Fishkin and Spiegelberg, 1976), or, rarely, primary extramedullary lymph node plasmacytoma (Addis et al, 1980). Kaposi's sarcoma–associated herpesvirus, the genome of which contains a homolog of human interleukin-6, a plasma cell growth factor, has recently been identified in the bone marrow stromal cells of patients with plasma cell myeloma (Rettig et al, 1997).

Histopathology

Lymph node involvement in plasmacytoma/plasma cell myeloma is characterized by focal or diffuse infiltrates of atypical plasma cells, with prominent nucleoli and eccentric amphophilic or basophilic cytoplasm with prominent perinuclear Golgi zone (Figs. 17.20 and 17.21). Binucleate or multinucleate forms are frequent. The plasma cells may be small and mature, or large and immature, with bizarre and pleomorphic forms. Dutcher bodies (intranuclear inclusions of dilated Golgi cisternae), Russell bodies (globular eosinophilic cytoplasmic immunoglobulin inclusions), or crystalline immunoglobulin inclusions may be present. Amyloid may be present in extramedullary plasmacytomas. Some plasmacytomas consist of poorly differentiated plasma cells with bizarre multinucleated giants cells (anaplastic plasmacytoma). Immunoblastic transformation of plasma cell myeloma has also been reported (Falini et al, 1982).

Differential Diagnosis

Plasmacytoma/plasma cell myeloma should be distinguished from lymphoplasmacytoid lymphoma and other B cell lymphomas with plasmacytoid differentiation. Plasmacytomas are characterized by a "pure" plasma cell population; the presence of lymphocytes

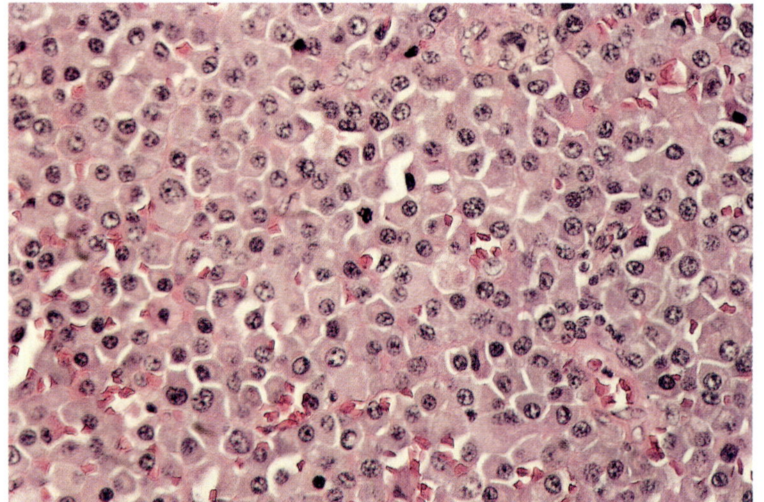

FIGURE 17.20

Plasmacytoma of cervical lymph node.

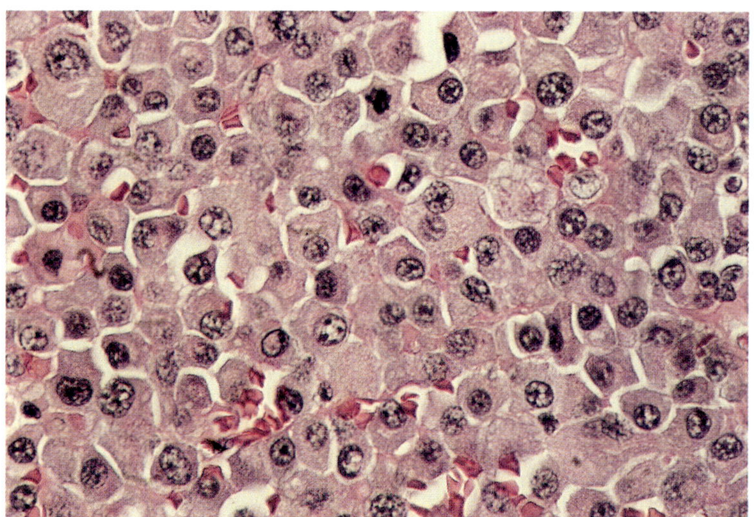

FIGURE 17.21

Plasmacytoma of cervical lymph node, higher magnification, showing sheets of atypical plasma cells with occasional Dutcher bodies.

and intermediate forms (plasmacytoid lymphocytes) should suggest a plasmacytoid lymphoma. Anaplastic plasmacytoma and immunoblastic transformation of plasma cell myeloma should be distinguished from immunoblastic diffuse large B cell lymphoma. Immunohistochemical studies are helpful. Plasmacytomas are characterized by loss of B cell antigens (CD19, CD20, CD22), leukocyte common antigen (CD45), and surface immunoglobulin; cytoplasmic immunoglobulin demonstrated in paraffin-embedded tissue and expression of plasma cell antigens (CD38, EMA, PCA-1) is frequent (Strickler et al, 1988).

Extramedullary lymph node plasmacytoma must be distinguished from benign lymph node hyperplasia with plasmacytosis, particularly the plasma cell variant of Castleman's disease. The plasma cells in Castleman's disease are usually mature and polyclonal; however, monoclonal plasma cells may be encountered in some cases (Radaszkiewicz et al, 1989). The development of plasmacytoma in lymph nodes with Castleman's disease has been described (Schlosnagle et al, 1982).

Extramedullary lymph node plasmacytoma should be distinguished from lymph node involvement in plasma cell myeloma and lymph node metastases from other extramedullary plasmacytoma (Fishkin and Spiegelberg, 1976). Careful clinical evaluation including skeletal survey, bone marrow biopsy, and serum protein studies should be performed to exclude plasma cell myeloma. Patients presenting with plasmacytoma of cervical lymph nodes should undergo thorough examination of the upper respiratory tract and nasopharynx to exclude metastases from other extramedullary plasmacytoma (Fishkin and Spiegelberg, 1976).

Course and Prognosis

Extramedullary plasmacytomas are treated with local radiation therapy. Regional lymph node involvement is present in 18% of extramedullary plasmacytomas; development of plasma cell myeloma is infrequent (Wiltshaw, 1976). Plasma cell myeloma may follow extramedullary plasmacytoma of mediastinal lymph nodes (Moran et al, 1995).

REFERENCES

Addis BJ, Isaacson P, Billings JA. Plasmacytoma of lymph nodes. Cancer 46:340–346, 1980.

Anderson KC, Boyd AW, Fisher DC, Leslie D, Schlossman SF, Nadler LF. Hairy cell leukemia: A tumor of pre-plasma cells. Blood 65:620, 1985.

Bailey EM, Ferry JA, Harris NL, Mihm MC, Jacobson JO, Duncan LM. Marginal zone lymphoma (low grade B cell lymphoma of mucosa associated lymphoid tissue type) of skin and subcutaneous tissue. A study of 15 patients. Am J Surg Pathol 20:1011–1023, 1996.

Catovsky D, Petit JE, Galton AG, Spiers ASD, Harrison CV. Leukemic reticuloendotheliosis ("hairy cell leukemia"): A distinct clinico-pathologic entity. Br J Haematol 26:9–27, 1974.

Cousar JB, McGinn DL, Glick AD, List AF, Collins RD. Report of an unusual lymphoma arising from parafollicular B-lymphocytes (PBLs) or so-called "monocytoid" lymphocytes. Am J Clin Pathol 87:121–128, 1987.

Dierlamm J, Pittaluga S, Wlodarska I, Stul M, Thomas J, Boogaerts M. Marginal zone B cell lymphomas of different sites share similar cytogenetic and morphologic features. Blood 87:299–307, 1996.

Diez Martin JL, Li C-Y, Banks PM. Blastic variant of hairy cell leukemia. Am J Clin Pathol 87:576–583, 1987.

Falini B, De Solas I, Levine A, Parker J, Lukes R, Taylor C. Emergence of B-immunoblastic sarcoma in patients with multiple myeloma: A clinicopathologic study of 10 cases. Blood 59:923, 1982.

Ferry JA, Yang W-I, Zukerberg LR, Wotherspoon A, Arnold A, Harris NL. CD5+ extranodal marginal zone B cell (MALT) lymphoma. A low grade neoplasm with a propensity for bone marrow involvement and relapse. Am J Clin Pathol 105:31–37, 1996.

Fisher RI, Dahlberg S, Nathwani BN, Banks PM, Miller TP, Grogan TM. A clinical analysis of two indolent lymphoma entities: Mantle cell lymphoma and marginal zone lymphoma (including the mucosa-associated lymphoid tissue and monocytoid B cell subcategories): A Southwest Oncology Group study. Blood 85:1075–1082, 1996.

Fishkin BG, Spiegelberg HI. Cervical lymph node metastases as the first manifestation of localised extramedullary plasmacytoma. Cancer 38:1641–1644, 1976.

Hammer RD, Glick AD, Greer JP, Collins RD, Cousar JB. Splenic marginal zone lymphoma. A distinct B cell neoplasm. Am J Surg Pathol 20:613–626, 1996.

Hsi ED, Eisbruch A, Greenson JK, Singleton TP, Ross CW, Schnitzer B. Classification of primary gastric lymphomas according to histologic features. Am J Surg Pathol 22:17–27, 1998.

Isaacson PG, Matutes E, Burke M, Catovsky D. The histopathology of splenic lymphoma with villous lymphocytes. Blood 84:3828–3834, 1994.

Kumar S, Kumar D, Kaldjian EP, Bauserman S, Raffeld M, Jaffe ES. Primary low grade B cell lymphoma of the dura. A mucosa associated lymphoid tissue-type lymphoma. Am J Surg Pathol 21:81–87, 1997.

Labouyrie E, Marit G, Vial JP, Lacombe F, Fialon P, Bernard P, de Mascarel A, Merlio JP. Intrasinusoidal bone marrow involvement by splenic lymphoma with villous lymphocytes: A helpful immunohistologic feature. Mod Pathol 10:1015–1020, 1997.

Matutes E, Morilla R, Owusu-Ankomah K, Houlihan A, Catovsky D. The immunophenotype of splenic lymphoma with villous lymphocytes and its relevance to the differential diagnosis with other B cell disorders. Blood 83:1558–1562, 1994.

Mollejo M, Lloret E, Menarguez J, Piris MA, Isaacson PG. Lymph node involvement by splenic marginal zone lymphoma: Morphological and immunohistochemical features. Am J Surg Pathol 21:772–780, 1997.

Moran CA, Suster S, Fishback NF, Koss MN. Extramedullary plasmacytomas presenting as mediastinal masses: Clinicopathologic study of two cases preceding the onset of multiple myeloma. Mod Pathol 8:257–259, 1995.

Piro LD, Carrera CJ, Carson D, Beutler E. Lasting remissions in hairy-cell leukemia induced by a single infusion of 2-chlorodeoxyadenosine. N Engl J Med 322:1117–1121, 1990.

Radaszkiewicz T, Hansmann ML, Lennert K. Monoclonality and polyclonality of plasma cells in Castleman's disease of the plasma cell variant. Histopathology 14:11–24, 1989.

Rettig MB, Ma HJ, Vescio RA, Pold M, Schiller G, Belson D, et al. Kaposi's sarcoma-associated herpesvirus infection of bone marrow dendritic cells from multiple myeloma patients. Science 276:1851–1854, 1997.

Robbins BA, Ellison DJ, Spinosa JC, Carey CA, Lukes RJ, Poppema S, Saven A, Piro LD. Diagnostic application of two-color flow cytometry in 161 cases of hairy cell leukemia. Blood 82:1277–1287, 1993.

Roggero E, Zucca E, Pinotti G, Pascarella A, Capella C, Savio A, et al. Eradication of Helicobacter pylori infection in primary low-grade gastric lymphoma of mucosa-associated lymphoid tissue. Ann Intern Med 122:767–769, 1995.

Schlosnagle DC, Chan WC, Hargreaves HK, Nolting SF, Brynes RK. Plasmacytoma in giant lymph node hyperplasia. Am J Clin Pathol 78:541–544, 1982.

Sheibani K, Burke JS, Swartz WG, Nademanee A, Winberg CD. Monocytoid B cell lymphoma. Clinicopathologic study of 21 cases of a unique type of low-grade lymphoma. Cancer 62:1531–1538, 1988.

Strickler J, Audel M, Copehaven C, Warnke R. Immunophenotypic differences between plasmacytoma/plasma cell myeloma and immunoblastic lymphoma. Cancer 61:1782–1786, 1988.

Wiltshaw E. The natural history of extramedullary plasmacytoma and its relation to solitary plasmacytoma of bone and myelomatosis. Medicine (Baltimore) 55:217–238, 1976.

Wotherspoon AC, Doglioni C, Diss TC, Pan L, Moschini A, De Boni M, Isaacson PG. Regression of primary low-grade B cell lymphoma of mucosa-associated lymphoid tissue after eradication of Helicobacter pylori. Lancet 342:575, 1993.

18

Peripheral B Cell Neoplasms: IV. Diffuse Large B Cell Lymphoma, Burkitt's Lymphoma, and Burkitt-Like Lymphoma

Diffuse large B cell lymphoma, Burkitt's lymphoma, and Burkitt-like lymphoma are tumors of transformed B lymphocytes. These are aggressive B cell lymphomas which are classified as intermediate to high grade in the WF. They are characterized by aggressive clinical course with potential curability with combination chemotherapy.

Diffuse Large B Cell Lymphoma

Classification

REAL: Diffuse large B cell lymphoma; subtype: primary mediastinal (thymic) B cell lymphoma.
WF: Malignant lymphoma, diffuse, large cell, cleaved cell, noncleaved cell; malignant lymphoma, large cell, immunoblastic.

Immunophenotype

CD19+, CD20+, CD22+, CD45+, SIg+ or −.

Molecular Pathology

BCL-2 oncogene rearrangement with t(14;18) chromosome translocation in 30%
BCL-6 oncogene rearrangement with t(3;x) chromosome translocation in 40%

Clinical Features

Diffuse large B cell lymphoma (DLBCL) is the final common pathway of transformation
of B cell neoplasms of varied origin. DLBCL is predominantly a disease of adults, but it
also occurs in children. Localized (Ann Arbor stage I and II) and advanced (Ann Arbor
stage III and IV) presentations occur with equal frequency; extranodal presentation is
frequent (40%). In contrast to low grade B cell lymphomas, bone marrow involvement
is uncommon (10%). BCL-2 oncogene rearrangement with t(14;18) chromosome translocation, found in follicle center lymphomas, is present in 30% of DLBCL; BCL-2 protein
expression, with or without the BCL-2 rearrangement, correlates with poorer prognosis
(Gascoyne et al, 1997; Hill et al, 1996). BCL-6 oncogene rearrangements with translocation involving chromosome 3 (3q27) are present in 40% (Lo Coco et al, 1994); the BCL-
6 rearrangement correlates with extranodal presentation, low incidence of bone marrow
involvement, and better prognosis (Offit et al, 1994). Although most DLBCLs occur de
novo; some DLBCLs develop by transformation of underlying low-grade B cell lymphomas (Strauchen et al, 1987).

Histopathology

Lymph node effacement in DLBCL is usually diffuse; occasionally sinusoidal or interfollicular patterns are encountered. DLBCL with tropism for follicular centers has been
rarely described (Suster, 1992). The lymphoma cells may be of any of several types,
including large cleaved cells, large noncleaved cells (centroblasts), immunoblasts, multilobated cells, and anaplastic cells (Figs. 18.1, 18.2, 18.3, and 18.4); frequently more than
one cell type is identified. Mitoses may be numerous; necrosis is frequently present as
single cell necrosis or zones of infarct-like necrosis. Admixed epithelioid histiocytes or
starry-sky macrophages may be present (Fig. 18.5). Sclerosis, in the form of delicate
compartmentalizing sclerosis or broad fibrous bands, may be present. Occasionally, a
component of simultaneous low-grade B cell lymphoma is evident (composite
lymphoma).

Subclassification of Diffuse Large B Cell Lymphoma

The existence of morphologically distinct forms of DLBCL is probable (Strauchen et al,
1978). The WF and Kiel classifications distinguish between DLBCL of follicle center type
(large cleaved and noncleaved cell, centroblastic) and DLBCL of immunoblastic type.
Large noncleaved cells (centroblasts) are characterized by scant basophilic cytoplasm
and paired nucleoli in apposition to the nuclear membrane (Fig. 18.1); immunoblasts
are characterized by more abundant amphophilic cytoplasm and prominent central
nucleoli (Figs. 18.2 and 18.3). Immunoblastic DLBCLs are characterized by a predominant population of immunoblasts; in the Kiel classification fewer than 10% of the cells
are centroblasts. Poorer survival for lymphomas of immunoblastic type has been shown

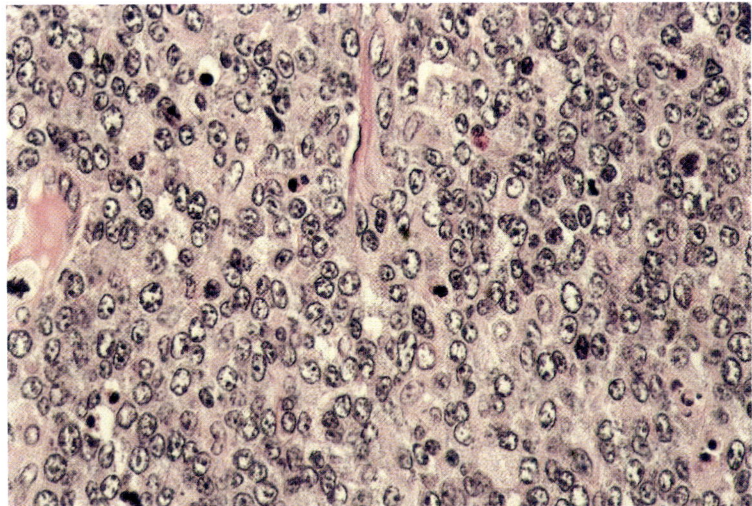

Diffuse large B cell lymphoma composed of large noncleaved cells.

FIGURE 18.1

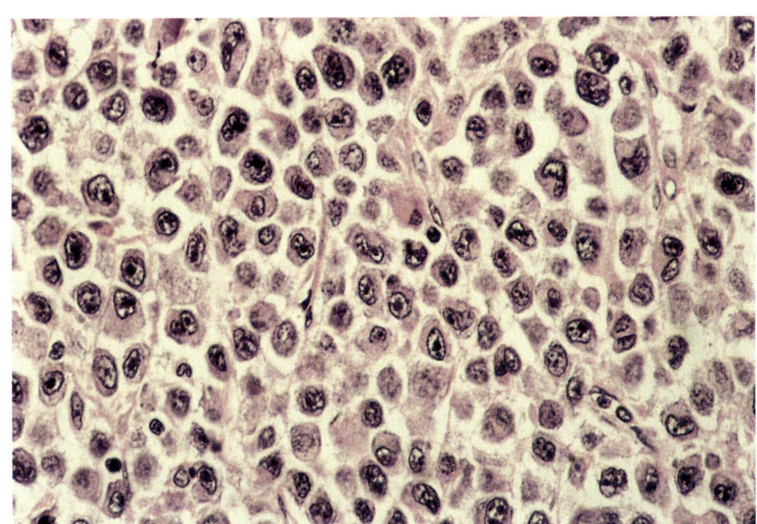

Diffuse large B cell lymphoma composed of plasmacytoid immuno-blasts.

FIGURE 18.2

in some (Engelhard et al, 1997; Strauchen et al, 1978; Warnke et al, 1982), but not all studies (Kwak et al, 1991; Nathwani et al, 1982). Because of lack of precise criteria for morphologic subclassification and poor reproducibility, the DLBCLs are not subclassified in the REAL classification; however, the likely heterogeneity of this category is acknowledged (Harris et al, 1994).

SUBTYPE: PRIMARY MEDIASTINAL (THYMIC) B CELL LYMPHOMA A clinicopathologically distinctive form of DLBCL occurs in the mediastinum (Perrone et al, 1986). Most patients are young women presenting with large, locally invasive mediastinal masses. The tumors are composed of large B cells with round to irregular, or multilobated, nuclei

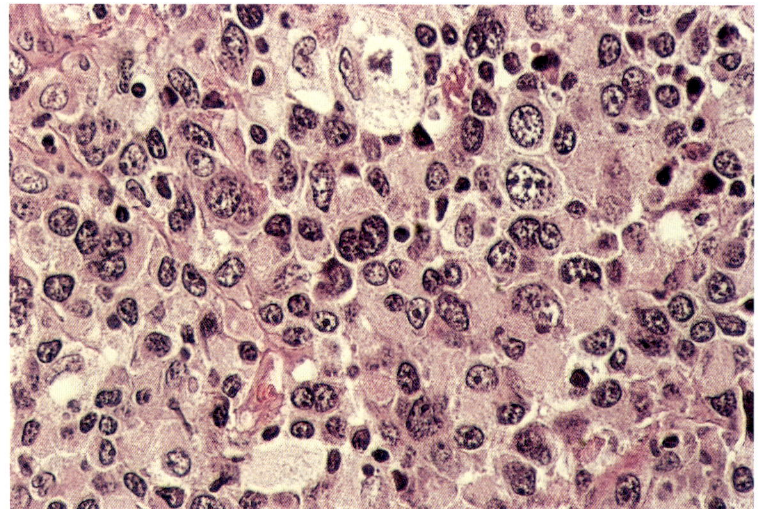

FIGURE
18.3

Diffuse large B cell lymphoma composed of pleomorphic immunoblasts.

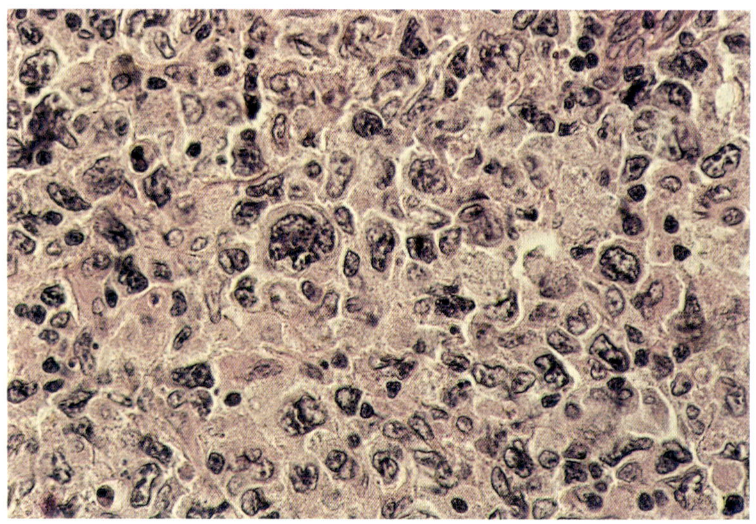

FIGURE
18.4

Diffuse large B cell lymphoma composed of pleomorphic cells resembling the cells of a peripheral T cell lymphoma.

and abundant, clear cytoplasm, with frequent compartmentalizing sclerosis (Figs. 18.6, 18.7, 18.8, and 18.9). Immunohistochemical studies aid in distinction from other mediastinal neoplasms (Suster and Moran, 1996). The tumor likely arises from a subset of thymic medullary B lymphocytes (Hofmann et al, 1988). BCL-2 and BCL-6 gene rearrangements are absent, suggesting a distinct molecular pathogenesis (Tsang et al, 1996). Recurrences are frequently extranodal (Perrone et al, 1986). Although some reported patients have had refractory disease, response to therapy in others has been similar to DLBCL at other sites treated with aggressive combination chemotherapy and radiotherapy (Jacobson et al, 1988; Lazzarino et al 1997; Sehn et al, 1998).

FIGURE
18.5

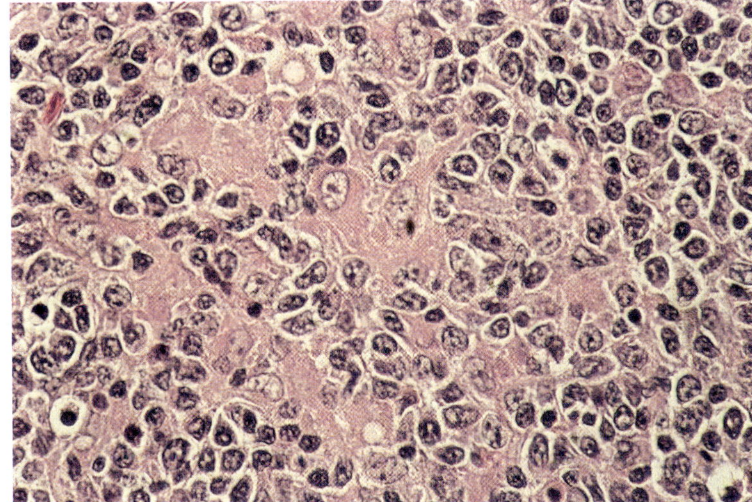

Diffuse large B cell lymphoma with admixture of epithelioid histiocytes.

FIGURE
18.6

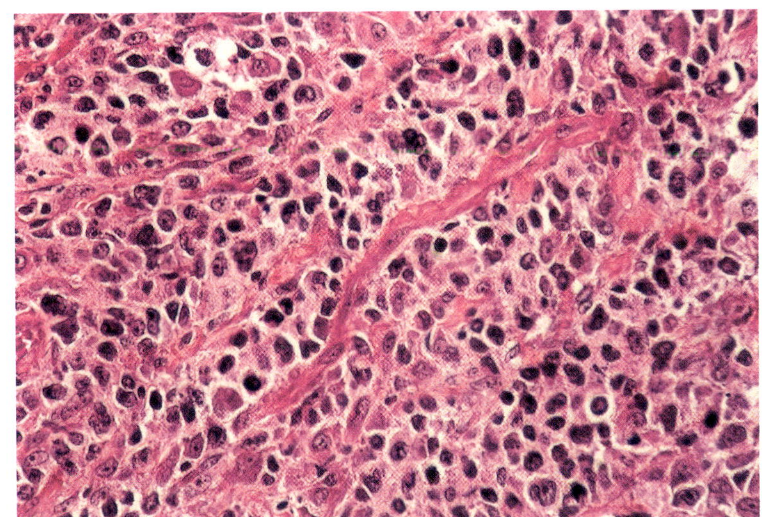

Primary mediastinal B cell lymphoma with sclerosis.

Histopathological Variants

MULTILOBATED CELL LYMPHOMA Multilobated cell lymphomas are DLBCLs characterized by cells with striking nuclear lobations; multiloblated cells with three or more nuclear lobes constitute 30% or more of the tumor cells (van Baarlen et al, 1988) (Fig. 18.10). Multilobated cell lymphomas are B cell neoplasms related to large cleaved follicle center cells and are associated with a high incidence of extranodal involvement and favorable prognosis (van Baarlen et al, 1988).

B CELL ANAPLASTIC LYMPHOMA Up to 20% of anaplastic large cell lymphomas (ALCLs) are of B cell phenotype (Filippa et al, 1996). B cell ALCLs are characterized by anaplas-

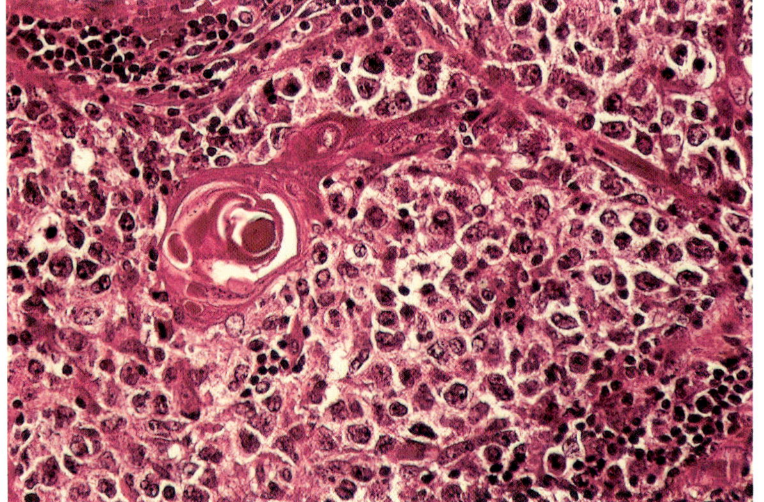

FIGURE 18.7

Primary mediastinal B cell lymphoma involving medulla of thymus and surrounding a Hassall's corpuscle. Mediastinal B cell lymphomas are derived from thymic medullary B lymphocytes.

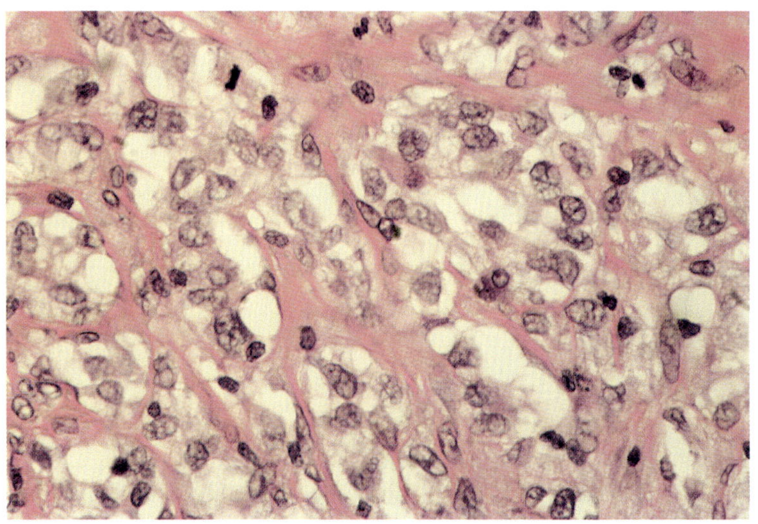

FIGURE 18.8

Primary mediastinal B cell lymphoma showing clear cytoplasm and compartmentalizing sclerosis.

tic morphology, with multinucleate Reed-Sternberg–like cells, sinusoidal involvement, and expression of the lymphoid activation antigen CD30 (Figs. 18.11, 18.12, and 18.13). In contrast to the more common T and null cell ALCL, the t(2;5) chromosome translocation and NPM/ALK oncogene rearrangement are absent. B cell ALCLs are associated with a high incidence of bone marrow involvement; in contrast to T and null cell ALCL, skin involvement is infrequent (Filippa et al, 1996). B cell ALCLs associated with HIV infection are EBV-related (Chadburn et al, 1993). A subtype of CD30-negative B cell

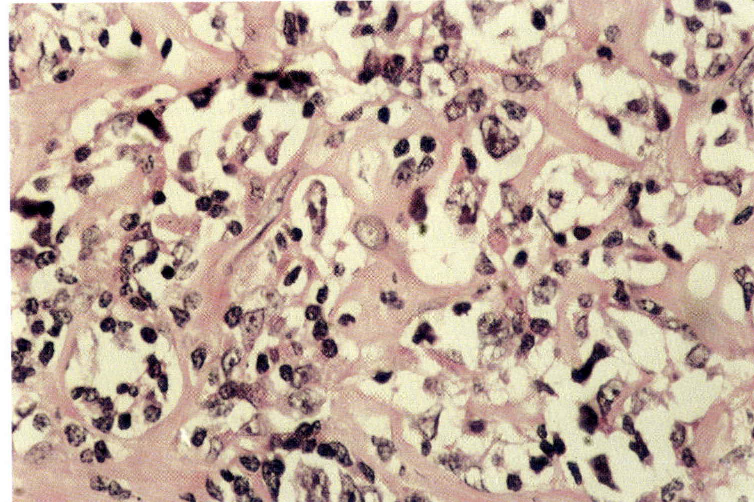

Primary mediastinal B cell lymphoma showing cytoplasmic retraction artifact and compartmentalizing sclerosis.

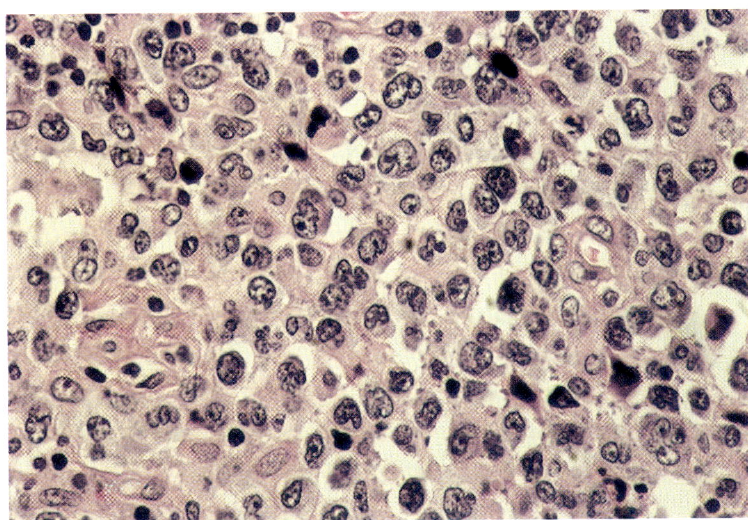

Diffuse large B cell lymphoma composed of multilobated cells.

ALCL has been reported with expression of the ALK kinase, in the absence of the t(2;5) chromosome translocation or NPM/ALK rearrangement (Delsol et al, 1997).

BODY-CAVITY-BASED B CELL LYMPHOMAS Body-cavity-based B cell lymphomas (primary effusion lymphomas, BCBLs) are a subset of DLBCLs associated with the Kaposi's sarcoma-associated herpesvirus (KSHV) (Cesarman et al, 1995; Nador et al, 1996) (Figs. 18.14, 18.15, and 18.16). BCBLs occur predominantly in patients with HIV infection; rare cases in the absence of HIV infection have been reported (Said et al, 1996; Strauchen et

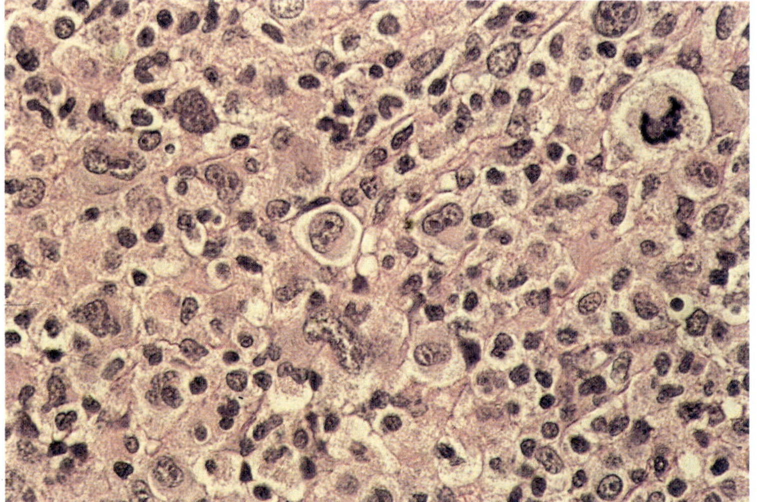

FIGURE
18.11

B cell anaplastic large cell lymphoma.

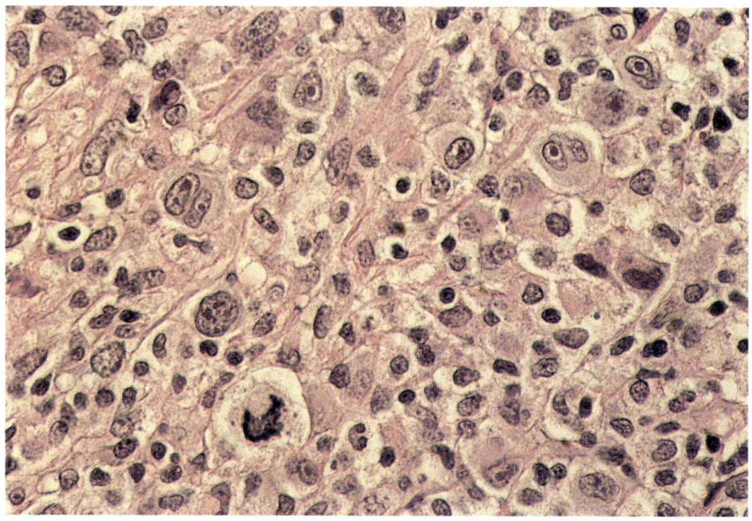

FIGURE
18.12

B cell anaplastic large cell lymphoma showing Reed-Sternberg–like cells.

al, 1996). HIV-related BCBLs also contain EBV; C-MYC rearrangements characteristic of other HIV-related lymphomas are absent (Cesarman et al, 1995). BCBLs frequently do not express surface B cell antigens; clonal immunoglobulin gene rearrangements are present, indicating B cell differentiation; CD45 and lymphoid activation antigens (CD30, CD38, EMA) are frequently expressed (Nador et al, 1996). Patients with BCBL present with malignant effusions (Figs. 18.14 and 18.15); lymph node involvement is infrequent but may be present in advanced cases (Nador et al, 1996); we have seen one case with sinusoidal lymph node involvement at autopsy (Fig. 18.16). Rare KSHV-associated

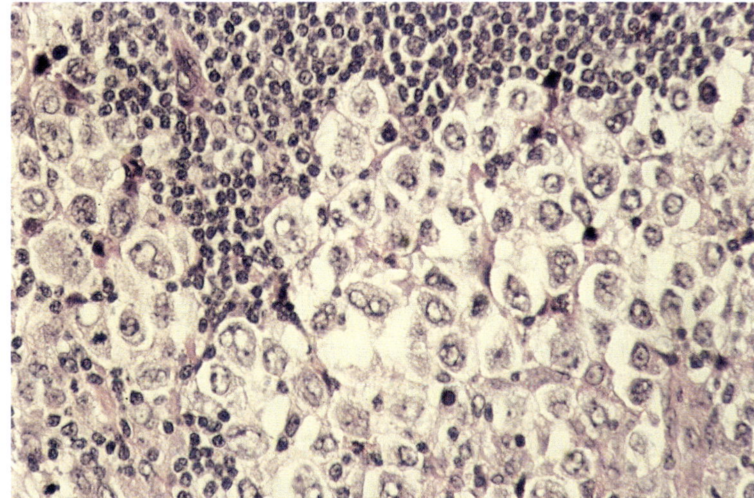

B cell anaplastic large cell lymphoma showing sinusoidal pattern of involvement.

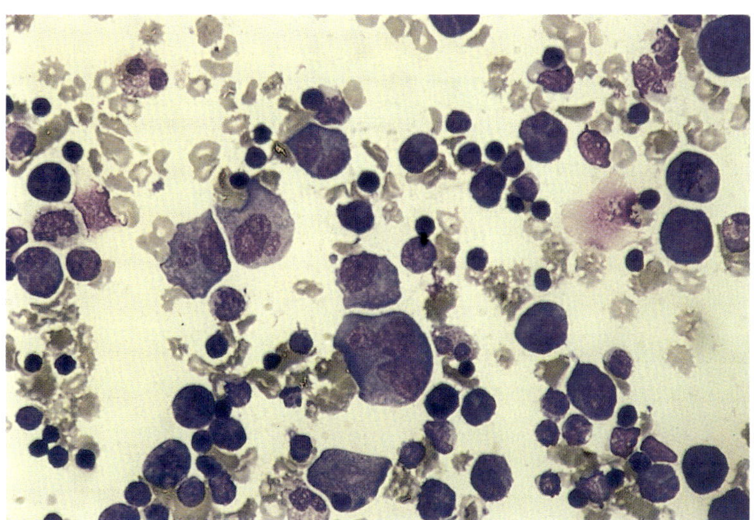

Body-cavity-based primary effusion B cell lymphoma. Cytospin preparation of malignant effusion stained with Giemsa.

lymphomas involving the gastrointestinal tract with secondary effusion lymphomas have been recognized (DePond et al, 1997). KSHV-associated BCBL are distinct from unrelated pleural cavity lymphomas arising in association with long-standing pyothorax (Iuchi et al, 1987).

T-CELL-RICH LARGE B CELL LYMPHOMA   T-cell-rich large B cell lymphoma (TCRBL) is a variant of DLBCL characterized by an extensive reactive T cell component (Krishnan et al, 1994; Macon et al 1992). TCRBL demonstrates a polymorphous histopathology, with admixture of small and large lymphoid cells; vascular proliferation and epithelioid his-

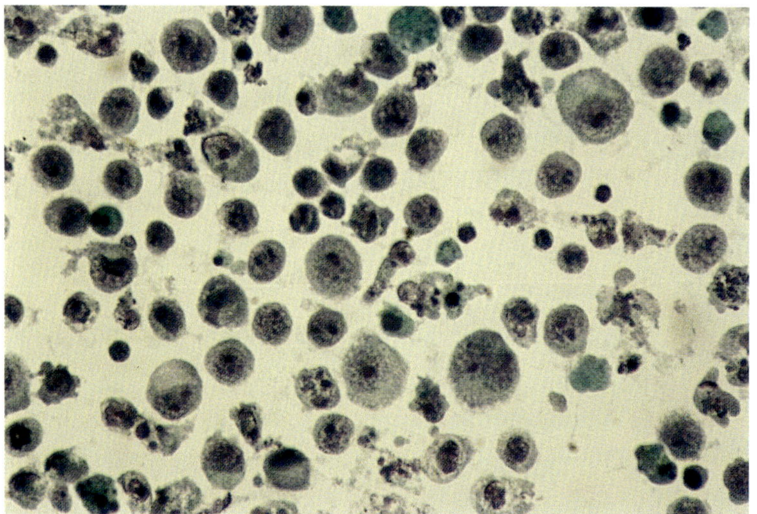

FIGURE 18.15

Body-cavity-based primary effusion B cell lymphoma. Cytospin preparation of malignant effusion stained with Papanicolaou stain.

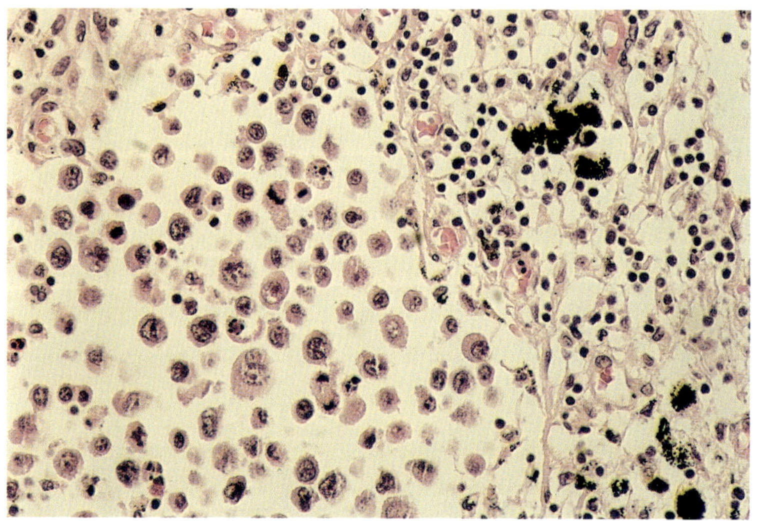

FIGURE 18.16

Body-cavity-based primary effusion B cell lymphoma. Autopsy lymph node showing sinusoidal involvement.

tiocytes are frequently present (Fig. 18.17). Reed-Sternberg–like cells may be present, mimicking Hodgkin's disease (Chittal et al, 1991; McBride et al, 1996) (Fig. 18.18). Immunohistochemical studies are necessary for diagnosis. Scattered CD20-positive large B cells, in a predominant population of small T lymphocytes, are characteristic (Krishnan et al, 1994; Macon et al, 1992) (Figs. 18.19 and 18.20). Immunoglobulin gene rearrangements are detected in the majority of cases. Response to therapy and prognosis is similar to other DLBCL (Krishnan et al, 1994). Bone marrow involvement may be more frequent than in other forms of DLBCL (Skinnider et al, 1997). Distinction from Hodgkin's disease may be difficult; in a recent series of 50 cases meeting the histologic

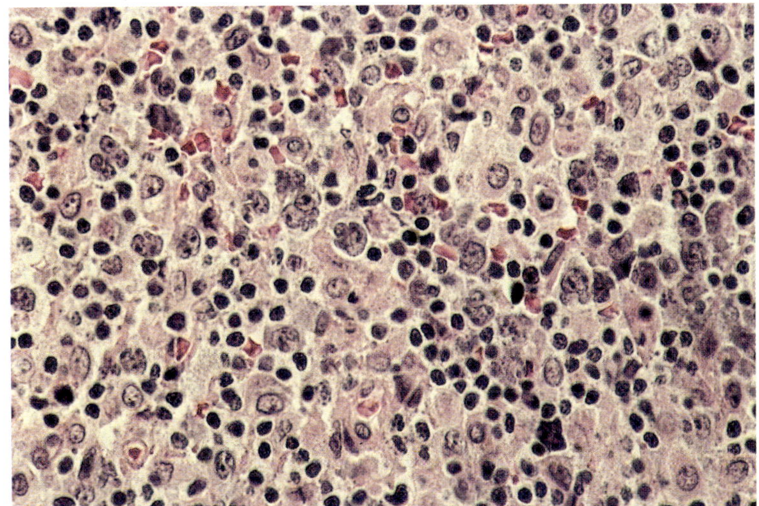

T-cell-rich large B cell lymphoma showing polymorphous histopathology.

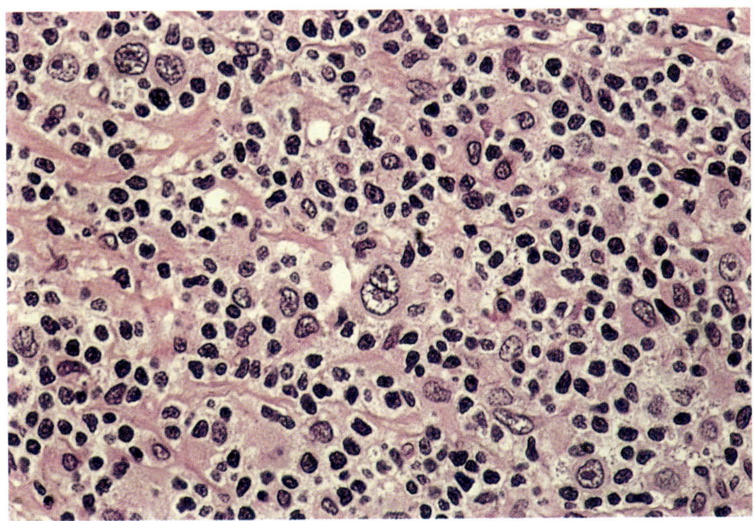

T-cell-rich large B cell lymphoma showing a Reed-Sternberg–like cell, mimicking Hodgkin's disease. Paucity of eosinophils and plasma cells is a clue to the correct diagnosis.

criteria for mixed cellularity Hodgkin's disease, nine cases were found to be TCRBL by immunohistochemical studies (McBride et al, 1996). Clues to the correct diagnosis were lymphocyte-rich background and paucity of eosinophils and plasma cells (Figs. 18.18 and 18.21). Correct diagnosis is important since TCRBL did not respond to therapies for Hodgkin's disease (McBride et al, 1996). Histiocyte-rich B cell lymphoma is probably a related disorder (Delabie et al, 1992).

ANGIOTROPHIC B CELL LYMPHOMA Angiotrophic B cell lymphoma (intravascular lymphomatosis, formerly malignant angioendotheliomatosis) is a rare systemic disorder

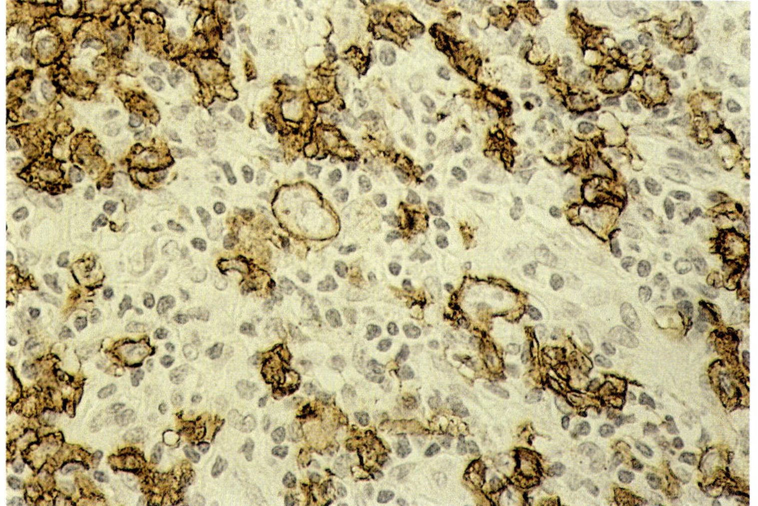

FIGURE
18.19

T-cell-rich large B cell lymphoma showing large cells staining for the B cell marker CD20.

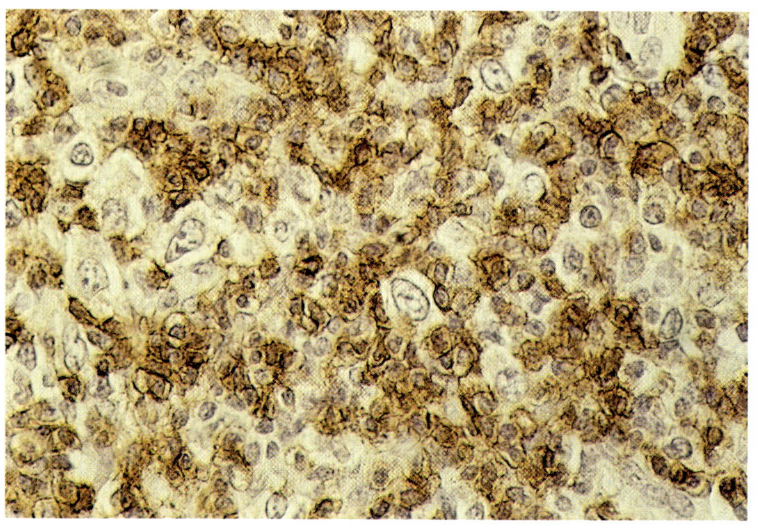

FIGURE
18.20

T-cell-rich large B cell lymphoma showing small lymphocytes staining for the T cell marker CD45RO.

with predominant central nervous system manifestations characterized by intravascular proliferation of large lymphoma cells (Sheibani et al, 1986) (Fig. 18.22). Involvement of the skin and central nervous system is frequent; renal and pulmonary involvement also occur; however, involvement of lymph nodes and bone marrow is infrequent (Demirer et al, 1994). Most cases are of B cell phenotype. Diagnosis is established by biopsy of the skin, brain, kidney, or other involved site. The prognosis is poor.

HIV-ASSOCIATED DIFFUSE LARGE B CELL LYMPHOMA   DLBCL and small noncleaved cell lymphomas (see below) constitute the principal forms of non-Hodgkin's lymphoma oc-

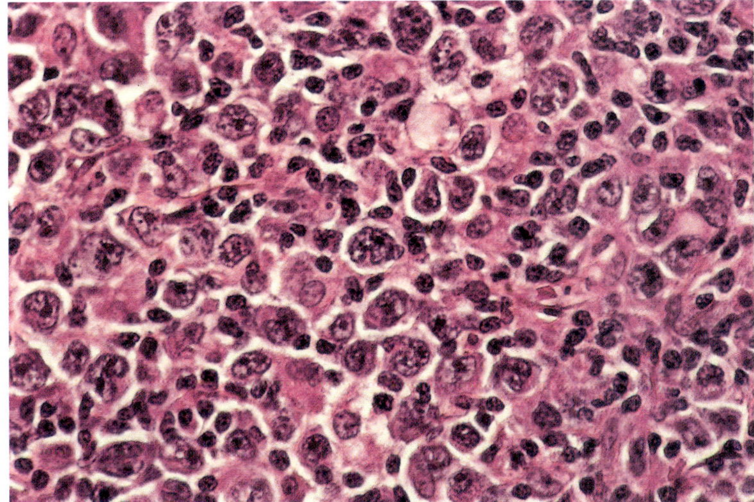

FIGURE 18.21

T-cell-rich large B cell lymphoma, which mimicked Hodgkin's disease, showing transformation to pleomorphic diffuse large B cell lymphoma (from same patient as Fig. 18.18).

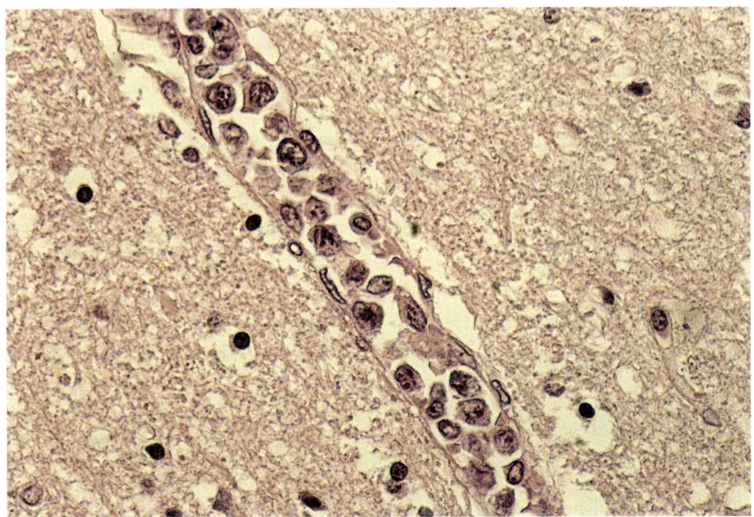

FIGURE 18.22

Angiotrophic B cell lymphoma showing intravascular proliferation of large cell lymphoma involving the central nervous system.

curring in association with HIV infection. The DLBCL may be of immunoblastic, large noncleaved, anaplastic, body-cavity-based, or plasmablastic type (Delecluse et al, 1997). EBV is frequently present (Ballerini et al, 1993).

OTHER VARIANTS OF DIFFUSE LARGE B CELL LYMPHOMA   DLBCLs with myxoid stroma, spindled cells (Fig. 18.23), fibrillary matrix and pseudorosettes (Fig 18.24), signet ring cells, microvillous cells, and cells with intercellular junctions have been rarely reported (Warnke et al, 1995).

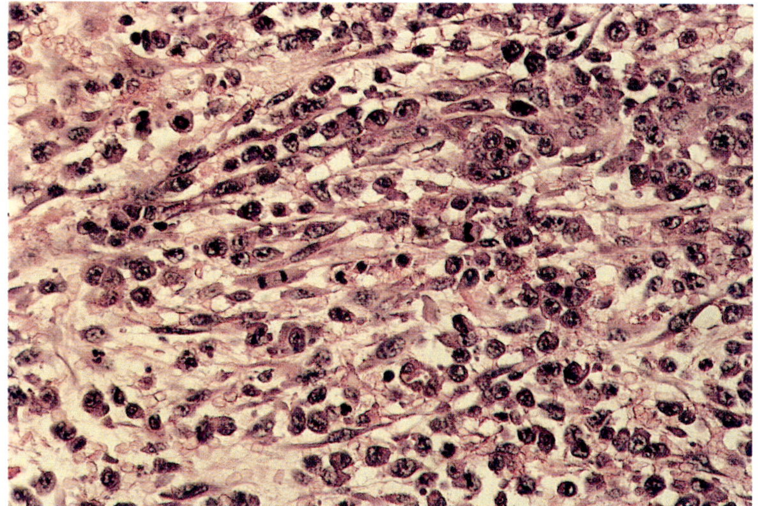

FIGURE
18.23

Diffuse large B cell lymphoma with spindled cells.

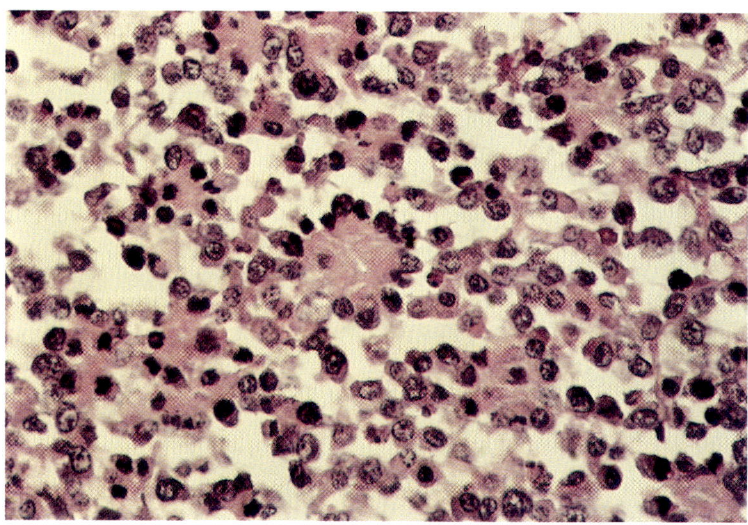

FIGURE
18.24

Diffuse large B cell lymphoma with pseudorosettes.

Differential Diagnosis

DLBCL should be distinguished from reactive lymphoid hyperplasia with prominent immunoblasts, from other lymphomas and hematopoietic neoplasms, and from nonhematopoietic neoplasms, especially metastatic carcinoma or melanoma. Distinction from reactive lymphoid hyperplasia with prominent immunoblasts in infectious mononucleosis, postvaccinial and hypersensitivity lymphadenopathy, and autoimmune disorders (Sjögren's syndrome) may be difficult. Attention to the polymorphous cell population and partial preservation of architecture in the latter conditions will be helpful. In difficult cases, application of immunophenotypic and gene rearrangement studies may be helpful. Distinction from low-grade B cell lymphomas is based principally on cell size. The cells of DLBCL are typically two to four times the size of a small lymphocyte; or the same size or larger than the nucleus of an admixed histiocyte or endothelial cell. Classification of B cell lymphomas composed of a mixture of small and large cells is, at times, arbitrary; the WF category of malignant lymphoma, diffuse, mixed, small and large cell is immunophenotypically and morphologically heterogenous and has no equivalent in the REAL classification (Harris et al, 1994). Distinction of DLBCL from other large cell hematopoietic neoplasms, including lymphocyte-depleted Hodgkin's disease, syncytial Hodgkin's disease, "true" histiocytic lymphoma, and granulocytic sarcoma depends largely on immunophenotypic studies. Distinction from nonhematopoietic neoplasms, particularly metastatic carcinoma and malignant melanoma, is critical, since DLBCL is treatable and potentially curable even when advanced. Immunohistochemical studies are helpful. The great majority of DLBCLs are CD45-positive in paraffin-embedded tissue or in frozen tissue. Some B cell anaplastic large cell lymphomas are CD45-negative (Filippa et al, 1996); anaplastic large cell lymphomas may be EMA-positive and rare anaplastic large cell lymphomas are positive for cytokeratin (Gustmann et al, 1991); immunohistochemical staining for CD30 is diagnostic.

Course and Prognosis

DLBCL is treated with aggressive combination chemotherapy. Responses to therapy are often durable. Disease-free survival is 70% or more in patients with localized (Ann Arbor stage I and II) disease and 40% in patients with advanced (Ann Arbor stage III and IV) disease. Large tumor masses (>10 cm), elevation of the serum lactate dehydrogenase, and bone marrow involvement are associated with a poorer prognosis. BCL-2 protein expression and mutations of the p53 gene also correlate with poorer prognosis (Gascoyne et al, 1997; Ichikawa et al, 1997). HIV-associated DLBCL may respond to dose-modified combination chemotherapy (Kaplan et al, 1997).

Burkitt's Lymphoma

Classification

REAL: Burkitt's lymphoma.
WF: Malignant lymphoma, small noncleaved cell, Burkitt's.

Immunophenotype

CD10+, CD19+, CD20+, CD22+, SIg+.

Molecular Pathology

C-MYC oncogene rearrangement with t(8;14), t(2;8), or t(8;22).

Clinical Features

Burkitt's lymphoma (BL) occurs in endemic and nonendemic forms. The endemic form occurs principally in Africa and affects children presenting with characteristic jaw and

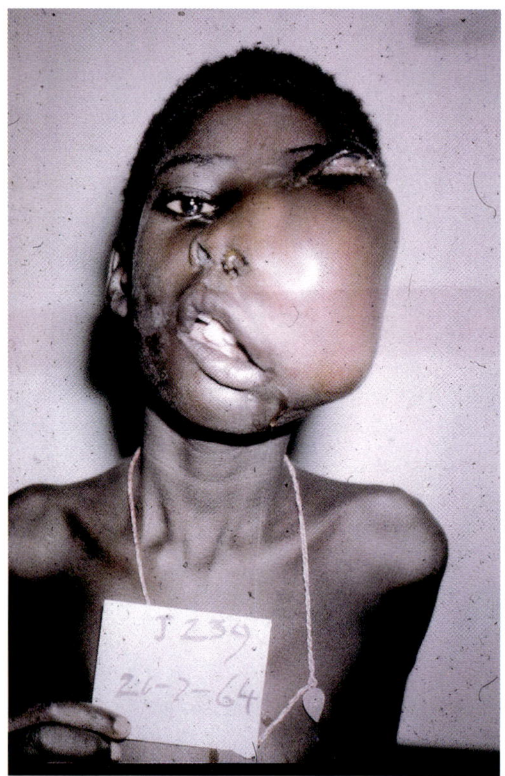

FIGURE 18.25

African Burkitt's lymphoma with characteristic jaw tumor.

ovarian tumors (Burkitt, 1958) (Fig. 18.25). The nonendemic form occurs in western countries and affects children presenting with abdominal (ileal) tumors and adults with HIV infection. The endemic form is highly associated with Epstein-Barr virus, which is present in the lymphoma cells in 90% of cases; the nonendemic form is less associated with EBV, which is found in 25–40% of cases. Burkitt's lymphoma consistently contains rearrangement of the C-MYC oncogene associated with the t(8;14), t(2;8), or t(8;22) chromosomal translocation; these translocations involve the C-MYC proto-oncogene on chromosome 8, and the immunoglobulin heavy chain, κ light chain, or λ light chain gene, on chromosome 14, 2, or 22, respectively. The resultant dysregulation of C-MYC expression is believed to play a key role in lymphomagenesis.

Histopathology

Burkitt's lymphoma is characterized by sheets of monotonous, round cells, with scant cytoplasm, moderately coarse chromatin, two to five distinct nucleoli, and numerous mitoses (Figs. 18.26 and 18.27). The cells of Burkitt's lymphoma are medium-sized ("small" noncleaved cells are small only in relation to large noncleaved cells) and have a distinct rim of basophilic cytoplasm, which typically "squares off" against the cytoplasm of adjacent cells. Admixed phagocytic macrophages are frequently present and impart a starry-sky appearance, characteristic of Burkitt's lymphoma, but also seen in other high-grade lymphomas. Burkitt's lymphoma cells characteristically vary little in size and shape and are approximately the same size as the nucleus of a starry-sky macrophage. Partial lymph node involvement in Burkitt's lymphoma may be characterized by selective involvment of follicular centers (Fig. 18.28). Burkitt's lymphoma cells in imprint or touch preparation stained with Giemsa have a characteristic appearance with coarsely reticular chromatin and deeply basophilic cytoplasm with neutral fat vacuoles (Fig. 18.29).

Differential Diagnosis

Burkitt's lymphoma should be distinguished from other high-grade lymphomas which may have a similar appearance. The cells of large cell lymphoma are larger (i.e., larger

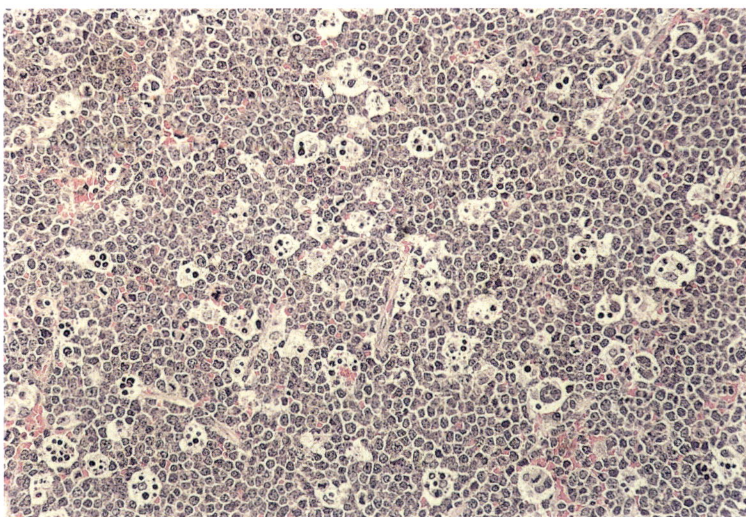

Burkitt's lymphoma consisting of sheets of monotonous round cells with interspersed starry-sky macrophages.

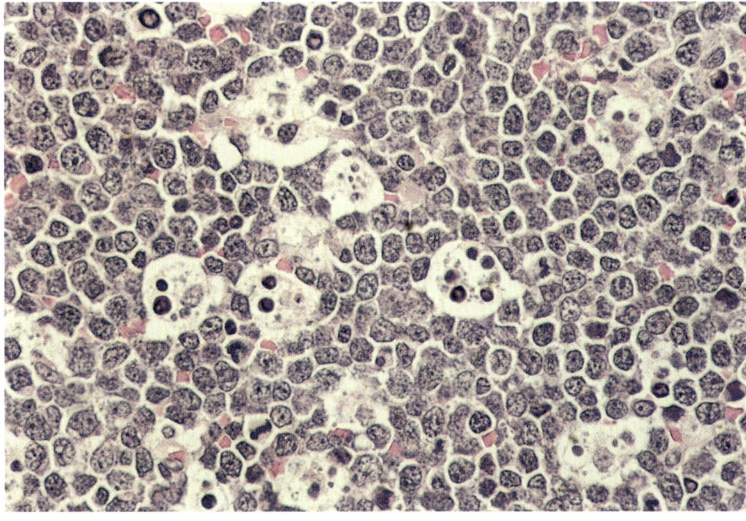

Burkitt's lymphoma, higher magnification, showing small noncleaved cells and starry-sky macrophages.

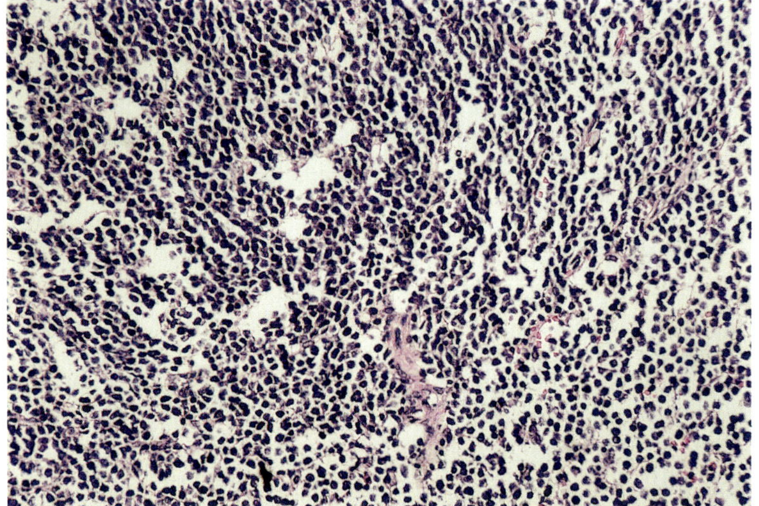

FIGURE 18.28

Burkitt's lymphoma showing selective involvement of a follicular center in a mesenteric lymph node from a western patient with an ileal tumor.

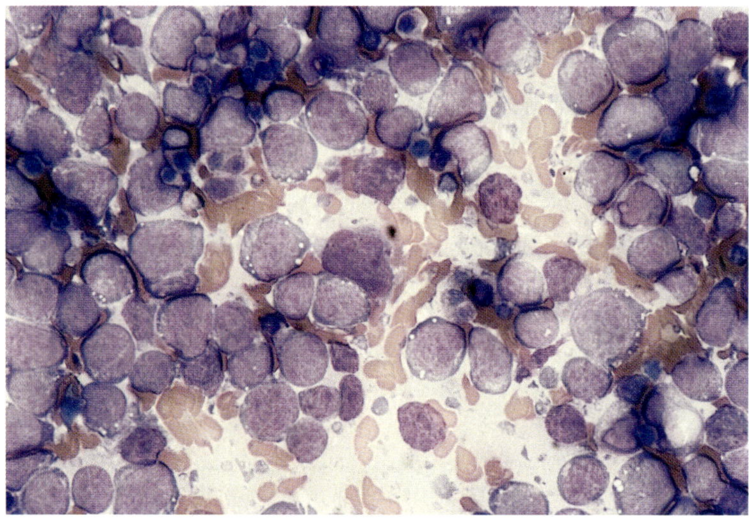

FIGURE 18.29

Burkitt's lymphoma cells, imprint preparation stained with Giemsa, showing basophilic cytoplasm containing neutral fat vacuoles.

than the nucleus of a starry-sky macrophage) and show greater pleomorphism. The cells of Burkitt-like lymphoma (see below) are approximately the same size but show greater pleomorphism and frequent admixture of cells with prominent central nucleoli. Lymphoblastic lymphoma is characterized by smaller cells (i.e., smaller than the nucleus of a starry-sky macrophage), with fine chromatin, inconspicuous nucleoli, and inconspicous cytoplasm. Lymphoblastic lymphoma is most frequently of T cell lineage; B lymphoblastic lymphoma differs from Burkitt's lymphoma immunphenotypically in that it is characteristically TdT-positive and SIg-negative. The cells of FAB L3 acute lymphoblastic leukemia are indistinguishable from the cells of Burkitt's lymphoma.

Course and Prognosis

Burkitt's lymphoma is a high-grade neoplasm which is rapidly progressive. Responses to chemotherapy are durable.

High-Grade B Cell Lymphoma, Burkitt-Like

Classification

REAL: Provisional entity: high-grade B cell lymphoma, Burkitt-like.
WF: Malignant lymphoma, small noncleaved cell.

Immunophenotype

CD19+, CD20+, CD22+, SIg+ or −.

Clinical Features

High-grade B cell lymphoma, Burkitt-like (Burkitt-like lymphoma) occurs in children and adults. Adult cases are frequently associated with HIV infection. Nodal presentations are more frequent than in Burkitt's lymphoma.

Histopathology

Burkitt-like lymphomas resemble Burkitt's lymphoma morphologically but are characterized by greater cellular pleomorphism with significant variation in cell size and shape, admixture of cells with prominent central nucleoli, and admixture of large or multinucleate cells (Figs. 18.30 and 18.31). The starry-sky pattern may or may not be present.

Differential Diagnosis

Burkitt-like lymphomas are a heterogenous group of B cell lymphomas which have morphologic features which overlap those of Burkitt's lymphoma and diffuse large B cell lymphoma (Harris et al, 1994). The immunophenotypic features of Burkitt-like lymphoma are more variable than those of Burkitt's lymphoma; the t(8;14) chromosomal translocation is frequently absent; C-MYC rearrangement is reported inconsistently but is frequently present in HIV-associated cases (Ballerini et al, 1993).

Course and Prognosis

Burkitt-like lymphoma is a high-grade neoplasm. Cases in children appear to behave similarly to Burkitt's lymphoma, with durable responses to chemotherapy; cases in adults appear to have poor prognosis (Harris et al, 1994).

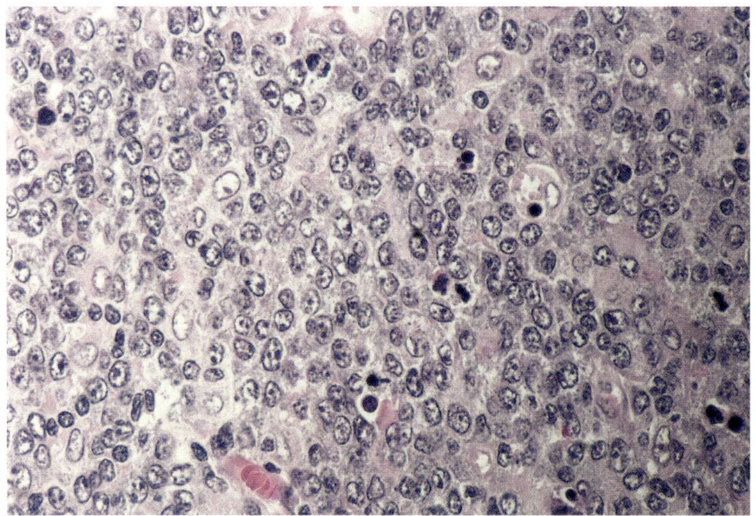

FIGURE
18.30

High-grade B cell lymphoma, Burkitt-like. Neoplastic cells resemble those of Burkitt's lymphoma but show a greater degree of pleomorphism.

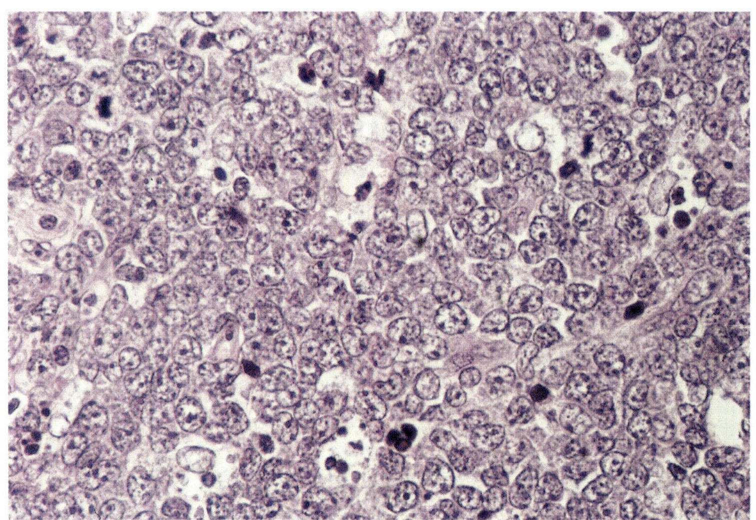

FIGURE
18.31

High-grade B cell lymphoma Burkitt-like. Neoplastic cells resemble those of Burkitt's lymphoma but show a greater degree of pleomorphism.

REFERENCES

Ballerini P, Gaidano G, Gong JZ, Tassi V, Saglio G, Knowles DM, Dalla-Favera R. Multiple genetic lesions in acquired immunodeficiency syndrome-related non-Hodgkin's lymphoma. Blood 81:166–176, 1993.

Burkitt D. A sarcoma involving the jaws in African children. BJ Surg 197:218–223, 1958

Cesarman E, Chang Y, Moore PS, Said JW, Knowles DM. Kaposi's sarcoma-associated herpesvirus-like DNA sequences in AIDS-related body-cavity-based lymphomas. N Engl J Med 332:1186–1191, 1995.

Chadburn A, Cesarman E, Jagirdar J, Subar M, Mir RN, Knowles DM. CD30(Ki-1) positive anaplastic large cell lymphoma in individuals infected with the human immunodeficiency virus. Cancer 72:3078–3090, 1993.

Chittal SM, Brousset P, Voigt J-J, Delsol G. Large B cell lymphoma rich in T-cells and simulating Hodgkin's disease. Histopathology 19:211–220, 1991.

Delabie J, Vandenberghe E, Kennes C, Verhoef G, Foschini MP, Stul M, Cassiman JJ, De Wolf-Peeters C. Histiocyte-rich B-cell lymphoma. A distinct clinicopathologic entity possibly related to lymphocyte predominant Hodgkin's disease, paragranuloma subtype. Am J Surg Pathol 16:37–48, 1992.

Delecluse HJ, Anagnostopoulos I, Dallenbach F, Hummel M, Marafioti T, Schneider U, et al. Plasmablastic lymphomas of the oral cavity: A new entity associated with the human immunodeficiency virus infection. Blood 1413–1420, 1997.

Delsol G, Lamant L, Mariame B, Pulford K, Dastugue N, Brousset P, et al. A new subtype of large B-cell lymphoma expressing the ALK kinase and lacking the 2;5 translocation. Blood 89:1483–1490, 1997.

Demirer T, Dail DH, Aboulafia DM. Four varied cases of intravascular lymphomatosis and a literature review. Cancer 73:1738–1745, 1994.

DePond W, Said JW, Tasaka T, de Vos S, Kahn D, Cesarman E, et al. Kaposi's sarcoma-associated herpesvirus and human herpesvirus 8 (KSHV/HHV8)-associated lymphoma of the bowel. Report of two cases in HIV-positive men with secondary effusion lymphomas. Am J Surg Pathol 21:719–724, 1997.

Engelhard M, Brittinger G, Huhn D, Gerhartz HH, Meusers P, Siegert W, et al. Subclassification of diffuse large B cell lymphomas according to the Kiel classification: Distinction of centroblastic and immunoblastic lymphomas is a significant prognostic risk factor. Blood 89:2291–2297, 1997.

Filippa DA, Ladanyi M, Wollner N, Straus DJ, O'Brien JP, Portlock C, Gangi M, Sun M. CD30 (Ki-1)-positive malignant lymphomas: Clinical, immunophenotypic, histologic, and genetic characteristics and differences with Hodgkin's disease. Blood 87:2905–2917, 1996.

Gascoyne RD, Adomat SA, Krajewski J, Krajewka M, Herjman DE, Tolcher AW, et al. Prognostic significance of Bcl-2 protein expression and Bcl-2 gene rearrangement in diffuse aggressive non-Hodgkin's lymphoma. Blood 90:244–251, 1997.

Gustmann C, Altmannsberger M, Osborn M, Griesser H, Feller AC. Cytokeratin expression and vimentin content in large cell anaplastic lymphomas and other non-Hodgkin's lymphomas. Am J Pathol 138:1413–1422, 1991.

Harris NL, Jaffe ES, Stein H, Banks PM, Chan JKC, Cleary ML, et al. A revised European-American classification of the lymphoid neoplasms: A proposal from the international lymphoma study group. Blood 84:1361–1392, 1994.

Hill ME, MacLennan KA, Cunningham DC, Hudson BV, Burke M, Clarke P et al. Prognositic significance of BCL-2 expression and bcl-2 major

breakpoint region rearrangements in diffuse large cell non-Hodgkin's lymphoma: A British National Lymphoma Investigation Study. Blood 88:1046–1051, 1996.

Hofmann WJ, Momburg F, Moller P. Thymic medullary cells expressing B lymphocyte antigens. Hum Pathol 19:1280–1287, 1988.

Ichikawa A, Kinoshita T, Watanabe I, Kato H, Nagai H, Tsushita K, et al. Mutations of the p53 gene as a prognostic factor in aggressive B-cell lymphoma. N Engl J Med 337:529–534, 1997.

Iuchi K, Ichimiya A, Akashi A, Mizuta A, Lee YE, Tada H, et al. Non-Hodgkin's lymphoma of the pleural cavity developing from long-standing pyothorax. Cancer 60:1771–1775, 1987.

Jacobson JO, Aisenberg AC, Lamarre L, Willett C, Linggood R, Miketic L, Harris N. Mediastinal large cell lymphoma: An uncommon subset of adult lymphoma curable with combined modality therapy. Cancer 62:1893–1808, 1988.

Kaplan LD, Straus DJ, Testa MA, Von Roenn J, Dezube BJ, Cooley TP et al. Low-dose compared with standard-dose m-BACOD chemotherapy for non-Hodgin's lymphoma associated with human immunodeficiency virus infection. N Engl J Med 336:1641–1648, 1997.

Krishnan J, Wallberg K, Frizzera G. T-cell-rich large B-cell lymphoma. A study of 30 cases, supporting its histologic heterogeneity and lack of clinical distinctiveness. Am J Surg Pathol 18:455–465, 1994.

Kwak LW, Wilson M, Weiss LM, Horning SJ, Warnke RA, Dorfman RF. Clinical significance of morphologic subdivision in diffuse large cell lymphoma. Cancer 68:1988–1993, 1991.

Lazzarino M, Orlandi E, Pauli M, Strater J, Klersy C, Gianelli U. Treatment outcome and prognostic factors for primary mediastinal (thymic) B-cell lymphoma: A multicenter study of 106 patients. J Clin Oncol 15:1646–1653, 1997.

Lo Coco F, Ye BH, Lista F, Corradini P, Offit K, Knowles DM, Chaganti RSK, Dalla-Favera R. Rearrangements of the BCL6 gene in diffuse large cell non-Hodgkin's lymphoma. Blood 83:1757–1759, 1994.

Macon WR, Williams ME, Greer JP, Stein RS, Collins RD. Cousar JB. T-cell-rich B-cell lymphomas. A clinicopathologic study of 19 cases. Am J Surg Pathol 16:351–363, 1992.

McBride JA, Rodriguez J, Luthra R, Ordonez NG, Cabanillas F, Pugh WC. T-cell-rich B large-cell lymphoma simulating lymphocyte-rich Hodgkin's disease. Am J Surg Pathol 20:193–201, 1996.

Nador RG, Cesarman E, Chadburn A, Dawson DB, Ansari MQ, Said J, Knowles DM. Primary effusion lymphoma: A distinct clinicopathologic entity associated with the Kaposi's sarcoma-associated herpes virus. Blood 88:645–656, 1996.

Nathwani BN, Dixon DO, Jones SE, et al. The clinical significance of the morphological subdivision of diffuse "histiocytic" lymphoma: A study of 162 patients treated by the Southwest Oncology Group. Blood 60:1068–1074, 1982.

Offit K, Lo Coco F, Louie DC, Parsa NZ, Leung D, Portlock C. Rearrangement of the bcl-6 gene as prognostic marker in diffuse large cell lymphoma. N Engl J Med 331:74–80, 1994.

Perrone T, Frizzera G, Rosai J. Mediastinal diffuse large-cell lymphoma with sclerosis. Am J Surg Pathol 10:176–191, 1986.

Said JW, Tasaka T, Takeuchi S, Asou H, de Vos S, Cesarman E, et al. Primary effusion lymphoma in women: Report of two cases of Kaposi's sarcoma herpes virus-associated effusion-based lymphoma in human · immunodeficiency virus-negative women. Blood 88:3124–3128, 1996.

Sehn LH, Antin JH, Shulman LN, Mauch P, Elias A, Kadin ME, Wheeler C. Primary diffuse large B-cell lymphoma of the mediastinum: Outcome following high-dose chemotherapy and autologous hematopoietic cell transplantation. Blood 91:717–723, 1998.

Sheibani K, Battifora H, Winberg C, Burke JS, Ben-Ezra J, Ellinger GM, et al. Further evidence that "malignant angioendotheliomatosis" is an angiotrophic large-cell lymphoma. N Engl J Med 314:943–948, 1986.

Skinnider BF, Connors JM, Gascoyne RD. Bone marrow involvement in T-cell-rich B-cell lymphoma. Am J Clin Pathol 108:570–578, 1997.

Strauchen JA, Young RC, DeVita VT, Anderson T, Fantone JC, Berard CW. Clinical relevance of the histopathological subclassification of diffuse "histiocytic" lymphoma. N Engl J Med 299:1382–1387, 1978.

Strauchen JA, May MM, Crown J. Large cell transformation of subclinical small lymphocytic leukemia/lymphoma: A variant of Richter's syndrome. Hematol Oncol 5:167–174, 1987.

Strauchen JA, Hauser AD, Burstein D, Jimenez R, Moore PS, Chang Y. Body cavity-based malignant lymphoma containing Kaposi sarcoma-associated herpesvirus in an HIV-negative man with previous Kaposi sarcoma. Ann Intern Med 125:822–825, 1996.

Suster S. Large cell lymphoma of the mediastinum with marked tropism for germinal centers. Cancer 69:2910–2916, 1992.

Suster S, Moran CA. Pleomorphic large cell lymphomas of the mediastinum. Am J Surg Pathol 20:224–232, 1996.

Tsang P, Cesarman E, Chadburn A, Liu YF, Knowles DM. Molecular characterization of primary mediastinal B cell lymphoma. Am J Pathol 148:2017–2025, 1996.

van Baarlen J, Schuurman H-J, van Unnik JAM. Multilobated non-Hodgkin's lymphoma. A clinicopathologic entity. Cancer 61:1371–1376, 1988.

Warnke RA, Strauchen JA, Burke JS, Hoppe RT, Campbell BA, Dorfman RF. Morphologic types of diffuse large cell lymphoma. Cancer 50:690–695, 1982.

Warnke RA, Weiss LM, Chan JKC, Cleary ML, Dorfman RF. Tumors of the lymph nodes and spleen. In: Atlas of Tumor Pathology, Third series, Fascicle 14. Rosai J, Sobin LH, eds. Washington, D.C., Armed Forces Institute of Pathology, 1995.

19

Peripheral T Cell and NK Cell Neoplasms: I. T Cell Chronic Lymphocytic Leukemia/ Prolymphocytic Leukemia, Large Granular Lymphocyte Leukemia, and Mycosis Fungoides/ Sézary's Syndrome

T cell chronic lymphocytic leukemia/prolymphocytic leukemia, large granular lymphocyte leukemia, and mycosis fungoides/Sézary's syndrome are systemic T cell lymphoproliferative disorders with predominantly extranodal involvement and frequent leukemic manifestations.

T Cell Chronic Lymphocytic Leukemia/Prolymphocytic Leukemia

Classification

REAL: T cell chronic lymphocytic leukemia/prolymphocytic leukemia.
WF: Malignant lymphoma, small lymphocytic.

Immunophenotype

CD2 +, CD3 +, CD4 +, CD5 +, CD7 +, CD8 − (rarely +), CD25 −.

Clinical Features

T cell chronic lymphocytic leukemia/prolymphocytic leukemia (T-CLL/PLL) is a systemic lymphoproliferative disorder characterized by peripheral lymphocytosis, which is frequently marked (>100,000 per mm^3), by mild or moderate generalized lymphadenopathy and hepatosplenomegaly, and by frequent cutaneous manifestations (Matutes et al, 1991). The abnormal lymphocytes in most cases have irregular nuclei, prominent nucleoli, and abundant cytoplasm—this is characterized as T cell prolymphocytic leukemia; rarely, the lymphocytes are small, with variably irregular nuclei and scant cytoplasm—this is characterized as the small cell variant of T cell prolymphocytic leukemia or T cell chronic lymphocytic leukemia (Hoyer et al, 1995). Dot-like paranuclear staining for acid phosphatase is frequently present (Matutes et al, 1991).

Histopathology

Lymph nodes in T-CLL/PLL show diffuse or paracortical infiltration by small irregular lymphocytes (Figs. 19.1 and 19.2). Preservation of the follicles may be present; pseudofollicular proliferation centers are absent. Proliferation of small vessels is a prominent feature and may be associated with sclerosis (Hoyer et al, 1995) (Figs. 19.3 and 19.4). Cutaneous involvement is frequent and characterized by nonepidermotrophic, dermal perivascular lymphocytic infiltrates.

Differential Diagnosis

T-CLL/PLL should be distinguished from other T lymphoproliferative disorders, including large granular lymphocyte leukemia, mycosis fungoides/Sézary's syndrome, and adult T cell lymphoma/leukemia. The cells of T-CLL/PLL are nongranular and differ phenotypically from the cells of large granular lymphocyte leukemia, which are CD16,

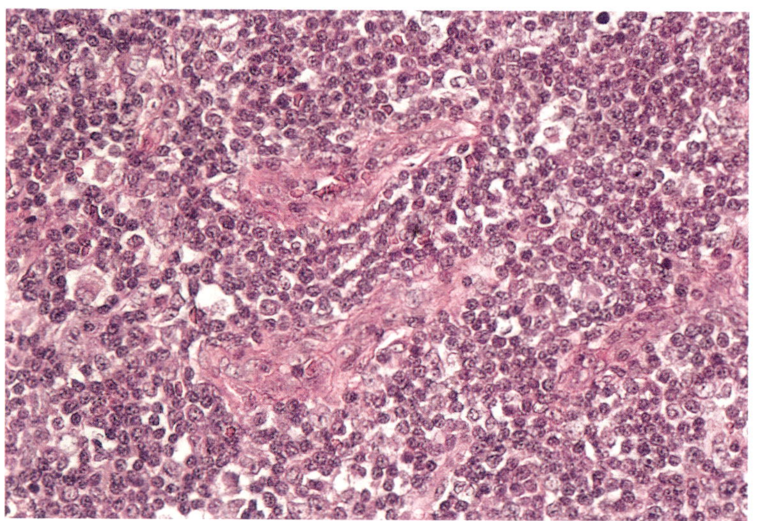

FIGURE 19.1

T cell chronic lymphocytic leukemia/prolymphocytic leukemia showing infiltration by small irregular lymphocytes and vascular proliferation.

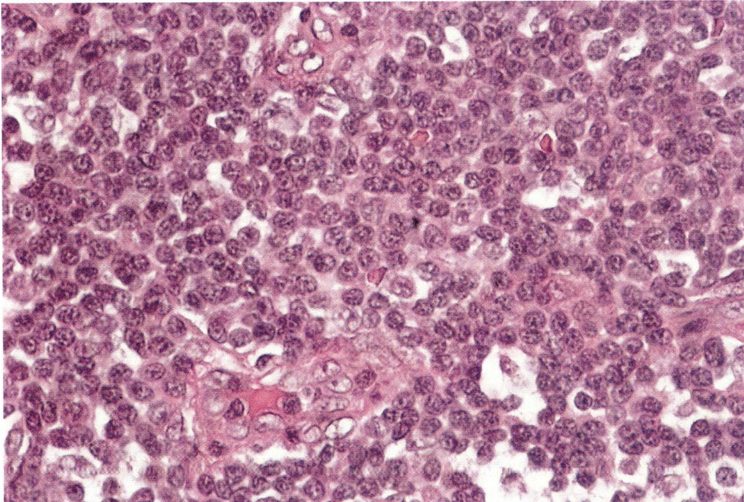

FIGURE 19.2

T cell chronic lymphocytic leukemia/prolymphocytic leukemia, higher magnification, showing atypical lymphocytes and absence of pseudofollicular proliferation centers.

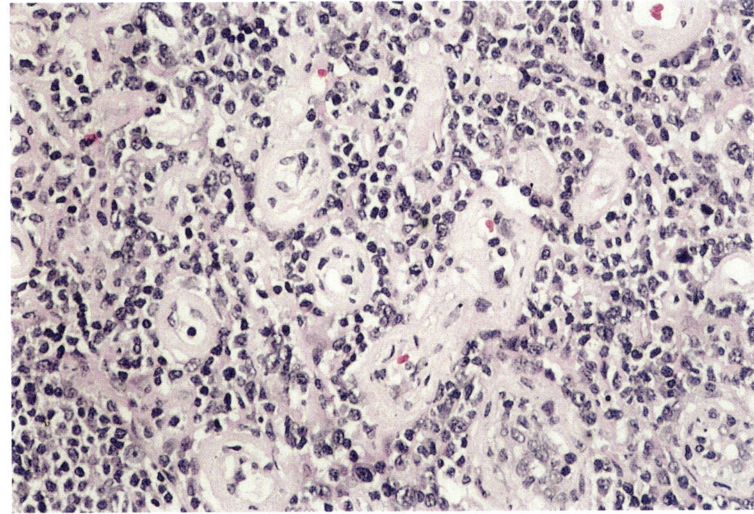

FIGURE 19.3

T cell chronic lymphocytic leukemia/prolymphocytic leukemia showing infiltration by small irregular lymphocytes and vascular proliferation with sclerosis.

CD56, or CD57 positive (Loughran, 1993). Sézary's syndrome is characterized by CD4-positive atypical lymphocytes and cutaneous manifestations but is distinguished by the marked epidermotrophism of the lymphocytic infiltrates in the skin and CD7-negative phenotype in most cases. Adult T cell lymphoma/leukemia is also characterized by CD4-positive atypical lymphocytes and cutaneous manifestations but is distinguished by the larger, more pleomorphic cells ("clover leaf" or "flower cells") and the CD7-negative, strongly CD25-positive phenotype. Distinction from B-CLL in the lymph node biopsy is

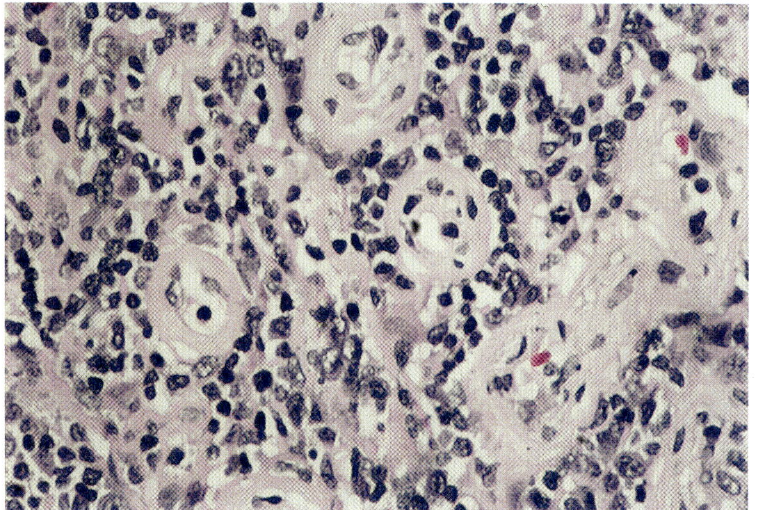

T cell chronic lymphocytic leukemia/prolymphocytic leukemia, higher magnification, showing atypical lymphocytes and sclerosis.

based on the absence of pseudofollicular proliferation centers and presence of cells with irregular nuclei and vascular proliferation.

Course and Prognosis

T-CLL/PLL is a progressive disorder which is refractory to therapy (Hoyer et al, 1995).

Large Granular Lymphocyte Leukemia

Classification

REAL: Large granular lymphocyte (LGL) leukemia, T cell and NK cell types.
WF: Malignant lymphoma, small lymphocytic.

Immunophenotype

T cell: CD2+, CD3+, CD8+, CD16+, CD56−, CD57+ or −
NK cell: CD2+, CD3−, CD8+, CD16+, CD56+ or −, CD57+ or −.

Clinical Features

Large granular lymphocyte leukemia (LGL) is a lymphoproliferative disorder character-ized morphologically by circulating atypical lymphocytes with abundant cytoplasm and coarse azurophilic granules. T cell and NK cell forms of the disease are recognized, with differing phenotypes and clinical features. The T cell form is more common in western countries and is a chronic disorder characterized by neutropenia, splenomegaly, rheu-matoid disease, and recurrent infections (Loughran, 1993). Anemia and thrombocyto-

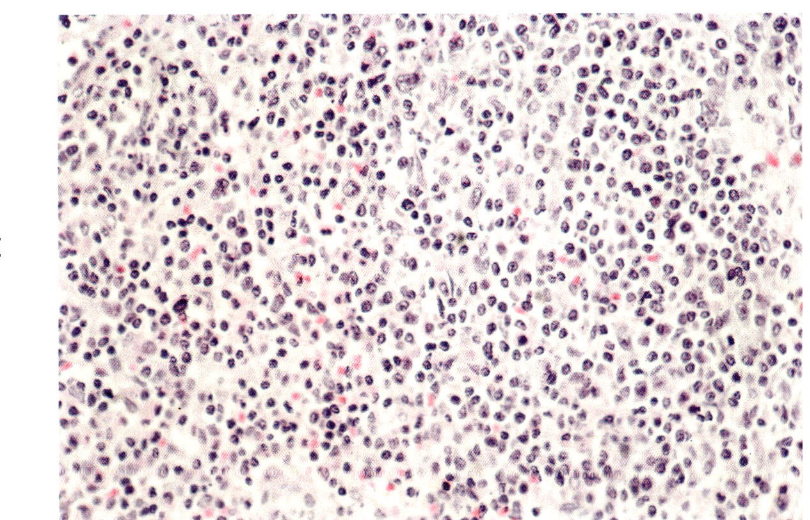

FIGURE 19.5

Large granular lymphocyte leukemia, T cell type, showing infiltration of splenic red pulp by atypical lymphocytes.

penia may also be present. The NK cell form is more common in Japan and is a fulminant disorder associated with Epstein-Barr virus, with less marked neutropenia and unassociated with rheumatoid disease (Loughran, 1993). The cells in the T cell form of the disease express T cell antigens (CD2, CD3, CD8) and NK cell antigens (CD16, CD57) and have clonal rearrangement of the T-cell antigen-receptor genes. The cells in the NK cell form of the disease express some T cell antigens (CD2, CD8) and NK cell antigens (CD16, CD56, CD57); CD3 is not expressed and the T-cell antigen-receptor genes are not rearranged.

Histopathology

Splenic involvement in LGL is characterized by infiltration of the red pulp by atypical lymphocytes (Figs. 19.5 and 19.6); the splenic white pulp is hyperplastic with prominent follicular centers (Loughran, 1993). Hepatic involvement is sinusoidal. The bone marrow shows diffuse interstitial lymphocytic infiltration; lymphoid aggregates resembling hyperplastic lymphoid follicles may also be present. Lymph node involvement is infrequent. NK cell cases may have involvement of the gastrointestinal tract (Loughran, 1993).

Differential Diagnosis

LGL should be distinguished from other lymphoproliferative disorders presenting with atypical lymphocytosis and splenomegaly, including infectious mononucleosis, hairy cell leukemia, and splenic lymphoma with villous lymphocytes. Immunophenotypic studies on peripheral blood are helpful, since the characteristic azurophilic granules may be sparse or absent. LGL may also be suspected in patients presenting with neutropenia and a small number of circulating large granular lymphocytes. Rearrangement of the T cell antigen-receptor β gene may be detected even when large granular lymphocytes are

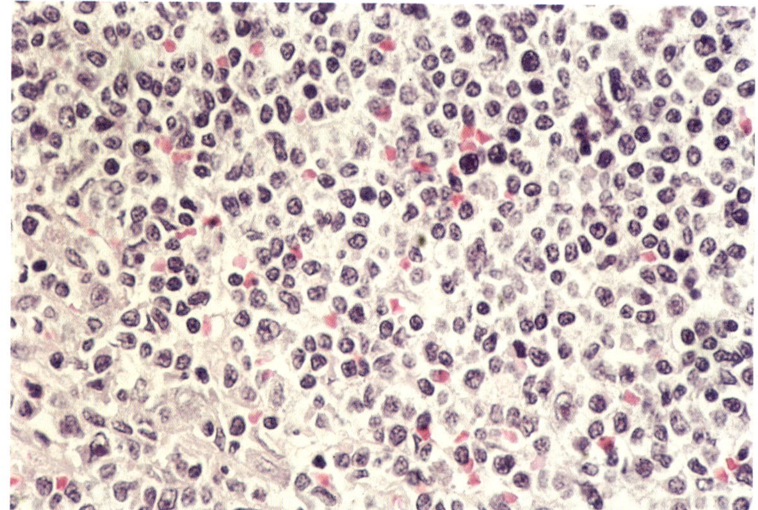

FIGURE
19.6

Large granular lymphocyte leukemia, T cell type, higher magnification,
showing atypical lymphocytes in splenic red pulp.

not numerous, and this is diagnostic (Semenzato et al, 1997). Cases of aggressive peripheral T cell lymphomas with an NK-like T cell phenotype have been reported and appear
to be a distinct disorder (Macon et al, 1996). Chronic reactive large granular lymphocytosis without evidence of clonality also occurs rarely (Loughran, 1993).

Course and Prognosis

LGL of T cell type is an indolent disorder; there is no specific treatment and therapy is
directed largely to correction of cytopenias. LGL of the NK cell type may be a fulminant
disorder; some cases have responded to combination chemotherapy.

Mycosis Fungoides/Sézary's Syndrome

Classification

REAL: Mycosis fungoides/Sézary's syndrome.
WF: Mycosis fungoides.

Immunophenotype

CD2+, CD3+, CD4+, CD5+, CD7− or +, CD8−, CD25− or +.

Clinical Features

Mycosis fungoides/Sézary's syndrome (MF/SS) is a cutaneous T cell lymphoma characterized by proliferation of epidermotrophic helper T cells in the skin and other sites
(Diamandidou et al, 1996). Patients with MF/SS are adults. The cutaneous lesions con-

sist of erythematous patches, plaques, or tumors in mycosis fungoides, and generalized erythroderma with circulating abnormal cells in Sézary's syndrome. Lymphadenopathy is frequent and may show the changes of dermatopathic lymphadenopathy or involvement by MF/SS. Lymph nodes showing the changes of dermatopathic lymphadenopathy frequently contain clonal rearrangements of the T-cell antigen-receptor genes, indicating occult involvement (Weiss et al, 1985). Transformation to diffuse large cell lymphoma or lymphoma resembling Hodgkin's disease may occur in the skin or extracutaneous lymph node sites (Scheen et al, 1984).

Histopathology

MF/SS in the skin is characterized by a band-like infiltrate of epidermotrophic T cells with nuclear irregularities and folds (cerebriform cells) (Fig. 19.7). The cells characteristically infiltrate the epidermis as single cells and as small clusters, referred to as Pautrier's microabscesses. The lymphocytes in the epidermis are frequently surrounded by a clear space or "halo," and the presence of "haloed" lymphocytes is a useful diagnostic feature (Smoller et al, 1995). Langerhans' cells are increased.

The lymph nodes in MF/SS frequently show the changes of dermatopathic lymphadenopathy, characterized by expansion of the paracortex by pale-staining histiocytes containing melanin, dendritic cells, and Langerhans' cells. Small clusters of irregular lymphocytes are frequently present in the paracortex in cases of dermatopathic lymphadenopathy, with or without associated MF/SS, and are a nonspecific finding. Infiltrates of irregular lymphocytes with effacement of the lymph node architecture, however, indicate involvement by MF/SS (Figs. 19.8 and 19.9). Transformation of MF/SS occurs and is characterized by cutaneous or extracutaneous large cell lymphoma with immunoblastic, anaplastic, or Hodgkin's-like features (Salhany et al 1988; Scheen et al, 1984) (Figs. 19.10 and 19.11).

FIGURE 19.7

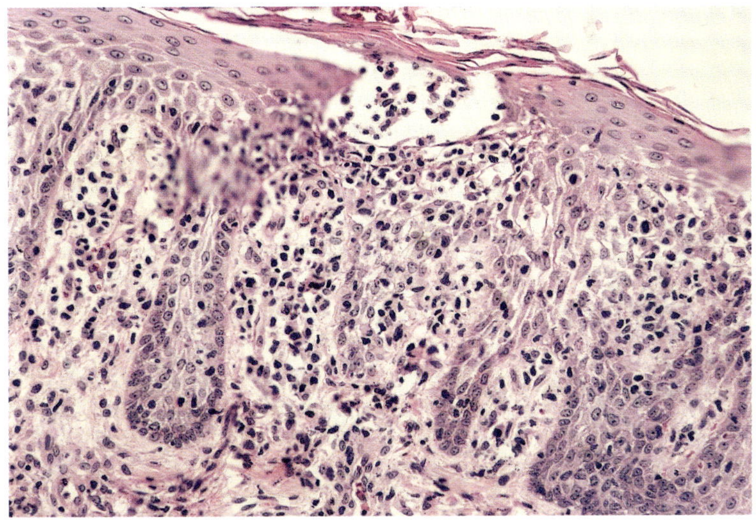

Mycosis fungoides/Sézary's syndrome, cutaneous involvement, showing band-like epidermotrophic infiltrate and Pautrier's microabscess.

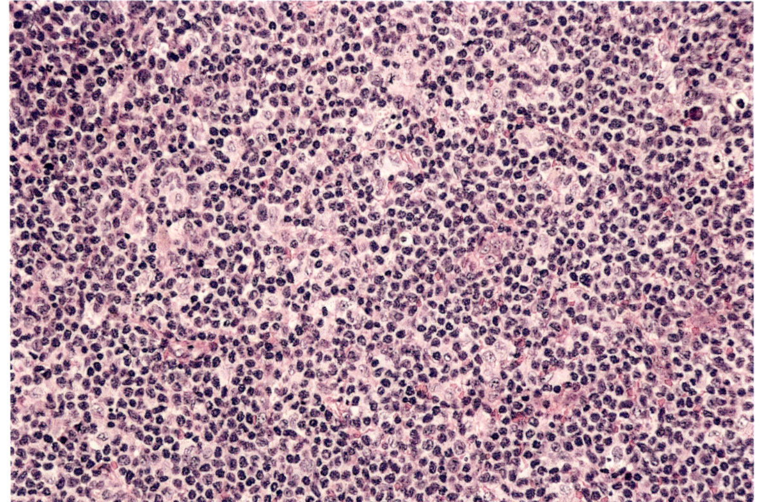

FIGURE 19.8

Mycosis fungoides/Sézary's syndrome, lymph node involvement, show-ing effacement of the lymph node architecture by infiltrates of small irregular lymphocytes.

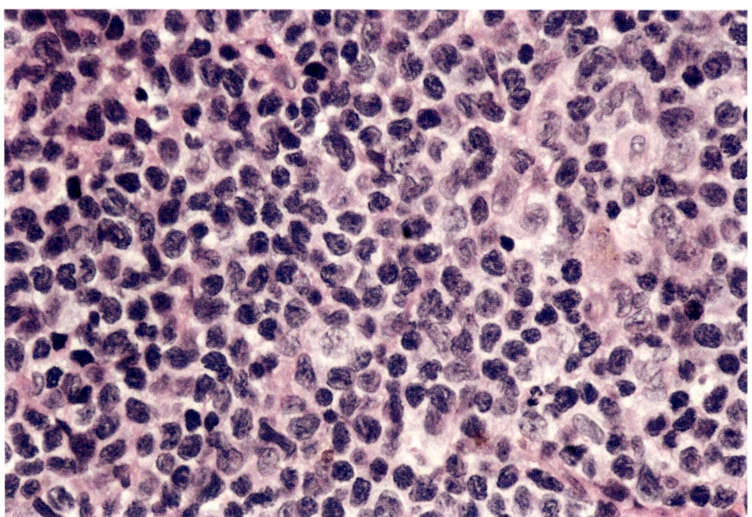

FIGURE 19.9

Mycosis fungoides/Sézary's syndrome, lymph node involvement, higher magnification, showing irregular cerebriform lymphocytes.

Differential Diagnosis

MF/SS must be distinguished from other cutaneous T lymphocytic infiltrates, including chronic dermatitis, actinic reticuloid and photodermatits, cutaneous pseudo–T cell lymphomas due to drug reactions, and lymphomatoid papulosis and primary cutaneous CD30-positive anaplastic large cell lymphoma. Lymphomatoid papulosis and primary cu-taneous CD30-positive anaplastic large cell lymphoma are closely related T cell prolifer-ations which may be associated with MF/SS and are characterized by CD30-positive

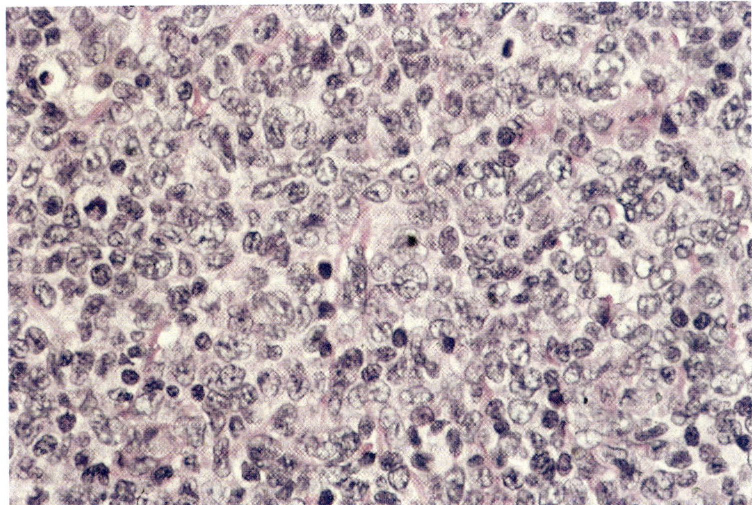

Mycosis fungoides/Sézary's syndrome, lymph node involvement, with transformation to large cell lymphoma.

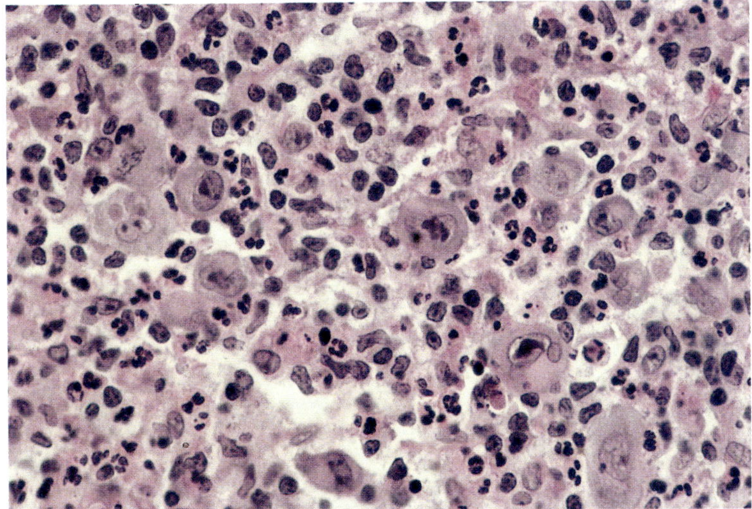

Mycosis fungoides/Sézary's syndrome, lymph node involvement, with transformation to Hodgkin's-like anaplastic large cell lymphoma.

cells and high frequency of spontaneous regression; clonal rearrangements of the T-cell antigen-receptor genes are frequently present (Weiss et al, 1986). Large plaque parapsoriasis *(parapsoriasis en plaque)*, alopecia mucinosa, and pagetoid reticulosis (Woringer Kolopp disease) are now considered to be variants of MF/SS by most authors (Diamandidou et al, 1996).

MF/SS should also be distinguished from other T cell lymphomas with cutaneous involvement, including peripheral T cell lymphoma, adult T cell lymphoma/leukemia, and granulomatous slack skin disease (Willemze et al, 1997). Adult T cell lymphoma/

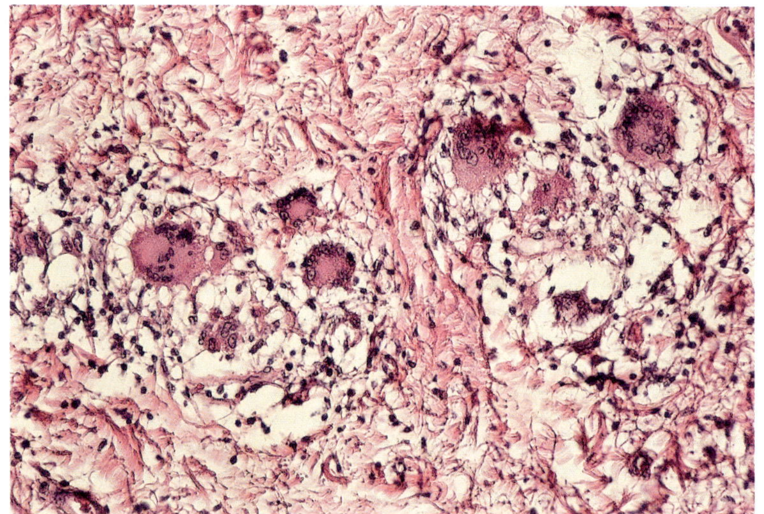

Granulomatous slack skin disease showing granulomatous dermal infiltrates and small lymphocytes. T-cell antigen-receptor gene is clonally rearranged, indicating a T cell lymphoproliferative disorder.

leukemia (ATLL) is characterized by cutaneous involvement and circulating abnormal lymphocytes, which may mimic MF/SS. The cutaneous infiltrates of ATLL are, however, less epidermotrophic than those of MF/SS and the circulating abnormal cells are frequently larger and more pleomorphic than those of Sézary's syndrome with clover leaf and flower cell forms. ATLL and MF/SS are both frequently CD4-positive and CD7-negative; ATLL characteristically shows strong CD25-positivity. Granulomatous slack skin disease is characterized by redundant skin folds in the axillae and groins, associated with a granulomatous dermal infiltrate (Fig. 19.12). Clonal T-cell antigen-receptor gene rearrangement is present, indicating a T cell lymphoproliferative disorder (Leboit et al, 1987).

Immunophenotypic studies are of limited diagnostic utility in MF/SS. Cutaneous MF/SS infiltrates are characteristically CD4-positive; CD8 cells are decreased and CD7 expression is frequently absent. These findings are, however, not specific for MF/SS and may be found in inflammatory dermatoses. T-cell antigen-receptor rearrangement studies are also of limited diagnostic value. Clonal T-cell antigen-receptor rearrangements are frequently not detected in early (patch stage) MF/SS; conversely clonal T-cell antigen-receptor rearrangements have been reported in cases of cutaneous pseudo–T cell lymphoma and in most cases of lymphomatoid papulosis (Weiss et al, 1986).

Lymph node involvement in MF/SS may be difficult to distinguish from the changes of dermatopathic lymphadenopathy. Small clusters of irregular lymphocytes may be present in dermatopathic lymphadenopathy unassociated with MF/SS; infiltrates of irregular lymphocytes with architectural effacement, however, indicate lymph node involvement. The histopathologic assessment of lymph node involvement in MF/SS may be of prognostic value (Sausville et al, 1988). Clonal rearrangement of the T-cell antigen-receptor genes is frequently present in lymph nodes showing dermatopathic lymphadenopathy from patients with MF/SS (Weiss et al, 1985).

Course and Prognosis

MF/SS is an indolent progressive disorder. MF/SS is managed with topical chemotherapy (mechlorethamine), oral psoralen and ultraviolet A light (PUVA), photophoresis, or electron beam irradiation (Diamandidou, 1996). Aggressive combination chemotherapy has not proven of benefit in randomized clinical trails.

REFERENCES

Diamandidou E, Cohen PR, Kurzrock R. Mycosis Fungoides and Sezary Syndrome. Blood 88:2385–2409, 1996.

Hoyer JD, Ross CW, Li C-Y, Witzig TE, Gascoyne RD, Dewald GW, Hanson CA. True T cell chronic lymphocytic leukemia: A morphologic and immunophenotypic study of 25 cases. Blood 86:1163–1169, 1995.

LeBoit PE, Beckstead JH, Bond B, Epstein WL, Frieden IJ, Parslow TG. Granulomatous slack skin: Clonal rearrangement of the T cell receptor beta gene is evidence for the lymphoproliferative nature of a cutaneous elastolytic disorder. J Invest Dermatol 89:183, 1987.

Loughran TP. Clonal diseases of large granular lymphocytes. Blood 82:1–14, 1993.

Macon WR, Williams JP, Hammer RD, Glick AD, Collins RD, Cousar JB. Natural killer-like T-cell lymphomas: Aggressive lymphomas of T-large granular lymphocytes. Blood 87:1474–1483, 1996.

Matutes E, Brito-Babapulle V, Swansbury J, Ellis J, Morilla R, Dearden C, Sempere A, Catovsky D. Clinical and laboratory features of 78 cases of T prolymphocytic leukemia. Blood 78:3269–3274, 1991.

Salhany KE, Cousar JB, Greer JB, Casey TT, Fields JP, Collins RD. Transformation of cutaneous T-cell lymphoma to large cell lymphoma: A clinicopathologic and immunohistologic study. Am J Pathol 132:265, 1988.

Sausville EA, Eddy JL, Makuch RW, Fischmann AB, Schecter GP, Matthews M, et al. Histopathologic staging at initial diagnosis of mycosis fungoides and Sezary syndrome. Definitions of three distinctive prognostic groups. Ann Intern Med 109:372, 1988.

Scheen SR, Banks PM, Winkelmann RK. Morphologic heterogeneity of malignant lymphomas developing in mycosis fungoides. Mayo Clin Proc 59:95–106, 1984.

Semenzato G, Zambello R, Starkebaum G, Oshimi K, Loughran TP. The lymphoproliferative disease of granular lymphocytes: Updated criteria for diagnosis. Blood 89:256–260, 1997.

Smoller BR, Bishop K, Glusac E, Kim YH, Hendrickson M. Reassessment of histologic parameters in the diagnosis of mycosis fungoides. Am J Surg Pathol 19:1423–1430, 1995.

Weiss LM, Hu E, Wood GS, Moulds C, Cleary ML, Warnke R, Sklar J. Clonal rearrangement of the T-cell receptor genes in mycosis fungoides and dermatopathic lymphadenopathy. N Engl J Med 313:539–544, 1985.

Weiss LM, Wood GS, Tela M, Warnke RA, Sklar J. Clonal T cell population in lymphomatoid papulosis: Evidence of a lymphoproliferative origin for a clinical benign disease. N Engl J Med 315:475, 1986.

Willemze R, Kerl H, Sterry W, Berti E, Cerroni L, Chimenti S, et al. EORTC classification for primary cutaneous lymphomas: A proposal from the Cutaneous Lymphoma Study Group of the European Organization for Research and Treatment of Cancer. Blood 90:354–371, 1997.

20

Peripheral T Cell and NK Cell Neoplasms: II. Peripheral T Cell Lymphomas

Peripheral T cell lymphomas include peripheral T cell lymphomas, unspecified, angioimmunoblastic T cell lymphoma, angiocentric lymphoma, intestinal T cell lymphoma, and adult T cell lymphoma/leukemia.

Peripheral T Cell Lymphomas, Unspecified

Classification

REAL: Peripheral T cell lymphomas, unspecified. Provisional cytologic categories: medium-sized cell, mixed medium and large cell, large cell, lymphoepithelioid cell. Provisional subtype: hepatosplenic γ-δ T cell lymphoma. Provisional subtype: subcutaneous panniculitic T cell lymphoma.
WF: Malignant lymphoma, diffuse, mixed small and large cell, epithelioid cell component. Malignant lymphoma, large cell, immunoblastic, clear cell, polymorphous, epithelioid cell component.

Immunophenotype

CD2+ or −, CD3+ or −, CD4+ or −, CD5+ or −, CD7− or +, CD8− or + (loss of one or more is frequent).

Clinical Features

Peripheral T cell lymphomas (PTCLs) are a heterogenous group of neoplasms which account for a minority (approximately 15%) of non-Hodgkin's lymphomas. In the WF most cases are found in the diffuse, mixed, small and large cell, and large cell, immunoblastic categories. Most patients are adults presenting with lymphadenopathy; advanced presentations (Ann Arbor stage III and IV), "B" symptoms, and extranodal involvement are frequent. Unusual manifestations, such as eosinophilia and lymphoma-associated hemophagocytosis may be present (Harris et al, 1994).

Histopathology

PTCLs are characterized by proliferation of small to large T cells with irregular nuclei (Figs. 20.1 and 20.2). Cellular pleomorphism and Reed-Sternberg–like cells may be prominent (Fig. 20.2). Vascular proliferation and admixture of inflammatory cells, including plasma cells, eosinophils, and epithelioid histiocytes, are frequent (Fig. 20.3). Lymph node involvement in PTCL is usually diffuse; an interfollicular or "T-zone" pattern may be present. Provisional cytologic categories of PTCL in the REAL classification are defined by the predominant cell type: medium-sized cell, mixed medium and large cell, large cell, and lymphoepithelioid cell (Harris et al, 1994). The last category refers to PTCL with a prominent component of epithelioid histiocytes, also referred to as Lennert's lymphoma (Patsouris et al, 1988) (Fig. 20.3). Lymphepithelioid cell lymphoma usually has a CD4-positive T cell phenotype (Spier et al, 1988).

Variants of Peripheral T Cell Lymphomas, Unspecified

PROVISIONAL SUBTYPE: HEPATOSPLENIC γ-δ T CELL LYMPHOMA Hepatosplenic γ-δ T cell lymphoma is a clinicopathologically distinct form of PTCL occurring in young adults

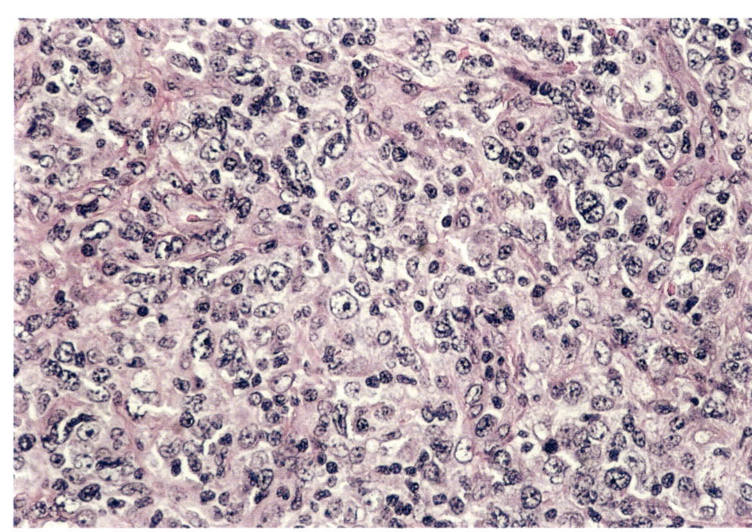

FIGURE 20.1

Peripheral T cell lymphoma showing small and large atypical lymphoid cells and admixture of plasma cells and epithelioid histiocytes.

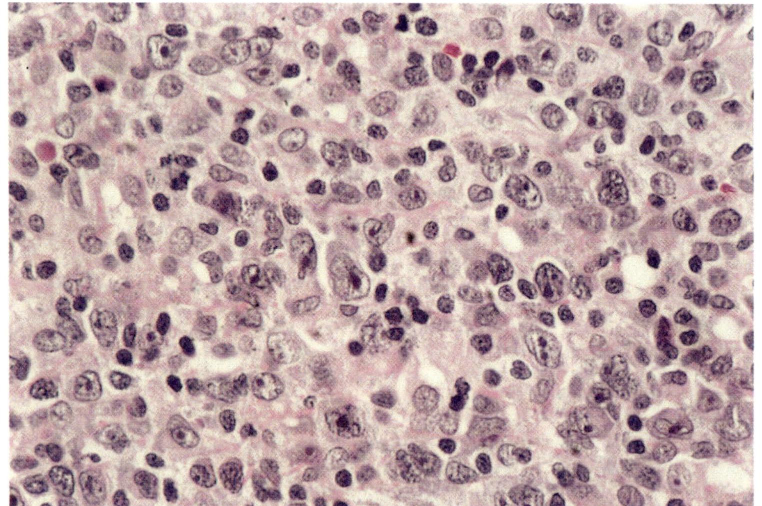

FIGURE
20.2

Peripheral T cell lymphoma showing pleomorphic Reed-Sternberg–like
cells.

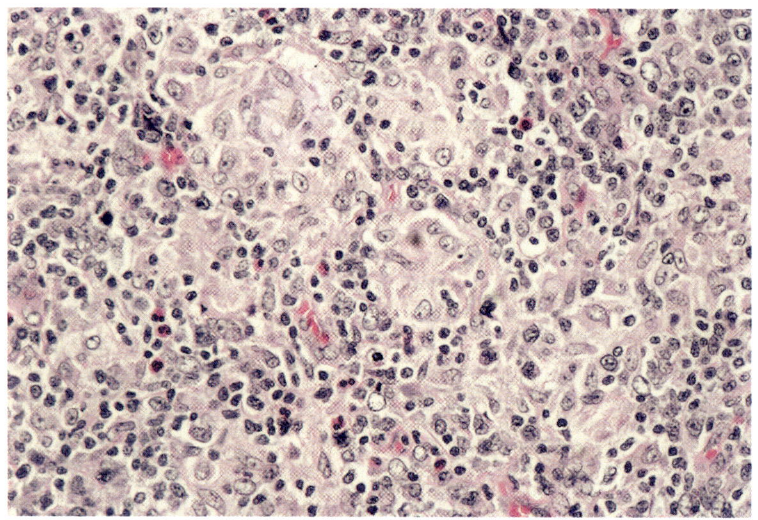

FIGURE
20.3

Lymphoepithelioid type of peripheral T cell lymphoma (Lennert's
lymphoma) showing irregular lymphocytes and numerous epithelioid
histiocytes.

presenting with hepatosplenomegaly and thrombocytopenia without lymphadenopathy.
Hepatosplenic T cell lymphoma is characterized by proliferation of cytotoxic γ-δ T cells
which exhibit a characteristic phenotype (CD2+, CD3+, CD4−, CD5−, CD7+, CD8+
or −, CD16+) and clonal rearrangement of the T-cell antigen-receptor γ gene (Cooke et
al, 1996). The lymphoma cells are medium sized cells with round nuclei and moderately
abundant cytoplasm and exhibit a characteristic sinusoidal pattern of involvement of
the red pulp of the spleen, liver, and bone marrow (Cooke et al, 1996) (Figs. 20.4 and
20.5). The prognosis is poor despite aggressive therapy.

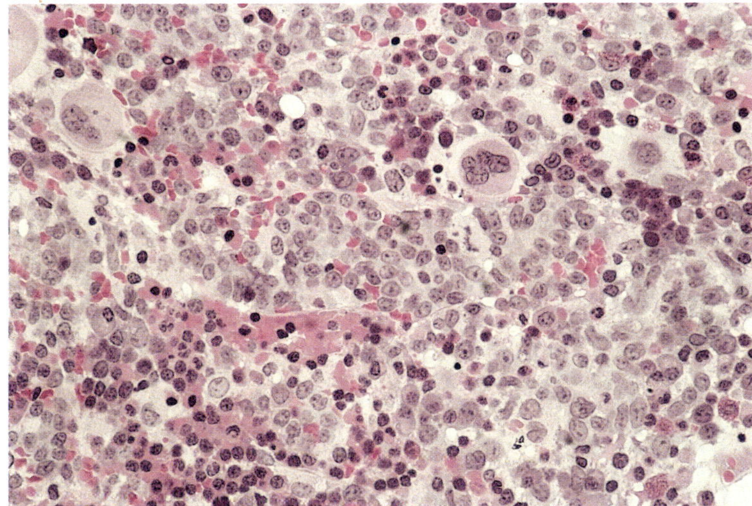

Hepatosplenic γ-δ T cell lymphoma, bone marrow, showing sinusoidal pattern of involvement.

FIGURE 20.4

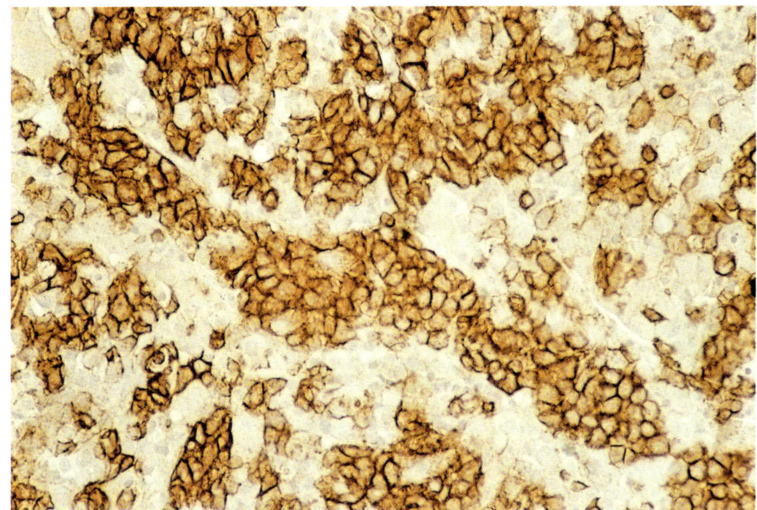

Hepatosplenic γ-δ T cell lymphoma, bone marrow stained for the T cell antigen CD3, showing sinusoidal pattern of involvement.

FIGURE 20.5

PROVISIONAL SUBTYPE: SUBCUTANEOUS PANNICULITIC T CELL LYMPHOMA Subcutaneous panniculitic T cell lymphoma is a clinicopathologically distinct form of T cell lymphoma presenting as subcutaneous fat necrosis (Gonzalez et al, 1991). Patients are adults presenting with subcutaneous nodules on the extremities which histologically mimic a panniculitis with infiltration of the subcutaneous fat by small and large irregular lymphocytes with associated fat necrosis (Figs. 20.6 and 20.7). Immunophenotypic studies show a T cell phenotype; clonal T-cell antigen-receptor gene rearrangement is identified in some patients (Gonzalez et al, 1991). Histiocytic cytophagic panniculitis (Fig.

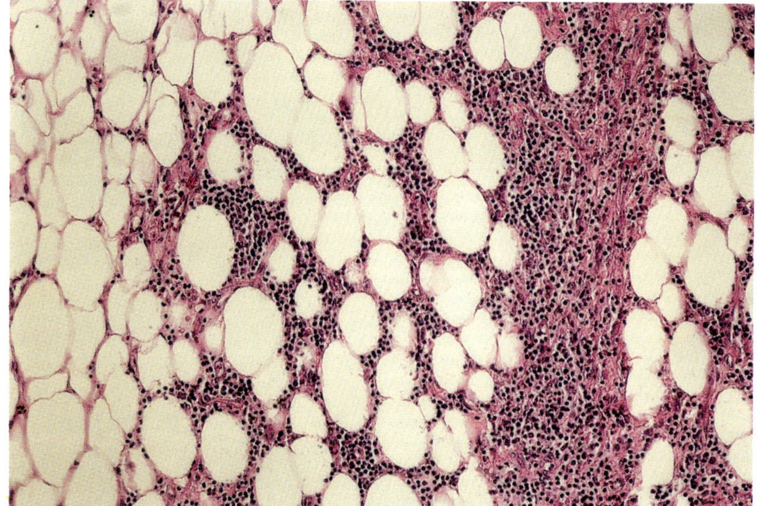

FIGURE 20.6

Subcutaneous panniculitic T cell lymphoma showing lace-like pattern of infiltration of subcutaneous fat.

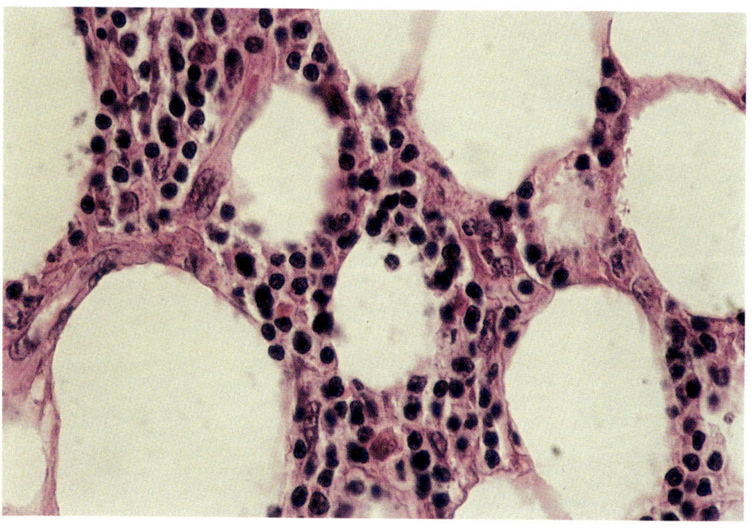

FIGURE 20.7

Subcutaneous panniculitic T cell lymphoma, higher magnification, showing atypical hyperchromatic lymphocytes.

20.8) is likely a related disorder (Hyteriglou et al, 1992). The clinical course is characterized by the frequent development of a hemophagocytic syndrome, which is often the cause of death. Dissemination of lymphoma to nonsubcutaneous sites is infrequent. Some patients have responded to aggressive combination chemotherapy (Gonzales et al, 1991).

Differential Diagnosis

PTCL must be distinguished from reactive lymphoid hyperplasias and from other lymphoproliferative disorders, including the more common B cell lymphomas and Hodgkin's

**FIGURE
20.8**

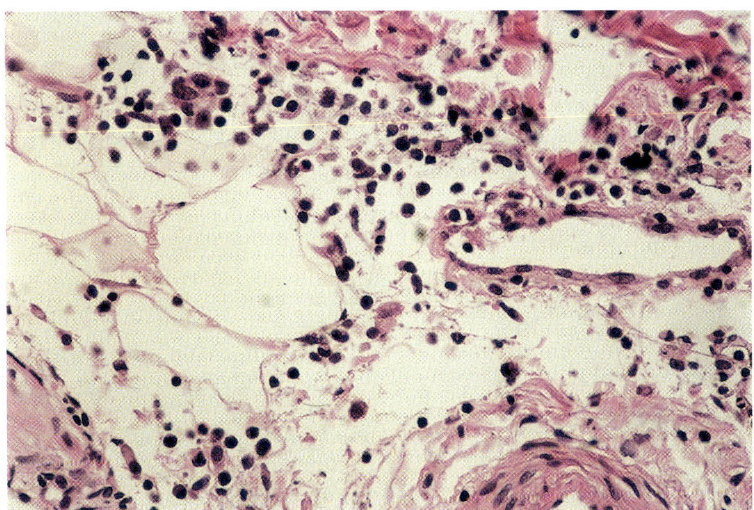

Histiocytic cytophagic panniculitis showing a mixed inflammatory infiltrate in the subcutaneous fat. Clonally rearranged T-cell antigen-receptor gene is present, indicating a T cell lymphoproliferative disorder.

disease. The frequent presence of inflammatory elements in PTCL, including plasma cells, eosinophils, and epithelioid histiocytes, may cause confusion with a reactive process. The presence of atypical small and large lymphocytes is a feature favoring PTCL. Immunohistochemical studies may be useful in differential diagnosis. The cells of PTCL frequently show loss of one or more pan–T cell antigens. The demonstration of an abnormal phenotype supports the diagnosis of PTCL. Gene rearrangement studies may also be useful. The demonstration of clonally rearranged T-cell antigen-receptor genes supports the diagnosis of PTCL.

Some B cell lymphomas exhibit features ordinarily associated with peripheral T cell lymphomas, including polymorphous cell population, vascular proliferation, and admixture of epithelioid histiocytes, and have been referred to as pseudo–T cell lymphomas. T-cell-rich B-large-cell lymphomas are regarded in this category. Cases of lymphoepithelioid cell lymphoma with B cell phenotype have been reported and have a better survival than cases with T cell phenotype (Spier et al, 1988).

PTCL with admixed inflammatory cells and Reed-Sternberg–like cells may be difficult to distinguish from Hodgkin's disease. Atypical small lymphocytes, intermediate forms between small and large cells, and atypical large cells with a paucity of diagnostic Reed-Sternberg cells are features favoring PTCL. In difficult cases, immunohistochemical studies may be helpful. The lymphoma cells in PTCL frequently demonstrate loss of one or more pan–T cell antigens; the lymphocytes in Hodgkin's disease are predominantly reactive helper T cells and demonstrate a normal phenotype. The Reed-Sternberg cells in Hodgkin's disease are consistently CD45-negative; most are CD15-positive (70%) and CD30-positive (90%). The atypical cells in PTCL are usually CD45-positive; a minority express CD15 or CD30. Hodgkin's disease usually lacks clonal T-cell antigen-receptor rearrangements.

Course and Prognosis

PTCLs are aggressive lymphomas which are treated with aggressive combination chemotherapy. Responses to therapy may be durable. The prognosis of PTCL may be less
favorable than that of comparable B cell lymphomas (Melnyk et al, 1997); but this has
not been a consistent finding in clinical trials.

Angioimmunoblastic T Cell Lymphoma

Classification

REAL: Angioimmunoblastic T cell lymphoma (AILD).
WF: Malignant lymphoma, diffuse, mixed small and large cell.

Immunophenotype

CD2+, CD3+, CD4+, CD5+, CD7+ or −, CD8−.

Clinical Features

Angioimmunoblastic T cell lymphoma includes the disorders also known as angioimmunoblastic lymphadenopathy with dysproteinemia (AILD), immunoblastic lymphadenopathy, and AILD-like T cell lymphoma. Patients are usually elderly, presenting with fever,
generalized lymphadenopathy, skin rash, and polyclonal hyperglobulinemia. A history of
drug or other exposure is obtained in nearly one-third of patients, suggesting an underlying abnormal immune response (Steinberg et al, 1988). The presence of clonal rearrangement of the T-cell antigen-receptor genes (Weiss et al, 1986) and clonal cytoge-

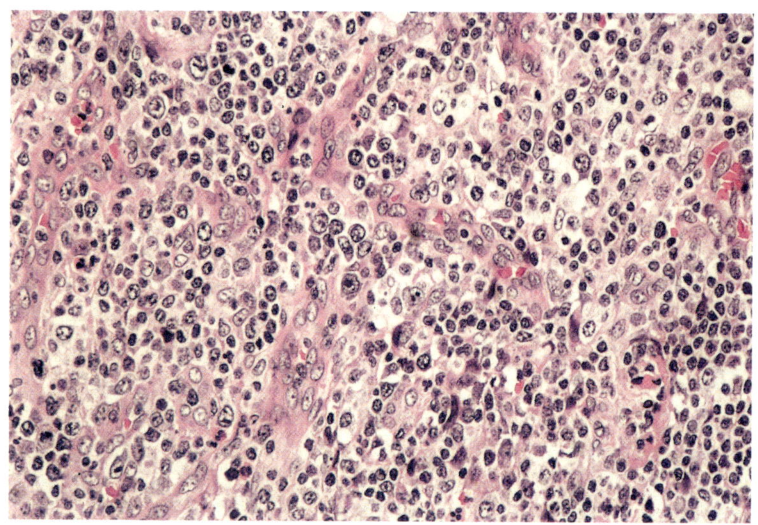

FIGURE
20.9

Angioimmunoblastic T cell lymphoma showing polymorphous lymphoid
proliferation and arborizing high endothelial venules.

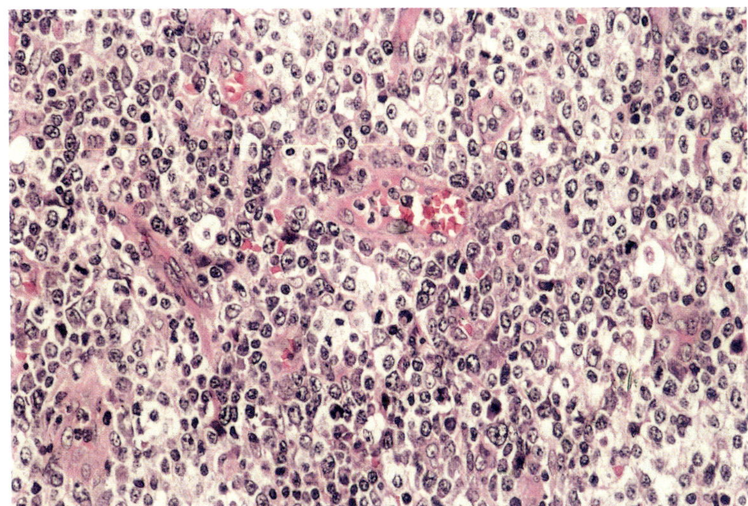

Angioimmunoblastic T cell lymphoma showing numerous clear cells.

netic abnormalities (Schlegelberger et al, 1994) indicate a T cell lymphoproliferative disorder. AILD is now accepted by most authors as a form of peripheral T cell lymphoma (Harris et al, 1994). Epstein-Barr Virus (EBV) is frequently detected in AILD (Weiss et al, 1992). Progression of AILD to diffuse large cell lymphoma of T or B cell phenotype may occur. Bone marrow involvement in AILD is frequent.

Histopathology

AILD is characterized by effacement of the lymph node architecture by a polymorphous proliferation of small and large lymphocytes, immunoblasts, "clear cells," plasma cells, eosinophils, and epithelioid histiocytes, with prominent proliferation of arborizing high endothelial venules (Figs. 20.9, 20.10, and 20.11). Involved lymph nodes have a characteristic hypocellular, depleted appearance at low magnification; the peripheral sinus is frequently intact or dilated, although lymphoid infiltration may extend beyond it. Involuted or "burnt out" follicular centers are often present and interstitial deposits of periodic acid–Schiff (PAS)-positive eosinophilic material are frequent. Bone marrow involvement is characterized by similarly hypocellular polymorphous lymphoid infiltrates.

Differential Diagnosis

The general acceptance of AILD as a form of peripheral T cell lymphoma has rendered moot a complex and confusing literature on malignant lymphoma developing in AILD. Some authors continue to distinguish between AILD and AILD-like T cell lymphoma, reserving the latter term for cases with greater hypercellularity and atypia of the small lymphocytes with prominent clear cells (Warnke et al, 1995).

AILD should be distinguished from reactive lymphoid hyperplasias which may mimic it. The involuted phase of persistent generalized lymphadenopathy associated with HIV infection may closely resemble AILD; typically, patients with AILD are elderly, in contrast to patients with HIV infection, who are younger. AILD should also be distinguished

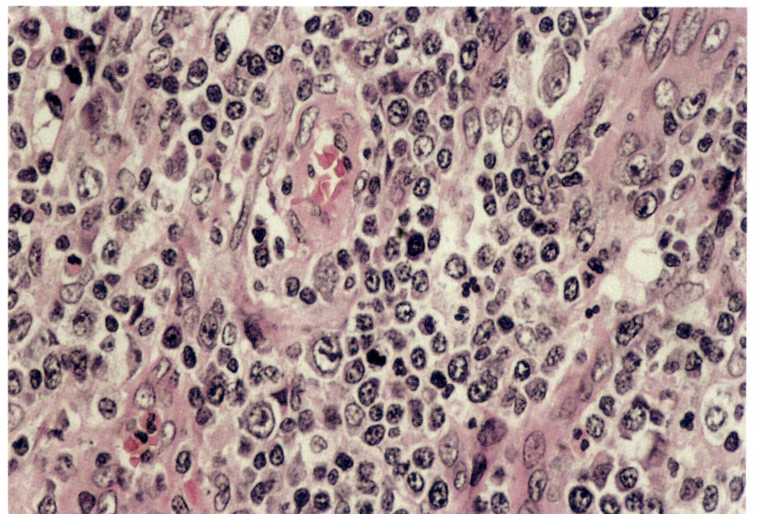

Angioimmunoblastic T cell lymphoma, higher magnification, showing polymorphous lymphoid proliferation.

from postvaccinial and hypersensitivity lymphadenopathy, which also show prominent vascular proliferation and numerous immunoblasts but lack the hypocellular, depleted appearance and PAS-positive interstitial deposits typical of AILD.

Course and Prognosis

AILD behaves as an indolent form of peripheral T cell lymphoma. There is no uniformly accepted therapy. Aggressive combination chemotherapy has not been of consistent benefit.

Angiocentric Lymphoma

Classification

REAL: Angiocentric lymphoma.
WF: Malignant lymphoma, diffuse, mixed small and large cell.

Immunophenotype

CD2+, CD3−, CD5−, CD7− or +, CD56+.

Clinical Features

Angiocentric lymphomas are extranodal lesions characterized by polymorphous lymphoid infiltrates with invasion of small blood vessels and necrosis. Two clinicopathologic forms are recognized: lymphomatoid granulomatosis and nasal T/NK cell lymphoma (also referred to as midline granuloma or polymorphic reticulosis). Although it had been suggested that these are closely related lesions and the term "angiocentric immunoproliferative lesion" has been applied to both, recent evidence suggests they are phenotypically distinct. Lymphomatoid granulomatosis presents with necrotizing lesions with predominantly pulmonary involvement; clonally rearranged immunoglobulin genes are frequently present and current evidence suggests lymphomatoid granulomatosis is T-cell-rich B cell proliferation related to Epstein-Barr virus infection (Wilson et al, 1996). T/NK cell nasal lymphoma (midline granuloma or polymorphic reticulosis) presents with necrotizing lesions involving the nose and paranasal sinuses; current evidence suggests this is a true T/NK cell lymphoma, also related to Epstein-Barr virus infection (Jaffe et al, 1996). T/NK cell nasal lymphoma most commonly expresses a phenotype consistent with NK cells (CD2+, CD3–, CD5–, CD56+); T-cell antigen-receptor genes are unrearranged (Emile et al, 1996). Cytoplasmic CD3 is detected in paraffin-embedded tissue with polyclonal anti-CD3 (CD3[P]) due to staining of the epsilon chain of the CD3 complex; CD3 epsilon is expressed in fetal and adult activated NK cells (Emile et al, 1996). CD45RO and CD43 are frequently also positive in paraffin-embedded tissue (Jaffe et al, 1996). Lymphomas with identical features occur at other extranodal sites (skin, subcutaneous tissue, gastrointestinal tract) and have been termed "nasal-type T/NK cell lymphomas"; the hemophagocytic syndrome may occur in these lymphomas (Jaffe et al, 1996).

Histopathology

Angiocentric T/NK cell lymphomas are characterized by an angiocentric pattern of growth with infiltration and destruction of the walls of small blood vessels and extensive necrosis (Fig. 20.12). Necrosis is coagulative with a zonal or infarct-like distribution. The extent of necrosis may obscure the underlying lymphoid proliferation; surviving lymphoid cells are frequently identified in islands surrounding small vessels The

FIGURE 20.12

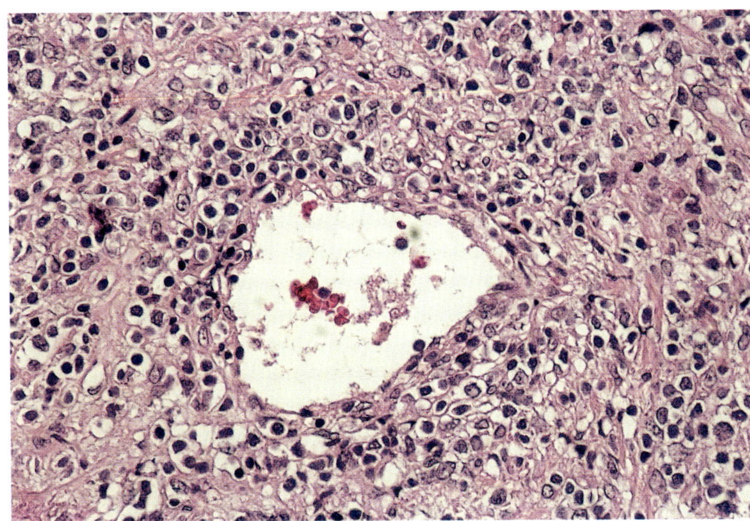

Angiocentric T/NK cell lymphoma of paranasal sinus showing infiltration of the wall of a small blood vessel by atypical lymphocytes. Immunophenotypic studies demonstrate a T/NK cell phenotype.

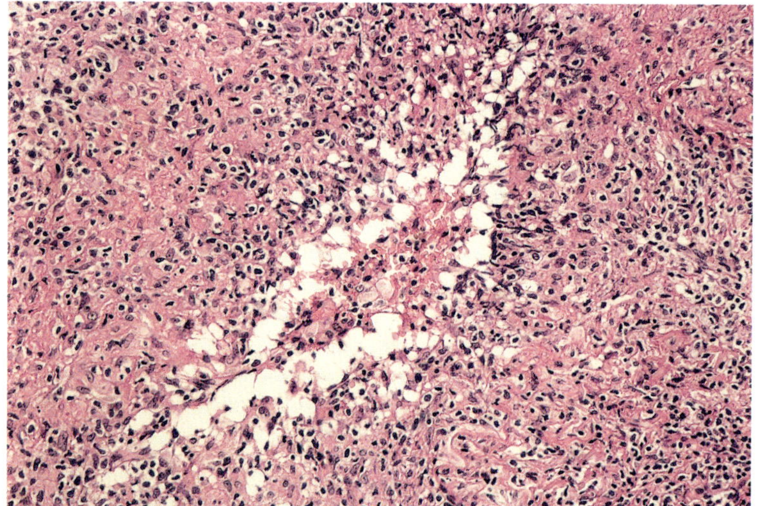

FIGURE 20.13

Lymphomatoid granulomatosis of the lung showing pulmonary vascular infiltration.

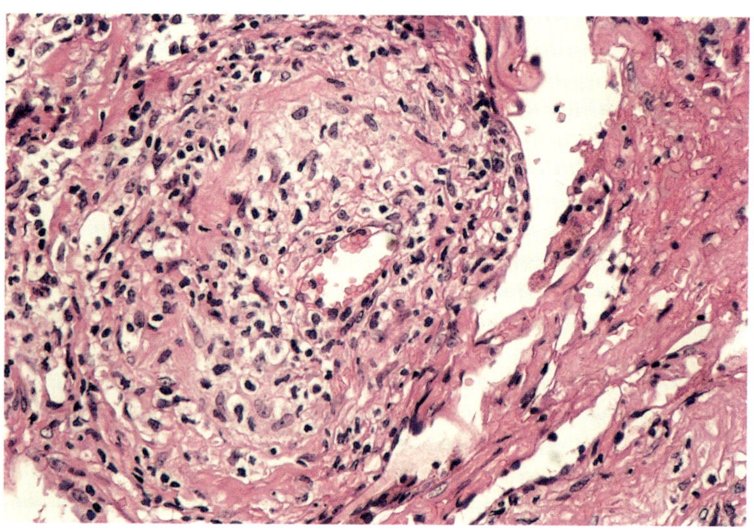

FIGURE 20.14

Lymphomatoid granulomatosis of the lung, higher magnification, showing infiltration of the wall of a small blood vessel by atypical lymphocytes. Although histologically resembling angiocentric T/NK cell lymphoma, immunophenotypic studies demonstrate a T cell-rich B cell proliferation.

angiocentric infiltrates are characteristically polymorphous with varying numbers of small and large atypical lymphoid cells; inflammatory cells are frequently admixed.

Differential Diagnosis

Angiocentric T/NK cell lymphomas must be distinguished from other necrotizing lesions involving the sinonasal tract, from other types of peripheral T cell lymphoma, and from lymphomatoid granulomatosis. The extensiveness of necrosis may make small biopsies from the sinonasal tract difficult to interpret. Granulomatous disease must be carefully excluded, in particular Wegener's granulomatosis, which may present with similar necrotizing lesions of the sinonasal tract (Crissman et al, 1982). Other peripheral T cell lymphomas may present with a CD56-positive NK-like T cell phenotype, but differ by CD3-positivity and the presence of clonally rearranged T-cell antigen-receptor genes (Emile et al, 1996; Macon et al, 1996). These lymphomas are also frequently extranodal but lack the characteristic clinicopathologic features of angiocentric T/NK lymphoma. Precursor T/NK cell lymphomas have the morphology of lymphoblastic lymphoma and should also be distinguished (Koita et al, 1997) as should a blastic or monomorphic form of NK cell leukemia/lymphoma occurring in the elderly (DiGiuseppe et al, 1997). Lymphomatoid granulomatosis may be morphologically indistinguishable from angiocentric T/NK cell lymphomas but is characterized by clonally rearranged immunoglobulin genes and a T-cell-rich B cell phenotype (Wilson et al, 1996) (Figs. 20.13 and 20.14). Pulmonary involvement is frequent in lymphomatoid granulomatosis, but rare in angiocentric T/NK cell lymphoma (Jaffe et al, 1996).

Course and Prognosis

Angiocentric T/NK cell lymphoma is an aggressive neoplasm. Localized sinonasal disease has responded to radiation therapy; disseminated disease may respond to aggressive combination chemotherapy (Crissman et al, 1982). Lymphomatoid granulomatosis may respond to therapy with α-interferon (Wilson et al, 1996).

Intestinal T Cell Lymphoma

Classification

REAL: Intestinal T cell lymphoma (with or without enteropathy).
WF: Malignant lymphoma, diffuse, mixed small and large cell. Malignant lymphoma, large cell, immunoblastic.

Immunophenotype

CD2 +, CD3 +, CD4 −, CD7 +, CD8 +.

Clinical Features

Intestinal T cell lymphoma occurs most frequently in adults with a history of celiac sprue (gluten-sensitive enteropathy) but may also occur de novo; the adjacent intestinal mucosa frequently shows villous atrophy. Intestinal T cell lymphoma was first reported as malignant histiocytosis of the intestine but has subsequently been shown to be of peripheral T cell phenotype (Isaacson et al, 1985). Patients frequently have a history of longstanding sprue, which has recently become refractory to therapy, or present with abdominal pain. Lymphoma may be preceded by the appearance of jejunal ulcerations (ulcerative jejunitis).

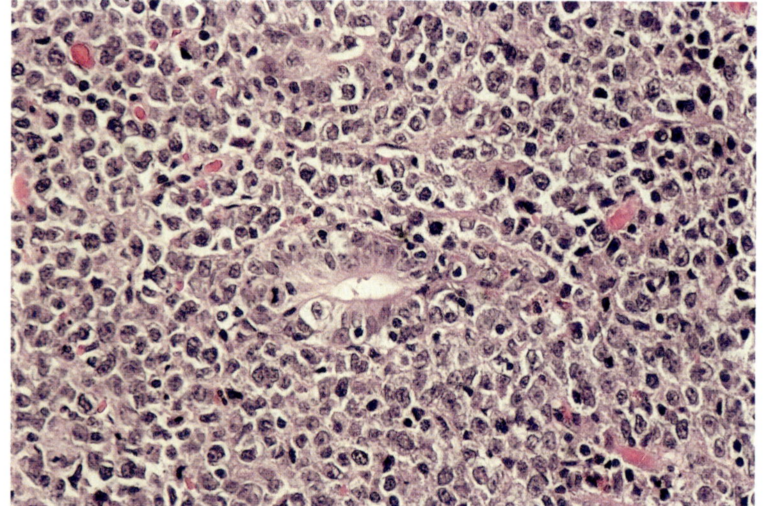

Intestinal T cell lymphoma showing infiltration of the mucosa by pleomorphic large cells.

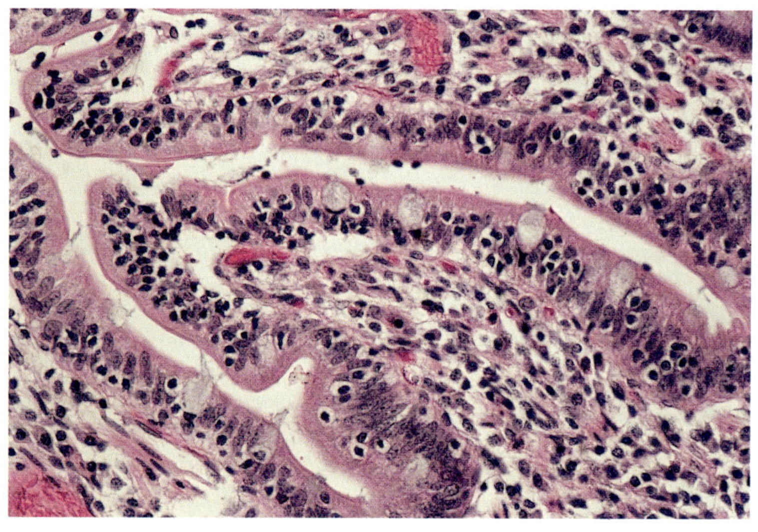

Intestinal T cell lymphoma, adjacent mucosa, showing intraepithelial lymphocytosis.

Histopathology

Multiple ulcerations of the small bowel are present and accompanied by a polymorphous infiltrate of small and large lymphoid cells (Chott et al, 1992) (Fig. 20.15). A mass may or may not be present. The adjacent intestinal mucosa frequently shows intraepithelial infiltration by atypical lymphocytes (Fig. 20.16); villous atrophy may be present.

Differential Diagnosis

Intestinal T cell lymphoma may be difficult to diagnose in endoscopic biopsies because of ulceration and superimposed inflammation. Ulcerative jejunitis in patients with celiac sprue may represent an early manifestation of lymphoma.

Course and Prognosis

Intestinal T cell lymphoma has a poor prognosis.

Adult T Cell Lymphoma/Leukemia

Classification

REAL: Adult T cell lymphoma/leukemia.
WF: Malignant lymphoma, diffuse, mixed small and large cell. Malignant lymphoma, large cell, immunoblastic.

Immunophenotype

CD2+, CD3+, CD4+, CD5+, CD7−, CD8− (rarely+), CD25+.

Clinical Features

Adult T cell lymphoma/leukemia (ATLL) results from infection with the human T lymphocytotrophic virus, type 1 (HTLV-1) (Broder et al, 1984). HTLV-1 infection is endemic in Japan and the Caribbean and occurs sporadically elsewhere, including the southeastern United States. HTLV-1 is trophic for T cells and infection results in a self-limited polyclonal T cell expansion which is mediated by interleukin-2. The integrated proviral form of HTLV-1 remains latent in infected T cells; in a small percentage of patients clonal proliferation gives rise to ATLL (Cavrois et al, 1996). ATLL is most frequently a fulminant disorder characterized by lymphadenopathy, skin lesions, hepatosplenomegaly, lytic bone lesions, hypercalcemia, and circulating abnormal T cells. The latter are characterized by multilobated clover leaf or flower cell nuclei (Fig. 20.17). Occasional patients exhibit a more indolent course characterized by isolated lymphadenopathy (lymphomatous form) or persistent lymphocytosis (chronic form).

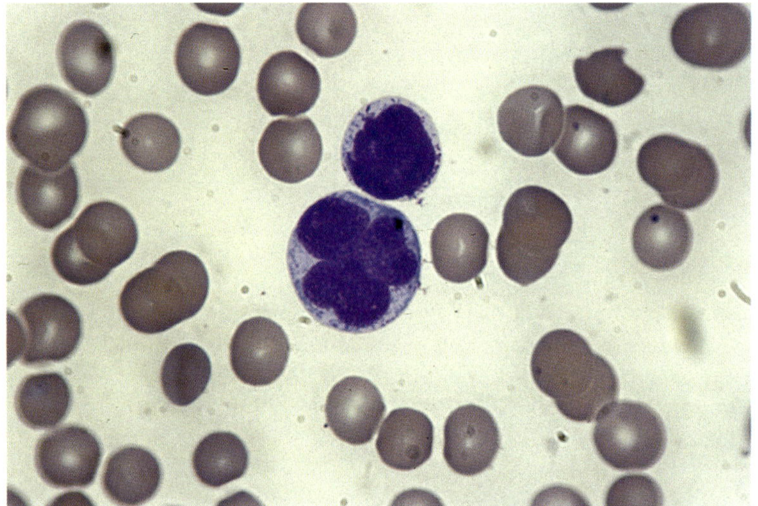

FIGURE
20.17

Adult T cell lymphoma/leukemia, peripheral blood smear, showing a clover leaf or flower cell.

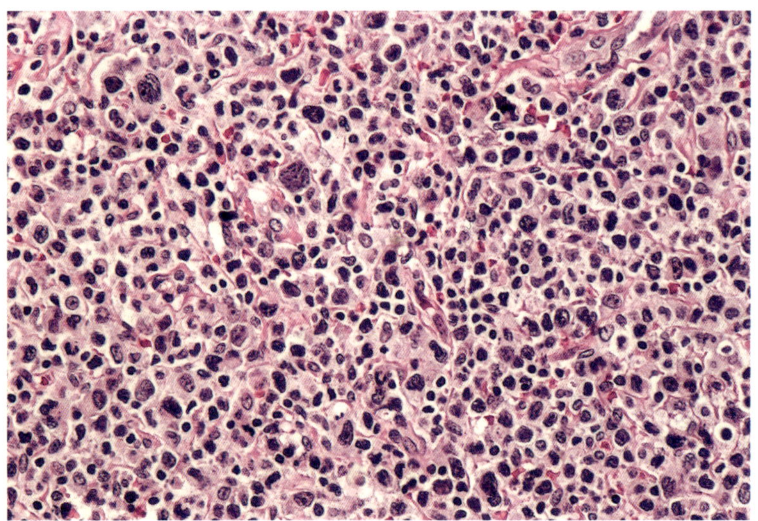

FIGURE
20.18

Adult T cell lymphoma/leukemia, involved lymph node, showing infiltrate of atypical pleomorphic lymphoid cells.

Histopathology

Lymph node involvement in ATLL is characterized by diffuse infiltration with large lymphoid cells with pleomorphic irregular nuclei and prominent nucleoli (Broder et al, 1984) (Figs. 20.18 and 20.19). In some patients atypical small or medium-sized cells predominate and a leukemic pattern of infiltration may be found with preservation of the lymph node sinuses (Jaffe et al, 1984). Pleomorphic Reed-Sternberg–like cells are present in some cases and may mimic Hodgkin's disease (Ohshima et al, 1991). Skin

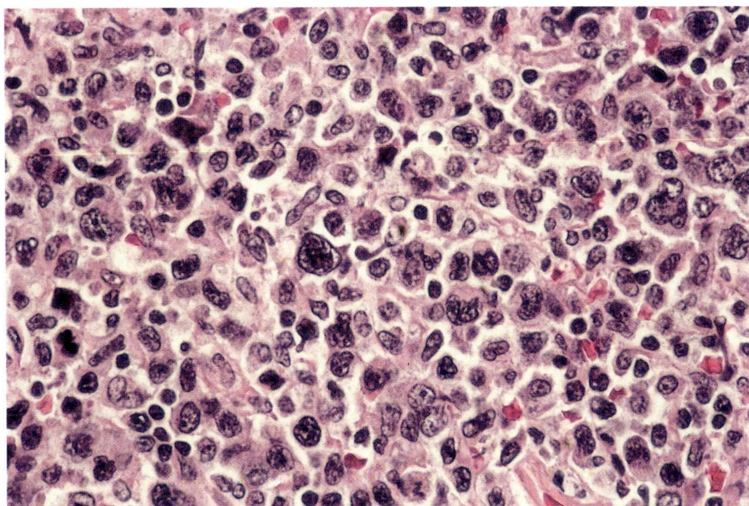

FIGURE 20.19

Adult T cell lymphoma/leukemia, higher magnification of involved lymph node, showing pleomorphic Reed-Sternberg–like cells.

involvement is characterized by dermal or dermal and epidermal lymphoid infiltrates with Pautrier's microabscess, which may mimic mycosis fungoides/Sézary's syndrome (Jaffe et al, 1984). The lytic bone lesions may show osteoclastic resorption of bone without lymphomatous infiltration; bone marrow involvement may be minimal despite overt leukemia.

Differential Diagnosis

ATLL should be distinguished from other peripheral T cell lymphomas and from mycosis fungoides/Sézary's syndrome. The presence of clover leaf or flower cells in the peripheral blood with CD4-positive T cell phenotype and strong positivity for CD25 is characteristic. Most patients will have antibodies to HTLV-1.

Course and Prognosis

ATLL is usually a fulminant disorder with poor prognosis. Responses to a combination of zidovudine and α-interferon have been reported (Gill et al, 1995).

REFERENCES

Broder S, Bunn PA, Jaffe ES, Blattner W, Gallo RC, Wong-Staal F, Waldmann TA, DeVita VT. T-cell lymphoproliferative syndrome associated with human T cell leukemia/lymphoma virus. Ann Intern Med 100:543–557, 1984.

Cavrois M, Wain-Hobson S, Gessain A, Plumelle Y, Wattel E. Adult T cell leukemia/lymphoma on a background of clonally expanded human T cell leukemia virus type 1 positive cells. Blood 88:4646–4650, 1996.

Chott A, Dragosics B, Radaszkiewcz T. Peripheral T cell lymphomas of the intestine. Am J Pathol 141:1361–1371, 1992.

Cooke CB, Krenacs L, Stetler-Stevenson M, Greiner TC, Raffeld M, Kingma DW, et al. Hepatosplenic T-cell lymphoma: A distinct clinicopathologic entity of cytotoxic gamma-delta T-cell origin. Blood 88:4265–4274, 1996.

Crissman JD, Weiss MA, Gluckman J. Midline granuloma syndrome. A clinicopathologic study of 13 patients. Am J Surg Pathol 6:335–346, 1982.

DiGiuseppe JA, Louie DC, Williams JE, Miller DT, Griffin CA, Mann RB, Borowitz MJ. Blastic natural killer cell leukemia/lymphoma: A clinicopathologic study. Am J Surg Pathol 21:1223–1230, 1997.

Emile J-F, Boulland M-L, Haioun C, Kanavaros P, Petrella T, Delfau-Larue M-H, et al. CD5-CD56+ T-cell receptor silent peripheral T-cell lymphomas are natural killer cell lymphomas. Blood 87:1466–1473, 1996.

Gill PS, Harrington W, Kaplan MH, Ribeiro RC, Bennet JM, Liebman HA et al. Treatment of adult T cell leukemia-lymphoma with a combination of interferon alfa and zidovudine. N Engl J Med 332:1744–1748, 1995.

Gonzalez CL, Medeiros LJ, Braziel RM, Jaffe ES. T cell lymphoma involving subcutaneous tissue. A clinicopathologic entity commonly associated with hemophagocytic syndrome. Am J Surg Pathol 15:17–27, 1991.

Harris NL, Jaffe ES, Stein H, Banks PM, Chan JKC, Cleary ML, et al. A revised European-American classification of lymphoid neoplasms: A proposal from the international lymphoma study group. Blood 84:1361–1392, 1994.

Hytiroglou P, Phelps RG, Wattenberg DJ, Strauchen JA. Histiocytic cytophagic panniculitis: Molecular evidence for a clonal T cell disorder. J Am Acad Dermatol 27:333–336, 1992.

Isaacson PG, O'Connor NT, Spencer J, Bevan DH, Connolly CE, Kirkham N, et al. Malignant histiocytosis of the intestine: A T cell lymphoma. Lancet 2:688–691, 1985.

Jaffe ES, Blattner WA, Blayney DW, Bunn PA, Cossman J, Robert-Guroff M, Gallo RC. The pathologic spectrum of adult T cell leukemia/lymphoma in the United States. Am J Surg Pathol 8:263–275, 1984.

Jaffe ES, Chan JKC, Su I-J, Frizzera G, Mori S, Feller AC, Ho FCS. Report of the workshop on nasal and related extranodal angiocentric T/Natural killer cell lymphomas. Definitions, differential diagnosis, and epidemiology. Am J Surg Pathol 20:103–111, 1996.

Koita H, Suzumiya J, Ohshima K, Takeshita M, Kimura N, Kikuchi M, Koono M. Lymphoblastic lymphoma expressing natural killer cell phenotype with involvement of the mediastinum and nasal cavity. Am J Surg Pathol 21:242–248, 1997.

Macon WR, Williams ME, Greer JP, Hammer RD,

Glick AD, Collins RD, Cousar JB. Natural killer-like T-cell lymphomas: Aggressive lymphomas of T-large granular lymphocytes. Blood 87:1474–1483, 1996.

Melnyk A, Rodriguez A, Pugh WC, Cabannillas F. Evaluation of the Revised European-American Lymphoma classification confirms the clinical relevance of immunophenotyping in 560 cases of aggressive non-Hodgkin's lymphoma. Blood 89:4514–4545, 1997.

Ohshima K, Kikuchi M, Yoshida T, Masuda Y, Kimura N. Lymph nodes in incipient adult T cell leukemia-lymphoma with Hodgkin's disease-like histologic features. Cancer 67:1622–1628, 1991.

Patsouris E, Noel H, Lennert K. Histological and immunohistological findings in lymphoepithelioid cell lymphoma (Lennert's lymphoma). Am J Surg Pathol 12:341–350, 1988.

Schlegelberger B, Zhang Y, Weber-Matthiesen K, Grote W. Detection of aberrant clones in nearly all cases of angioimmunoblastic lymphadenopathy with dysproteinemia-type T cell lymphoma by combined interphase and metaphase cytogenetics. Blood 84:2640–2648, 1994.

Spier CM, Lippman SM, Miller TP, Grogan TM. Lennert's lymphoma. A clinicopathologic study with emphasis on phenotype and its relationship to survival. Cancer 61:517–524, 1988.

Steinberg AD, Seldin MF, Jaffe ES, Smith HR, Klinman DM, Krieg AM, Cossman J. Angioimmunoblastic lymphadenopathy with dysproteinemia. Ann Intern Med 108:575–584, 1988.

Warnke RA, Weiss LM, Chan JKC, Cleary ML, Dorfman RF. Tumors of the lymph nodes and spleen. In: Atlas of Tumor Pathology, Third Series, Fascicle 14. Rosai J, Sobin LH, eds. Washington, D.C., Armed Forces Institute of Pathology, 1995.

Weiss LM, Strickler JG, Dorfman RF, Horning SJ, Warnke RA, Sklar J. Clonal T cell populations in angioimmunoblastic lymphadenopathy and angioimmunoblastic lymphadenopathy-like lymphoma. Am J Pathol 122:392–397, 1986.

Weiss LM, Jaffe ES, Liu XF, Chen Y, Shibata D, Medeiros L. Detection and localization of Epstein-Barr virus genomes in angioimmunoblastic lymphadenopathy and angioimmunoblastic lymphadenopathy-like lymphomas. Blood 79:1789–1795, 1992.

Wilson WH, Kingma DW, Raffeld M, Wittes RE, Jaffe ES. Association of lymphomatoid granulomatosis with Epstein-Barr viral infection of B lymphocytes and response to interferon alpha2b. Blood 87:4531–4537, 1996.

21

Peripheral T Cell and NK Cell Neoplasms: III. Anaplastic Large Cell Lymphomas

The anaplastic large cell lymphomas include anaplastic large cell lymphoma (CD30 +) of T and null cell types, primary cutaneous anaplastic large cell lymphoma, and anaplastic large cell lymphoma, Hodgkin's-like. Anaplastic large cell lymphomas of B cell type are considered with the diffuse large B cell lymphomas in Chapter 18.

Anaplastic Large Cell Lymphoma (CD30 +), T and Null Cell Types

Classification

REAL: Anaplastic large cell lymphoma (CD30 +), T and null cell types.
WF: Malignant lymphoma, large cell, immunoblastic.

Immunophenotype

CD2 − or +, CD3 − or +, CD30 +, CD45 + or −, EMA + or −.

Molecular Pathology

NPM/ALK oncogene rearrangement with t(2;5) in 50%.

Clinical Features

Anaplastic large cell lymphoma (ALCL) occurs in children and adults as a systemic disorder and in a primary cutaneous form (see below). ALCL are associated with a high incidence of extranodal involvement (61%) and cutaneous involvement (25%) at presentation (Filippa et al, 1996). ALCL occurs in a primary form, arising de novo, and in a secondary form, following other lymphomas, including mycosis fungoides/Sézary's syndrome and Hodgkin's disease. Epstein-Barr virus is present in a minority of ALCL (Lopategui et al, 1995); ALCL may occur in patients with HIV infection (Chadburn et al, 1993). ALCL's are characterized by the t(2;5) chromosomal translocation, resulting in fusion of the anaplastic lymphoma kinase gene (ALK) with the nucleolar protein nucleophosmin gene (NPM) (Morris et al, 1994). The resulting fusion transcript, NPM/ALK, is detected in 65% of cases of classical ALCL, but not in cases of primary cutaneous or HIV-associated ALCL, other peripheral T cell lymphomas, or Hodgkin's disease (Wellman et al, 1995; Wood et al, 1996). The NPM/ALK fusion gene results in production of a novel chimeric protein, p80 NPM/ALK, which has ALK kinase activity and likely plays a role in lymphomagenesis; p80 NPM/ALK can be detected by immunohistochemical staining (Pulford et al, 1997; Shiota et al, 1995). Some ALCL also express BCL-6 protein (Carbone et al, 1997).

ALCLs are characterized by expression of CD30 (Ki-1), a cell surface cytokine receptor belonging to the tumor necrosis factor (TNF) receptor superfamily (Falini et al, 1995). CD30 is expressed on the cells of ALCL, Hodgkin's disease, lymphomatoid papulosis, infectious mononucleosis, and activated lymphocytes; CD30 is frequently present on the cells of embryonal carcinoma but rarely on the cell of other nonhematopoietic tumors (Falini et al, 1995). CD30 is detected in frozen tissue with the monoclonal antibody Ki-1 or in paraffin embedded tissue with the monoclonal antibody Ber-H2; staining for CD30 is characteristically membranous, cytoplasmic, or paranuclear (Golgi). ALCLs frequently express epithelial membrane antigen (EMA) and vimentin and may express cytokeratins (Gustmann et al, 1991).

The majority of ALCLs are of T cell (50%) or null cell (30%) phenotypes. Clonal T-cell antigen-receptor gene rearrangements are present in 50–60% (Harris et al, 1994).

Histopathology

ALCLs are characterized by diffuse infiltrates of large, pleomorphic cells, with prominent nucleoli, single "horseshoe-shaped," or multiple nuclei, arranged in a "ring" or "wreath," and abundant cytoplasm (Figs. 21.1, 21.2, 21.3, and 21.4). Cohesive growth and sinusoidal involvement are characteristic features (Figs. 21.1 and 21.2). Reed-Sternberg–like cells and inflammatory cell infiltrate may be present (Fig. 21.3). Histopathologic variants of ALCL include a sarcomatoid variant with myxoid stroma and spindled cells (Chan et al, 1990) (Figs. 21.5 and 21.6); a small cell variant (Kinney et al, 1993); a variant with numerous histiocytes (Pileri et al, 1990); and a variant with numerous neutrophils (Mann et al, 1995).

Variants of Anaplastic Large Cell Lymphoma

PRIMARY CUTANEOUS ANAPLASTIC LARGE CELL LYMPHOMA   Primary cutaneous ALCL is likely a distinct entity which is closely related to lymphomatoid papulosis and differs

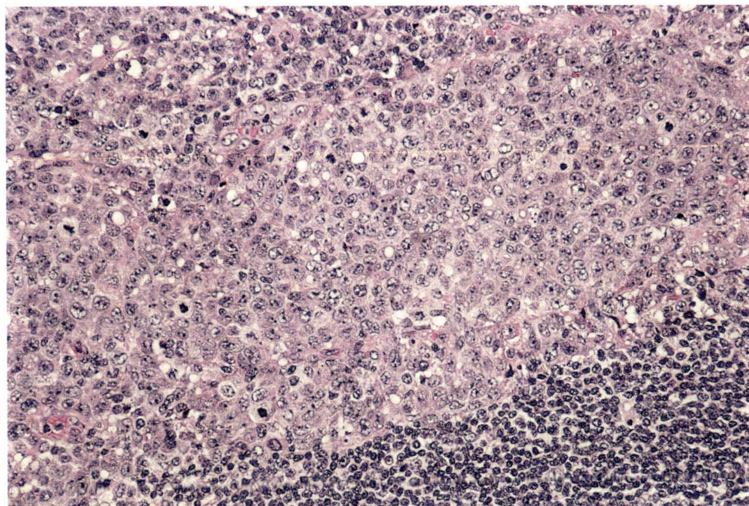

Anaplastic large cell lymphoma showing sinusoidal pattern of involvement.

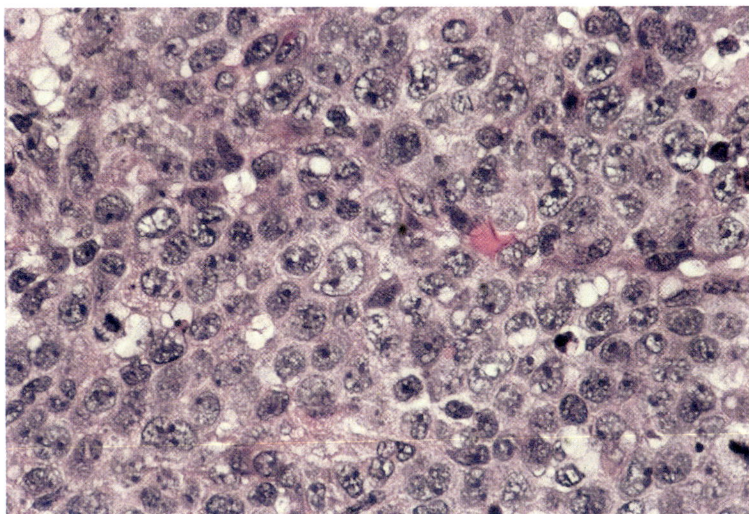

Anaplastic large cell lymphoma showing cohesive growth pattern and horseshoe nuclei.

clinically and biologically from systemic forms of ALCL (Fig. 21.7). Primary cutaneous ALCL is confined to the skin and is distinguished by an indolent natural history with frequent spontaneous regression; patients may develop typical lymphomatoid papulosis (Fig. 21.8). The histopathology of primary cutaneous ALCL is characterized by a dermal infiltrate of large, pleomorphic, CD30-positive cells; EMA, in contrast to systemic ALCL, is negative. Primary cutaneous ALCL lacks the t(2;5) and NPM/ALK rearrangements characteristic of systemic ALCL (Wellman et al, 1995; Wood et al, 1996). Primary cutaneous ALCL is distinguished from lymphomatoid papulosis principally by the smaller number and larger size of the lesions. Regressing atypical histiocytosis is likely a closely

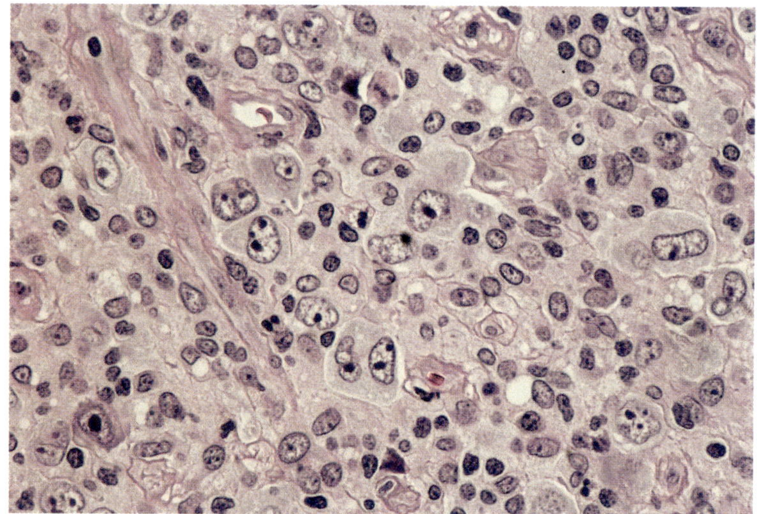

**FIGURE
21.3**

Anaplastic large cell lymphoma showing Reed-Sternberg–like cells.

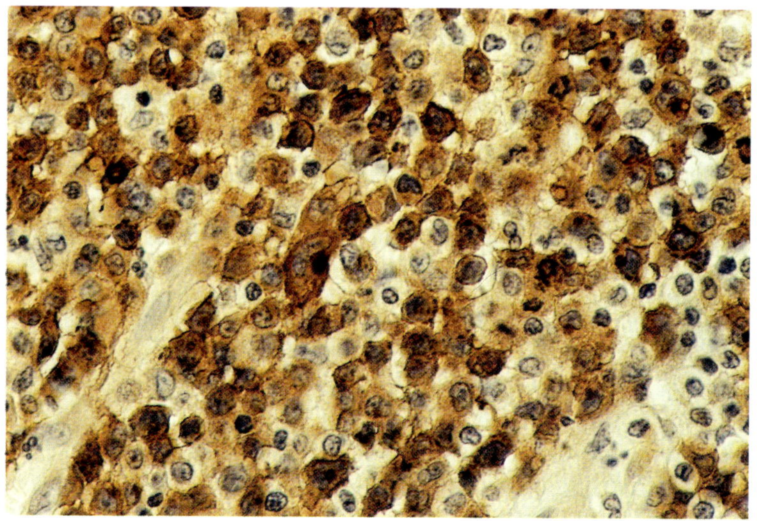

**FIGURE
21.4**

Anaplastic large cell lymphoma showing positive staining for CD30. Paranuclear (Golgi) pattern of staining is present in the cell at center.

related lesion. Primary cutaneous ALCL should be distinguished from the frequent cutaneous involvement in systemic ALCL.

PROVISIONAL ENTITY: ANAPLASTIC LARGE CELL LYMPHOMA, HODGKIN'S-LIKE Anaplastic large cell lymphoma, Hodgkin's-like is a controversial entity which shares features
of Hodgkin's disease and non-Hodgkin's lymphoma (Harris et al, 1994). Patients are
typically young adults presenting with mediastinal involvement. The histopathologic fea-

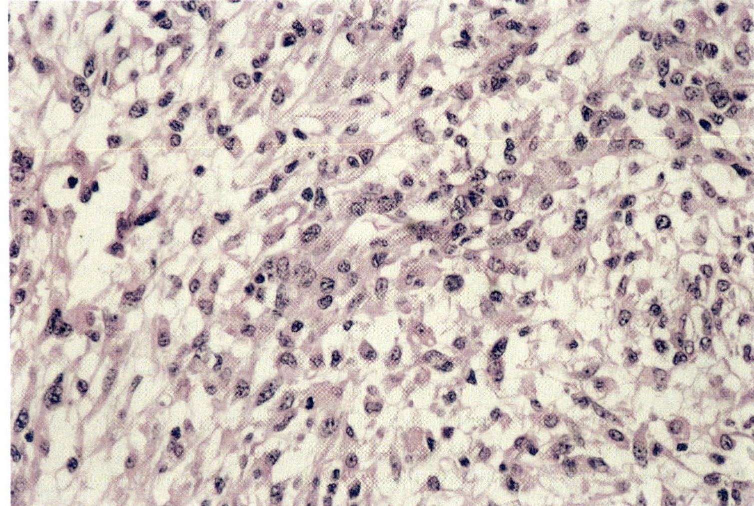

FIGURE
21.5

Anaplastic large cell lymphoma, variant with myxoid stroma and spindled cells.

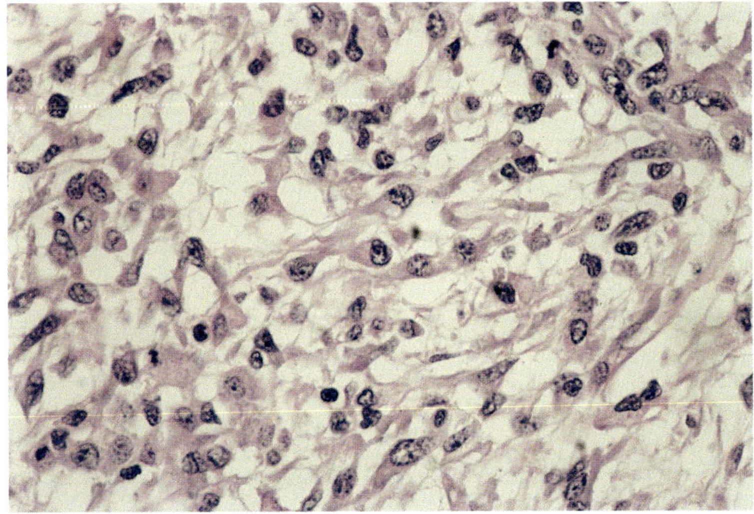

FIGURE
21.6

Anaplastic large cell lymphoma, variant with myxoid stroma and spindled cells, higher magnification, showing sarcomatoid appearance.

tures resemble those of the syncytial variant of nodular sclerosis Hodgkin's disease,
with sheets of large pleomorphic lacunar-like cells; cohesive growth pattern and sinusoidal involvement may be present (Figs. 21.9 and 21.10). Distinction from Hodgkin's disease may be extremely difficult or impossible (see Differential Diagnosis, below). The
natural history is uncertain. In the European literature, response to therapy for Hodgkin's disease has been poor; however, response to aggressive therapy for non-Hodgkin's
lymphoma has been reported (Pileri et al, 1994).

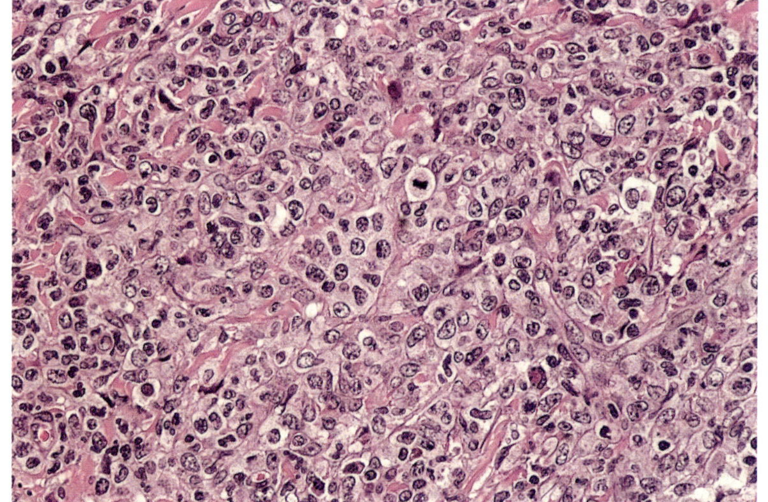

Primary cutaneous anaplastic large cell lymphoma showing dermal infiltration with large atypical lymphoid cells. Primary cutaneous anaplastic large cell lymphoma is closely related to lymphomatoid papulosis and should be distinguished from cutaneous involvement in systemic anaplastic large cell lymphoma.

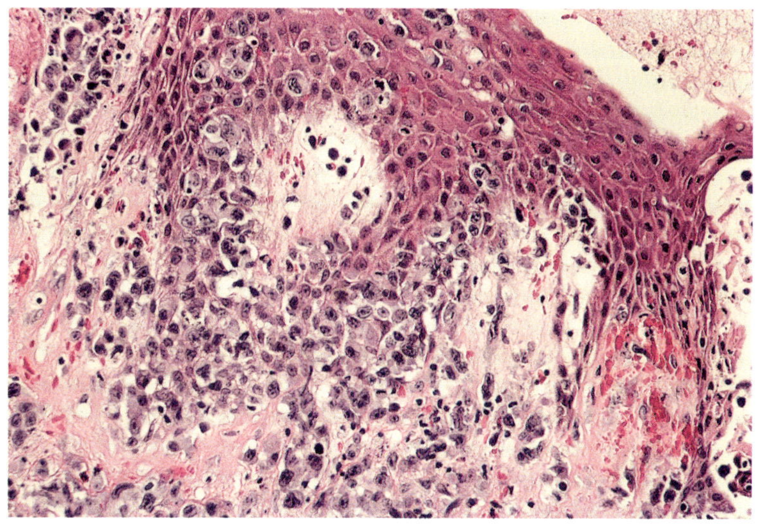

Lymphomatoid papulosis showing superficial infiltrate of large atypical cells at the dermal–epidermal junction. Lymphomatoid papulosis is closely related to primary cutaneous anaplastic large cell lymphoma.

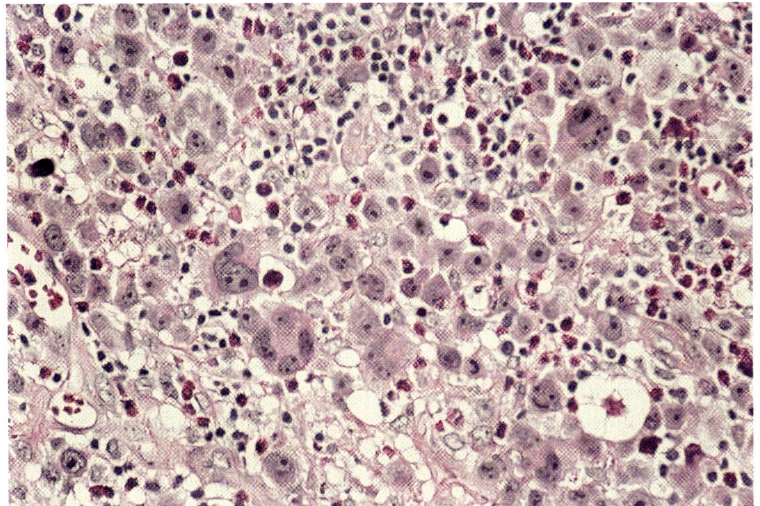

Anaplastic large cell lymphoma, Hodgkin's like, showing sinusoidal involvement with pleomorphic Reed-Sternberg–like cells. Distinction from Hodgkin's disease may be difficult.

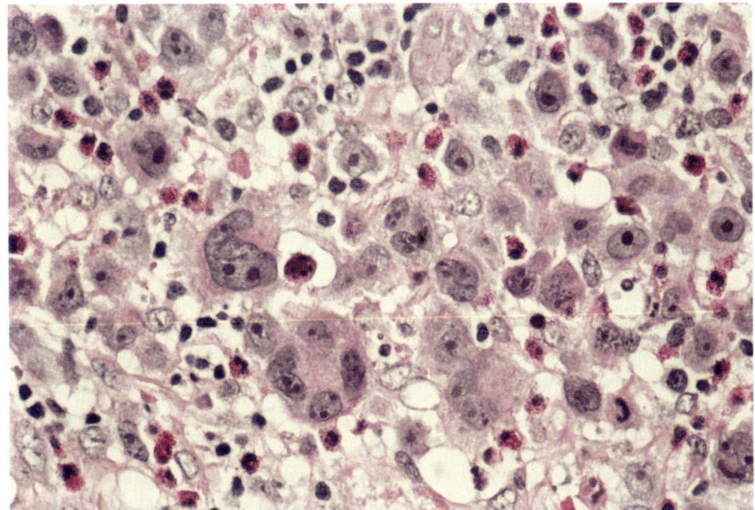

Anaplastic large cell lymphoma, Hodgkin's like, showing pleomorphic Reed-Sternberg–like cells.

Differential Diagnosis

ALCL must be distinguished from other hematopoietic and nonhematopoietic neoplasms. The sinusoidal growth pattern has in the past been misinterpreted as evidence of histiocytic origin; most cases of malignant histiocytosis reported prior to the advent of immunophenotypic studies have been found to be ALCL (Wilson et al, 1990). Some ALCLs stain for the histiocytic antigen CD68 with the frequently used monoclonal antibody KP-1 but not with the more specific monoclonal antibody PG-M1 (Falini et al, 1993).

The sinusoidal growth pattern and cohesiveness of the cells in ALCL may cause confusion with metastatic carcinoma. Immunohistochemical findings may cause further confusion, since ALCL may be negative for CD45 and may express EMA and even cytokeratin (Gustmann et al, 1991). Staining for CD30 will usually resolve the issue; however, embryonal carcinoma is also CD30 positive (Falini et al, 1995).

ALCL may be extremely difficult to distinguish from some cases of Hodgkin's disease, particularly variants with numerous Reed-Sternberg and Reed-Sternberg–variant cells, including the syncytial variant of nodular sclerosis (Harris et al, 1994). The lack of the t(2;5) chromosomal translocation and NPM/ALK rearrangement in most cases of Hodgkin's disease suggests that these disorders are not closely related (Wellman et al, 1995; Wood et al, 1996). Immunohistochemical studies may be helpful in distinction. ALCL, in contrast to Hodgkin's disease, was found to express one or more lymphocyte antigens (CD45, CD45RO, CD43, CD20) or EMA, in addition to CD30, in all cases (Filippa et al, 1996). Hodgkin's disease, in contrast, frequently expressed CD15, which was rarely expressed in ALCL.

Course and Prognosis

Systemic ALCL is an aggressive disorder with durable responses to aggressive combination chemotherapy. The prognosis of systemic ALCL is comparable to that of other diffuse large cell lymphomas (Tilly et al, 1997); in children the prognosis of ALCL appears to be more favorable than for B cell tumors. Primary cutaneous ALCL, in contrast, is an indolent disorder with high frequency of spontaneous regression; cases not undergoing regression have been treated with radiation therapy. Primary cutaneous ALCL may recur as ALCL or as lymphomatoid papulosis.

REFERENCES

Carbone A, Gloghini A, Gaidano G, Dalla-Favev R, Falini B. BCL-6 protein expression in human peripheral T-cell neoplasms is restricted to CD30+ anaplastic large-cell lymphomas. Blood 90:2445–2450, 1997.

Chadburn A, Cesarman E, Jagirdar J, Subar M, Mir RN, Knowles DM. CD30 (Ki-1) positive anaplastic large cell lymphomas in individuals infected with the human immunodeficiency virus. Cancer 72:3078–3090, 1993.

Chan JKC, Buchanan R, Fletcher CDM. Sarcomatoid variant of anaplastic large-cell Ki-1 lymphoma. Am J Surg Pathol 14:983–988, 1990.

Falini B, Flenghi L, Pileri S, Gambacorta M, Bigerna B, Durkop H, et al. PG-M1: A new monoclonal antibody directed against a fixative-resistant epitope on the macrophage restricted form of the CD68 molecule. Am J Pathol 142:1359, 1993.

Falini B, Pileri S, Pizzolo G, Durkop H, Flenghi L, Stirpe F, Martelli MF, Stein H. CD30 (Ki-1) molecule: A new cytokine receptor of the tumor necrosis factor receptor superfamily as a tool for diagnosis and immunotherapy. Blood 85:1–14, 1995.

Filippa DA, Ladanyi M, Wollner N, Straus DJ, O'Brien JP, Portlock C, et al. CD30 (Ki-1)-positive malignant lymphomas: Clinical, immunophenotypic, histologic, and genetic characteristics and differences with Hodgkin's disease. Blood 87:2905–2917, 1996.

Gustmann C, Altmannsberger M, Osborn M, Griesser H, Feller AC. Cytokeratin expression and vimentin content in large cell anaplastic and other non-Hodgkin's lymphomas. Am J Pathol 138:1413–1422, 1991.

Harris NL, Jaffe ES, Stein H, Banks PM, Chan JKC, Cleary ML. A revised European-American classification of lymphoid neoplasms: A proposal from the International Lymphoma Study Group. Blood 84:1361–1392, 1994.

Kinney MC, Collins RD, Greer JP, Whitlock JA, Sioutos N, Kadin ME. A small-cell-predominant variant of primary Ki-1 (CD30)+ T-cell lymphoma. Am J Surg Pathol 17:859–868, 1993.

Lopategui JR, Gaffey MJ, Chan JKC, Frierson HF, Sun L-H, Bellafiore FJ, Chang KL, Weiss LR. Infrequent association of Epstein-Barr virus with CD30-positive anaplastic large cell lymphomas from American and Asian patients. Am J Surg Pathol 19:42–49, 1995.

Mann KP, Hall B, Kamino H, Borowitz MJ, Ratech H. Neutrophil-rich, Ki-1 positive anaplastic large-cell malignant lymphoma. Am J Surg Pathol 19:407–416, 1995.

Morris SW, Kirstein MN, Valentine MB, Dittmer KG, Shapiro DN, Saltman DL, Look AT. Fusion of a kinase gene, ALK, to a nucleolar protein gene, NPM, in non-Hodgkin's lymphoma. Science 263:1281–1284, 1994.

Pileri S, Bocchia M, Baroni C, Martinelli M, Falini B, Sabatini E, et al. Anaplastic large cell lymphoma (CD30+/Ki-1+): Results of a prospective clinicopathologic study of 69 cases. Br J Haematol 86:513, 1994.

Pileri S, Falini B, Delsol G, Stein H, Baglioni P, Poggi S, et al. Lymphohistiocytic T cell lymphoma (anaplastic large cell lymphoma CD30+/Ki-1+ with a high content of reactive histiocytes). Histopathology 16:383, 1990.

Pulford K, Lamant L, Morris SW, Butler L, Wood KM, Stroud D, Delsol G, Mason DY. Detection of anaplastic lymphoma kinase (ALK) and nucleolar protein nucleophosmin (NPM)-ALK proteins in normal and neoplastic cells with the monoclonal antibody ALK1. Blood 89:1394–1404, 1997.

Shiota M, Nakamura S, Ichinohasama R, Abe M, Akagi T, Takeshita M, et al. Anaplastic large cell lymphomas expressing the novel chimeric protein p80 NPM/ALK: A distinct clinicopathologic entity. Blood 86:1954–1960, 1995.

Tilly H, Gaulard P, Lepage E, Dumontet C, Diebold J, Plantier I, et al. Primary anaplastic large-cell lymphoma in adults: Clinical presentation, immunophenotype, and outcome. Blood 90:3727–3734, 1997.

Wellman A, Otsuki T, Vogelbruch M, Clark HM, Jaffe ES, Raffeld M. Analysis of the t(2;5)(p23;q35) translocation by reverse transcription-polymerase chain reaction in CD30+ anaplastic large cell lymphomas, in other non-Hodgkin's lymphomas of T cell phenotype and in Hodgkin's disease. Blood 86:2321–2328, 1995.

Wilson MS, Weiss LM, Gatter KC, Mason DY, Dorfman RF, Warnke RA. Malignant histiocytosis: A reassessment of cases previously reported in 1975 based on paraffin section immunophenotyping studies. Cancer 66:530–536, 1990.

Wood GS, Hardman DL, Boni R, Dummer R, Kin Y-H, Smoller R, et al. Lack of the t(2;5) or other mutations resulting in expression of the anaplastic lymphoma kinase catalytic domain in CD30+ primary cutaneous lymphoproliferative disorders and Hodgkin's disease. Blood 88:1765–1770, 1996.

22

Hodgkin's Disease: I. Lymphocyte Predominance Hodgkin's Disease

Lymphocyte predominance Hodgkin's disease is considered separately from other forms of Hodgkin's disease because the most frequent, nodular, form of the disease exhibits a distinct immunophenotype and characteristic natural history which distinguishes it from other forms of Hodgkin's disease (Mason et al, 1994). To emphasize the distinctiveness of this form of Hodgkin's disease and probable unrelatedness to other forms of Hodgkin's disease, the term "paragranuloma" has been proposed, the original term for this form of Hodgkin's disease in the Jackson and Parker classification (Jackson and Parker, 1944). In contrast to other forms of Hodgkin's disease, nodular lymphocyte predominance Hodgkin's disease is of consistent B cell phenotype (Pinkus and Said, 1988).

Nodular Lymphocyte Predominance Hodgkin's Disease

Classification

REAL: Lymphocyte predominance (paragranuloma).
Rye: Lymphocyte predominance.
Lukes and Butler: Lymphocytic and/or histiocytic, nodular.

Immunophenotype

CD45 +, EMA +, CD20 +, CD15 −, CD30 − (or faint +), SIg usually −, EBV −.

Clinical Features

Nodular lymphocyte predominance Hodgkin's disease (NLPHD, paragranuloma) occurs in children and adults. Patients typically present with localized (Ann Arbor stage I or II) disease; "B" symptoms (fever, night sweats, and weight loss) are usually absent. Cervical lymph nodes are most frequently involved; inguinal lymph node involvement may also occur. Frequently only a single enlarged lymph node is present. Mediastinal involvement, in contrast to other forms of Hodgkin's disease, is unusual. Extranodal involvement occurs occasionally (Chang et al, 1995). Bone marrow involvement is infrequent. Patients may have had prior enlarged lymph nodes showing progressive transformation of germinal centers (Burns et al, 1984). Subsequent development of enlarged lymph nodes showing progressive transformation of germinal centers or diffuse large B cell non-Hodgkin's lymphoma may occur (Greiner et al, 1996).

Histopathology

NLPHD is characterized by effacement of the lymph node architecture by proliferation of ill-defined, vague nodules, which are larger than normal follicles and are composed predominantly of small mature lymphocytes (Figs. 22.1 and 22.2). A rim of preserved normal lymph node may be present. The characteristic cells of NLPHD are scattered within the nodules and consist of "L&H" (from the Lukes and Butler term for this form of Hodgkin's disease) Reed-Sternberg–variant cells or "popcorn" cells. These are characterized by a delicately lobulated nucleus with one or more inconspicuous nucleoli and relatively abundant pale cytoplasm (Figs. 22.3 and 22.4). Diagnostic Reed-Sternberg cells are uncharacteristic and, if present in significant numbers, should suggest an alternative diagnosis of one of the forms of classical Hodgkin's disease (Mason et al, 1994). Epithelioid histiocytes are frequently present (Fig. 22.5); epithelioid granulomata are occasionally present and may form "wreathes" around the nodules. Delicate fibrosis may be present around the nodules. In contrast to other forms of Hodgkin's disease, eosinophils and plasma cells are scarce. In some cases of NLPHD, L&H cells are relatively numerous and may form nodules consisting predominantly of L&H cells (Greiner et al, 1996). Progressively transformed germinal centers may be present within the same lymph node (Burns et al, 1984).

Immunopathology

The L&H cells of NLPHD exhibit a B cell phenotype distinct from other forms of Hodgkin's disease (Pinkus and Said, 1988; von Wasielewski et al, 1997). L&H cells are strongly positive for CD45, EMA, and B cell antigens, including CD20, which is readily demonstrable in paraffin-embedded tissue (Figs. 22.6 and 22.7). CD15 and CD30, characteristic of classical Hodgkin's disease, are typically absent; however weak staining for CD30 may be present, particularly in frozen tissue. Surface immunoglobulin is not detected in most cases; clonally restricted surface immunoglobulin with κ light chain expression has been reported in some cases, however (Schmid et al, 1991; Stoler et al, 1995) (Fig. 22.8). Paradoxically, clonal rearrangement of the immunoglobulin genes is not detected in most cases of NLPHD but is detected in diffuse large B cell non-Hodgkin's lymphoma

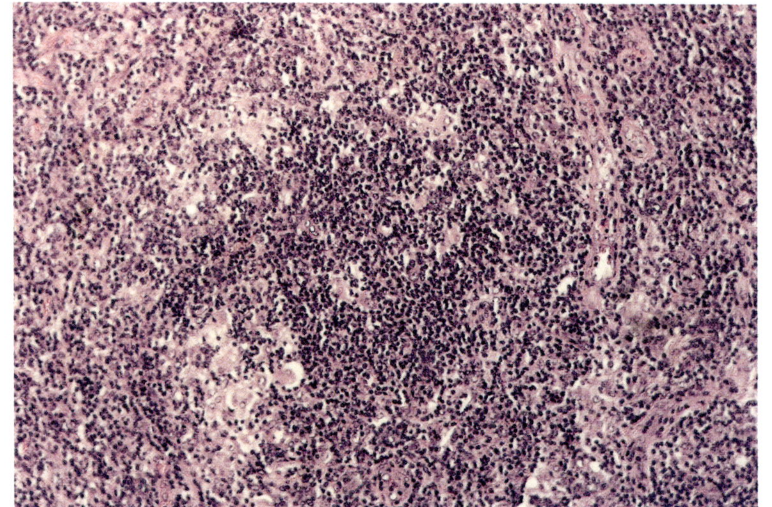

Nodular lymphocyte predominance Hodgkin's disease, low magnification, showing ill-defined nodule composed of small mature lymphocytes and epithelioid histiocytes.

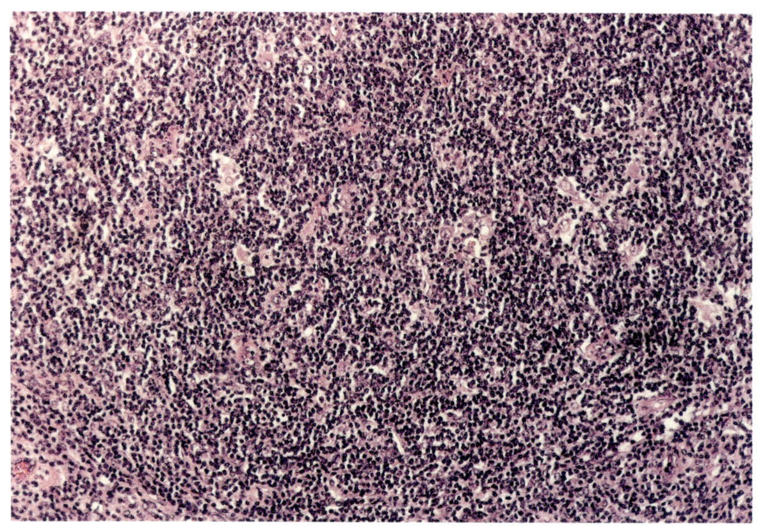

Nodular lymphocyte predominance Hodgkin's disease, low magnification, showing ill-defined nodule composed predominantly of small mature lymphocytes.

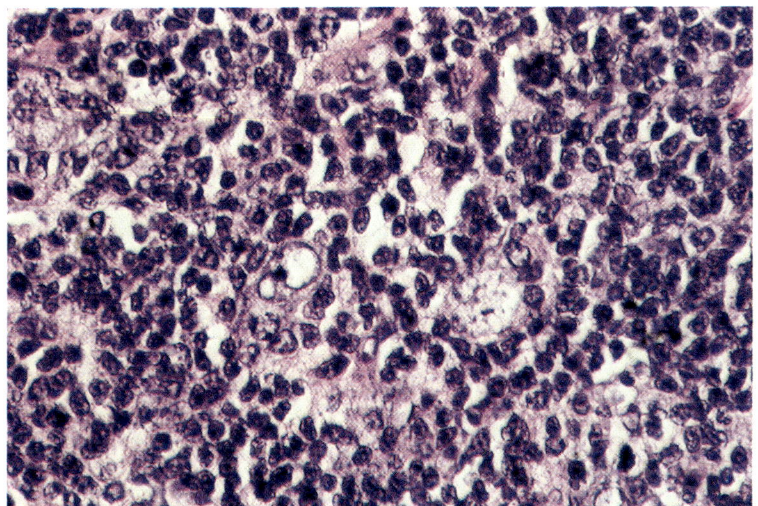

Nodular lymphocyte predominance Hodgkin's disease, higher magnification, showing L&H Reed-Sternberg–variant cells.

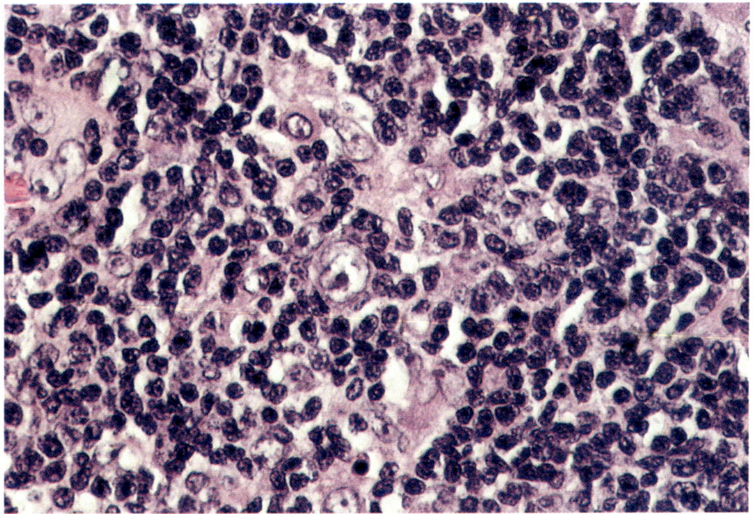

Nodular lymphocyte predominance Hodgkin's disease, higher magnification, showing L&H Reed-Sternberg–variant cell.

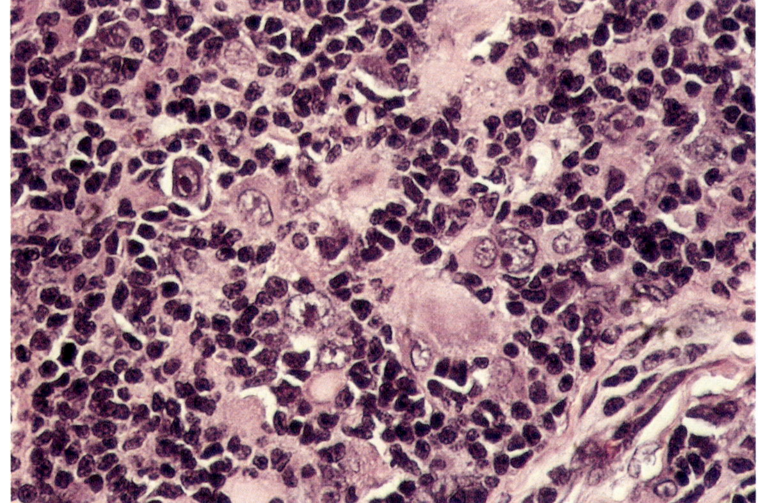

FIGURE
22.5

Nodular lymphocyte predominance Hodgkin's disease, higher magnification, showing epithelioid histiocytes admixed with L&H Reed-Sternberg–variant cells.

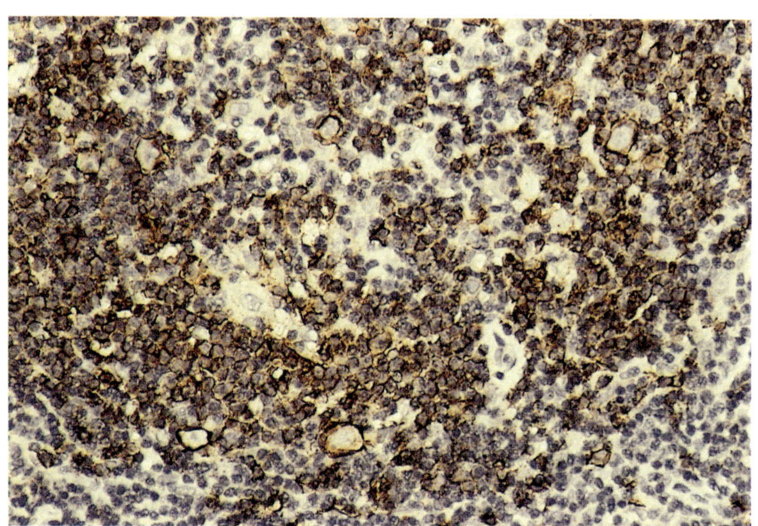

FIGURE
22.6

Nodular lymphocyte predominance Hodgkin's disease, stained with monoclonal antibody to CD20 in paraffin embedded tissue, showing numerous small B lymphocytes within the nodule and strong staining of the larger L&H Reed-Sternberg–variant cells.

complicating NLPHD (Greiner et al, 1996). This finding has been interpreted to suggest that NLPHD may be a polyclonal process (Pan et al, 1996). Clonal populations have, however, recently been identified by PCR analysis of single L&H cells isolated by microdissection (Marafioti et al, 1997; Ohno et al, 1997). Epstein-Barr virus is not associated with NLPHD, in contrast to other forms of Hodgkin's disease, and the BCL-2 oncoprotein, associated with follicular lymphomas, is absent (Alkan et al, 1995). BCL-6 protein,

FIGURE
22.7

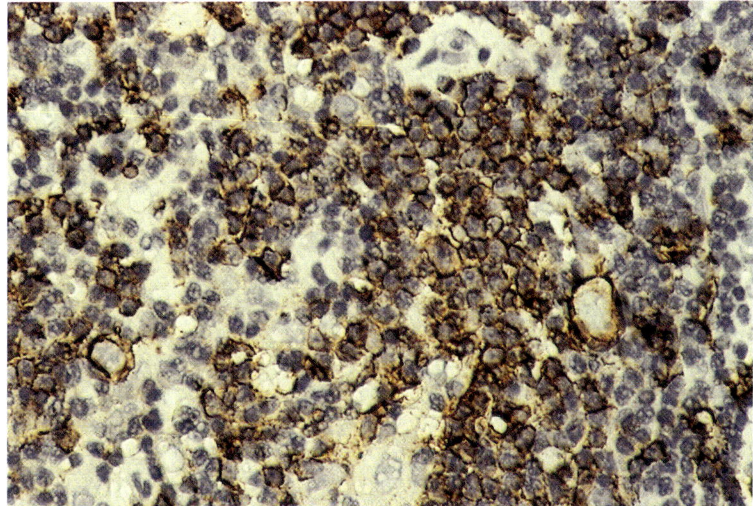

Nodular lymphocyte predominance Hodgkin's disease, stained with monoclonal antibody to CD20 in paraffin-embedded tissue, higher magnification, showing strong staining of L&H Reed-Sternberg–variant cells.

associated with normal follicular center cells and found in some diffuse large B cell lymphomas, is also present in L&H cells (Falini et al, 1996). The small lymphocytes in the nodules of NLPHD consist of numerous polyclonal B lymphocytes and CD57-positive T cells. The latter are frequently arranged in rosettes or rings around the L&H cells (Fig. 22.9). A meshwork of follicular dendritic cells is present within the nodules (Fig. 22.10).

Differential Diagnosis

NLPHD must be distinguished from reactive lymphoid hyperplasia, other forms of Hodgkin's disease, and non-Hodgkin's lymphomas. Progressive transformation of germinal centers may closely simulate the low-magnification appearance of NLPHD; however, the characteristic L&H cells are absent. NLPHD and progressive transformation of germinal centers may be present simultaneously in the same lymph node (Burns et al, 1984). Distinction from other forms of Hodgkin's disease is aided by immunophenotypic findings. The characteristic CD45-positive, CD20-positive, CD15-negative, and CD30-negative phenotype of NLPHD is distinct from that observed in other forms of Hodgkin's disease (von Wasielewski et al, 1997). Rarely, NLPHD and classical Hodgkin's disease coexist in the same patient (Gelb et al, 1993). Distinction from non-Hodgkin's lymphomas, particularly T-cell-rich large B cell lymphoma may be difficult, since the large cells in both may demonstrate a similar B cell phenotype. The demonstration of the characteristic abundant CD57-positive cells in NLPHD is a helpful diagnostic feature. Distinction between L&H cell-rich variants of NLPHD and NLPHD with simultaneous diffuse large B cell non-Hodgkin's lymphoma may also be difficult (Fig. 22.11) The presence of clonal rearrangement of the immunoglobulin genes may be helpful in equivocal cases (Greiner et al, 1996).

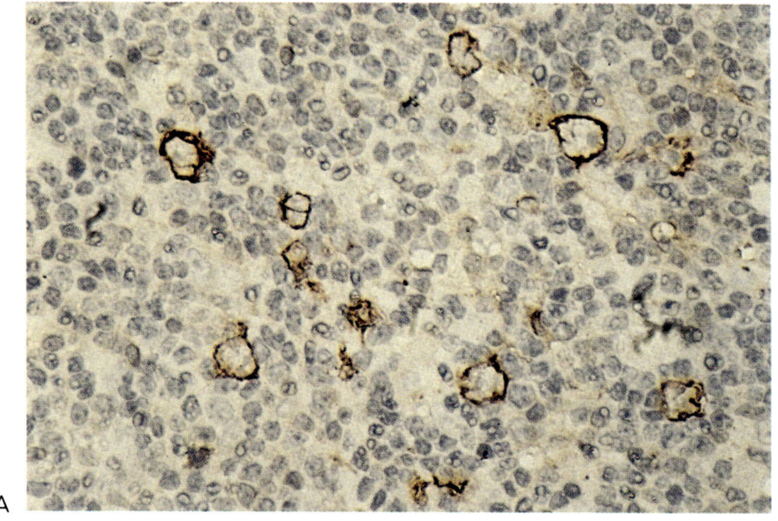

A

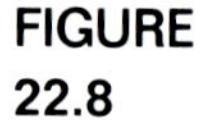

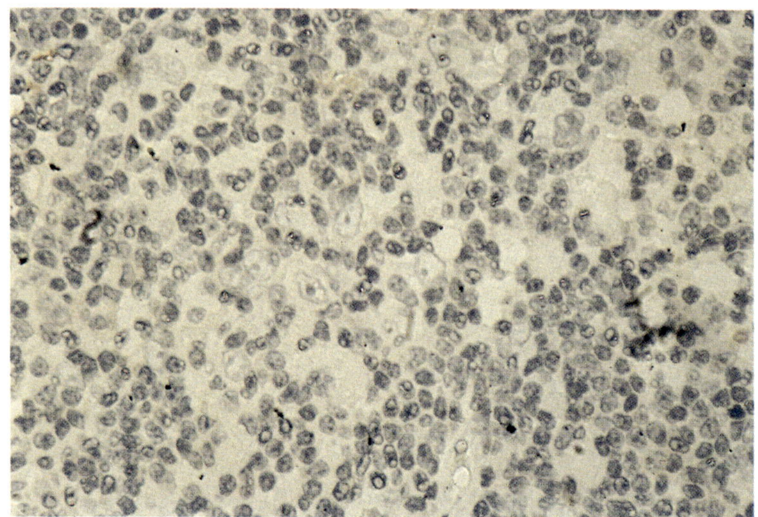

B

Nodular lymphocyte predominance Hodgkin's disease demonstrating clonal light chain restriction within a nodule. A. Paraffin-mbedded tissue stained for κ light chain showing positive staining of L&H cells. B. Paraffin-embedded tissue stained for λ light chain showing negative staining of L&H cells. Clonal light chain restriction is demonstrated in a minority of cases of nodular lymphocyte predominance Hodgkin's disease; clonal immunoglobulin gene rearrangements are not detected by conventional techniques.

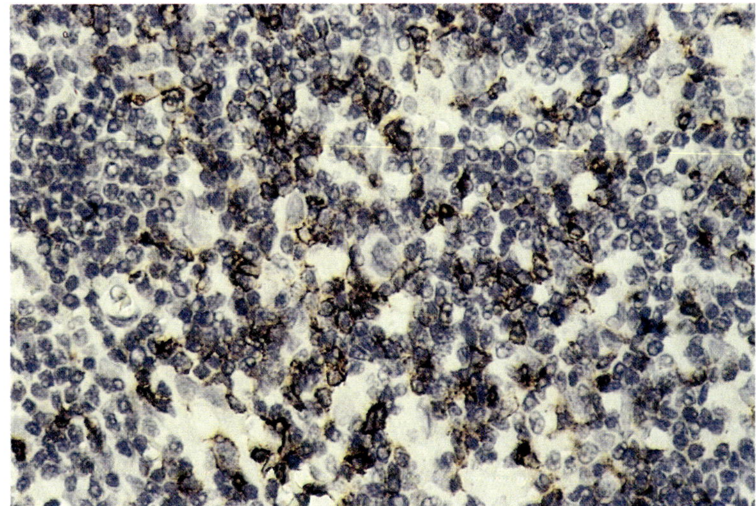

FIGURE 22.9

Nodular lymphocyte predominance Hodgkin's disease stained with monoclonal antibody to CD57 (Leu-7) showing numerous CD57–positive T lymphocytes within the nodules forming rosettes around L&H cells.

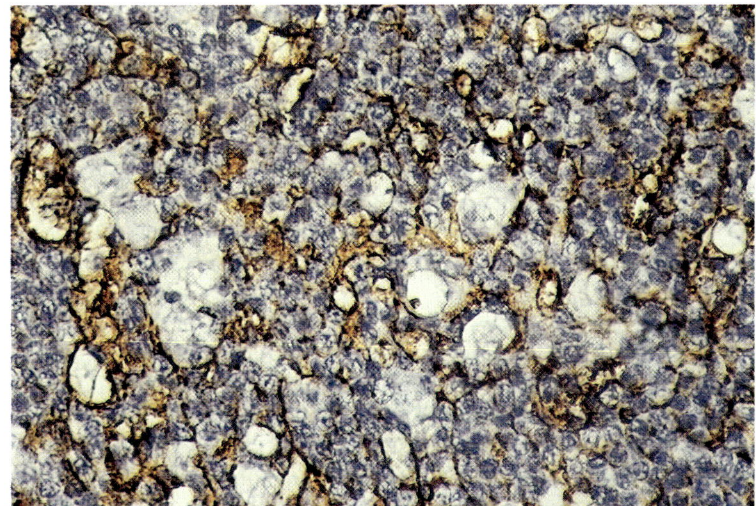

FIGURE 22.10

Nodular lymphocyte predominance Hodgkin's disease stained with monoclonal antibody to CD21 showing meshwork of CD21–positive follicular dendritic cells.

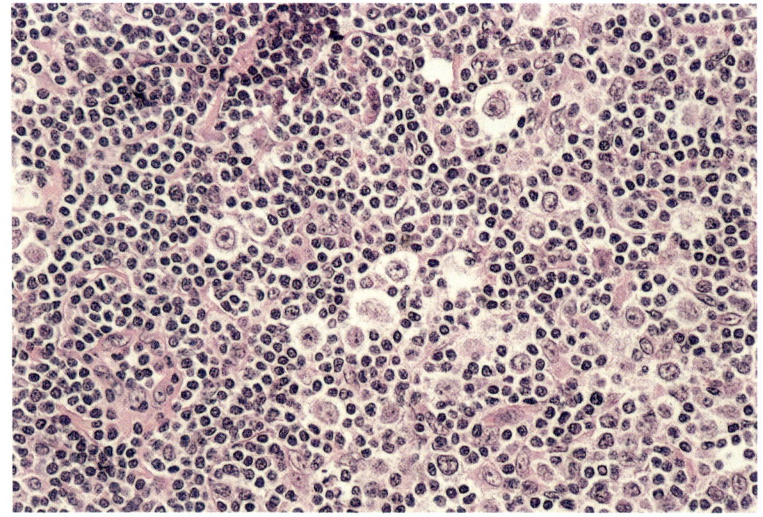

A

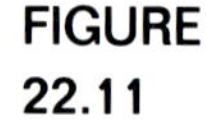

FIGURE
22.11

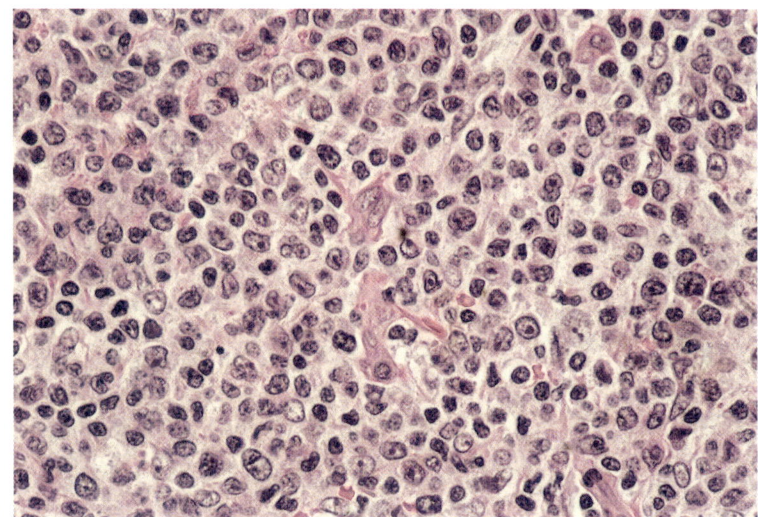

B

Nodular lymphocyte predominance Hodgkin's disease with simultaneous diffuse large B cell non-Hodgkin's lymphoma. A. Area of nodular lymphocyte predominance Hodgkin's disease showing L&H Reed-Sternberg–variant cells and small mature lymphocytes. B. Area of diffuse large B cell lymphoma.

Course and Prognosis

NLPHD is an indolent disorder with prolonged survival and low mortality (Bodis et al, 1997). An incidence of late relapses (up to 10 years) has been noted in some series (Regula et al, 1988). Treatment is controversial because of the indolent natural history. Limited or involved field radiotherapy has been recommended. The subsequent development of progressive transformation of germinal centers or diffuse large B cell non-Hodgkin's lymphoma is infrequent (Bodis et al, 1997).

Diffuse Lymphocyte Predominance Hodgkin's Disease

Diffuse lymphocyte predominance Hodgkin's disease (DLPHD) is distinctly uncommon. Some cases of DLPHD exhibit immunophenotypic findings indistinguishable from NLPHD; these cases frequently exhibit subtle nodularity and there is little reason to separate them from NLPHD. Other cases of DLPHD demonstrate the immunophenotypic features of classical Hodgkin's disease, with CD15- and CD30-positive Reed-Sternberg cells. These cases are more likely closely related to classical Hodgkin's disease than to NLPHD. The provisional designation "lymphocyte-rich classical Hodgkin's disease" has been proposed for these cases in the REAL classification (Harris et al, 1994).

REFERENCES

Alkan S, Ross CW, Hanson CA, Schnitizer B. Epstein-Barr virus and bcl-2 protein overexpression are not detected in the neoplastic cells of lymphocyte predominance Hodgkin's disease. Mod Pathol 8:544–547, 1995.

Bodis S, Kraus MD, Pinkus G, Silver R, Kadin ME, Canellos GP, Shulman LN, Tarbell NJ, Mauch PM. Clinical presentation and outcome in lymphocyte predominant Hodgkin's disease. J Clin Oncol 15: 3060–3066, 1997.

Burns BF, Colby TV, Dorfman RF. Differential diagnostic features of nodular L&H Hodgkin's disease, including progressive transformation of germinal centers. Am J Surg Pathol 8:253–261, 1984.

Chang KL, Kamel OW, Arber DA, Horyd ID, Weiss LM. Pathologic features of nodular lymphocyte predominance Hodgkin's disease in extranodal sites. Am J Surg Pathol 19:1313–1324, 1995.

Falini B, Bigerna B, Pasqualucci L, Fizzotti M, Martelli MF, Pileri S, et al. Distinctive expression of the BCL-6 protein in nodular lymphocyte predominance Hodgkin's disease. Blood 87:465–471, 1996.

Gelb AB, Dorfman RF, Warnke RA. Coexistence of nodular lymphocyte predominance Hodgkin's disease and Hodgkin's disease of the usual type. Am J Surg Pathol 17:364–374, 1993.

Greiner TC, Gascoyne RD, Anderson ME, Kingma DW, Adomat SA, Said J, Jaffe ES. Nodular lymphocyte predominant Hodgkin's disease associated with large cell lymphoma: analysis of Ig gene rearrangements by V-J polymerase chain reaction. Blood 88:657–666, 1996.

Harris NK, Jaffe ES, Stein H, Banks PM, Chan JKC, Cleary ML. A revised European-American classification of lymphoid neoplasms: A proposal from the international lymphoma study group. Blood 84:1361–1392, 1994.

Jackson H, Parker F. Hodgkin's disease. II. Pathology. N Engl J Med 231:35–44, 1944.

Marafioti T, Hummel M, Anagnostopoulos I, Foss H-D, Falini B, Delsol G, et al. Origin of nodular lymphocyte-predominant Hodgkin's disease from a clonal expansion of highly mutated germinal-center B cells. N Engl J Med 337:453–458, 1997.

Mason DY, Banks PM, Chan J, Cleary ML, Delsol G, de Wolf Peeters C, et al. Nodular lymphocyte predominance Hodgkin's disease. A distinct clinicopathologic entity. Am J Surg Pathol 18:526–530, 1994.

Ohno T, Strigley JA, Wu G, Hinrichs SH, Weisenburger D, Chan WC. Clonality in nodular lymphocyte-predominant Hodgkin's disease. N Engl J Med 337:459–465, 1997.

Pan LX, Diss TC, Peng HZ, Norton AJ, Isaacson PG. Nodular lymphocyte predominance Hodgkin's disease: a monoclonal or polyclonal B cell disorder. Blood 87:2428–2434, 1996.

Pinkus GS, Said JW. Hodgkin's disease, lymphocyte predominance type, nodular—further evidence for a B cell derivation. L&H variants of Reed-Sternberg cells express L26, a pan B cell marker. Am J Pathol 133:211–217, 1988.

Regula DP, Hoppe RT, Weiss LM. Nodular and diffuse types of lymphocyte predominance Hodgkin's disease. N Engl J Med 318:214–219, 1988.

Schmid C, Sargent C, Isaacson PG. L and H cells of nodular lymphocyte predominant Hodgkin's disease show immunoglobulin light chain restriction. Am J Pathol 139:1281–1289, 1991.

Stoler MH, Nichols GE, Symbula M, Weiss LM. Lymphocyte predominance Hodgkin's disease. Evidence for a kappa light chain-restricted monotypic B cell neoplasm. Am J Pathol 146:812–818, 1995.

von Wasielewski R, Werner M, Fischer R, Hansmann M-L, Hubner K, Hasenclever D, et al. Lymphocyte-predominant Hodgin's disease. An immunohistochemical analysis of 208 reviewed Hodgkin's disease cases from the German Hodgkin study group. Am J Pathol 150:793–803, 1997.

23

Hodgkin's Disease: II. Classical Hodgkin's Disease

Classical Hodgkin's Disease (HD) is characterized by proliferation of Reed-Sternberg (RS) and Reed-Sternberg–variant cells in an inflammatory background. Although several histopathologic variants are recognized, the RS and RS-variant cells demonstrate a uniform immunophenotype, characterized by CD15 and CD30 positivity and lack of specific B or T cell antigens.

Classification

REAL: Nodular sclerosis, mixed cellularity, lymphocyte depletion; provisional entity: lymphocyte-rich classical Hodgkin's disease.
Rye: Nodular sclerosis, mixed cellularity, lymphocyte depletion.
Lukes and Butler: Nodular sclerosis, mixed cellularity, diffuse fibrosis, reticular.

Immunophenotype

CD45 − (or weakly +), EMA −, CD20 − (or focally +), CD15 +, CD30 +, EBV − or +

The Reed-Sternberg Cell

The RS cell and RS mononuclear-variant cells (sometimes referred to as "Hodgkin's cells") are the neoplastic cells of classical HD. The diagnostic RS cell is found in all histopathologic variants of classical HD and is a requirement for diagnosis. The diagnos-

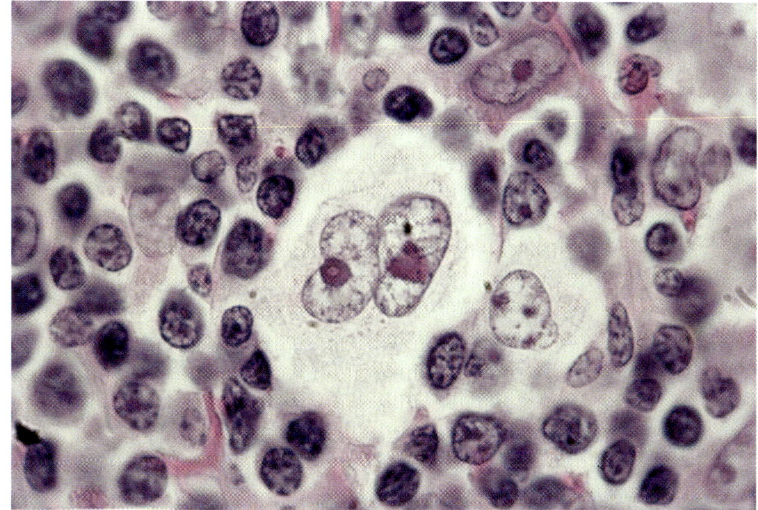

FIGURE
23.1

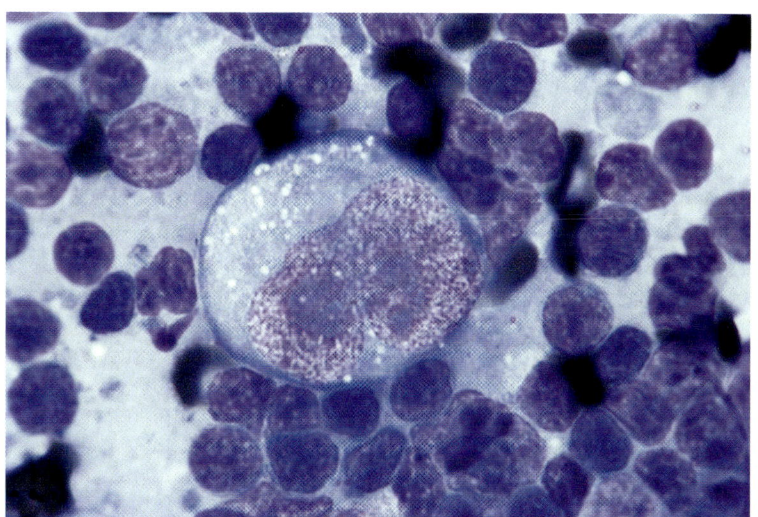

Diagnostic Reed-Sternberg cell of classical Hodgkin's disease showing bilobed nucleus, marginated chromatin, eosinophilic inclusion-like nucleoli, and abundant pale cytoplasm (A) and Giemsa-stained touch preparation (B). Identification of diagnostic Reed-Sternberg cells is a requirement for the initial diagnosis of classical Hodgkin's disease. (From same case as Figs. 23.12 and 23.13.)

tic RS cell is a large cell with bilobed nucleus, prominent inclusion-like eosinophilic nucleoli, marginated chromatin, and abundant eosinophilic cytoplasm (Fig. 23.1). The origin of the RS cell of classical HD remains undetermined. Origin from transformed lymphocytes, histiocytes, and interdigitating reticulum cells has been proposed in the past (Kadin, 1982). RS cells exhibit a characteristic phenotype with absent (or faint expression) CD45, expression of the granulocyte antigen CD15 (Leu M1), and expression of the lymphoid activation antigen CD30 (Ki-1) (Haluska et al, 1994; Urba and Longo, 1992). Other activation antigens, including HLA-DR, CD71 (transferrin receptor),

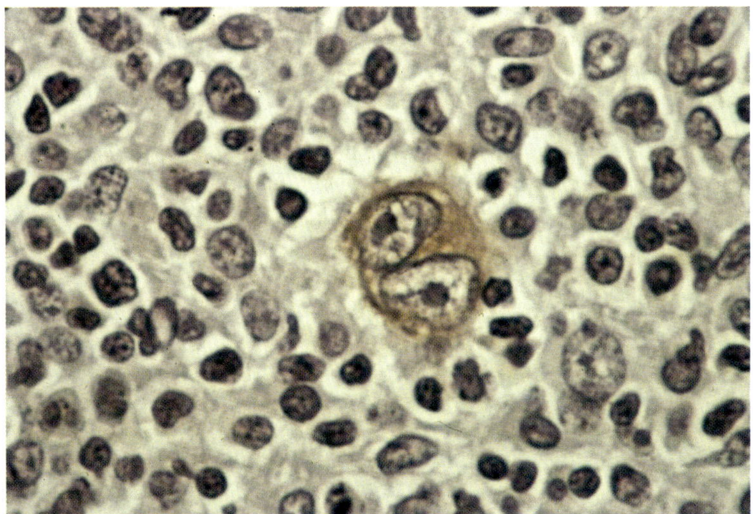

FIGURE
23.2

Reed-Sternberg cell of classical Hodgkin's disease showing positive cytoplasmic staining for Epstein-Barr virus latent membrane protein.

and CD25 (interleukin-2 receptor), are also expressed. Lineage specific markers are generally not expressed; however, variable staining for the B cell antigen CD20 is present in some cases (Schmid et al, 1991; Zukerberg et al, 1991). Several lines of evidence support a relation of Reed-Sternberg cells to transformed lymphoid cells of B or T cell lineage. These include the high frequency of EBV infection (Herndier et al, 1993; Khan et al, 1993; Weiss et al, 1989) (Fig. 23.2); the immunophenotypic similarities of RS cells to the transformed lymphoid cells of infectious mononucleosis (Reynolds et al, 1995); the common clonal derivation of Hodgkin's disease and lymphomatoid papulosis/cutaneous T cell lymphoma in the same patient (Davis et al, 1992); the presence of clonal immunoglobulin gene rearrangements in Hodgkin's tissue (Kamel et al, 1995); and the identification of immunoglobulin gene rearrangements in single Reed-Sternberg cells isolated by microdissection (Hummel et al, 1995; Kuppers et al, 1994).

Clinical Features

Hodgkin's disease exhibits a bimodal age distribution with an early peak in adolescents and young adults and a second peak in middle or older age. The early peak is predominantly of favorable histopathologic type (nodular sclerosis) and early presentations (Ann Arbor stage I and II) with a high incidence of mediastinal involvement. The later peak is predominantly of unfavorable histopathologic type (mixed cellularity and lymphocyte depletion) with advanced presentations (Ann Arbor stage III and IV) and a high incidence of abdominal involvement. "B" symptoms (fevers, night sweats, weight loss) frequently accompany advanced disease.

Hodgkin's disease is predominantly a nodal disease, although extranodal involvement occasionally occurs. Hodgkin's disease, unlike non-Hodgkin's lymphomas, tends to involve contiguous lymph node groups. Involvement is frequently confined to axial lymph nodes (cervical, axillary, mediastinal, retroperitoneal, and inguinal) with sparing of peripheral (epitrochlear, mesenteric) lymph nodes. Splenic involvement is not infrequent and precedes hepatic involvement. Bone marrow involvement is uncommon at presentation in young patients with early stage disease but is more common in older patients with advanced-stage disease and in HIV-associated Hodgkin's disease.

The etiology of Hodgkin's disease is unknown. Epstein-Barr virus is present in the Reed-Sternberg cells of 30–50% of cases (Khan et al, 1993) and in almost all cases of HIV-associated Hodgkin's disease (Herndier et al, 1993). Identical twin studies have suggested a role of genetic susceptibility in young adult cases (Mack et al, 1995). Hodgkin's disease occasionally follows non-Hodgkin's lymphoma (Zarate-Osorno et al, 1993).

Histopathology

Nodular Sclerosis Hodgkin's Disease

Nodular sclerosis is the most common form of Hodgkin's disease, accounting for up to 70% of cases, and it is particularly prevalent in young adults with a high incidence of mediastinal involvement. Nodular sclerosis is characterized by formation of nodules separated by collagenous fibrous bands (Figs. 23.3) and a particular type of RS-variant cell, referred to as a "lacunar" cell (Figs. 23.4, 23.5, and 23.6). The latter are large cells, with a multilobed nucleus, one or more prominent eosinophilic nucleoli, and abundant pale cytoplasm, which retracts from the cell membrane, giving the appearance of an empty space or "lacune." The space is an artifact of fixation and is not seen in frozen sections or well-fixed material. The characteristic fibrous bands extend from a thickened lymph node capsule and are composed of birefringent collagen. The nodules contain a mixed cellular population, containing varying numbers of small lymphocytes, eosinophils, plasma cells, histiocytes, and lacunar cells. Subcategorization of nodular sclerosis HD according to the relative number of lymphocytes within the nodules has

FIGURE
23.3

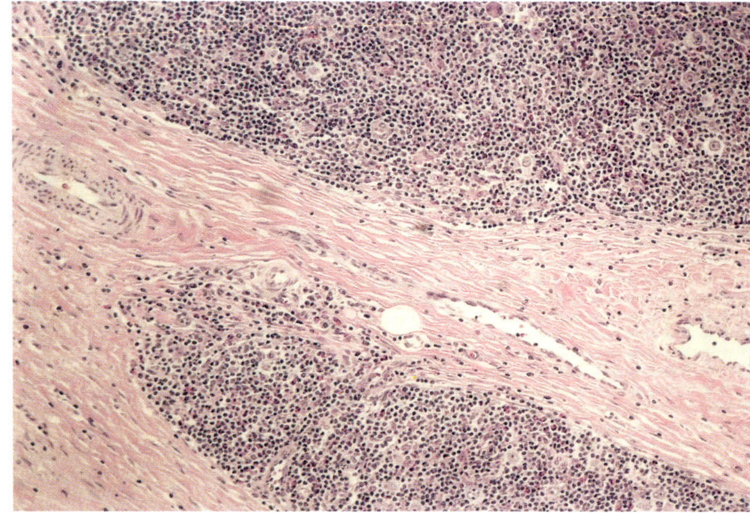

Nodular sclerosis Hodgkin's disease showing collagenous fibrous bands.

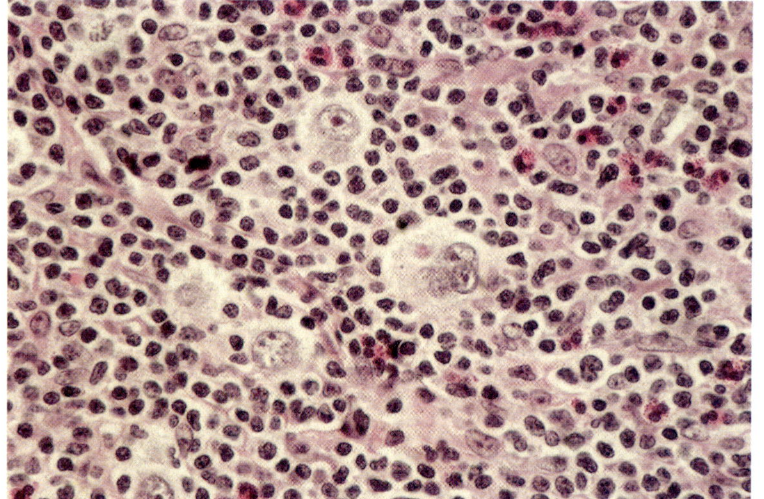

FIGURE 23.4

Nodular sclerosis Hodgkin's disease showing lacunar Reed-Sternberg–
variant cells with abundant pale cytoplasm and multilobed nucleus. The
lacunar space is an artifact which is not seen in well-fixed material.

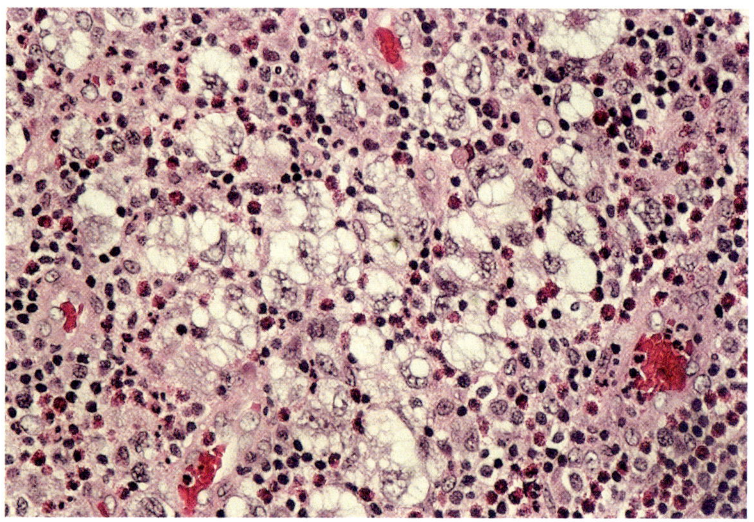

FIGURE 23.5

Nodular sclerosis Hodgkin's disease showing lacunar Reed-Sternberg–
variant cells with cytoplasmic retraction artifact.

not proven to have independent prognostic value. Subcategorization of nodular sclerosis
HD into NS I and NS II categories, according to the number of atypical cells, has been
proposed by the British National Lymphoma Investigation (BNLI) but has not been of
consistent prognostic value (MacLennan et al, 1989; Hess et al, 1994).

Variants

CELLULAR PHASE OF NODULAR SCLEROSIS Some cases of Hodgkin's disease resemble
nodular sclerosis in having lacunar RS-variant cells but have few or no fibrous bands.

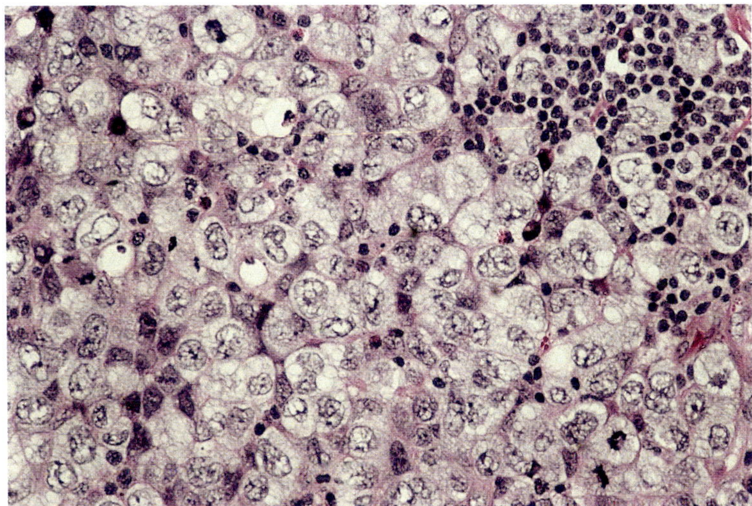

FIGURE 23.6

Nodular sclerosis Hodgkin's disease showing an aggregate of lacunar Reed-Sternberg–variant cells.

Typical nodular sclerosis HD may be present in other lymph nodes. These cases have been referred to as the cellular phase of nodular sclerosis; other authors prefer to classify them as mixed cellularity HD with lacunar cells. The prognosis appears to be intermediate between typical nodular sclerosis HD and mixed cellularity HD.

SYNCYTIAL VARIANT OF NODULAR SCLEROSIS Some cases of nodular sclerosis HD have a distinctive morphology characterized by cohesive sheets and masses of lacunar-like cells with central necrosis and frequent neutrophilic infiltration (Figs. 23.7 and 23.8). These have been referred to as lacunar cell predominant Hodgkin's disease or as the syncytial variant of nodular sclerosis (Strickler et al, 1986). The cohesive masses of atypical cells may mimic metastatic carcinoma or melanoma or non-Hodgkin's lymphoma. Diagnosis is aided by identification of areas of more typical nodular sclerosis HD or by immunohistochemical studies demonstrating the Hodgkin's phenotype (CD15-positive, CD30-positive). Distinction from Hodgkin's-like anaplastic large cell lymphoma may be difficult or in some cases impossible (Harris et al, 1994). The clinical behavior of syncytial HD is not well documented but seems to be similar to conventional nodular sclerosis HD.

Mixed Cellularity Hodgkin's Disease

Mixed cellularity Hodgkin's disease follows nodular sclerosis HD in frequency and is particularly prevalent in older patients and in HIV-associated HD (Mir et al, 1993; Ree et al, 1991). Mixed cellularity HD is defined strictly as HD without specific features of other forms of HD and is therefore a category of exclusion. Most cases demonstrate numerous diagnostic RS cells in a mixed inflammatory background (Figs. 23.9 and 23.10). Fibrosis may be present, but it is not in the form of birefringent collagenous bands.

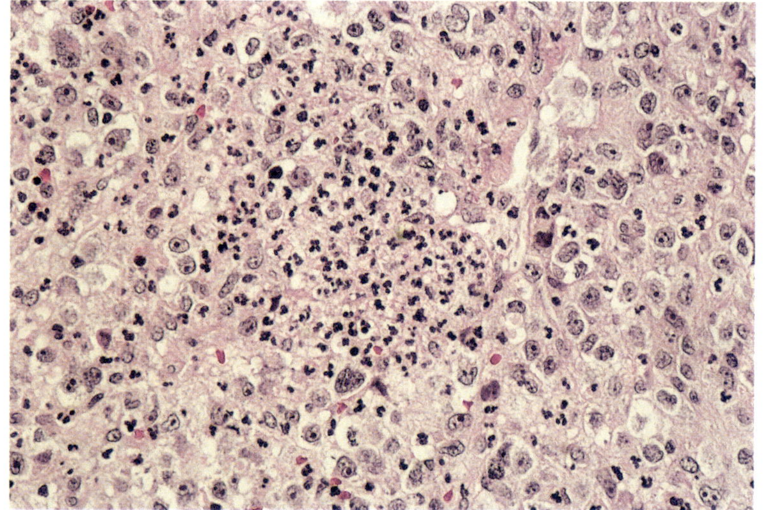

Syncytial variant of nodular sclerosis Hodgkin's disease showing a cohesive sheet of lacunar-variant cells with central necrosis and neutrophilic infiltration. The histology may be unfamiliar as Hodgkin's disease and suggest a diagnosis of non-Hodgkin's lymphoma or metastatic carcinoma or melanoma. Immunohistochemical studies and search for areas of typical nodular sclerosis Hodgkin's disease will lead to the correct diagnosis.

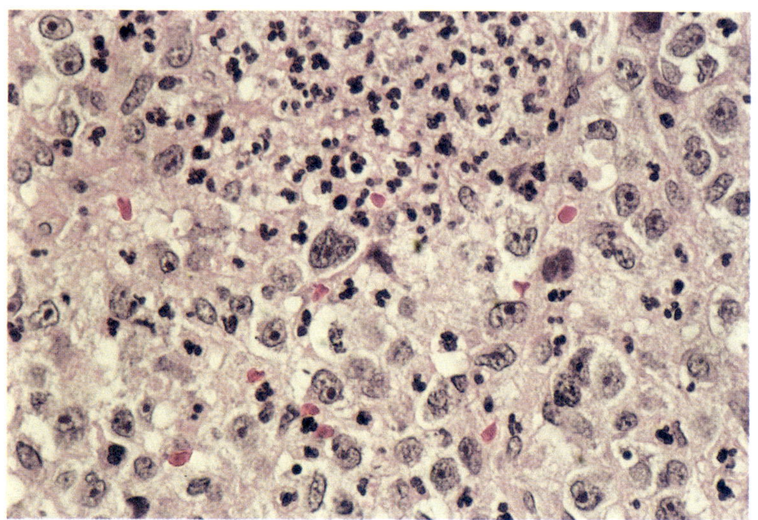

Syncytial variant of nodular sclerosis Hodgkin's disease, higher magnification, showing cytologic detail of lacunar-variant cells.

FIGURE
23.9

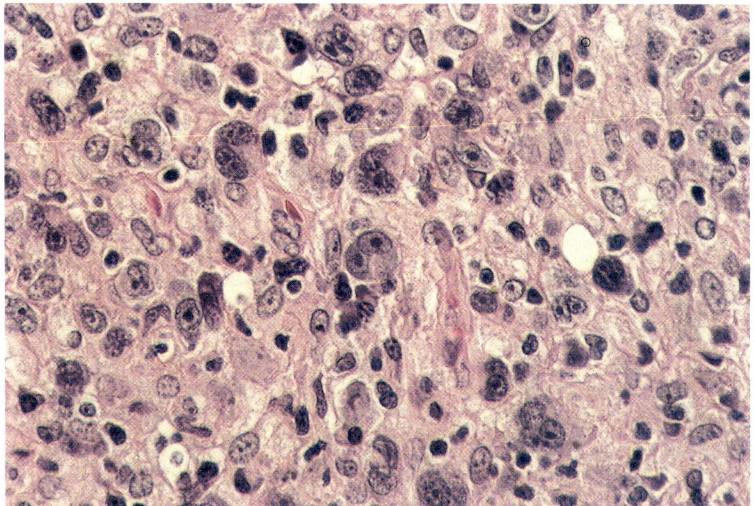

Mixed cellularity Hodgkin's disease showing numerous Reed-Sternberg cells.

FIGURE
23.10

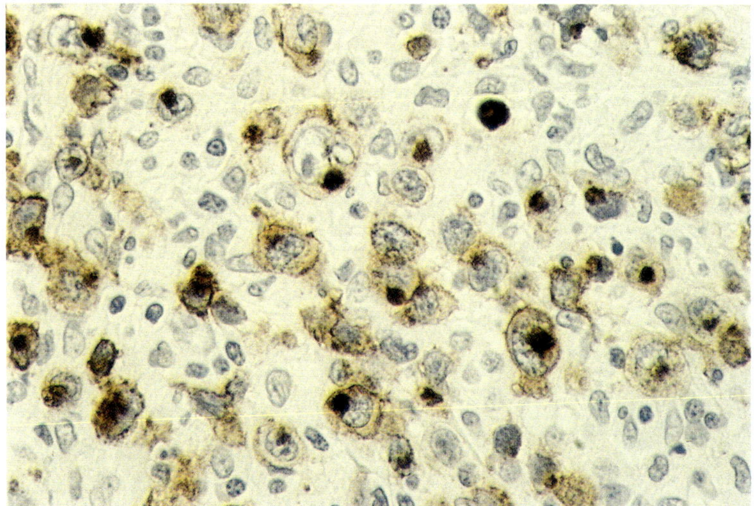

Mixed cellularity Hodgkin's disease showing staining of Reed-Sternberg and mononuclear Reed-Sternberg–like cells for CD15. Membranous and paranuclear (Golgi) pattern is typical.

Variants

HODGKIN'S DISEASE WITH A HIGH EPITHELIOID CELL CONTENT Some cases of mixed cellularity HD demonstrate large numbers of epithelioid histiocytes and may mimic lymphoepithelioid cell lymphoma (Lennert's lymphoma) (Patsouris et al, 1989). Diagnosis is based on identification of diagnostic RS cells amongst the epithelioid histiocytes (Fig. 23.11).

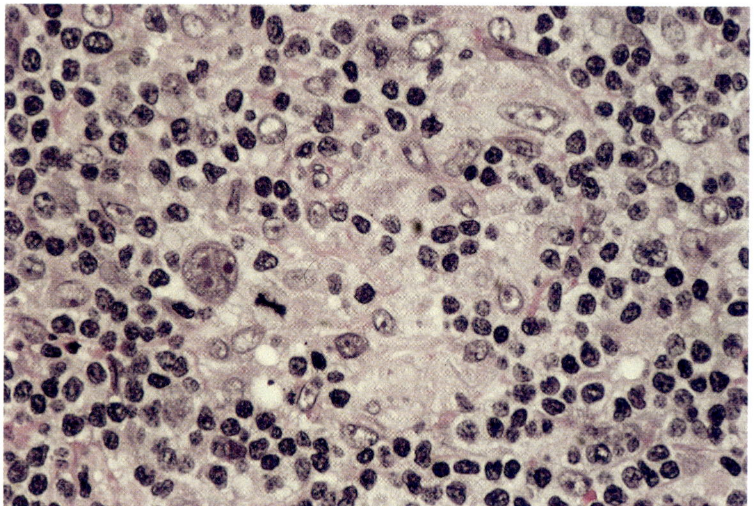

Mixed cellularity Hodgkin's disease with a high content of epithelioid histiocytes may be confused with lymphoepithelioid cell lymphoma (Lennert's lymphoma) or granulomatous disease. The presence of Reed-Sternberg cells amongst the epithelioid histiocytes is diagnostic.

INTERFOLLICULAR HODGKIN'S DISEASE Interfollicular Hodgkin's disease is characterized by reactive follicular lymphoid hyperplasia; scattered Reed-Sternberg cells are present in the interfollicular zone (Doggett et al, 1983) (Figs. 23.12 and 23.13). Interfollicular Hodgkin's disease appears not to be a specific histopathologic type of HD but to be a distinctive pattern of early lymph node involvement. Most cases prove to be of mixed cellularity, or occasionally of nodular sclerosis, type.

Lymphocyte Depletion Hodgkin's Disease

Lymphocyte depletion HD is the least common of the major forms of classical HD and includes the diffuse fibrosis and reticular subtypes of Lukes and Butler. The former subtype is characterized by relatively acellular fibrosis containing scattered RS and RS-variant cells (Fig. 23.14); the latter subtype is characterized by sheets of RS and pleomorphic RS-variant cells. On critical examination, many cases of lymphocyte depletion HD have proven to be other entities, particularly pleomorphic non-Hodgkin's lymphomas (Kant et al, 1986). Immunophenotypic studies are therefore essential for accurate diagnosis.

Provisional Entity: Lymphocyte-Rich Classical Hodgkin's Disease

Lymphocyte-rich classical Hodgkin's disease is the proposed designation in the REAL classification for those cases of lymphocyte predominance HD in which the RS cells demonstrate the CD15-positive, CD30-positive phenotype of classical Hodgkin's disease (Harris et al, 1994). Although few large studies are available, it is likely that these cases are more closely related to classical HD than to nodular lymphocyte predominance HD (Regula et al, 1988).

FIGURE 23.12

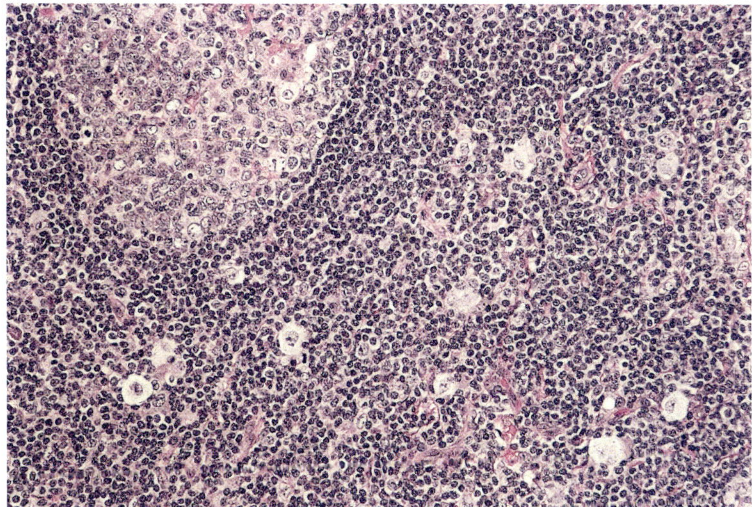

Interfollicular Hodgkin's disease showing follicular hyperplasia with scattered Reed-Sternberg and mononuclear Reed-Sternberg–like cells in the interfollicular zone. This form of Hodgkin's disease appears to be a pattern of early lymph node involvement rather than a specific histopathologic subtype of Hodgkin's disease; most cases are of mixed cellularity type.

FIGURE 23.13

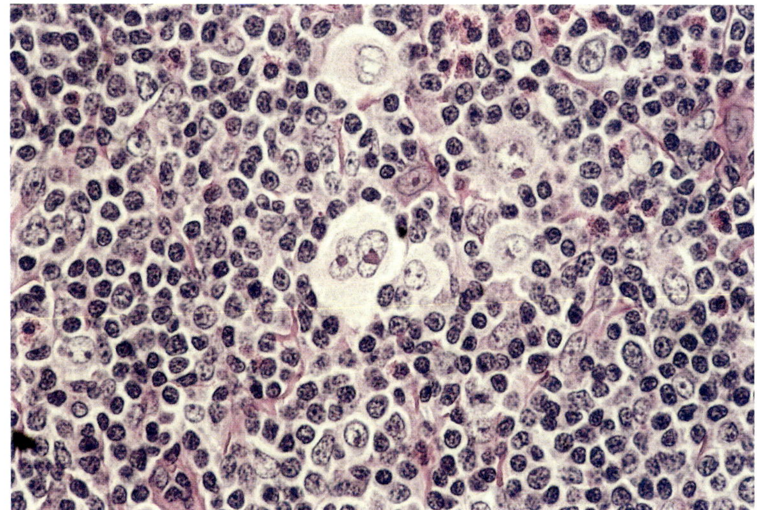

Intefollicular Hodgkin's disease, higher magnification, showing a diagnostic Reed-Sternberg cell.

HIV-Associated Hodgkin's Disease

Hodgkin's disease may occur with increased frequency in patients with HIV infection (Serraino et al, 1997). HIV-associated HD exhibits characteristic clinicopathologic features, including advanced stage at presentation, frequent "B" symptoms, high incidence of bone marrow involvement, and poor prognosis (Ree et al, 1991). Most cases are of

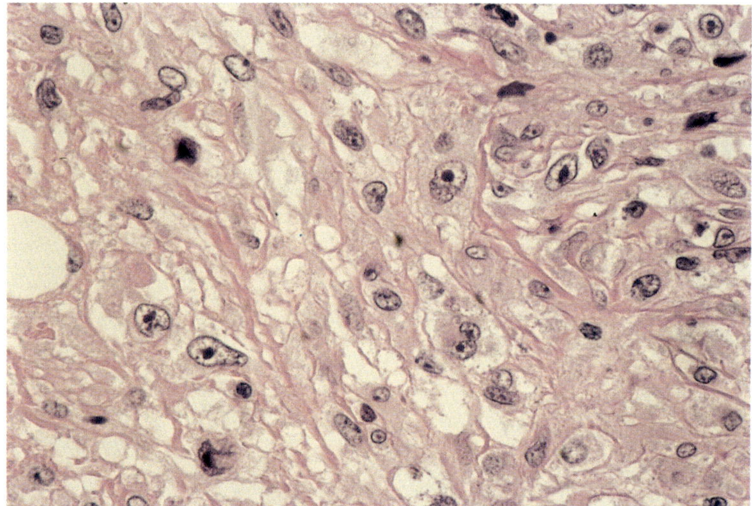

FIGURE
23.14

Lymphocyte depletion Hodgkin's disease, diffuse fibrosis form of Lukes
and Butler, showing scattered Reed-Sternberg and mononuclear Reed-
Sternberg–like cells in a background of acellular fibrosis.

mixed cellularity type and may demonstrate unusual pathologic features, including relative lymphocyte depletion and prominent fibrohistiocytoid stromal cells (Ree et al, 1991)
(Fig. 23.15). Epstein-Barr virus is present in nearly all cases (Herndier et al, 1993). In
contrast to Hodgkin's disease in normal hosts, in which the small lymphocytes consist
predominantly of CD4-positive helper T cells, the small lymphocytes in HIV-associated
HD consist predominantly of CD8-positive suppressor T cells (Unger and Strauchen,
1986).

Differential Diagnosis

Hodgkin's disease is usually not a difficult diagnosis. In typical cases, the diagnosis is
established morphologically based on the identification of diagnostic Reed-Sternberg
cells in the appropriate cellular background; immunophenotypic studies in typical cases
are not necessary and are, at best, an adjunct to diagnosis. In atypical cases, however,
immunophenotypic studies may be valuable, since cells morphologically resembling RS
cells are seen in a variety of other conditions (vide infra). CD30 is detected in paraffin
embedded tissue in 90% or more of cases of classical HD; CD15 is detected in 70%.
Staining may be membranous, cytoplasmic, or paranuclear (Golgi zone) in distribution.

Diagnostic RS cells are a requirement for the initial diagnosis of Hodgkin's disease. In
patients with an established diagnosis of Hodgkin's disease, however, the diagnosis of
involvement at other sites (bone marrow, liver, lung, etc.) may be established by the
presence of atypical mononuclear cells in the appropriate cellular background.

Reed-Sternberg–Like Cells in Other Conditions

Reed-Sternberg–like cells may be seen in a variety of conditions other than Hodgkin's
disease, including viral lymphadenitis and infectious mononucleosis, non-Hodgkin's

lymphomas, and metastatic carcinoma or malignant melanoma. Distinction of these conditions from Hodgkin's disease is clinically important and is aided by immunophenotypic studies.

VIRAL LYMPHADENITIS AND INFECTIOUS MONONUCLEOSIS Reed-Sternberg–like cells may be prominent in viral lymphadenitis and infectious mononucleosis and frequently surround foci of necrosis. RS-like cells in infectious mononucleosis share immunophenotypic features with RS cells in HD, including lack of CD45, expression of CD30, and expression of EBV latent membrane protein, but differ by lack of expression of CD15 (Reynolds et al, 1995). The partial preservation of the architecture, presence of immunoblasts with paracortical "mottling" or "moth-eaten" appearance, and presence of lymphocytes at all stages of transformation usually permit morphologic distinction of infectious mononucleosis from Hodgkin's disease.

PERIPHERAL T CELL LYMPHOMAS Peripheral T cell lymphomas frequently contain Reed-Sternberg–like cells. Distinction from Hodgkin's disease is based on the presence of atypia of the small as well as large cells and paucity of diagnostic RS cells. Immunophenotypic studies are of limited utility since the majority of small lymphocytes in Hodgkin's disease are T cells, and the RS-like cells in peripheral T cell lymphomas may express HD-associated antigens CD15 and CD30. Demonstration of an abnormal T cell phenotype or clonal T-cell antigen-receptor rearrangement, however, favors a peripheral T cell lymphoma.

ANAPLASTIC LARGE CELL LYMPHOMAS Anaplastic large cell lymphomas (ALCL) may closely resemble Hodgkin's disease and distinction of RS cell-rich variants of Hodgkin's disease (e.g., syncytial variant of nodular sclerosis) from Hodgkin's-like ALCL may be difficult or, in some cases, impossible (Harris et al, 1994). The presence of sinusoidal involvement or cells with "horseshoe-shaped" or "wreath-like" nuclei are features fa-

FIGURE 23.15

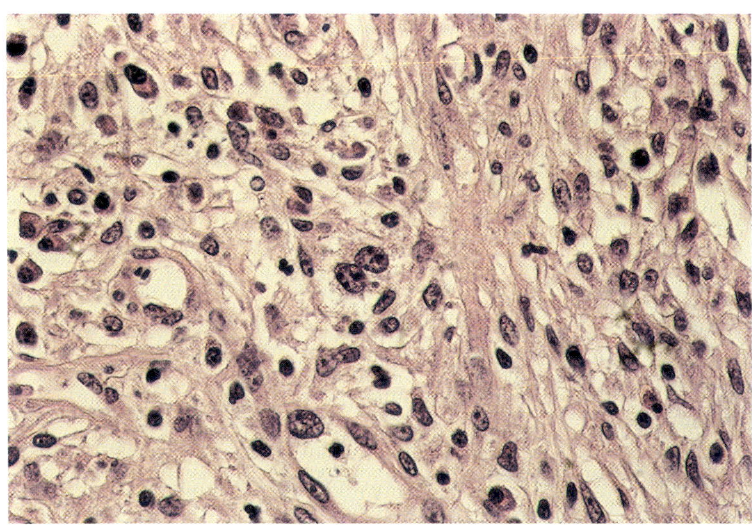

Human immunodeficiency virus-associated Hodgkin's disease showing atypical Reed-Sternberg cell and prominent fibrohistiocytoid stromal cells.

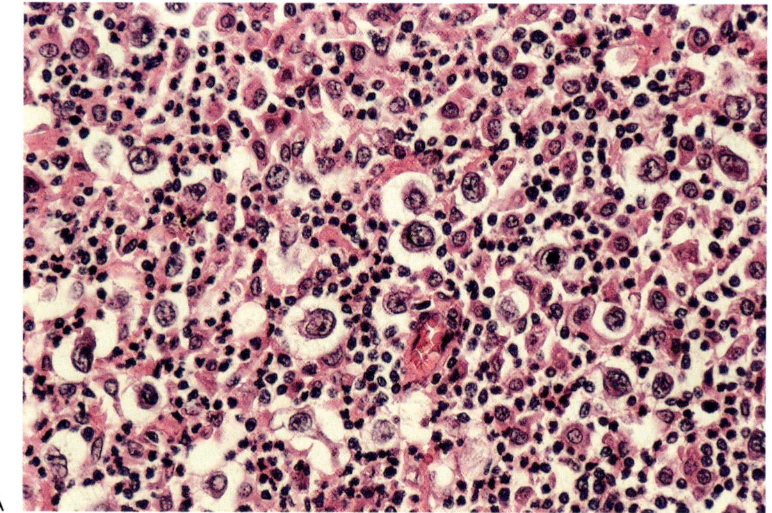

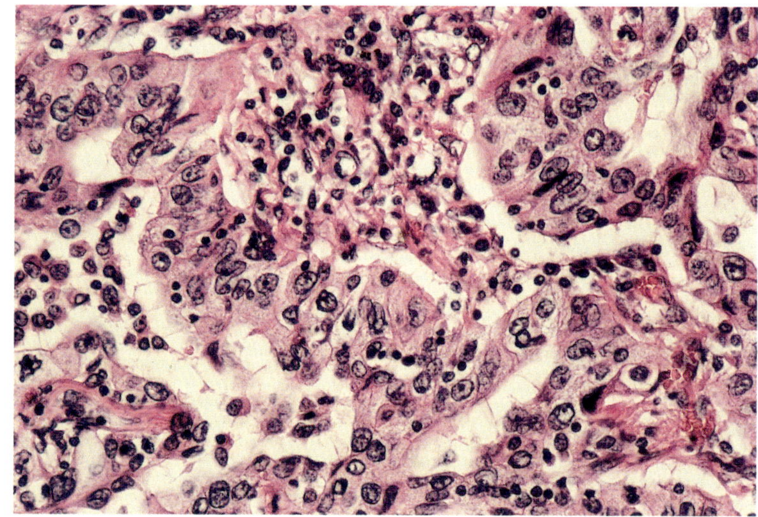

FIGURE 23.16

Metastatic large cell undifferentiated carcinoma of the lung mimicking Hodgkin's disease. A. Large atypical cells in an inflammatory background mimic Hodgkin's disease. B. Another area of the tumor showing glandular differentiation.

voring ALCL. Immunophenotypic studies are helpful in some cases. CD30 is expressed in both HD and ALCL; expression of CD15 favors HD, while expression of EMA favors ALCL.

T-CELL-RICH B LARGE CELL LYMPHOMA   T-cell-rich B large cell lymphoma (TCRBL) may closely simulate Hodgkin's disease with RS-like cells in a background of small T lymphocytes (McBride et al, 1996). The presence of a lymphocyte-rich background and a paucity of plasma cells and eosinophils are clues to the correct diagnosis. Distinction is aided by immunophenotypic studies (Wang et al, 1997). In contrast to Hodgkin's disease,

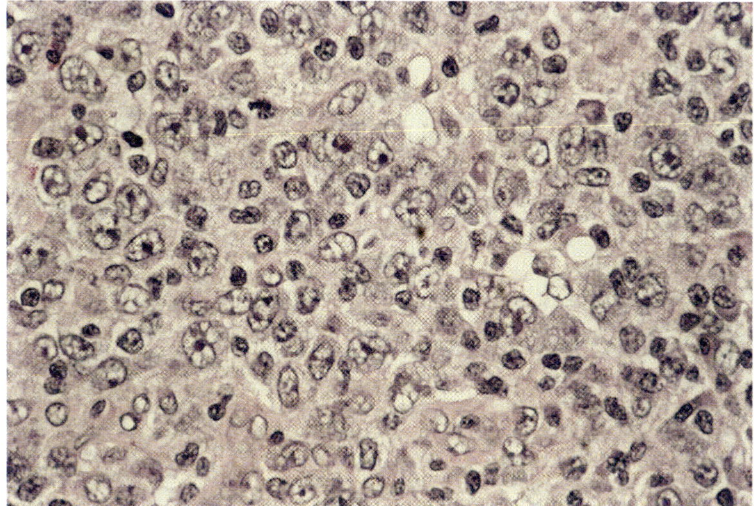

Diffuse large B cell non-Hodgkin's lymphoma following Hodgkin's disease.

the RS-like cells in TCRBL are CD45-positive, CD15- and CD30-negative, and strongly positive for CD20. Distinction appears to be clinically relevant: Four patients with TCRBL treated on protocols for Hodgkin's disease relapsed and died, whereas four of five patients treated on protocols for non-Hodgkin's lymphoma were alive and free of disease (McBride et al, 1996).

METASTATIC CARCINOMA AND MELANOMA RS-like cells may be seen in non-hematopoietic malignant neoplasms including metastatic carcinoma and malignant melanoma. Metastatic nasopharyngeal carcinoma with lymphoid stroma (so called "lympho-epithelioma") in particular mimics the appearance of Hodgkin's disease. Metastatic squamous carcinoma from other sites and metastatic large cell undifferentiated carcinoma of the lung may also have an inflammatory component and mimic Hodgkin's disease (Fig. 23.16). Distinction is aided by immunohistochemical studies for cytokeratins, present in carcinomas, and S-100 protein or HMB-45, present in melanoma. CD15 is frequently present in adenocarcinoma as well as Hodgkin's disease (Sheibani et al, 1986).

Course and Prognosis

The therapy of Hodgkin's disease is gratifying, with a high frequency of durable complete responses (Urba and Longo, 1992). Early stage Hodgkin's disease (Ann Arbor stage I and II) is treated primarily with radiotherapy to extended or subtotal nodal fields. Staging laparotomy for treatment planning in early stage Hodgkin's disease is performed less frequently than in the past. Advanced Hodgkin's disease (Ann Arbor stage III and IV) is treated with combination chemotherapy. Disease-free survivals range from 50 to 90%. Patients failing conventional therapy may sometimes be salvaged with bone marrow transplantation. Advanced age and massive mediastinal disease (mediastinal mass greater than one-third of the thoracic diameter) remain poor prognostic features. Patients successfully treated for Hodgkin's disease have an increased incidence of non-Hodgkin's lymphomas and other neoplasms, including acute granulocytic leukemia and cutaneous malignant melanoma (Urba and Longo, 1992; Zarate-Osorno et al, 1992) (Fig. 23.17).

REFERENCES

Davis TH, Morton CC, Miller-Cassman R, Balk S, Kadin ME. Hodgkin's disease, lymphomatoid papulosis, and cutaneous T cell lymphoma derived from a common T cell clone. N Engl J Med 326:1115–1122, 1992.

Doggett RS, Colby TV, Dorfman RF. Interfollicular Hodgkin's disease. Am J Surg Pathol 7:145–149, 1983.

Haluska FG, Brufsky AM, Canellos GP. The cellular biology of the Reed-Sternberg cell. Blood 84:1005–1019, 1994.

Harris NL, Jaffe ES, Stein H, Banks PM, Chan JKC, Cleary ML, et al. A revised European-American classification of lymphoid neoplasms: A proposal from the international lymphoma study group. Blood 84:1361–1392, 1994.

Herndier BG, Sanchez HC, Chang KL, Chen YY, Weiss LM. High prevalence of Epstein-Barr virus in the Reed-Sternberg cells of HIV-associated Hodgkin's disease. Am J Pathol 142:1073–1079, 1993.

Hess JL, Bodis S, Pinkus G, Silver B, Mauch P. Histopathologic grading of nodular sclerosis Hodgkin's disease. Lack of prognostic significance in 254 surgically staged patients. Cancer 74:708–714, 1994.

Hummel M, Ziemann K, Lammert H, Pileri S, Sabattini E, Stein H. Hodgkin's disease with monoclonal and polyclonal populations of Reed-Sternberg cells. N Engl J Med 333:901–906, 1995.

Kadin ME. Possible origin of the Reed-Sternberg cell from an interdigitating reticulum cell. Cancer Treat Rep 66:601–608, 1982.

Kamel OW, Chang PP, Hsu FJ, Dolezal MV, Warnke RA, van de Rijn M. Clonal VDJ recombinations of the immunoglobulin heavy chain gene by PCR in classical Hodgkin's disease. Am J Clin Pathol 104:419–423, 1995.

Kant JA, Hubbard SM, Longo DL, Simon RM, DeVita VT, Jaffe ES. The pathologic and clinical heterogeneity of lymphocyte-depleted Hodgkin's disease. J Clin Oncol 4:284–294, 1986.

Khan G, Norton AJ, Slavin G. Epstein-Barr virus in Hodgkin's disease. Relation to age and subtype. Cancer 71:3124–3129, 1993.

Kuppers R, Rajewsky K, Zhao M, Simons G, Laumann R, Fischer R, Hansmann ML. Hodgkin's disease: Hodgkin and Reed-Sternberg cells picked from histological sections show clonal immunoglobulin gene rearrangements and appear to be derived from B cells at various stages of development. Proc Natl Acad Sci USA 91:10962–10966, 1994.

Mack TM, Cozen W, Shibata D, Weiss LM, Nathwani BN, Hernandez AM, et al. Concordance for Hodgkin's disease in identical twins suggesting genetic susceptibility to the young-adult form of the disease. N Engl J Med 332:413–418, 1995.

MacLennan KA, Bennett MH, Tu A, Hudson BV, Easterling J, Hudson GV, Jelliffe AM. Relationship of histopathologic features to survival and relapse in nodular sclerosing Hodgkin's disease: A study of 1,659 patients. Cancer 64:1686–1693, 1989.

McBride JA, Rodriguez J, Luthra R, Ordonez NG, Cabanillas F, Pugh WC. T-cell-rich B large cell lymphoma simulating lymphocyte-rich Hodgkin's disease. Am J Surg Pathol 20:193–201, 1996.

Mir R, Anderson J, Strauchen J, Nissen NI, Cooper R, Rafla S, et al. Hodgkin's disease in patients 60 years of age or older. Histologic and clinical features of advanced stage disease. Cancer 71:1857–1866, 1993.

Patsouris E, Noel H, Lennert K. Cytologic and immunohistochemical findings in Hodgkin's disease, mixed cellularity type, with a high content of epithelioid cells. Am J Surg Pathol 13:1014–1022, 1989.

Ree HJ, Strauchen JA, Khan AA, Gold JE, Crowley JP, Kahn H, Zalusky R. Human immunodeficiency virus-associated Hodgkin's disease. Clinicopathologic studies of 24 cases and preponderance of mixed cellularity type characterized by the occurrence of fibrohistiocytoid stroma cells. Cancer 67:1614–1621, 1991.

Regula DP, Hoppe RT, Weiss LM. Nodular and diffuse types of lymphocyte predominance Hodgkin's disease. N Engl J Med 318:214–219, 1988.

Reynolds DJ, Banks PM, Gulley ML. New characterization of infectious mononucleosis and a phenotypic comparision with Hodgkin's disease. Am J Pathol 146:379–388, 1995.

Schmid C, Pan L, Diss T, Isaacson PG. Expression of B cell antigens by Hodgkin's and Reed-Sternberg cells. Am J Pathol 139:701–707, 1991.

Serraino D, Pezzotti P, Dorrucci M, Alliegro MB, Sinicco A, Rezza G. Cancer incidence in a cohort of human immunodeficiency virus seroconverters. Cancer 79:1004–1008, 1997.

Sheibani K, Battifora H, Burke JS, Rappaport H. Leu-M1 antigen in human neoplasms. An immunohistologic study of 400 cases. Am J Surg Pathol 10:227–236, 1986.

Strickler JG, Michie SA, Warnke RA, Dorfman RF. The "syncytial variant" of nodular sclerosing Hodgkin's disease. Am J Surg Pathol 10:470–477, 1986.

Unger PD, Strauchen JA. Hodgkin's disease in AIDS-complex patients: Report of four cases and tissue immunologic marker studies. Cancer 58:821–825, 1986.

Urba WJ, Longo DL. Hodgkin's disease. N Engl J Med 326:678–687, 1992.

Wang Q, Unger PD, Strauchen JA. T-cell-rich B-large-cell lymphoma simulating Hodgkin's disease: Report of two cases with transformation to pleomorphic B-large-cell lymphoma. Int J Surg Pathol 5:31–36, 1997.

Weiss LM, Mohaved LA, Warnke RA, Sklar J. Detec-tion of Epstein-Barr viral genomes in Reed-Sternberg cells of Hodgkin's disease. N Engl J Med 320:502–506, 1989.

Zarate-Osorno A, Medeiros LJ, Longo DL, Jaffe ES. Non-Hodgkin's lymphomas arising in patients successfully treated for Hodgkin's disease. A clinical, histologic, and immunophenotypic study of 14 cases. Am J Surg Pathol 16:885–895, 1992.

Zarate-Osorno A, Medeiros LJ, Kingma DW, Longo DL, Jaffe ES. Hodgkin's disease following non-Hodgkin's lymphoma. A clinicopathologic and immunophenotypic study of nine cases. Am J Surg Pathol 17:123–132, 1993.

Zukerberg LR, Collins AB, Ferry JA, Harris NL. Coexpression of CD15 and CD20 by Reed-Sternberg cells in Hodgkin's disease. Am J Pathol 139:475–483, 1991.

Lymphoproliferative Disorders Associated with Immunosuppression

Lymphoproliferative disorders develop with increased frequency in patients receiving immunosuppressive therapy for prevention of rejection of transplanted organs (post-transplant lymphoproliferative disorder) or for the management of chronic autoimmune disease. A striking feature of these disorders is the frequent association with Epstein-Barr virus (EBV) infection and spontaneous regression with reduction or withdrawal of the immunosuppressive therapy.

Post-transplant Lymphoproliferative Disorder

An increased incidence of malignant lymphoma has been known to follow solid organ transplants, including transplants of the kidney, heart, lung, and liver (Frizzera et al, 1981; Nalesnik et al, 1988). A striking feature of these lesions is association with EBV infection and frequent spontaneous regression following reduction or withdrawal of immunosuppressive therapy. These lesions constitute a spectrum of EBV-associated B cell proliferations, which are referred to as post-transplant lymphoproliferative disorders (PTLDs).

Clinical Features

Post-transplant lymphoproliferative disorder may follow any organ transplantation. Risk factors include heart or heart-lung transplantation and therapy with cyclosporine A or monoclonal antibody OKT3 (Knowles et al, 1995). PTLDs are frequently extranodal and may be rapidly progressive, appearing as early as 60 days following transplantation. PTLDs are invariably associated with EBV. Adult patients with PTLD usually show serologic evidence of past infection; pediatric patients previously negative for EBV may undergo seroconversion following transplantation from an EBV-positive donor. PTLDs demonstrated a range of morphological appearances and may appear polyclonal or monoclonal by immunophenotypic analysis; however, most demonstrate molecular evidence for a clonal proliferation (Cleary et al, 1984). Diverse monoclonal and polyclonal proliferations may coexist at different sites in the same patient (Shearer et al, 1985). The observations are most consistent with the hypothesis that PTLD results from an EBV-induced B cell proliferation, which evolves from polyclonal to oligoclonal to monoclonal (Knowles et al, 1995). Morphologic subclassification of PTLD has been proposed, with categories of polymorphic B cell hyperplasia and polymorphic B cell lymphoma (Frizzera et al, 1981) and polymorphic and monomorphic PTLD (Nalesnik et al, 1988). Morphologic and molecular genetic analysis of PTLD suggests the existence of three distinct categories: plasmacytic hyperplasia, polymorphic B cell hyperplasia/polymorphic B cell lymphoma, and immunoblastic lymphoma/multiple myeloma (Knowles et al, 1995). These lesions constitute a spectrum of PTLD of low, intermediate, and high grade.

Histopathology

PLASMACYTIC HYPERPLASIA (LOW-GRADE PTLD) Plasmacytic hyperplasia (PH) is a low-grade form of PTLD with frequent involvement of tonsils, Waldeyer's ring, and lymph nodes (Knowles et al, 1995). PH is polyclonal by immunoglobulin gene rearrangement and contains multiple forms of Epstein-Barr virus. Microscopic examination of affected tonsils or lymph nodes shows preservation of the architecture with expansion of the interfollicular zone by infiltrates of plasmacytoid lymphocytes and plasma cells, with few immunoblasts. Follicular centers may be hyperplastic or involuted.

POLYMORPHIC B CELL HYPERPLASIA/POLYMORPHIC B CELL LYMPHOMA (INTERMEDIATE GRADE PTLD) Polymorphic B cell hyperplasia/polymorphic B cell lymphoma (PBCH/L) is an intermediate grade of PTLD corresponding to the polymorphic PTLD of Nalesnik and colleagues (Nalesnik et al, 1988). Nearly all cases are monoclonal by immunoglobulin gene rearrangement and contain a single form of Epstein-Barr virus; however, oncogene and tumor suppressor gene mutations are not identified (Knowles et al, 1995). PBCH/L may be nodal or extranodal and is characterized by effacement of architecture by a polymorphous proliferation of lymphocytes and immunoblasts with varying degrees of plasmacytoid differentiation (Figs. 24.1 and 24.2). PBCH/L includes lesions previously designated polymorphic B cell hyperplasia and polymorphic B cell lymphoma; the latter is distinguished by incomplete plasmacytoid differentiation, greater cytologic atypia, and confluent areas of necrosis (Frizzera et al, 1981).

IMMUNOBLASTIC LYMPHOMA/MULTIPLE MYELOMA (HIGH-GRADE PTLD) Immunoblastic lymphoma/multiple myeloma (IBL/MM) is a high-grade form of PTLD characterized by the monomorphic proliferation of immunoblasts or atypical plasma cells, corresponding to the monomorphic PTLD of Nalesnik and colleagues (Nalesnik et al, 1988). IBL/MM is monoclonal by immunoglobulin gene rearrangement, contains a single form of Epstein-

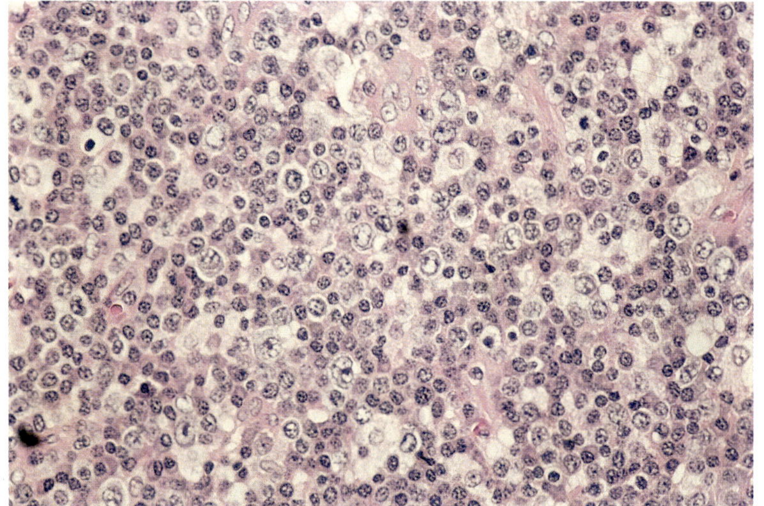

Post-transplant lymphoproliferative disorder, polymorphic type (polymorphic B cell hyperplasia/polymorphic B cell lymphoma), showing polymorphous proliferation of lymphocytes, plasma cells, and immunoblasts.

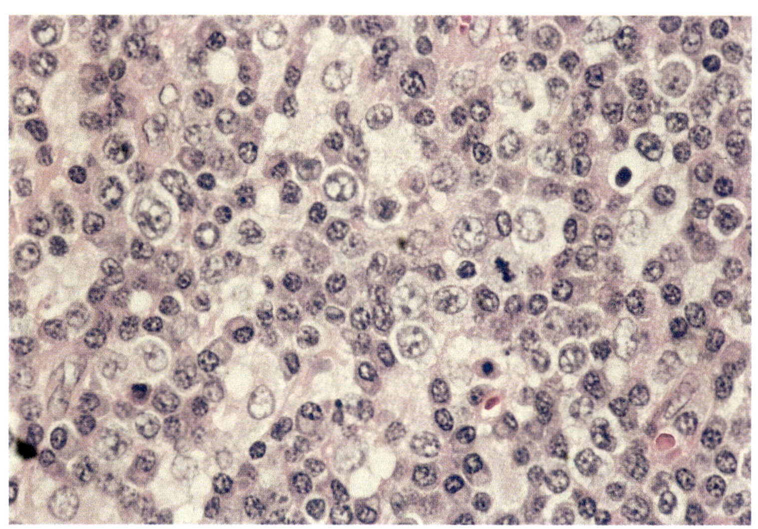

Post-transplant lymphoproliferative disorder, polymorphic type (polymorphic B cell hyperplasia/polymorphic B cell lymphoma), higher magnification, showing plasma cells and immunoblasts.

Barr virus, and, in addition, contains mutations of one or more oncogenes or tumor suppressor genes (N-RAS, p53, or C-MYC) (Knowles et al, 1995).

Differential Diagnosis

PTLD should be distinguished from nonspecific reactive lymphoid hyperplasia and from other post-transplant neoplasms, including Kaposi's sarcoma and rare lymphomas of donor origin (Spiro et al, 1993). A post-transplant syndrome related to Kaposi's sarcoma-associated herpesvirus should also be distinguished (Strauchen et al, 1997).

Course and Prognosis

The management of PTLD is largely independent of the histopathologic classification or determination of clonality and is based on reduction or withdrawal of immunosuppressive therapy. Acyclovir and α-interferon have been used adjunctively; however, the former is likely only useful in cases of primary EBV infection (Sullivan et al, 1984). Patients failing to respond to withdrawal of immunosuppression may benefit from radiation or combination chemotherapy (Garrett et al, 1993).

Lymphoproliferative Disorders Associated With Chronic Immunosuppression

Lymphoproliferative disorders, including diffuse large B cell lymphomas, Hodgkin's disease, and Hodgkin's-like lymphomas have been reported in patients undergoing long-term immunosuppressive therapy for autoimmune and rheumatologic disorders (Kamel et al, 1993; Kamel et al, 1996) (Figs. 24.3 and 24.4). The underlying disorders have included rheumatoid arthritis, psoriasis, juvenile rheumatoid arthritis, dermatomyositis, and polymyositis. Reported cases have occurred in association with long-term methotrexate therapy; however, we have seen similar cases following long-term therapy with azathioprine (Imuran). Epstein-Barr virus is frequently present; spontaneous regression may follow withdrawal of immunosuppressive therapy (Kamel et al, 1993; Kamel et al, 1996).

Lymphoproliferative Disorders Associated With Immunodeficiency Syndromes

An increased incidence of lymphoproliferative disorders is associated with acquired and congenital primary immunodeficiency syndromes. Lymphoproliferative disorders associated with the acquired immunodeficiency syndrome due to HIV are considered in Chapter 5. Primary immunodeficiency disorders associated with the development of lymphoproliferative disorders include ataxia telangiectasia, Wiskott-Aldrich syndrome, common variable immunodeficiency, severe combined immunodeficiency, X-linked hypogammaglobulinemia, and selective IgA and IgM deficiency (Frizzera et al, 1980). The lymphoproliferative disorders developing in the setting of primary immunodeficiency are pre-

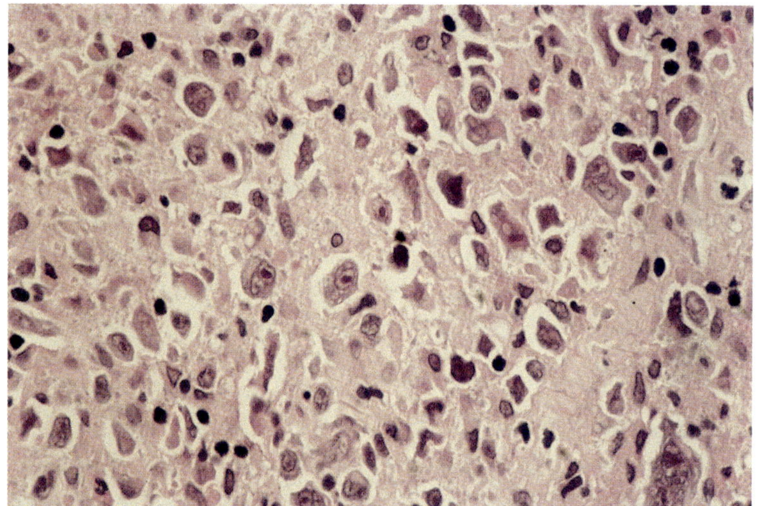

FIGURE 24.3

Epstein-Barr virus (EBV)-positive Hodgkin's-like lymphoma in a patient receiving long term methotrexate therapy for psoriatic arthritis.

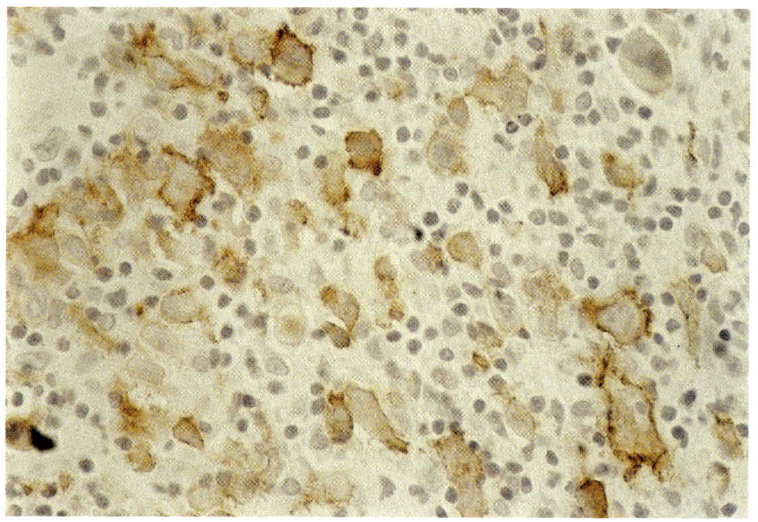

FIGURE 24.4

EBV-positive Hodgkin's-like lymphoma in a patient receiving long-term methotrexate therapy for psoriatic arthritis showing positive staining for CD30.

dominantly of non-Hodgkin's or unclassified type; however, an increased incidence of Hodgkin's disease, frequently of lymphocyte depletion type, is associated with ataxia-telangiectasia (Frizzera et al, 1980). The X-linked lymphoproliferative syndrome is a familial disorder characterized by an impaired host response to Epstein-Barr virus, with frequent fatal infectious mononucleosis, acquired agammaglobulinemia, and development of malignant lymphoma (Grierson and Purtilo, 1987; Harrington et al, 1987).

REFERENCES

Cleary ML, Warnke R, Sklar J. Monoclonality of lymphoproliferative lesions in cardiac-transplant patients. N Engl J Med 310: 477, 1984.

Frizzera G, Rosai J, Dehner LP, Spector BD, Kersey JH. Lymphoreticular disorders in primary immuno-deficiencies: New findings based on an up-to-date histologic classification of 35 cases. Cancer 46:692–699, 1980.

Frizzera G, Hanto DW, Gajl-Peczalska KJ, Rosai J, McKenna RW, Sibley RK, et al. Polymorphic diffuse B cell hyperplasias and lymphomas in renal transplant recipients. Cancer Res 41:4262, 1981.

Garrett TJ, Chadburn A, Barr ML, Drusin RE, Chen JM, Schulman LL, et al. Posttransplantation lymph-oproliferative disorders treated with cyclophos-phamide-doxorubicin-vincristine-prednisone chemotherapy. Cancer 72:2782–2785, 1993.

Grierson H, Purtilo DT. Epstein-Barr virus infections in males with the X-linked lymphoproliferative syndrome. Ann Intern Med 106:538–545, 1987.

Harrington DS, Weisenberger DD, Purtilo DT, et al. Malignant lymphoma in the X-linked lymphoproli-ferative syndrome. Cancer 59:1419–1429, 1987.

Kamel OW, van de Rijn M, Weiss LW, Del Zoppo GJ, Hench PK, Robbins BA, et al. Brief report: Reversible lymphomas associated with Epstein-Barr virus occurring during methotrexate therapy for rheumatoid arthritis and dermatomyositis. N Engl J Med 328:1317–1321, 1993.

Kamel OW, Weiss LW, van de Rijn M, Colby TV, Kingma DW, Jaffe ES. Hodgkin's disease and lymphoproliferations resembling Hodgkin's disease in patients receiving long term low-dose meth-otrexate therapy. Am J Surg Pathol 20:1279–1287, 1996.

Knowles DM, Cesarman E, Chadburn A, Frizzera G, Chen J, Rose EA, Michler RE. Correlative morpho-logic and molecular genetic analysis demonstrates three distinct categories of posttransplantation lymphoproliferative disorders. Blood 85:552–565, 1995.

Nalesnik MA, Jaffe R, Starzl TE, Demetris AJ, Porter K, Burnham JA, et al. The pathology of posttrans-plant lymphoproliferative disorders occurring in the setting of cyclosporine A-prednisone immuno-suppression. Am J Pathol 133:173, 1988.

Shearer WT, Ritz J, Finegold MJ, Guerra IC, Rosen-blatt HM, Lewis DE, et al. Epstein-Barr virus-associated B-cell proliferations of diverse clonal origins after bone marrow transplantation in a 12 year old patient with severe combined immunode-ficiency. N Engl J Med 312:1151, 1985.

Spiro IJ, Yandell DW, Li C, Saini S, Ferry J, Powelson J, et al. Brief report: Lymphoma of donor origin occurring in the porta hepatis of a transplanted liver. N Engl J Med 329:27–29, 1993.

Strauchen JA, Matsushima A, Lee G, Scigliano E, Hale E, Weisse M, Burstein D, Moore PS, Chang Y. Posttransplantation lymphoproliferative syn-dromes related to Kaposi's sarcoma-associated herpesvirus (abstract). Blood 90 (suppl 1): 270b, 1997.

Sullivan JL, Medveczky P, Forman SJ, Baker SM, Monroe JE, Mulder C. Epstein-Barr virus induced lymphoproliferation. Implications for antiviral che-motherapy. N Engl J Med 311:1163–1167, 1984.

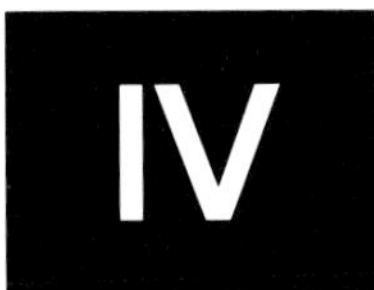

IV

Proliferations of Other Elements

25

Storage and Deposition Disorders

Several disorders are characterized by abnormal deposits of lipids, proteins, or foreign materials in lymph nodes. Deposits in these disorders may be intracellular or extracellular and may be associated with characteristic histopathologic changes.

Lipid Deposits

Lipid deposits in lymph nodes include lipogranulomata and the lipidoses, storage disorders due to hereditary lysosomal enzyme deficiencies.

Lipogranulomata

Lipogranulomata are frequently found as an incidental finding in upper abdominal (celiac and porta hepatis) lymph nodes removed during abdominal surgery. Lipogranulomata consist of aggregates of vacuolated, lipid-laden histocytes which are found in the sinuses or interfollicular areas (Fig. 25.1). The lipid vacuoles may be single or multiple; multinucleate histiocytes or epithelioid cells may be admixed. The origin of the lipid in lipogranulomata is unestablished; a reaction to ingested mineral oil has been suggested in some cases (Boitnott and Margolis, 1966; Liber and Rose, 1967).

Differential Diagnosis

Lipogranulomata must be distinguished from infectious or sarcoidal granulomata. The presence of vacuolated histiocytes and absence of necrosis is characteristic of lipogranulomata. Whipple's disease may closely resemble lipogranulomata in abdominal, or less frequently, peripheral lymph nodes. PAS stain, electron microscopy, or PCR for *Tropheryma whippelii* is diagnostic (see Chapter 8).

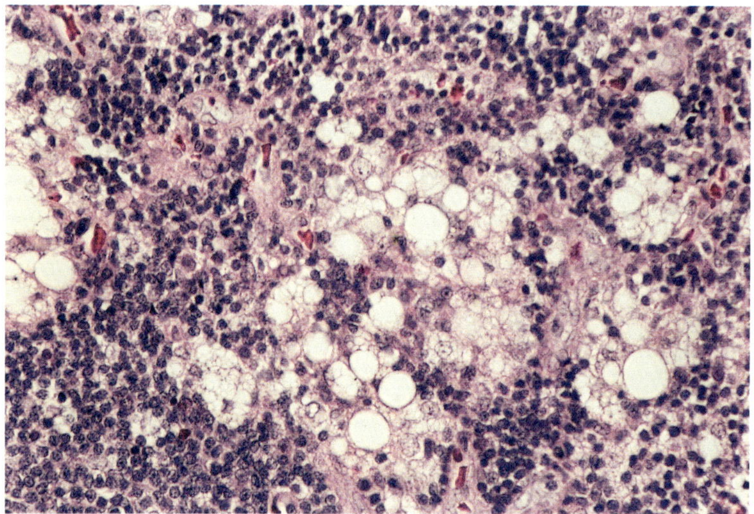

FIGURE
25.1

Lipogranuloma in a porta hepatis lymph node showing vacuolated histiocytes.

Lipidoses

The lipidoses are storage disorders which are due to inherited deficiencies of lysosomal enzymes resulting in accumulation of lipid material in macrophages in the liver, spleen, bone marrow, lymph nodes, and other organs. The lipidoses include Gaucher's disease, due to deficiency of glucocerebrosidase, and Niemann-Pick disease, due to deficiency of sphingomyelinase. The "sea-blue" histiocyte syndrome, also considered amongst the lipidoses, is a heterogenous group of disorders characterized by accumulation of ceroid, a lipofuscin-like material, in macrophages in the liver, spleen, bone marrow, and lymph nodes. Patients with acquired sea-blue histiocyte syndrome frequently have an underlying hematologic disorder with increased membrane turnover (e.g., idiopathic thrombocytopenic purpura); patients with primary sea-blue histiocyte syndrome may have an adult form of Niemann-Pick disease (Landas et al, 1985).

Gaucher's Disease

Gaucher's disease is the most frequent of the lipidoses. The most common form, type I or non-neuropathic (adult) form, occurs in both children and adults and frequently presents with splenomegaly and hematologic manifestations. Lymphadenopathy is infrequent; however, lymph node involvement may be found in incidentally removed lymph nodes. Gaucher's disease is associated with an increased incidence of monoclonal gammopathy, plasma cell dyscrasias, and B lymphoproliferative disorders (Shoenfeld et al, 1980).

Histopathology

Lymph node involvement in Gaucher's disease is characterized by sinusoidal infiltrates of Gaucher's cells. The latter are large histiocytes with abundant clear to faintly eosinophilic cytoplasm and distinctive cytoplasmic striations which are likened to wrinkled cigarette paper. Gaucher's cells stain weakly positive with PAS and iron stains.

Differential Diagnosis

Gaucher's disease should be distinguished from other storage disorders. The cytoplasmic striations are a characteristic feature. Specific diagnosis is established by demonstration of glucocerebrosidase (β-glucosidase) deficiency in peripheral blood leukocytes (Beutler and Kuhl, 1970). Gaucher's disease should be distinguished from disorders characterized by pseudo-Gaucher's cells. The latter are morphologically similar histiocytes which occur in the bone marrow in patients with chronic granulocytic leukemia and other hematologic disorders. A distinct form of pseudo-Gaucher's cell occurs in the lymph nodes and other organs in patients with AIDS and *Mycobacterium avium-intracellulare* infection (Solis et al, 1986). These are characterized by histiocytes filled with mycobacterial organisms, the nonstaining bacilli mimicking the cytoplasmic striations of Gaucher's cells. PAS or AFB stain is diagnostic, demonstrating bundles of intracellular mycobacteria; touch or imprint preparations will frequently also demonstrate numerous extracellular bacilli.

Niemann-Pick Disease

Niemann-Pick disease classically presents in infants with central nervous system involvement (type A); however, variants may present in adults without central nervous system involvement, or as the sea-blue histiocyte syndrome (Landas et al, 1985). Lymphadenopathy may be present.

Histopathology

Niemann-Pick disease is characterized by foamy macrophages with multivacuolated or bubbly cytoplasm, which lack the characteristic cytoplasmic striations of Gaucher's cells. Yellow-brown ceroid pigment, resulting from oxidation of sphingomyelin, may be present and is PAS and acid-fast positive. Niemann-Pick cells are positive for oil red O and Sudan B black in appropriately processed material.

Differential Diagnosis

Foamy macrophages are not specific for Niemann-Pick disease and may be found in a wide variety of lipid storage disorders and other conditions. Specific diagnosis of Neimann-Pick disease is established by demonstration of sphingomyelinase deficiency in peripheral blood leukocytes (Gal et al, 1975).

Proteinaceous Deposits

Several distinct disorders are characterized by abnormal deposits of proteinaceous material in lymph nodes. These include amyloidosis, systemic light chain deposition disease, and proteinaceous lymphadenopathy.

Amyloidosis

Amyloidosis results from deposition of insoluble fibrillary proteins of diverse origins which are characterized by the β-pleated sheet configuration, rendering them resistant to metabolic degradation and resulting in characteristic birefringence with Congo Red (Glenner, 1980). The most frequent types of amyloid are designated AL (primary or light chain amyloid), derived from monoclonal immunoglobulin light chains, and AA (secondary amyloid), derived from a serum acute phase reactant, serum amyloid A protein. Rarer, familial types of amyloidosis are derived from a variety of other proteins (Falk et al, 1997). AL amyloidosis is associated with an underlying plasma cell dyscrasia or multiple myeloma, most frequently of λ light chain type; AA amyloidosis is associated with chronic inflammatory disorders, including rheumatoid arthritis, inflammatory bowel disease, familial Mediterranean fever, and chronic tuberculosis. Lymph node involvement may occur in either type of amyloidosis and, rarely, is the presenting manifestation of amyloidosis (Kahn et al, 1991).

Histopathology

Lymph node involvement in amyloidosis is characterized by amorphous deposits of eosinophilic hyaline amyloid material. Deposits are frequently perivascular and interfollicular and may be associated with a foreign-body giant cell reaction. Identification of amyloid is aided by special stains. Amyloid is characteristically congophilic, demonstrating salmon pink staining with Congo red stain and characteristic apple green birefringence on examination with polarized light. Crystal violet and thioflavin T staining are useful in cases which do not stain with Congo red; amyloid demonstrates characteristic metachromasia with crystal violet and fluorescence with thioflavin T. In rare cases, electron microscopy may be used to demonstrate the characteristic amyloid fibrils.

Differential Diagnosis

The diagnosis of amyloidosis is established by histopathologic identification of amyloid. Localized forms of amyloidosis (as in metastatic medullary carcinoma of the thyroid with amyloid stroma) should be ruled out. Sarcoidosis with extensive lymph node fibrosis and hyalinization may mimic amyloidosis with foreign-body reaction; stains for amyloid permit distinction. AL amyloidosis may be distinguished from AA amyloidosis by immunohistochemical staining for immunoglobulin light chains and AA protein or by Congo red staining following treatment with potassium permanganate; AL amyloid retains congophilia, while AA amyloid does not (Feiner, 1988).

Systemic Light Chain Deposition Disease

Disorders associated with monoclonal gammopathy may rarely be associated with light chain deposits, which lack the histochemical and ultrastructural features of amyloid. These have been referred to as light chain deposition disease. The kidney is most frequently affected; however, rare cases of light chain deposition disease with systemic manifestations have been described (Kijner and Yousem, 1988). Deposits are perivascular and resemble amyloid histologically, but are ultrastructurally and immunohistochemically distinct.

Proteinaceous Lymphadenopathy

Proteinaceous lymphadenopathy is a rare systemic disorder characterized by nonamyloid perivascular proteinaceous deposits in the lymph nodes and other organs (Osborne et al, 1979). Although some of these patients may have systemic light chain deposition disease, others have an apparently distinct disorder with constitutional symptoms, generalized lymphadenopathy, hypocomplementemia, cryoglobulinemia, and lack evidence for a monoclonal serum immunoglobulin (Michaeli et al, 1995). Lymph node involvement is characterized by perivascular hyaline sclerosis with an onion-skin appearance. The nature of the hyaline material is unestablished; one patient responded to corticosteroid therapy (Michaeli et al, 1995).

Deposits of Foreign Material

A number of foreign materials are deposited in the lymph nodes and may be associated with a characteristic cellular reaction. These include lymphangiogram contrast material, silicone, polyvinylpyrrolidone, and material from prosthetic joints.

Lymphangiogram Effect

Lymphangiography is a radiologic technique for imaging of retroperitoneal lymph nodes. It has largely been replaced by computerized tomography and magnetic resonance imaging but is still occasionally utilized in the staging of Hodgkin's disease and testicular germ cell tumors. The lymphangiographic contrast material is an iodized oil (Ethiodol) which is injected into the lymphatics of the dorsum of the foot and drains to and opacifies the pelvic and retroperitoneal lymph nodes. Patients undergoing subsequent surgical staging are found to have changes in the lymph nodes referred to as lymphangiogram effect. Lymphangiogram effect is characterized by pools of iodized oil in the lymph node sinuses; the oil is dissolved out in processing, leaving large clear spaces surrounded by histiocytes and multinucleated giant cells. Lymphangiogram effect may mimic the appearance of lipogranulomata or Whipple's disease and should not be confused with lymphomatous involvement or metastatic tumor. The deposits of iodized oil may persist in lymph nodes for several months following lymphangiography.

Silicone

Silicone used in breast prostheses may find its way to axillary lymph nodes as a result of rupture or leakage of the prosthesis. Silicone in tissue appears as clear, refractile, nonbirefringent material which elicits little cellular reaction (Bleiweiss et al, 1996; Travis et al, 1985). A case of follicular lymphoma has been reported in association with leakage of silicone from a breast prosthesis; however, a causal relationship is unestablished (Cook et al, 1995).

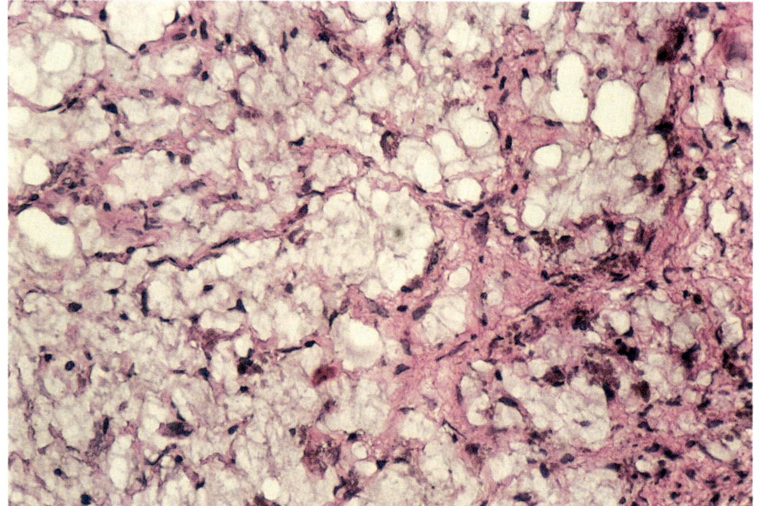

FIGURE
25.2

Polyvinylpyrrolidone granuloma showing deposits of basophilic material. Histiocytes containing polyvinylpyrrolidone mimic signet ring cells.

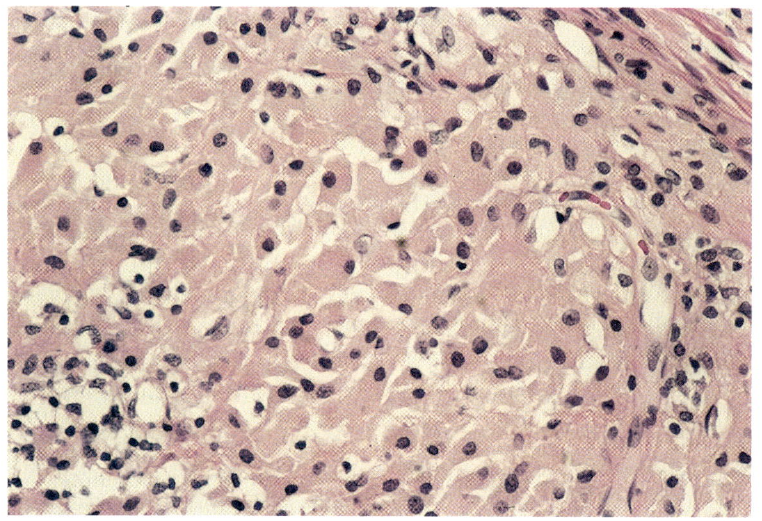

FIGURE
25.3

Hip prosthesis histiocytes in a pelvic lymph node from a patient who had undergone hip replacement surgery showing distention of the subcapsular sinus by histiocytes with abundant eosinophilic cytoplasm.

Polyvinylpyrrolidone

Polyvinylpyrrolidone (PVP), a synthetic polymer which was widely used as plasma expander and vehicle for intravenous pharmaceuticals in the Far East, is deposited in histiocytes in the liver, spleen, bone marrow, and lymph nodes (Kuo and Hsueh, 1984). PVP in tissue appears as basophilic material, which is characteristically intensely Congo red and mucicarmine positive (Fig. 25.2). PVP-containing histiocytes may mimic the appearance of signet ring cells or hereditary storage disorders (Kuo et al, 1997).

FIGURE
25.4

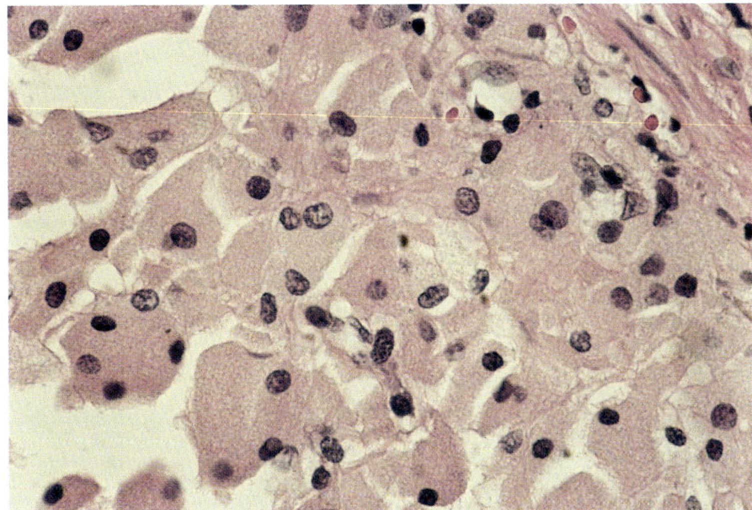

Hip prosthesis histiocytes, higher magnification, showing histiocytes with abundant, finely granular, eosinophilic cytoplasm.

Hip Prosthesis Histiocytes

Lymph nodes draining the sites of prosthetic joints may show characteristic large granular histiocytes containing material released from the prosthetic joints (Albores-Saavedra et al, 1994). Pelvic lymph nodes in patients who have undergone hip replacement surgery are predominantly affected. The involved lymph nodes show sinusoidal proliferation of large foamy histiocytes with abundant granular eosinophilic cytoplasm, which may resemble Gaucher's cells (Figs. 25.3 and 25.4). X-ray dispersive analysis demonstrates cobalt-chromium and titanium particles within the histiocytes; polyethylene particles may also be present (Albores-Saavedra et al, 1994). Affected pelvic lymph nodes have been encountered predominantly during resections for prostatic or bladder carcinomas; distinction from metastatic tumor is critical.

REFERENCES

Albores-Saavedra J, Vuitch F, Delgado R, Wiley E, Hagler H. Sinus histiocytosis of pelvic lymph nodes after hip replacement: A histiocytic proliferation induced by cobalt-chromium and titanium. Am J Surg Pathol 18:83–90, 1994.

Beutler E, Kuhl W. The diagnosis of adult type of Gaucher's disease and its carrier state by demonstration of deficiency of beta-glucosidase activity in peripheral blood leukocytes. J Lab Clin Med 76:747, 1970.

Bleiweiss IJ, Klein MJ, Copeland M. Breast prosthesis reaction (letter). Am J Surg Pathol 20:505–506, 1996.

Boitnottt JK, Margolis S. Mineral oil in human tissues. II. Oil droplets in lymph nodes of the porta hepatis. Bull Johns Hopkins Hosp 118:414, 1966.

Cook PD, Osborne BM, Connor RL, Strauss JF. Follicular lymphoma adjacent to foreign body granulomatous inflammation and fibrosis surrounding silicone breast prosthesis. Am J Surg Pathol 19:712–717, 1995.

Falk RH, Comenzo RL, Skinner M. The systemic amyloidoses. N Engl J Med 337:898–909, 1997.

Feiner HD. Pathology of dysproteinemia: Light chain amyloidosis, non-amyloid immunoglobulin deposition disease, cryoglobulinemia syndromes and macroglobulinemia of Waldenstrom. Hum Pathol 19:1255–1272, 1988.

Gal AE, Brady RO, Hibberg SR, Pentchev PG. A practical chromogenic procedure for the detection of homozygotes and heterozygous carriers of Niemann-Pick disease. N Engl J Med 293:632, 1975.

Glenner GG. Amyloid deposits and amyloidosis: The beta fibrilloses. N Engl J Med 302:1283–1292, 1980.

Kahn H, Strauchen JA, Gilbert H, Fuchs A. Immunoglobulin-related amyloidosis presenting as recurrent lymph node involvement. Arch Pathol Lab Med 115:948–950, 1991.

Kijner CH, Yousem SA. Systemic light chain deposition disease presenting as multiple pulmonary nodules. A case report and review of the literature. Am J Surg Pathol 12:405–413, 1988.

Kuo T-T, Hsueh S. Mucicarminophilic histiocytosis: A polyvinylpyrrolidone ({PVP) storage disease simulating signet ring carcinoma. Am J Surg Pathol 8:419, 1984.

Kuo T-T, Hu S, Huang C-L, Chan H-L, Chang MJW, Dunn P, Chen Y-J. Cutaneous involvement in polyvinylpyrrolidone storage disease: A clinicopathologic study of five patients, including two patients with severe anemia. Am J Surg Pathol 21:1361–1367, 1997.

Landas S, Foucar K, Sando GN, et al. Adult Niemann-Pick disease masquerading as sea blue histiocyte syndrome: Report of a case confirmed by lipid analysis and enzyme assays. Am J Hematol 20:391, 1985.

Liber AF, Rose HG. Saturated hydrocarbons in follicular lipidosis of the spleen. Arch Pathol 83:116, 1967.

Michaeli J, Niesvizky R, Siegel D, Ladanyi M, Lieberman PH, Filippa DA. Proteinaceous (angiocentric sclerosing) lymphadenopathy: A polyclonal systemic, nonamyloid deposition disorder. Blood 86:1159–1162, 1995.

Osborne BA, Butler JJ, Mackay B. Proteinaceous lymphadenopathy with hypergammglobulinemia. Am J Surg Pathol 3:137, 1979.

Shoenfeld Y, Berliner S, Pinkhas J, Beutler E. The association of Gaucher's disease and dysproteinemia. Acta Haematol 64:241, 1980.

Solis OG, Belmonte HH, Ramaswamy G, Tchertkoff V. Pseudo-Gaucher cells in Mycobacterium avium-intracellulare infection in acquired immunodeficiency syndrome (AIDS). Am J Clin Pathol 85:233, 1986.

Travis WD, Balogh K, Abraham JL. Silicone granulomas: report of three cases and review of the literature. Hum Pathol 16:19–27, 1985.

26

Proliferations of Histiocytes and Dendritic Cells

The term "histiocyte" is applied to two distinct cell types: monocyte-macrophages and dendritic cells (Cline, 1994; van Voorhis et al, 1983). Monocyte-macrophages are derived from blood monocytes, are actively phagocytic, are rich in lysosomal enzymes, and play their major role in antigen processing. Monocyte-macrophages in the lymph node include the sinus and tingible body macrophages. Dendritic cells, in contrast, are of uncertain derivation, weakly phagocytic, poor in lysosomal enzymes, and play their major role in antigen presentation. Dendritic cells in the lymph node include the Langerhans' cells, follicular dendritic cells, and interdigitating reticulum cells. Recent evidence suggests that both monocyte-macrophages and dendritic cells are derived from a common monocyte-dendritic cell precursor in the bone marrow (Santiago-Schwartz et al, 1994). Proliferations of monocyte-macrophages include "true" histiocytic lymphoma and "malignant histiocytosis," virus-associated and reactive hemophagocytic syndromes, and sinus histiocytosis with massive lymphadenopathy. Proliferations of dendritic cells include Langerhans' cell histiocytosis, follicular dendritic cell tumors, and interdigitating reticulum cell tumors; the latter two tumors constitute "true" reticulum cell sarcomas of lymph nodes (Weiss et al, 1990).

"True" Histiocytic Lymphoma and "Malignant Histiocytosis"

True histiocytic lymphoma (THL) and malignant histiocytosis refer to localized and systemic forms, respectively, of a malignant proliferation of monocyte-macrophages. The existence of the systemic form of the disease (malignant histiocytosis) is now doubtful; most cases reported prior to the advent of immunophenotypic studies are reclassified as anaplastic large cell lymphoma or virus-associated hemophagocytic syndrome on review

(Wilson et al, 1990). Malignant neoplasms of monocyte-macrophages, termed true histiocytic lymphomas, undoubtedly occur, but they are infrequent (Kamel et al, 1995; Turner et al, 1984). Diagnosis of THL is established by the identification of cytologically malignant cells expressing unequivocal macrophage markers in the absence of B- or T-lineage-specific markers.

Clinical Features

THL exhibits no specific clinical features. THL may occur with increased incidence in patients with previous lymphoblastic leukemia or lymphoma; however, the nature of the association is uncertain (Soslow et al, 1996). THL may present with nodal or extranodal involvement; involvement of bone, gastrointestinal tract, salivary gland, or breast may occur (Kamel et al, 1995). Bone marrow involvement is not infrequent (Turner et al, 1984).

Histopathology

THL is characterized by diffuse infiltrates of large, pleomorphic cells with ovoid or indented nuclei, prominent nucleoli, and abundant eosinophilic cytoplasm with well-defined cytoplasmic borders (Kamel et al, 1995) (Figs. 26.1 and 26.2). Erythrophagocytosis is frequently present. Sarcomatoid features may be present in rare cases (Strauchen, 1991) (Figs. 26.3 and 26.4).

Immunopathology

THL is characterized by expression of one or more monocyte-macrophage markers, including CD15, CD68, lysozyme, and S100 protein in paraffin-embedded tissue and CD4, CD11c, and CD14 in frozen tissue (Kamel et al, 1995). CD43, CD45RO, and CD45RB may also be positive (Kamel et al, 1995). Lineage-specific T and B cell markers are characteristically absent. Immunoglobulin and T-cell antigen-receptor genes are usually in the germline configuration; however, rearrangements are found in some cases (Kamel et al, 1995; Soslow et al, 1996).

Differential Diagnosis

THL must be distinguished from non-Hodgkin's lymphomas, particularly anaplastic large cell lymphoma, and from non-neoplastic reactive histiocytic proliferations. Distinction from non-Hodgkin's lymphoma may be difficult. Features previously considered characteristic of histiocytic neoplasms, including sinusoidal involvement and erythrophagocytosis, are now appreciated to occur frequently in T cell and anaplastic large cell non-Hodgkin's lymphomas. Distinction is therefore based on immunophenotypic studies. THLs are characterized by expression of one or more monocyte-macrophage markers, including CD68, in paraffin-embedded tissue, and CD14, in frozen tissue, and the absence of T- or B-lineage-specific markers. Anaplastic large cell lymphomas are characterized by expression of CD30 and, frequently, by expression of one or more T-lineage-specific markers. Anaplastic large cell lymphomas are usually negative for CD68; occasional cases are positive with the monoclonal antibody KP-1 but are negative with the

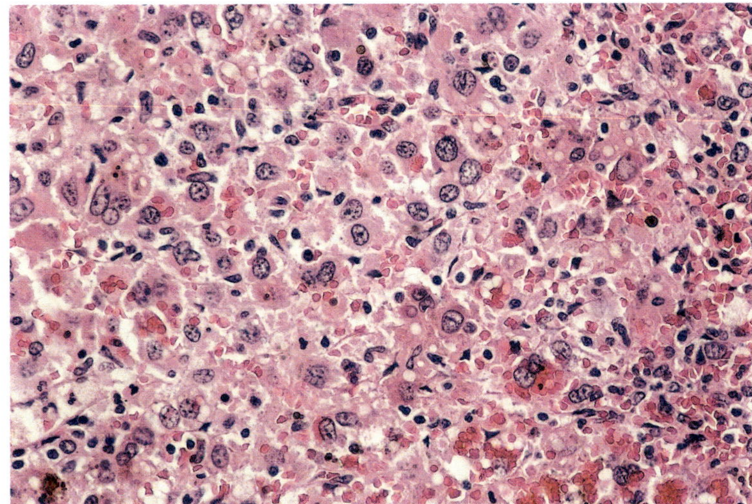

FIGURE 26.1

True histiocytic lymphoma showing proliferation of atypical histiocytes with large nuclei and abundant eosinophilic cytoplasm.

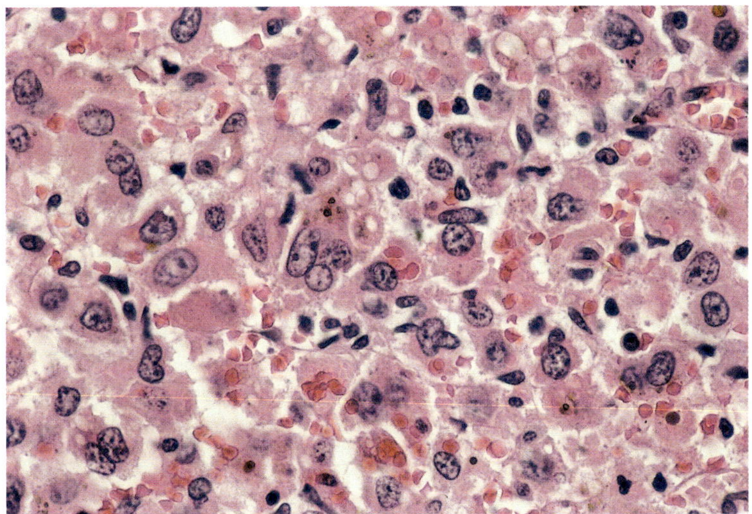

FIGURE 26.2

True histiocytic lymphoma, higher magnification, showing proliferation of atypical histiocytes with erythrophagocytosis.

monoclonal antibody PG-M1 (Falini et al, 1993). Immunoglobulin and T-cell antigen-receptor genes are frequently rearranged in lymphoid neoplasms and in the germline configuration in THL; however, rearrangement may be present in some THL (Kamel et al 1995; Soslow et al, 1996).

THL must also be distinguished from reactive histiocytic proliferations, including virus-associated hemophagocytic syndrome and other reactive hemophagocytic syndromes. Distinction is based on the absence of cytologic atypia of the histiocytes in the latter syndromes. THL should be distinguished from Langerhans' cell histiocytosis (LCH). Distinction is based on the typical morphologic features of LCH, with delicately

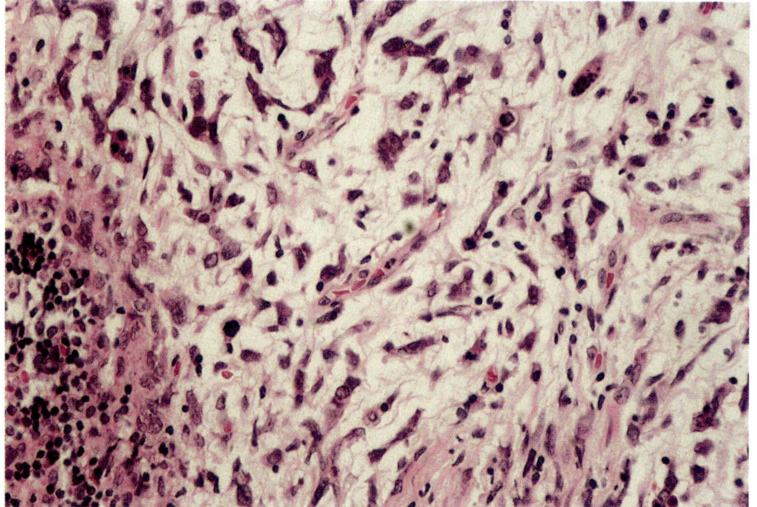

FIGURE 26.3

Sarcomatoid monocytic neoplasm showing spindled cells and myxoid stroma.

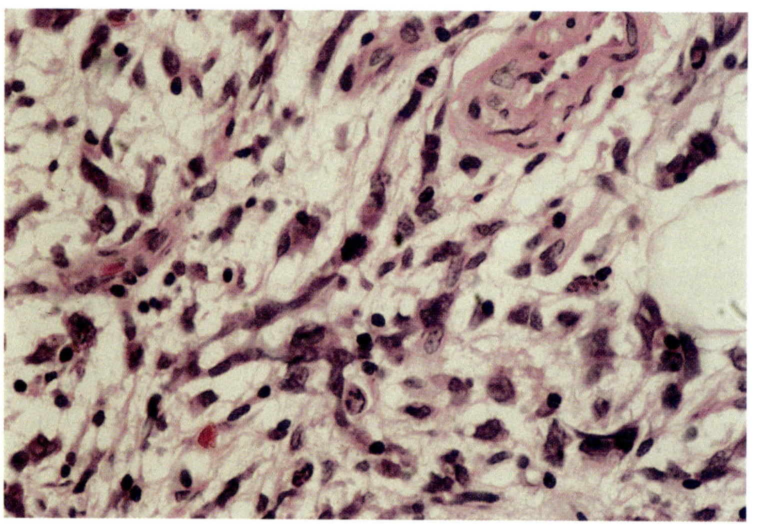

FIGURE 26.4

Sarcomatoid monocytic neoplasm, higher magnification, showing cord-like arrangement of neoplastic cells. Immunophenotypic studies demonstrated a monocyte–macrophage phenotype.

grooved and folded nuclei, and the presence of CD1a positivity and Birbeck granules in cases of LCH. THL may be morphologically and immunophenotypically indistinguishable from extramedullary infiltrates of acute monocytic leukemia; distinction is based on the clinical features at presentation.

Course and Prognosis

THL is treated with combination chemotherapy, similar to that used for aggressive non-Hodgkin's lymphoma. The prognosis is poor.

Hemophagocytic Syndromes

Hemophagocytic syndromes (HS's, reactive hemophagocytic syndromes) are non-neoplastic proliferations of monocyte-macrophages frequently associated with prominent hemophagocytosis which are triggered by an infectious or other stimulus. Familial erythrophagocytic lymphohistiocytosis (FEL) is likely closely related (Gaffey et al, 1993).

Clinical Features

HS's were first recognized in association with viral infections (Risdall et al, 1979) but are now recognized to occur in the course of a wide variety of bacterial, mycobacterial, fungal, and protozoan infections (Risdall et al, 1984). HS's are particularly frequent in association with Epstein-Barr virus infection (Gaffey et al, 1993). HS also occurs in association with peripheral T cell lymphomas (Gonzalez et al, 1991; Hyteriglou et al, 1992). The common feature in these disorders appears to be excessive activation of monocyte-macrophages by cytokines released by activated T cells. FEL is a familial disorder which shares features with infection-associated HS (Gaffey et al, 1993). HS is characterized clinically by the abrupt onset of fever, constitutional symptoms, hepatosplenomegaly, anemia, and thrombocytopenia. Lymphadenopathy may be present. Liver function abnormalities and coagulopathy are frequent. Hypertriglyceridemia frequently accompanies the familial form of the disease (FEL).

Histopathology

The lymph nodes in HS frequently have a depleted appearance. The sinusoids contain increased numbers of histiocytes with little or no cytologic atypia (Fig. 26.5); erythro-

FIGURE 26.5

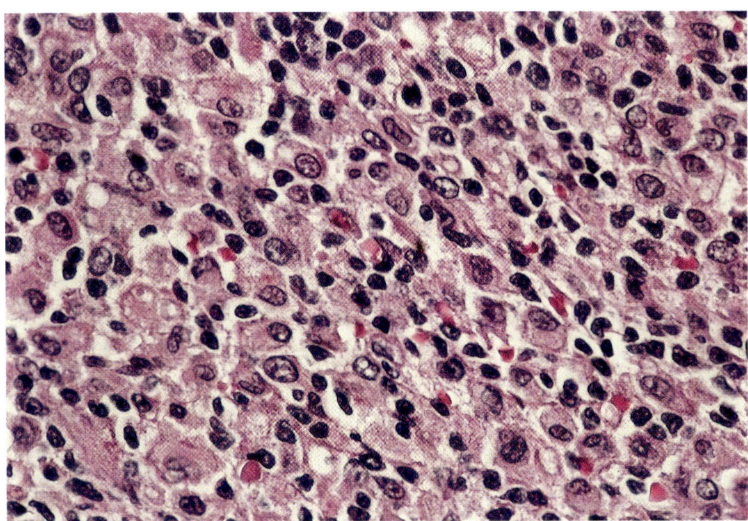

Hemophagocytic syndrome, associated with peripheral T cell lymphoma, showing proliferation of histiocytes with minimal cytologic atypia and erythrophagocytosis.

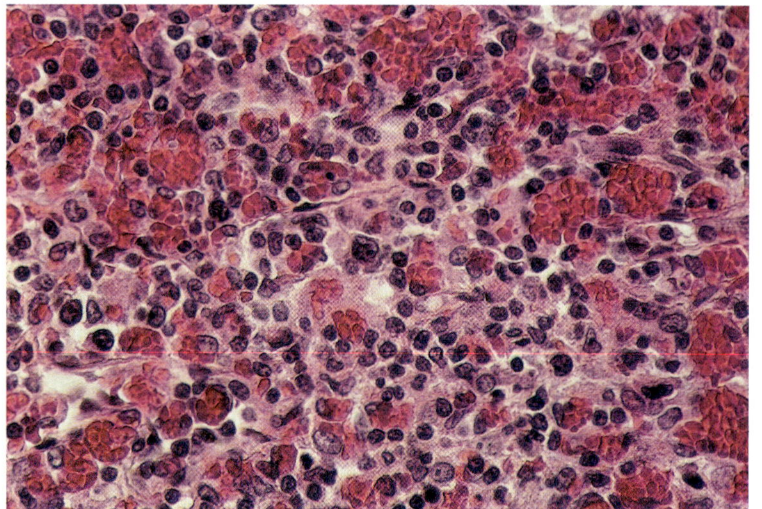

FIGURE 26.6

Hematophagocytic syndrome, associated with peripheral T cell lymphoma, showing prominent erythrophagocytosis.

phagocytosis may be prominent (Fig. 26.6). The bone marrow and spleen, similarly, are depleted and contain large numbers of phagocytic histiocytes. Imprint or touch preparations show phagocytosis of erythrocytes, platelets, and neutrophils.

Differential Diagnosis

HS should be distinguished from THL; the distinction is based principally on the lack of cytologic atypia of the histiocytes in HS.

Course and Prognosis

HS is frequently an acute, fulminant disorder. Therapy is directed to treatment of the underlying disorder; single agent chemotherapy with etoposide (VP-16) has been used to suppress the histiocytic proliferation. The prognosis is poor; recurrent HS may develop, particularly in familial cases.

Sinus Histiocytosis With Massive Lymphadenopathy

Sinus histiocytosis with massive lymphadenopathy (SHML, Rosai-Dorfman disease) is a peculiar, histologically distinctive, non-neoplastic proliferation of monocyte-macrophages of undetermined etiology (Rosai and Dorfman, 1969; Rosai and Dorfman, 1972).

Clinical Features

SHML is predominantly a disease of young people. Cervical lymph nodes are most commonly affected; extranodal involvement is not infrequent and may involve the upper airway, skin, orbit, or meninges (Song et al, 1989; Wenig et al, 1993). Although initially reported cases occurred predominantly in black children, Caucasians are equally affected. Patients typically present with massive, bilateral, cervical lymphadenopathy with a "bull neck" appearance. Fever, usually low grade; elevated erythrocyte sedimentation rate; and polyclonal hypergammaglobulinemia may be present. The etiology of SHML is undetermined; features suggest an infectious or viral etiology; however, no organism has been consistently identified.

Histopathology

Lymph nodes in SHML show marked dilation of the sinuses, which are filled with large, distinctive appearing histiocytes, with prominent nucleoli and abundant, finely vacuolated, clear to eosinophilic cytoplasm (Figs. 26.7 and 26.8). The histiocytes contain numerous ingested lymphocytes and occasionally plasma cells and other hematologic elements, a phenomenon referred to as emperipolesis (Fig. 26.9). The lymph node capsule is characteristically fibrotic and thickened; the intersinusoidal tissue contains numerous plasma cells. Extranodal involvement in SHML is characterized by infiltrates of morphologically similar histiocytes and plasma cells; the presence of emperipolesis is a distinctive feature (Song et al, 1989).

Immunopathology

The histiocytes in SHML demonstrate a phenotype consistent with monocyte-macrophages (Paulli et al, 1992). The cells are positive for S100 protein and CD68 in paraffin-embedded tissue and for CD11c, CD14, and CD33 in frozen tissue. Lysozyme and α-1–antichymotrypsin are frequently positive in some cells; CD1a and HLA-DR are usually negative (Paulli et al, 1992).

**FIGURE
26.7**

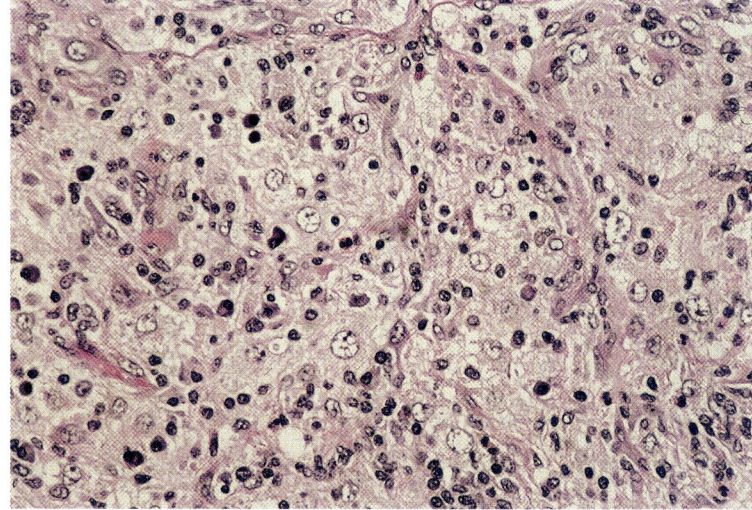

Sinus histiocytosis with massive lymphadenopathy showing distention of the sinuses by large histiocytes with abundant pale cytoplasm.

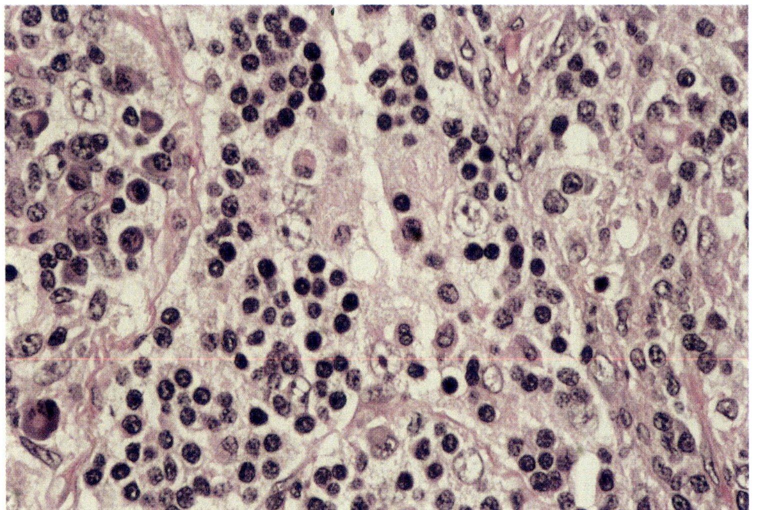

FIGURE
26.8

Sinus histiocytosis with massive lymphadenopathy, higher magnification, showing characteristic histiocytes with admixed lymphocytes and inter-sinusoidal plasma cells.

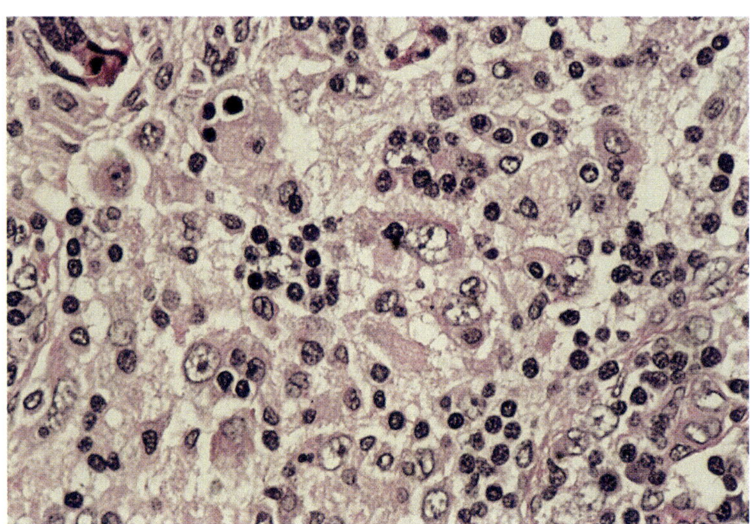

FIGURE
26.9

Sinus histiocytosis with massive lymphadenopathy showing characteristic histiocytes with intracytoplasmic lymphocytes, a phenomenon referred to as "emperipolesis."

Differential Diagnosis

SHML should be distinguished from other histiocytic proliferations. Morphologically distinctive histiocytes, emperipolesis, and plasmacytosis are characteristic features.

Course and Prognosis

SHML has a protracted, but generally benign, course with eventual spontaneous resolution of the lymphadenopathy. Recurrent or persistent disease occurs in some patients.

Treatment, in persistent cases, has included surgical resection, radiation therapy, corticosteroids, and chemotherapy (Wenig et al, 1993).

Langerhans' Cell Histiocytosis

Langerhans' cell histiocytosis (LCH) is a proliferation of dendritic cells which includes disorders previously referred to as eosinophilic granuloma, histiocytosis-X, Letterer-Siwe disease, and Hand-Schuller-Christian disease; Langerhans' cell granulomatosis is preferred by some authors (Lieberman et al, 1996). The disorder is of uncertain etiology; recent evidence suggests it is a clonal proliferative process (Willman et al, 1994).

Clinical Features

LCH is principally a disease of childhood; occasional cases are seen in adults. Involvement may be localized (eosinophilic granuloma), multifocal (Hand-Schuller-Christian disease), or systemic (Letter-Siwe disease); the use of the eponymic terminology is discouraged (Lieberman et al, 1996). Skin and bone involvement are most frequent; lymph node involvement is also frequent and occurs in lymph nodes draining sites of localized skin or bone involvement, and in systemic disease. Isolated foci indistinguishable from LCH are occasionally encountered in lymph nodes containing malignant lymphoma (Burns et al, 1983). The existence of a malignant form of LCH, with cytologically atypical cells, is controversial (Ben-Ezra et al, 1991); cases of histiocytosis with an indeterminate, or precursor Langerhans' cell phenotype, also occur (Segal et al, 1992).

Histopathology

Lymph node involvement in LCH is characterized by sinusoidal infiltrates of Langerhans' cells and admixed eosinophils (Figs. 26.10 and 26.11). Langerhans' cells are large mononuclear cells with inconspicuous nucleoli, delicately folded or "grooved" nuclei, and abundant pale cytoplasm (Figs. 26.12 and 26.13) Multinucleated cells with similar features are frequently present. The Langerhans' cells show little cytologic atypia in typical cases; cytologic atypia may be present in some cases (Ben Ezra et al, 1991) (Fig. 26.14). Inflammatory cells, including eosinophils, neutrophils, lymphocytes, and plasma cells are frequently admixed. Older lesions frequently show fibrosis and foamy macrophages.

Immunopathology

Langerhans' cells in LCH demonstrate a phenotype indistinguishable from normal Langerhans' cells. The cells are positive for S100 protein and CD68 and demonstrate characteristic membrane and Golgi staining with peanut agglutinin (PNA) in paraffin-embedded tissue (Ree and Kadin, 1986) (Fig. 26.15). The cells are positive for CD1a, CD4, CD11c, and CD14 in frozen tissue. S-100, PNA, and CD1a are the most consistently useful markers. A monoclonal antibody recognizing an epitope of CD1a which is preserved in formalin-fixed paraffin-embedded tissue has recently become available (Clone 010, Immunotech, Marseille, France) (Fig. 26.16). Langerhans cells also are positive for the enzymes adenosine triphosphatase and α-D-mannosidase.

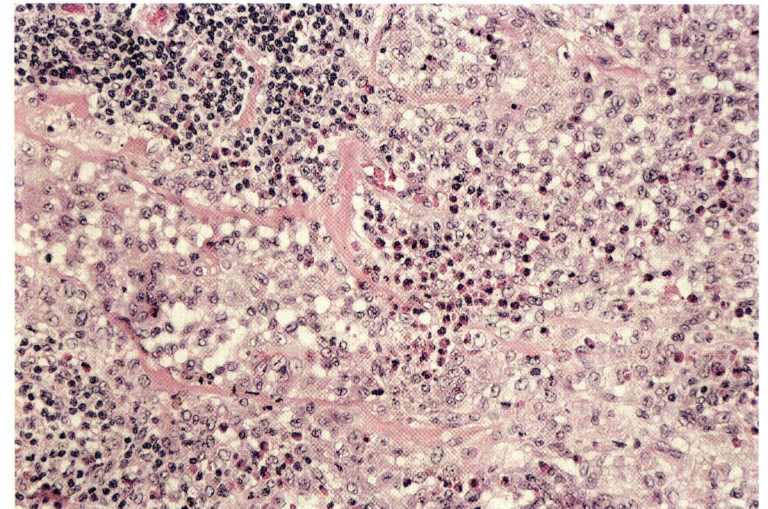

FIGURE 26.10

Langerhans' cell histiocytosis showing sinusoidal pattern of involvement.

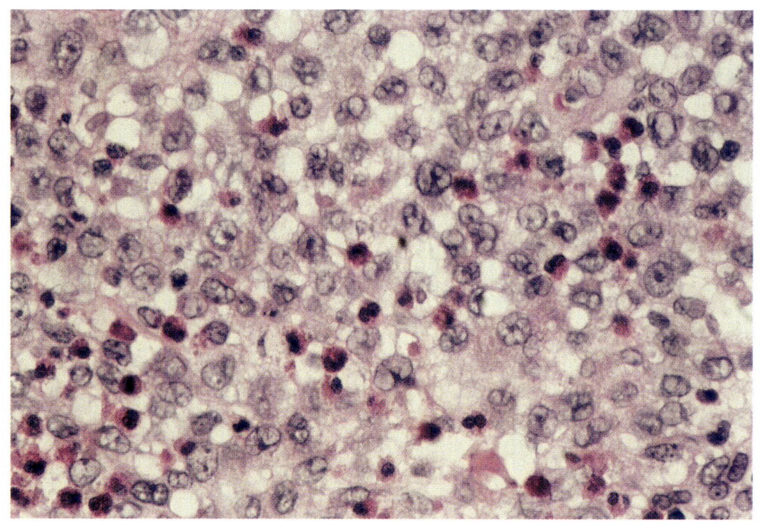

FIGURE 26.11

Langerhans' cell histiocytosis, higher magnification, showing Langerhans' cells with delicately folded nuclei and admixed eosinophils.

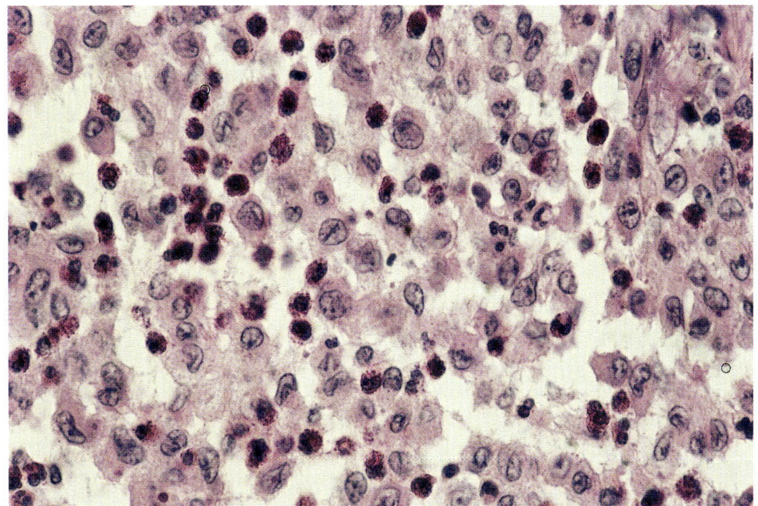

Langerhans' cell histiocytosis showing Langerhans' cells with characteristic "grooved" nuclei.

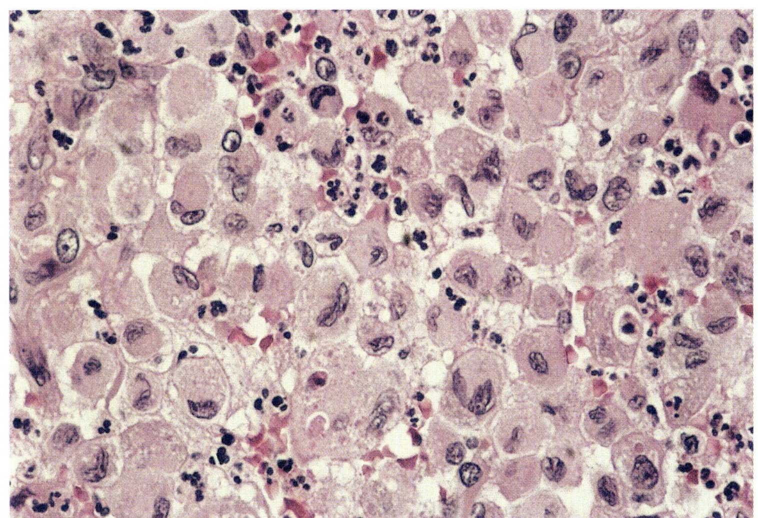

Langerhans' cell histiocytosis showing Langerhans' cells with folded nuclei, abundant eosinophilic cytoplasm, and admixed neutrophils.

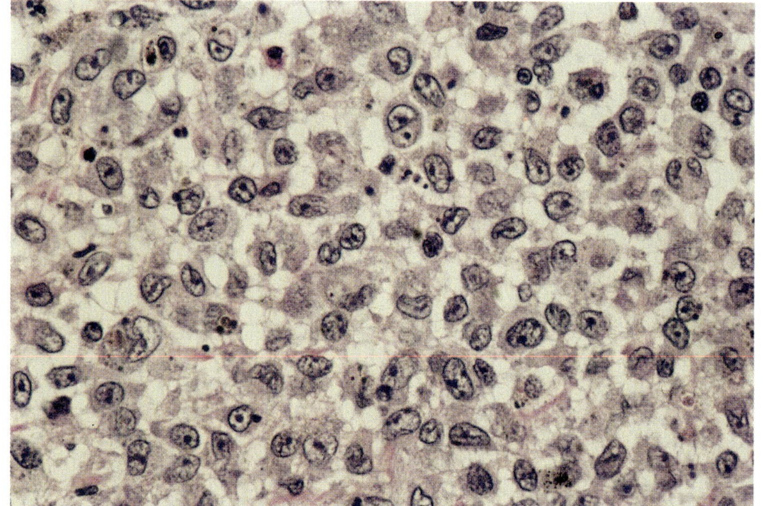

Langerhans' cell histiocytosis showing Langerhans' cells with cytologic atypia.

FIGURE 26.14

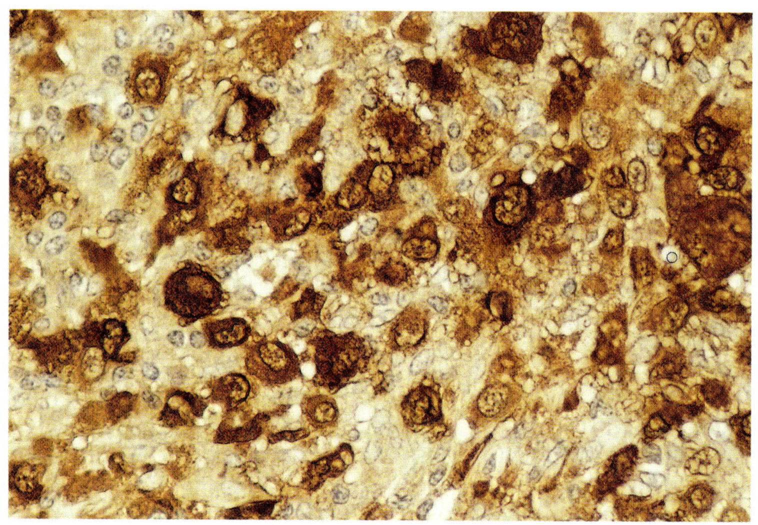

Langerhans' cell histiocytosis showing staining with antibody to S100 protein.

FIGURE 26.15

FIGURE 26.16

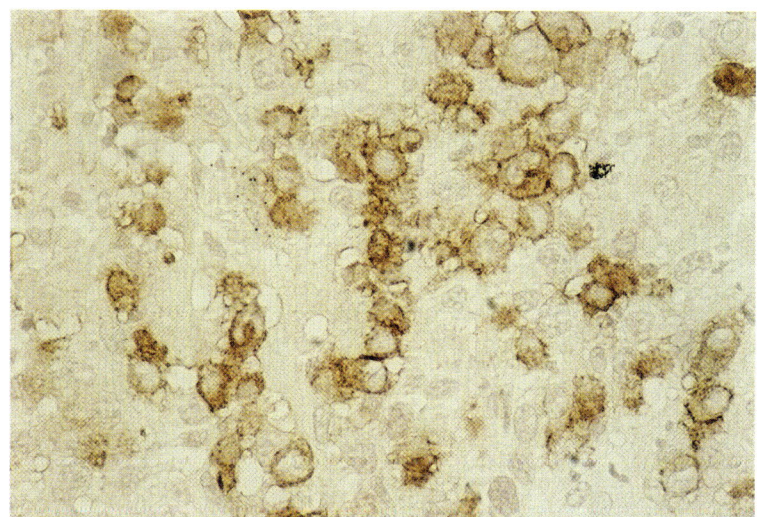

Langerhans' cell histiocytosis showing staining with monoclonal antibody to CD1a in paraffin embedded tissue.

Ultrastructural Pathology

Normal and pathologic Langerhans' cells are characterized by the presence of Birbeck granules, pentilaminar cytoplasmic rod-like structures, found in continuity with the plasma membrane. A dilated "tennis-racquet-like" end is frequently present. Birbeck granules are identified ultrastructurally; their presence is diagnostic of LCH.

Differential Diagnosis

LCH should be distinguished from other histiocytic proliferations and storage disorders. The presence of cells with delicate grooved and folded nuclei is characteristic. Demonstration of S100 protein, characteristic staining with PNA, or positivity for adenosine triphosphatase or α-D-mannosidase supports the diagnosis; demonstration of CD1a positivity or Birbeck granules is definitively diagnostic of LCH.

Course and Prognosis

LCH exhibits a characteristic waxing and waning course, making evaluation of therapeutic interventions difficult. The prognosis is related to the number of organs systems involved. Localized lesions are frequently treated with radiation therapy. Multifocal and systemic involvement has been treated with corticosteroids and a variety of chemotherapeutic agents, singly and in combination; 2-chlorodeoxyadenosine has recently been shown to be active in adults with LCH (Saven et al, 1994). The prognosis in most patients is favorable with eventual regression of the lesions (Lieberman et al, 1996).

Follicular Dendritic Cell Tumor

Follicular dendritic cell (FDC) tumors are spindle cell tumors of lymph nodes which have the phenotype of follicular dendritic cells, the specialized antigen-presenting cells of the follicle center (Weiss et al, 1990). Extranodal FDC tumors also occur (Chan et al, 1994b) and may mimic inflammatory pseudotumor (Selves et al, 1996).

Clinical Features

FDC tumors present as a localized enlarged lymph node or soft tissue mass without distinctive clinical features; some cases have arisen in association with Castleman's disease (Chan et al, 1994a; Saiz et al, 1997).

Histopathology

FDC tumors are spindle cell neoplasms, characterized by sheets of plump spindle cells with vesicular nuclei, inconspicuous nucleoli, and eosinophilic cytoplasm (Figs. 26.17 and 26.18). A focal storiform arrangement and meningioma-like whorls are frequently present (Figs. 26.19 and 26.20); the latter are reminiscent of follicle-like formations. The presence of interstitial small lymphocytes is a constant feature; perivascular cuffing is frequently present. Multinucleated giant cells, mitoses, and foci of necrosis are present in some cases (Perez-Ordonez et al, 1996).

Immunopathology

FDC tumors demonstrate the phenotypic features of follicular dendritic cells. FDC tumors are positive for CD21 and CD35 (Fig. 26.21) and may be positive for vimentin and S100 protein (Perez-Ordonez et al, 1996). LCA in paraffin-embedded tissue is usually negative.

Ultrastructural Pathology

FDC tumors demonstrate the presence of long, complex cytoplasmic processes with desmosomal attachments (Perez-Ordonez et al, 1996) (Fig. 26.22).

Differential Diagnosis

FDC tumors should be distinguished from other spindle cell tumors which may involve lymph nodes, including Kaposi's sarcoma, intranodal hemorrhagic spindle cell tumor with "amianthoid" fibers (palisaded myofibroblastoma), inflammatory lymph node pseudotumor, and metastatic spindle cell tumors. Interstitial small lymphocytes and meningioma-like whorls are characteristic. CD21 and CD35 positivity on immunohistochemical staining and long branching processes with desmosomes on ultrastructural study are diagnostic (Perez-Ordonez et al, 1996).

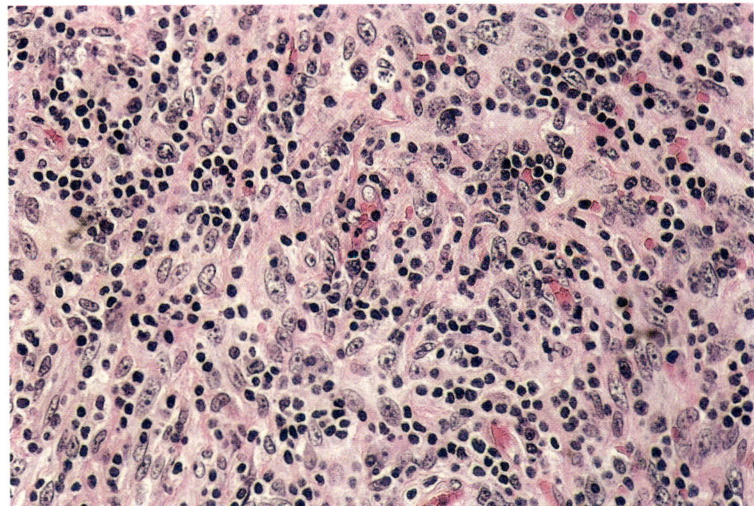

Follicular dendritic cell tumor showing spindle cells and admixed lymphocytes.

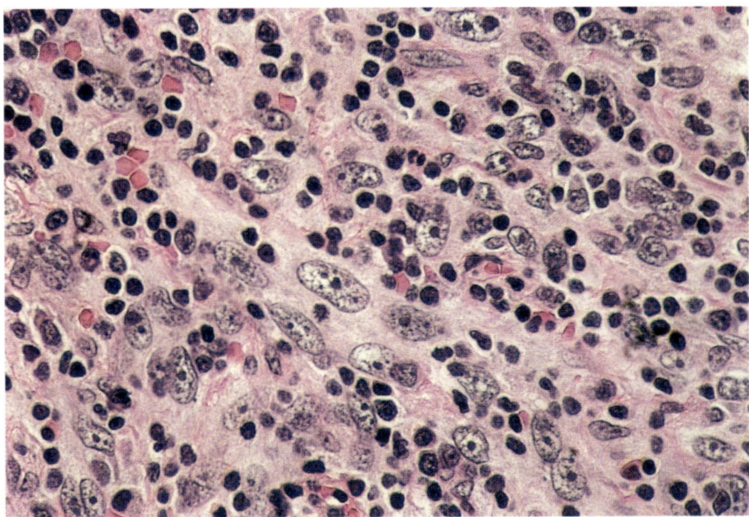

Follicular dendritic cell tumor, higher magnification, showing spindle cells with vesicular nuclei, small nucleoli, and interstitial small lymphocytes.

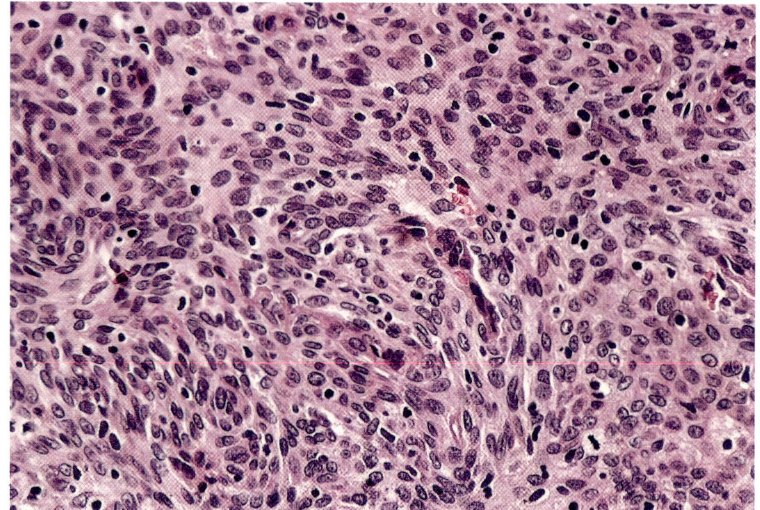

Follicular dendritic cell tumor showing spindle cells with meningioma-like whorls.

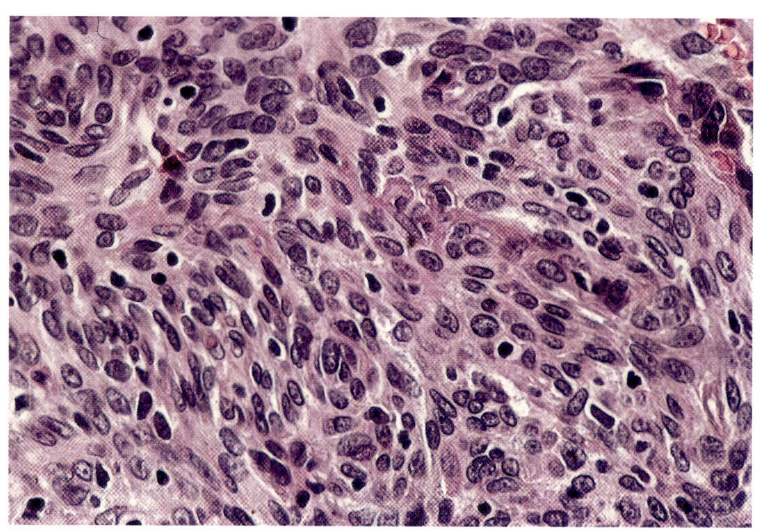

Follicular dendritic cell tumor, higher magnification, showing spindle cells with meningioma-like whorls, inconspicuous nucleoli, and scattered interstitial lymphocytes.

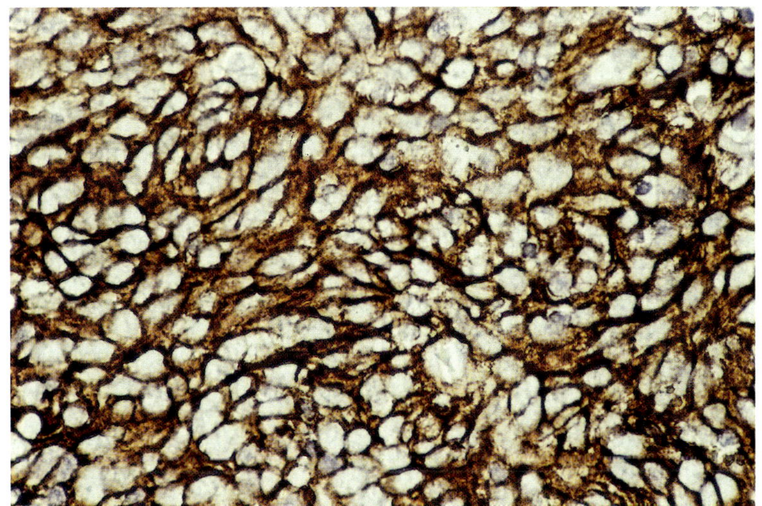

Follicular dendritic cell tumor showing staining for CD21.

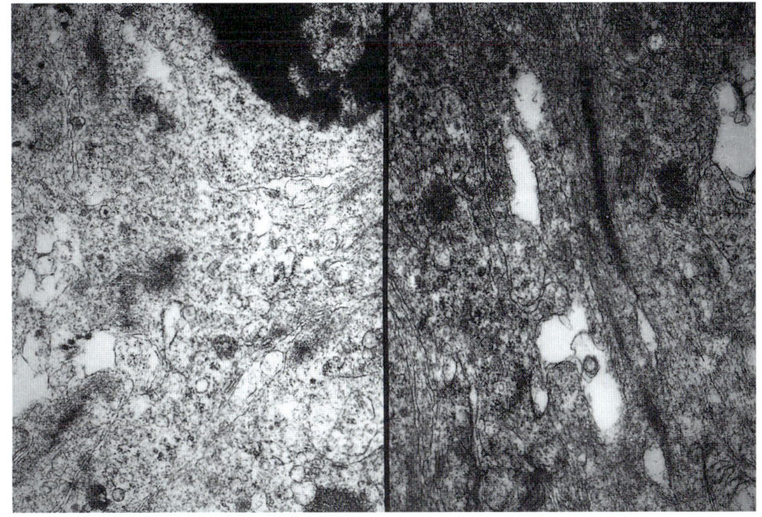

Follicular dendritic cell tumor, electron microscopy, showing interdigitating cell processes (left) and desmosomal attachments (right).

Course and Prognosis

FDC tumors behave as low-grade malignant neoplasms, with frequent local recurrence. Therapy has consisted of surgical resection and postoperative radiation therapy. Distant metastases have occasionally developed.

Interdigitating Reticulum Cell Tumor

Interdigitating reticulum cell (IRC) tumors are tumors of lymph nodes which have the phenotype of interdigitating reticulum cells, the specialized antigen presenting cells of the paracortex. IRC and FDC tumors constitute "true" reticulum cell sarcomas of lymph nodes (Weiss et al, 1990).

Clinical Features

IRC tumors present with nodal or extranodal involvement. In contrast to FDC tumors, disseminated disease is not infrequently present at presentation. Constitutional symptoms may be present.

Histopathology

IRC tumors are morphologically heterogenous, ranging from spindle cell neoplasms, resembling FDC tumors, to pleomorphic large cell neoplasms, resembling pleomorphic large cell lymphoma (Weiss et al 1990) (Fig. 26.23).

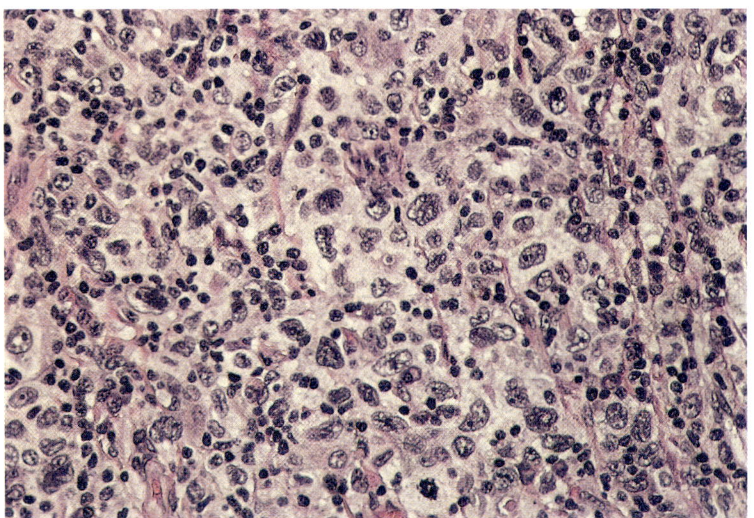

FIGURE 26.23

Interdigitating reticulum cell tumor showing pleomorphic lymphoma-like cells with irregular nuclei and abundant pale cytoplasm.

**FIGURE
26.24**

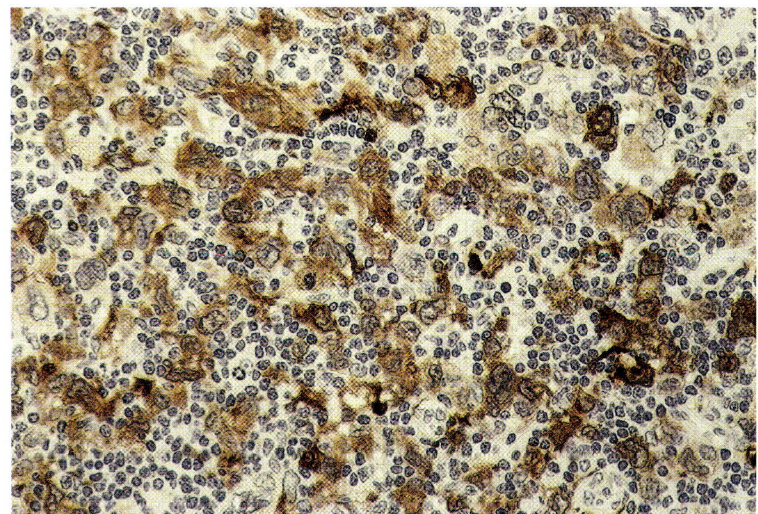

Interdigitating reticulum cell tumor showing staining for S100 protein.

Immunopathology

IRC tumors phenotypically resemble interdigitating reticulum cells. IRC tumors are positive for S100 protein, LCA, and CD68 (Weiss et al, 1990) (Fig. 26.24). CD1a, characteristic of Langerhans' cells, and CD21 and CD35, characteristic of FDC, are negative. B- and T-lineage-specific antigens are also negative.

Ultrastructural Pathology

IRC tumors demonstrate interdigitating cytoplasmic processes; however, in contrast to FDC tumors, desmosomes are not present.

Differential Diagnosis

IRC tumors may be difficult to distinguish from other poorly differentiated tumors, including pleomorphic large cell lymphoma and metastatic melanoma. Immunohistochemical studies may be helpful in diagnosis (Weiss et al, 1990). IRC tumors are distinguished from FDC tumors by the lack of CD21 and CD35 and absence of desmosomes.

Course and Prognosis

IRC tumors are aggressive neoplasms, with disseminated disease in up to 50% of patients. Treatment has included surgery, radiation, and combination chemotherapy.

REFERENCES

Ben-Ezra J, Bailey A, Azumi N, et al. Malignant histiocytosis X: A distinct clinicopathologic entity. Cancer 68:1050–1060, 1991.

Burns BF, Colby TV, Dorfman RF. Langerhans' cell granulomatosis (histiocytosis X) associated with malignant lymphomas. Am J Surg Pathol 7:529–533, 1983.

Chan JKC, Tsang WYW, Ng CS. Follicular dendritic cell tumor and vascular neoplasm complicating hyaline-vascular Castleman's disease. Am J Surg Pathol 18:517–525, 1994a.

Chan JKC, Tsang WYW, Ng CS, Tang SK, Yu HC, Lee AW. Follicular dendritic cell tumors of the oral cavity. Am J Surg Pathol 18:148–157, 1994b.

Cline MJ. Histiocytes and histiocytosis. Blood 84:2840–2853, 1994.

Falini B, Flenghi L, Pileri S, Gambacorta M, Bigerna B, Durkop H, et al. PG-M1: A new monoclonal antibody directed against a fixative-resistant epitope on the macrophage-restricted form of the CD68 molecule. Am J Pathol 142:1359–1372, 1993.

Gaffey MJ, Frierson HF, Medeiros LJ, Weiss LM. The relationship of Epstein-Barr virus to infection related (sporadic) and familial hemophagocytic syndrome and secondary (lymphoma-related) hemophagocytosis: An in situ hybridization study. Hum Pathol 24:657–667, 1993.

Gonzalez CL, Medeiros LJ, Braziel RM, Jaffe ES. T cell lymphoma involving subcutaneous tissue: A clinicopathologic entity commonly associated with hemophagocytic syndrome. Am J Surg Pathol 15:17–27, 1991.

Hyteriglou P, Phelps RG, Wattenberg DJ, Strauchen JA. Histiocytic cytophagic panniculitis: Molecular evidence for a clonal T cell disorder. J Am Acad Dermatol 27:333–336, 1992.

Kamel OW, Gocke CD, Kell DL, Cleary ML, Warnke RA. True histiocytic lymphoma: A study of 12 cases based on current definition. Leuk Lymphoma 18:81–86, 1995.

Lieberman PH, Jones CR, Steinman PM, Erlandson RA, Smith J, Gee T, et al. Langerhans cell (eosinophilic) granulomatosis. A clinicopathologic study encompassing 50 years. Am J Surg Pathol 20:519–552, 1996.

Paulli M, Rosso R, Kindl S, Boveri E, Marocolo D, Chioda C, et al. Immunophenotypic characterization of the cell infiltrate in five cases of sinus histiocytosis with massive lymphadenopathy (Rosai-Dorfman disease). Hum Pathol 23:647–654, 1992.

Perez-Ordonez B, Erlandson RA, Rosai J. Follicular dendritic cell tumor: Report of 13 additional cases of a distinctive entity. Am J Surg Pathol 20:944–955, 1996.

Ree HJ, Kadin ME. Peanut agglutinin: A useful marker for histiocytosis X and interdigitating reticulum cells. Cancer 57:282–287, 1986.

Risdall RJ, McKenna RW, Nesbit ME, et al. Virus-associated hemophagocytic syndrome: A benign histiocytic proliferation distinct from malignant histiocytosis. Cancer 44:993–1002, 1979.

Risdall RJ, Brunning RD, Hernandez JI, Gordon DH. Bacteria-associated hemophagocytic syndrome. Cancer 54:2968–2972, 1984.

Rosai J, Dorfman RF. Sinus histiocytosis with massive lymphadenopathy: A new recognized benign clinicopathologic entity. Arch Pathol 87:63–70, 1969.

Rosai J, Dorfman RF. Sinus histiocytosis with massive lymphadenopathy—A pseudolymphomatous benign disorder: Analysis of 34 cases. Cancer 30:1174–1188, 1972.

Saiz AS, Chan OW, Strauchen JA. Follicular dendritic cell tumor in Castleman's disease: A report of two cases. Int J Surg Pathol 5:25–30, 1997.

Santiago-Schwartz F, Coppock DL, Hindenburg AA, Kern J. Identification of a malignant counterpart of the monocytic-dendritic cell progenitor in an acute myeloid leukemia. Blood 84:3054–3062, 1994.

Saven A, Foon KA, Piro LD. 2-chlorodeoxyadenosine-induced complete remissions in Langerhans' cell histiocytosis. Ann Intern Med 121:430–432, 1994.

Segal GH, Mesa MV, Fishleder AJ, et al. Precursor Langerhans' cell histiocytosis. An unusual histiocytic proliferation in a patient with persistent non-Hodgkin's lymphoma and terminal acute monocytic leukemia. Cancer 70:547–553, 1992.

Selves J, Meggetto F, Brousset P, Voight J-J, Pradere B, Grasset D, et al. Inflammatory pseudotumor of the liver. Evidence for follicular dendritic cell proliferation associated with clonal Epstein-Barr virus. Am J Surg Pathol 20:747–753, 1996.

Song SK, Schwartz IS, Strauchen JA, Huang YP, Sachdev V, Daftary DR, Vas CJ. Meningeal nodules with features of extranodal sinus histiocytosis with massive lymphadenopathy. Am J Surg Pathol 13:406–412, 1989.

Soslow RA, Davis RE, Warnke RA, Cleary ML, Kamel OW. True histiocytic lymphoma following therapy for lymphoblastic neoplasms. Blood 87:5207–5212, 1996.

Strauchen JA. Sarcomatoid neoplasm of monocytic lineage (letter). Am J Surg Pathol 15:1206–1208, 1991.

Turner RR, Wood GS, Beckstead JH, Colby TV, Horning SJ, Warnke RA. Histiocytic malignancies: Morphologic, immunologic, and enzymatic heterogeneity. Am J Surg Pathol 8:485–500, 1984.

van Voorhis WC, Witmer MD, Steinman RM. The phenotype of dendritic cells and macrophages. Federation Proc 42:3114–3118, 1983.

Weiss LM, Berry GJ, Dorfman RF, Banks PM, Kaiserling E, Curtis J, Rosai J, Warnke RA. Spindle cell neoplasms of lymph nodes of probably reticulum cell lineage. True reticulum cell sarcoma? Am J Surg Pathol 14:405–414, 1990.

Wenig BM, Abbondanzo SL, Childers EL, Kapadia SB, Heffner DR. Extranodal sinus histiocytosis with massive lymphadenopathy (Rosai-Dorfman disease) of the head and neck. Hum Pathol 24:483–492, 1993.

Willman CL, Busque L, Griffith BB, Favara BE, McClain KL, Duncan MH, Gilliland DG. Langerhans'-cell histiocytosis (histiocytosis-X)—A clonal proliferative disease. N Engl J Med 331:154–160, 1994.

Wilson MS, Weiss LM, Gatter KC, Mason DY, Dorfman RF. Malignant histiocytosis: A reassessment of cases previously reported in 1975 based on paraffin section immunophenotyping studies. Cancer 66:530–536, 1990.

27

Myeloproliferative Disorders and Mastocytosis

Myeloproliferative disorders which may involve the lymph node include granulocytic sarcoma (extramedullary myeloid cell tumor or chloroma), plasmacytoid monocytic proliferation (plasmacytoid T cell lymphoma), and the chronic myeloproliferative diseases, including chronic granulocytic leukemia and myeloid metaplasia-myelofibrosis. Mastocytosis, which is related to the myeloproliferative disorders, is also considered in this chapter.

Granulocytic Sarcoma

Granulocytic sarcoma (GS) is also referred to as extramedullary myeloid cell tumor, myeloblastoma, and chloroma, the last term descriptive of the green color imparted to some tumors by the enzyme myeloperoxidase. GS is an extramedullary manifestation of acute granulocytic leukemia (AGL). GS may precede, accompany, or follow AGL; GS may also occur as a manifestation of leukemic transformation of an underlying myelodysplastic syndrome, chronic myeloproliferative disorder, or blast crisis of chronic granulocytic leukemia.

Clinical Features

Patients with GS may have been previously healthy or may have a history of previous AGL or hematologic disorder predisposing to AGL, including myelodysplastic syndromes and chronic myeloproliferative disorders (Elenitoba-Johnson et al, 1996). Hematologic abnormalities may or may not be present at presentation. GS may involve skin, bone, soft tissues, lymph nodes, breast, central nervous system, and other sites (Neiman et al, 1981). An increased incidence of GS has been reported in AGL with t(8;21) chromosome translocation (Tallman et al, 1993). T cell lymphoblastic lymphoma with eosinophilia is a distinct syndrome associated with a high incidence of subsequent myeloid neoplasia and may be a related disorder (Abruzzo et al, 1992).

Histopathology

GS's are characterized by infiltrates of immature granulocytic cells. These have been characterized as well differentiated extramedullary myeloid cell tumor (EMT), with readily evident granulocytic differentiation on hematoxylin-and-eosin-stained sections (Fig. 27.1); poorly differentiated EMT, without readily evident granulocytic differentiation on routinely stained sections (Fig. 27.2); and blastic EMT, resembling the cells of lymphoblastic lymphoma (Fig. 27.3) (Traweek et al, 1993). Most cases of GS fall into the poorly differentiated EMT category, consisting of large cells with vesicular chromatin, round to irregular or folded nuclei, prominent nucleoli, and moderately abundant cytoplasm (Fig. 27.2). Distinction from large cell non-Hodgkin's lymphoma is difficult, and may be impossible on morphologic grounds alone. Careful examination may reveal rare cells with cytoplasmic granules (eosinophilic myelocytes), indicating the correct diagnosis. Histochemical staining for chloroacetate esterase (Leder stain) demonstrates characteristic cytoplasmic positivity in up to two thirds of cases, including all well-differentiated EMT, 65% of poorly differentiated EMT, and 20% of blastic EMT (Traweek et al, 1993) (Fig. 27.4). Imprints or touch preparations stained with Giemsa may also be helpful, demonstrating characteristic Auer rods or azurophilic cytoplasmic granules in progranulocytes. Cytochemical staining for myeloperoxidase (MPO) in imprint or touch preparations is frequently positive.

FIGURE 27.1

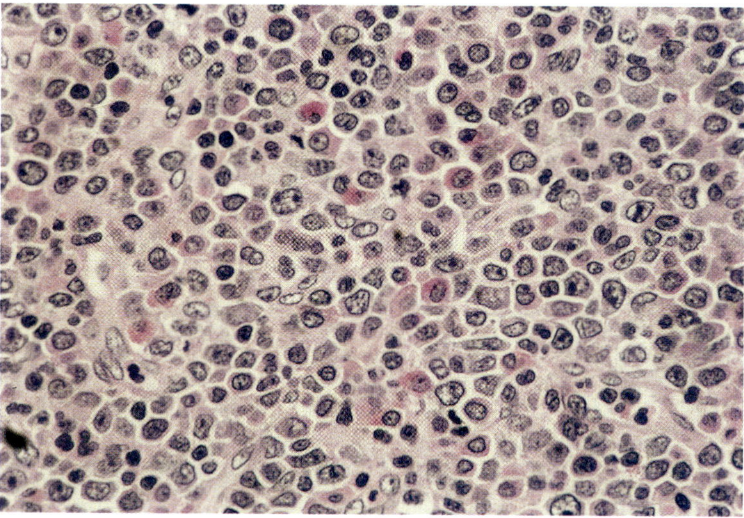

Granulocytic sarcoma, well-differentiated extramedullary myeloid tumor type, showing numerous eosinophilic myelocytes.

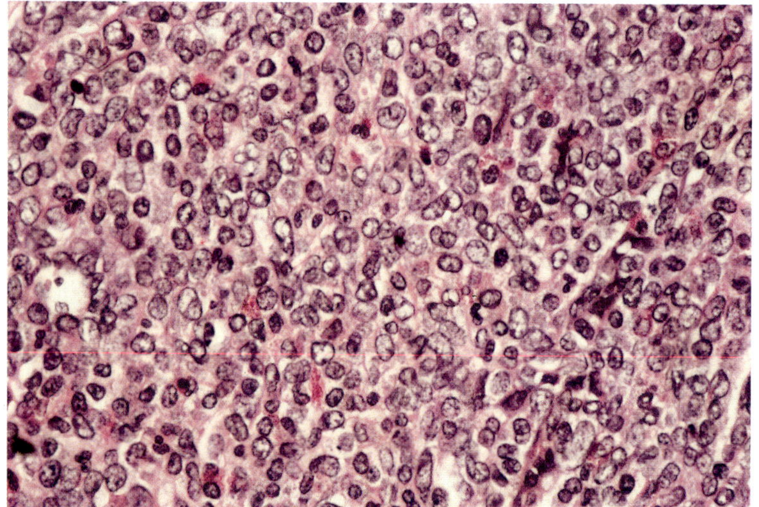

FIGURE 27.2

Granulocytic sarcoma, poorly differentiated extramedullary myeloid tumor type, showing ovoid vesicular nuclei and moderately abundant agranular cytoplasm.

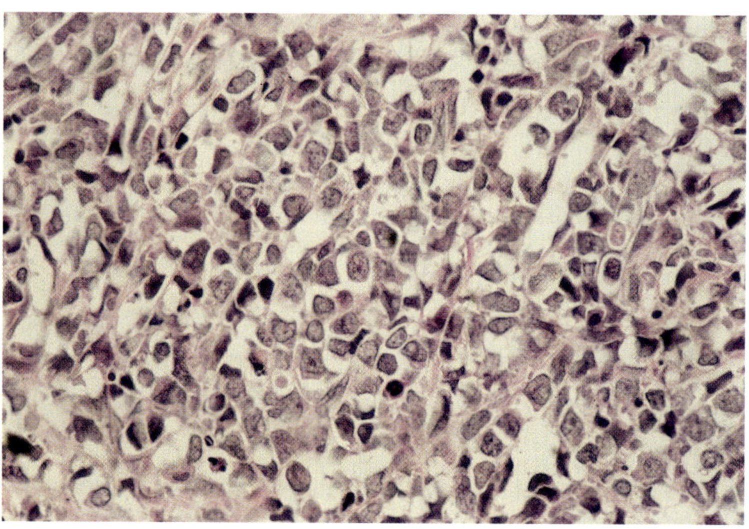

FIGURE 27.3

Granulocytic sarcoma, blastic extramedullary myeloid tumor type, showing cells with finely dispersed chromatin and scant cytoplasm.

Immunopathology

The diagnosis of GS is aided by immunohistochemical studies. GS's are positive for one or more granulocytic antigens in paraffin-embedded tissue, including MPO, CD68, lysozyme, CD15, and elastase (Traweek et al, 1993). Immunohistochemical staining for MPO is the most sensitive marker and is positive in greater than 90% of cases. CD34, the human progenitor cell antigen, a marker for immature hematopoietic cells and stem cells, is positive in one-third of cases (Traweek et al, 1993). CD45 is positive in most

**FIGURE
27.4**

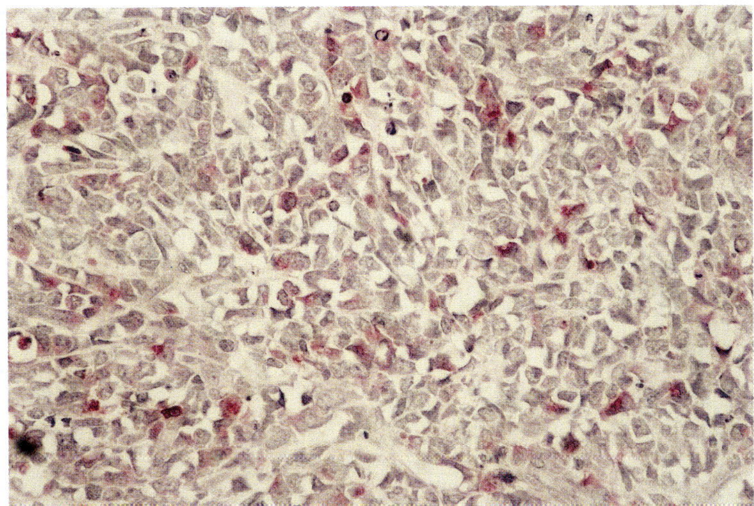

Granulocytic sarcoma stained for chloroacetate esterase (Leder stain) showing positive cells.

cases and CD43 is positive in nearly all cases; confusion with T cell non-Hodgkin's lymphoma may result. CD30 is negative. In frozen tissue, GS's are positive for myeloid antigens CD13 and CD33.

Differential Diagnosis

Distinction from non-Hodgkin's lymphoma may be difficult. Misdiagnosis usually results from failure to consider GS in the differential diagnosis. The diagnosis of GS should be suggested by a clinical history of previous myelodysplastic syndrome or myeloproliferative disorder, by the presence of eosinophilic myelocytes, or by a lymphoma with non-B, non-T or CD43-only phenotype. Histochemical staining for chloroacetate esterase (Leder stain) or immunohistochemical staining for MPO in these circumstances will frequently lead to the correct diagnosis. Care must be taken in interpreting the Leder stain, since mast cells, frequently present in a variety of neoplasms, are also positive. GS's with monocytic differentiation, arising in the setting of chronic myelomonocytic leukemia, are frequently chloroacetate esterase negative and may be particularly difficult to recognize (Elenitoba-Johnson et al, 1996).

Course and Prognosis

Patients with GS are treated for acute granulocytic leukemia with aggressive cytotoxic chemotherapy. Radiation therapy to bulky or symptomatic masses may also be given. Patients with GS and the t(8;21) chromosome translocation appear to have a poorer prognosis than other patients with AGL (Tallman et al, 1993). Patients presenting with GS, without AGL at presentation, will almost invariably progress to AGL, and should therefore receive systemic therapy for AGL in addition to radiation therapy. Patients with GS occurring in the course of myelodysplastic syndrome or chronic myeloproliferative disease have a poor prognosis.

Plasmacytoid Monocytic Proliferation (Plasmacytoid T Cell Lymphoma)

Plasmacytoid monocytic proliferation (PMP), formerly referred to as plasmacytoid T cell lymphoma, occurs in the course of chronic myeloproliferative disorders and chronic myelomonocytic leukemia (Baddoura et al, 1992; Harris and Demirjian, 1991).

Clinical Features

Patients with PMP are typically elderly, presenting with generalized lymphadenopathy and hepatosplenomegaly. Usually there is hematologic evidence of underlying chronic myelomonocytic leukemia (Facchetti et al, 1990; Harris and Demirjian, 1991).

Histopathology

Affected lymph nodes show paracortical infiltrates of medium sized cells, with eccentric, round to ovoid nuclei, and a moderate amount of amphophilic cytoplasm (Figs. 27.5 and 27.6). These cells resemble the so called "plasmacytoid T cells" found in clusters in the paracortex of some reactive lymph nodes and shown to be of myelomonocytic lineage (Facchetti et al, 1988) (Fig. 27.7). These cells and the cells of PMP are now considered to be plasmacytoid monocytes. Infiltrates of morphologically distinct leukemic cells have also been present in some cases (Facchetti et al, 1990; Harris and Demirjian, 1991).

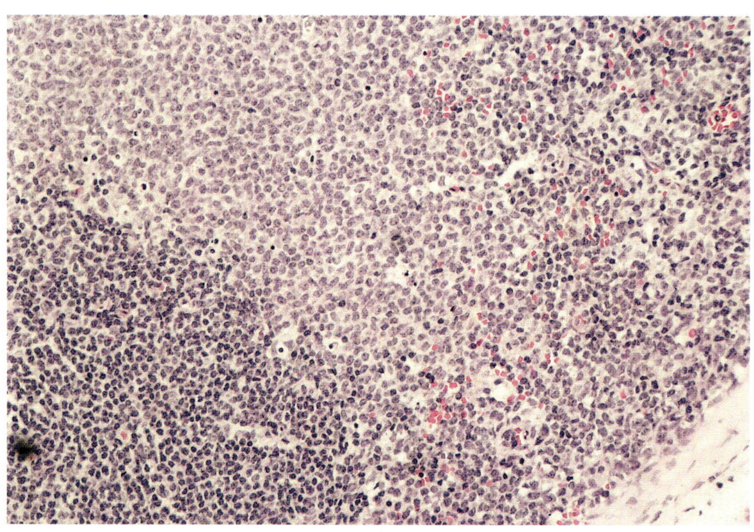

FIGURE 27.5

Plasmacytoid monocytic proliferation in chronic myelomonocytic leukemia showing paracortical infiltrates of plasmacytoid monocytes.

**FIGURE
27.6**

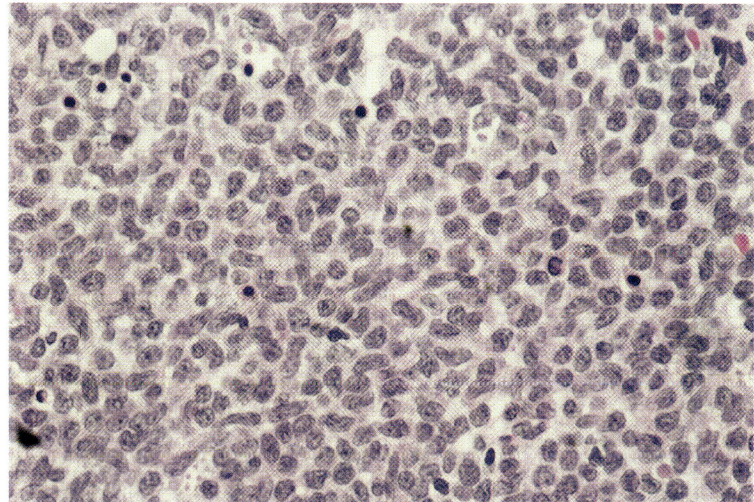

Plasmacytoid monocytic proliferation in chronic myelomonocytic leukemia, higher magnification, showing plasmacytoid monocytes with ovoid
nuclei and amphophilic cytoplasm.

**FIGURE
27.7**

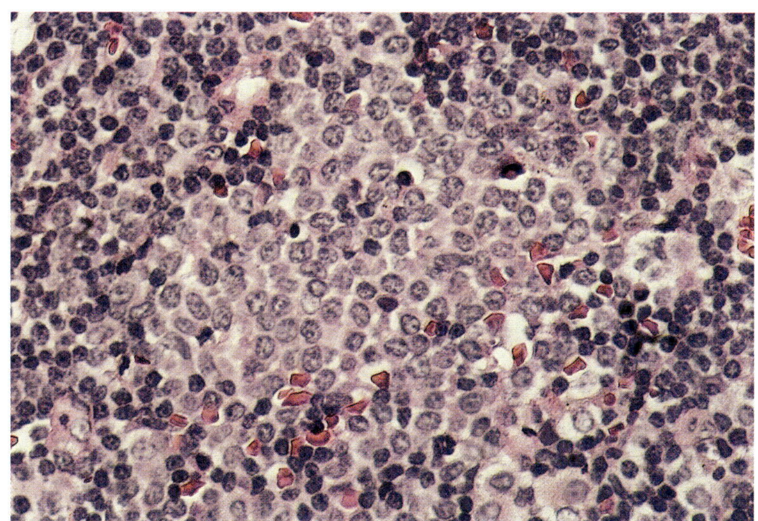

Plasmacytoid monocytes in a reactive lymph node.

Immunopathology

Plasmacytoid monocytes in reactive lymph nodes and plasmacytoid monocytic proliferations demonstrate a similar phenotype. The cells are positive for CD43 and CD68 in
paraffin-embedded tissue, and positive for CD4 in frozen tissue; CD14 and CD15 may be
positive or negative (Facchetti et al, 1990; Facchetti et al, 1988).

Differential Diagnosis

PMPs are closely related to myeloproliferative disorders and chronic myelomonocytic leukemia and should be distinguished from conventional non-Hodgkin's lymphomas. The myelomonocytic phenotype is distinctive. The nature of the cellular proliferation in PMP is uncertain; in some cases the PMP appears to be part of the leukemic clone; in others it appears distinct and may be reactive (Facchetti et al, 1990; Harris and Demirjian, 1991). Some authors consider PMP a form of granulocytic sarcoma (Baddoura et al, 1992).

Course and Prognosis

Therapy for PMP is directed to the underlying leukemic process. The prognosis is poor.

Chronic Myeloproliferative Diseases

Extramedullary involvement may be a feature of chronic myeloproliferative diseases (MPDs), including myeloid metaplasia-myelofibrosis (MMM), polycythemia vera, essential thrombocythemia, and chronic granulocytic leukemia (CGL). Leukemic infiltrates in CGL consist of mature and immature granulocytes and usually involve the medullary cords and sinuses and interfollicular regions. Blast crisis of CGL may be indistinguishable from granulocytic sarcoma. Lymph node involvement in other MPD ranges from sinusoidal foci of extramedullary hematopoiesis (EM) (Figs. 27.8 and 27.9) to extensive replacement by tumoral masses of EM; the latter is frequent in cases of MMM. Giant, cytologically atypical megakaryocytes may be present in MMM and may cause confusion with Hodgkin's disease (Fig. 27.10). The presence of immature granulocytes and erythroid precursors and the characteristic thick, ropy chromatin of megakaryocytes usu-

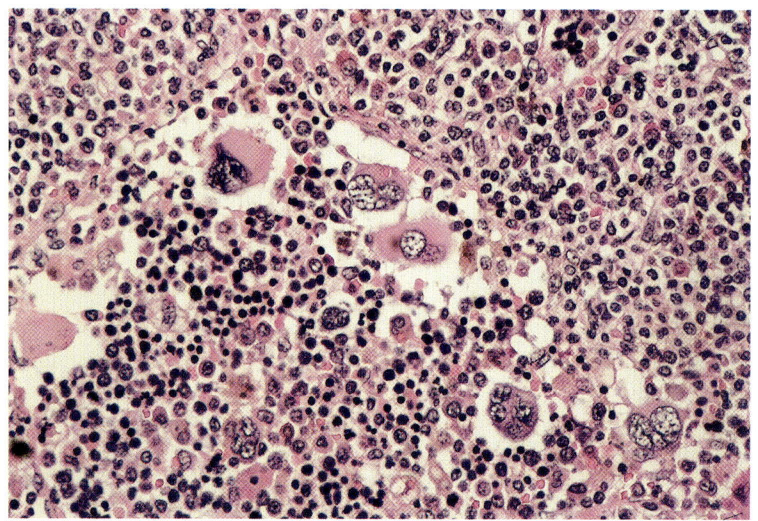

FIGURE 27.8

Extramedullary hematopoiesis in a lymph node in chronic myeloproliferative disease.

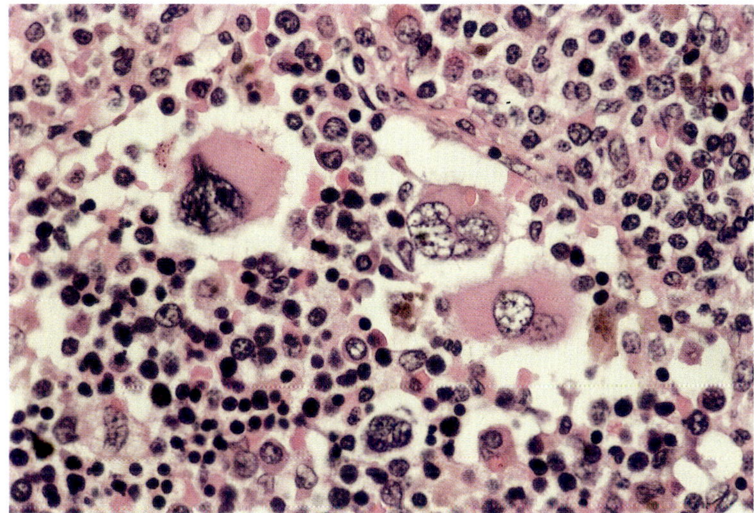

Extramedullary hematopoiesis in chronic myeloproliferative disease, higher magnification, showing sinusoidal megakaryocytes, immature granulocytes, and erythroid precursors.

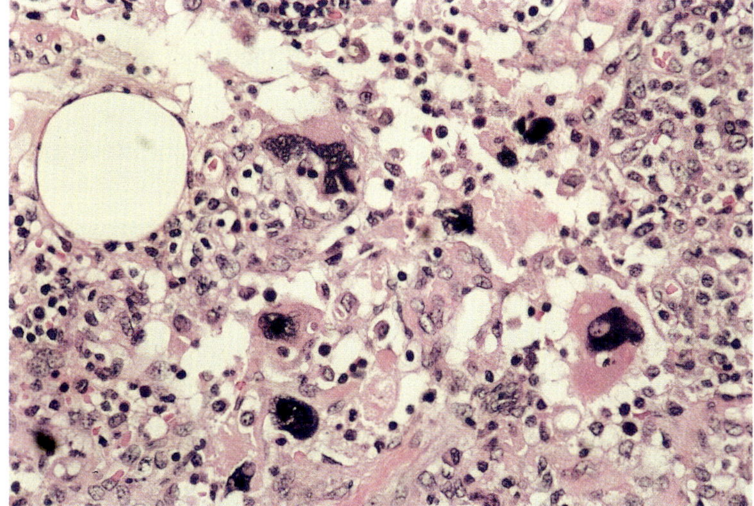

Extramedullary hematopoiesis in chronic myeloproliferative disease showing cytologically atypical megakaryocytes. These should not be confused with Reed-Sternberg cells or metastatic tumor cells.

ally permit distinction. Megakaryocytes can also be identified by immunohistochemical positivity for factor VIII–related antigen and platelet glycoprotein IIb/IIIa (CD41) or IIIa (CD61). Megakaryocytes are also frequently PAS-positive.

Mastocytosis

Mastocytosis refers to proliferation of mast cells, which may be confined to the skin (urticaria pigmentosa) or involve the bone marrow, liver, spleen, lymph nodes, and other organs (systemic mastocytosis, systemic mast cell disease). Mastocytosis may be considered a form of myeloproliferative disease, since mast cells are derived from the bone marrow, and mastocytosis is not infrequently associated with underlying myeloproliferative or myelodysplastic disorders (Travis et al, 1988).

Clinical Features

Mastocytosis confined to the skin (urticaria pigmentosa) occurs most frequently in children; systemic mastocytosis, with or without skin involvement, occurs in adults and is characterized by symptoms of histamine release, including flushing, hypotension, and diarrhea (Webb et al, 1982). Hepatosplenomegaly, lymphadenopathy, and skeletal lesions (osteoporosis and/or osteosclerosis) are frequently present (Webb et al, 1982). One third of patients show evidence of an underlying hematologic disorder, including myelodysplastic syndromes, myeloproliferative disease, acute granulocytic leukemia, or malignant lymphoma (Travis et al, 1988). Malignant mastocytosis or mast cell leukemia is a rare manifestation of systemic mast cell disease (Baghestanian et al, 1996).

Histopathology

Lymph node involvement in mastocytosis is characterized by infiltrates of mast cells, small to medium-sized, ovoid to spindled cells, with indented or bilobed nuclei, inconspicuous nucleoli, and abundant, pale cytoplasm (Figs. 27.11 and 27.12). Cytoplasmic granules are often not evident in hematoxylin and eosin-stained sections. The mast cell infiltrates are characteristically perifollicular (Webb et al, 1982) or involve the medullary cords and sinuses (Horny et al, 1992a). The mast cell infiltrates are frequently admixed with eosinophils and associated with vascular proliferation and delicate lamellar fibrosis. Splenic involvement is characterized by mast cell infiltrates involving the perifollicular white pulp, fibrous trabeculae, and red pulp (Horny et al, 1992b; Webb et al, 1982). Bone marrow involvement is characterized by peritrabecular and perivascular infiltrates of mast cells and eosinophils. Aggregates of spindled mast cells and eosinophils (so called "eosinophilic fibrohistiocytic lesions") are frequently present. The presence of numerous spindled mast cells may mimic myelofibrosis (Webb et al, 1982).

Cytochemical and Immunohistochemical Studies

The mast cells in mastocytosis are usually sparsely granulated, and characteristic mast cell granules are frequently not evident in hematoxylin and eosin-stained sections. The mast cell granules are readily demonstrated, however, in sections stained with Giemsa

FIGURE 27.11

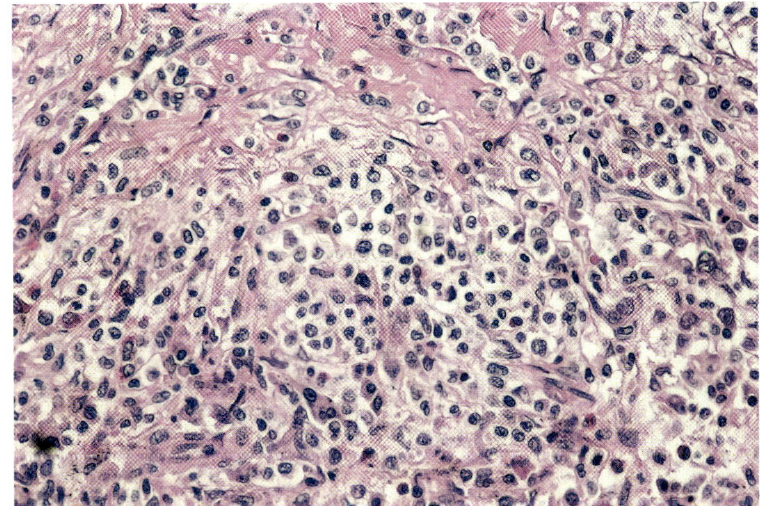

Mastocytosis showing mast cell infiltrates with characteristic fibrosis.

FIGURE 27.12

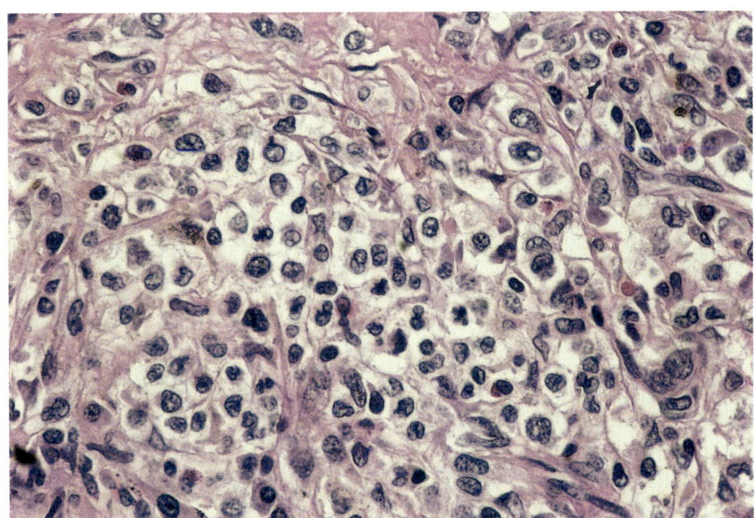

Mastocytosis, higher magnification, showing mast cells with ovoid or indented nuclei, abundant pale cytoplasm, and delicate fibrosis.

or toluidine blue, demonstrating characteristic metachromasia. Mast cell granules are also demonstrated by the chloroacetate esterase (Leder) stain. Mast cells are positive for CD68 and for tryptase by immunohistochemistry (Li et al, 1996).

Differential Diagnosis

Misdiagnosis usually results from failure to consider mastocytosis in the differential diagnosis. Mast cells may resemble the cells of monocytoid B cell lymphoma or hairy cell leukemia. The presence of eosinophils, vascular proliferation, and lamellar fibrosis, however, should suggest the correct diagnosis. The absence of lymphoid markers and demonstration of characteristic mast cell granules by Giemsa, toluidine blue, or chloroacetate esterase (Leder) stain is diagnostic. A rare solitary spindle mast cell tumor of lymph nodes has been described and should be distinguished from systemic mastocytosis (Horny et al, 1994).

Course and Prognosis

The course of mastocytosis is variable but frequently indolent. Aggressive forms of mastocytosis, including mast cell leukemia and mastocytosis associated with underlying hematologic disorders, have a poorer prognosis. Antihistamines may be helpful in controlling symptoms of hyperhistaminemia. Responses to α-interferon have been reported (Kluin-Nelemans et al, 1992; Petit et al, 1995).

REFERENCES

Abruzzo LV, Jaffe ES, Cotelingam JD, Whang-Peng J, Del Duca V, Medeiros LJ. T cell lymphoblastic lymphoma with eosinophilia associated with subsequent myeloid malignancy. Am J Surg Pathol 16:236–245, 1992.

Baddoura FK, Hanson C, Chan WC. Plasmacytoid monocytic proliferation associated with myeloproliferative disorders. Cancer 69:1457–1467, 1992.

Baghestanian M, Bankl HC, Sillaber C, Beil WJ, Radaszkiewicz T, Fureder W, et al. A case of malignant mastocytosis with circulating mast cell precursors: biologic and phenotypic characterization of the malignant clone. Leukemia 10:159–166, 1996.

Elenitoba-Johnson K, Hodges GF, King TC, Wu CD, Medeiros LJ. Extramedullary myeloid cell tumors arising in the setting of chronic myelomonocytic leukemia. Arch Pathol Lab Med 120:62–67, 1996.

Facchetti F, De Wolf-Peeters C, Mason DY, Pulford K, van den Oord JJ, Desmet VJ. Plasmacytoid T cells. Immunohistochemical evidence for their monocyte/macrophage origin. Am J Pathol 133:15–21, 1988.

Facchetti F, De Wolf-Peeters C, Kennes C, Rossi G, De Vos R, van den Oord JJ, Desmet VJ. Leukemia-associated lymph node infiltrates of plasmacytoid monocytes (so called plasmacytoid T cells). Evidence for two distinct histological and immunophenotypical patterns. Am J Surg Pathol 14:101–112, 1990.

Harris NL, Demirjian Z. Plasmacytoid T-zone proliferation in patients with chronic myelomonocytic leukemia. Histologic and immunohistologic characterization. Am J Surg Pathol 15:87–95, 1991.

Horny HP, Kaiserling E, Parwaresch MR, Lennert K. Lymph node findings in generalized mastocytosis. Histopathology 21:439–446, 1992a.

Horny HP, Ruck MT, Kaiserling E. Spleen findings in generalized mastocytosis. A clinicopathologic study. Cancer 70:459–468, 1992b.

Horny HP, Rabenhorst G, Loffler H, Kaiserling E. Solitary fibromastocytic tumor arising in an inguinal lymph node: the first description of a unique spindle cell tumor simulating mastocytosis. Mod Pathol 7:962–966, 1994.

Kluin-Nelemans HC, Jansen JH, Breukelman H, et al. Response to interferon alfa-2b in a patient with systemic mastocytosis. N Engl J Med 326:619–623, 1992.

Li WV, Kapadia SB, Sonmez-Alpan E, Swerdlow SH. Immunohistochemical characterization of mast cell disease in paraffin sections using tryptase, CD68, myeloperoxidase, lysozyme, and CD20 antibodies. Mod Pathol 9:982–988, 1996.

Neiman RS, Barcos M, Berard C, et al. Granulocytic sarcoma: a clinicopathologic study of 61 biopsied cases. Cancer 48:1426–1437, 1981.

Petit A, Pulik M, Gaulier A, Lionnet F, Mahe A, Sigal M. Systemic mastocytosis with chronic myelomonocytic leukemia: Clinical features and response to interferon alfa therapy. J Am Acad Dermatol 32:850–853, 1995.

Tallman MS, Hakimian D, Shaw JM, Lissner GS, Russell EJ, Variakojis D. Granulocytic sarcoma is associated with the 8;21 translocation in acute myeloid leukemia. J Clin Oncol 11:690–697, 1993.

Travis WD, Li C-Y, Yam LT, Bergstralh EJ, Swee RG. Significance of systemic mast cell disease with associated hematologic disorders. Cancer 62:965–972, 1988.

Traweek ST, Arber DA, Rappaport H, Brynes RK. Extramedullary myeloid cell tumors. An immunohistochemical and morphologic study of 28 cases. Am J Surg Pathol 17:1011–1019, 1993.

Webb TA, Li C-Y, Yam LT. Systemic mast cell disease: A clinical and hematopathologic study of 26 cases. Cancer 49:927–938, 1982.

28

Proliferations of Mesenchymal Elements

Normal lymph nodes contain a variety of mesenchymal elements, including fibrous tissue in the lymph node capsule, trabeculae, and hilum; smooth muscle; blood vessels; lymphatics; and fat. Proliferations of these elements occasionally occur. Additionally, lymph nodes may be the site of hamartomatous proliferations containing several mesenchymal elements.

Fibroblastic Proliferations

Fibroblastic proliferations which may involve the lymph node include fibrosis, inflammatory pseudotumor, and intranodal hemorrhagic spindle cell tumor (palisaded myofibroblastoma).

Fibrosis

Fibrosis is a frequent feature of inguinal and pelvic lymph nodes, which often contain foci of densely hyalinized collagen, frequently in a perivascular distribution with varying degrees of replacement of the lymph node parenchyma. The etiology is obscure. Fibrosis in inguinal and pelvic lymph nodes has been attributed to recurrent infections; however, there is little direct evidence to support this. Proliferation of smooth muscle in the hilum of inguinal lymph nodes is occasionally seen in association with fibrosis and vascular proliferation and has also been attributed to previous inflammation (Channer and Davies, 1985).

Inflammatory Pseudotumor

Inflammatory pseudotumor (IPT) is a distinctive pattern of lymph node reaction with spindle cell proliferation which resembles inflammatory pseudotumor (plasma cell granuloma) of the lung and other sites (Perrone et al, 1988). The etiology is obscure. The spindle cells are of fibrohistiocytic (Facchetti et al, 1990) or myofibroblastic origin (Davis et al, 1991).

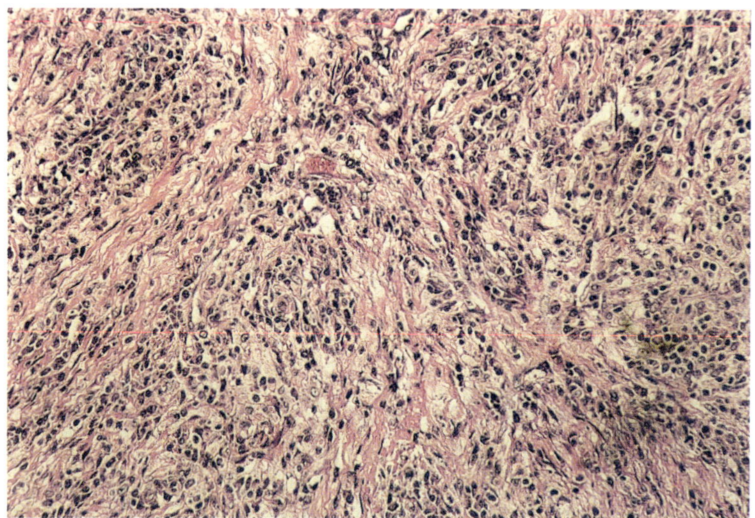

FIGURE 28.1

Inflammatory pseudotumor showing spindle cell proliferation arising from the supporting structures of the lymph node.

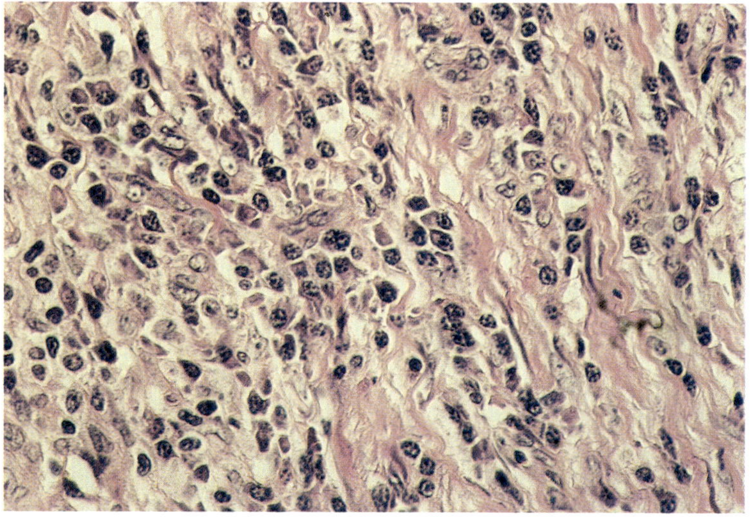

FIGURE 28.2

Inflammatory pseudotumor, higher magnification, showing spindle cells admixed with numerous plasma cells.

**FIGURE
28.3**

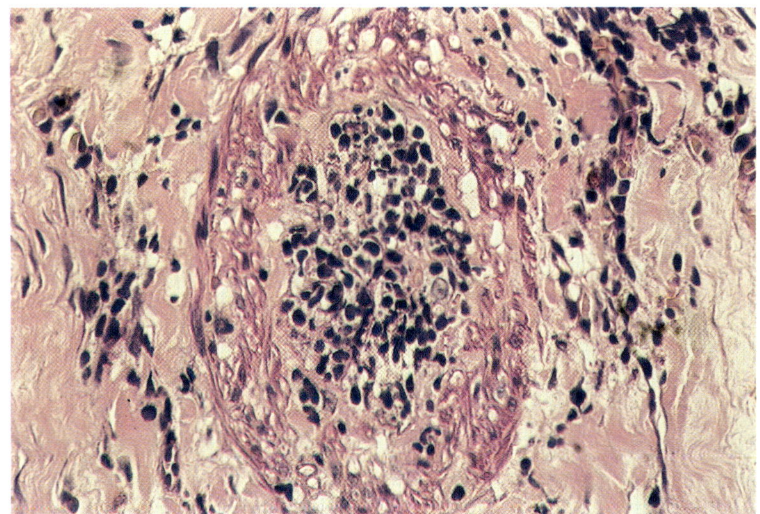

Inflammatory pseudotumor showing vasculitis in perinodal soft tissue.

Clinical Features

Inflammatory pseudotumor of lymph nodes may occur at any age. Most patients have been young or middle-aged adults, presenting with localized or regional lymphadenopathy. Constitutional symptoms, including fever and fatiguability, are frequently present and may be accompanied by laboratory evidence of an inflammatory process with elevated erythrocyte sedimentation rate, anemia, and polyclonal hypergammaglobulinemia (Perrone et al, 1988).

Histopathology

IPT is characterized by a collagenous spindle cell proliferation predominantly affecting the supporting structures of the lymph node, including the capsule, trabeculae, and hilum, with secondary involvement of the lymph node parenchyma (Perrone et al, 1988) (Figs. 28.1 and 28.2). The spindle cell proliferation is characterized by a storiform growth pattern, varying degrees of collagen deposition, vascular proliferation, and admixture of numerous inflammatory cells, including prominent plasma cells, small and large lymphocytes without atypia, and scattered neutrophils. Involvement of perinodal soft tissue is characteristic. Evidence of small vessel vasculitis, with vascular infiltration and fibrinoid necrosis, is frequently present (Davis et al, 1991; Perrone et al, 1988) (Fig. 28.3).

Immunopathology

The spindle cells in IPT demonstrate the phenotype of myofibroblasts, staining for α smooth muscle actin, but not for desmin, and spindled histiocytes, staining for CD68 (Davis et al, 1991; Facchetti et al, 1990). The lymphocytic cells consist predominantly of reactive T cell; the plasma cells are polyclonal by immunoglobulin light chain staining (Davis et al, 1991).

Differential Diagnosis

IPT must be distinguished from other spindle cell tumors which may involve lymph nodes. The predominant involvement of the supporting structures of the lymph node and perinodal soft tissue, admixture of inflammatory cells, and evidence of vasculitis are characteristic features. Mycobacterial spindle cell pseudotumor is a distinct entity which occurs in patients with AIDS and is characterized by proliferation of spindled histiocytes containing numerous intracellular *Mycobacterium avium-intracellulare* organisms (Chen, 1992). PAS and AFB stains are diagnostic.

Course and Prognosis

The course of IPT is generally benign and self limited; there is no specific therapy. Constitutional symptoms may remit following excision of involved lymph nodes. Some patients have received corticosteroids or nonsteroidal antiinflammatory drugs; rare patients have received chemotherapy (Perrone et al, 1988). Recurrences may occur.

Intranodal Hemorrhagic Spindle Cell Tumor

Intranodal hemorrhagic spindle cell tumor with amianthoid fibers, also known as palisaded myofibroblastoma, is a rare mesenchymal tumor with myofibroblastic differentiation (Suster et al, 1989; Weiss et al, 1989). The histogenesis is uncertain; there is a predilection for inguinal lymph node involvement.

Clinical Features

Intranodal hemorrhagic spindle cell tumor (IHST) is a rare mesenchymal neoplasm affecting predominantly inguinal lymph nodes. Most patients have been middle aged adults presenting with an inguinal mass with a history of recent growth. IHST of other lymph nodes also occurs (Alguacil-Garcia, 1992).

Histopathology

IHST is characterized by replacement of the lymph node parenchyma by a proliferation of interlacing fascicles of spindle cells with a surrounding zone of sclerosis and hemorrhage (Fig. 28.4). A compressed rim of residual uninvolved lymph node is frequently identified at the periphery. A characteristic feature of IHST is the presence of amianthoid fibers, stellate aggregates of eosinophilic fibrillar collagen and actin, which may be organized around small blood vessels (Suster et al, 1989; Weiss et al, 1989) (Figs. 28.5 and 28.6).

Immunopathology

The spindle cells in IHST are positive for actin, myosin, and vimentin, consistent with myofibroblastic or modified smooth muscle differentiation (Suster et al, 1989; Weiss et al, 1989). The tumor cells are negative for S100 protein.

FIGURE 28.4

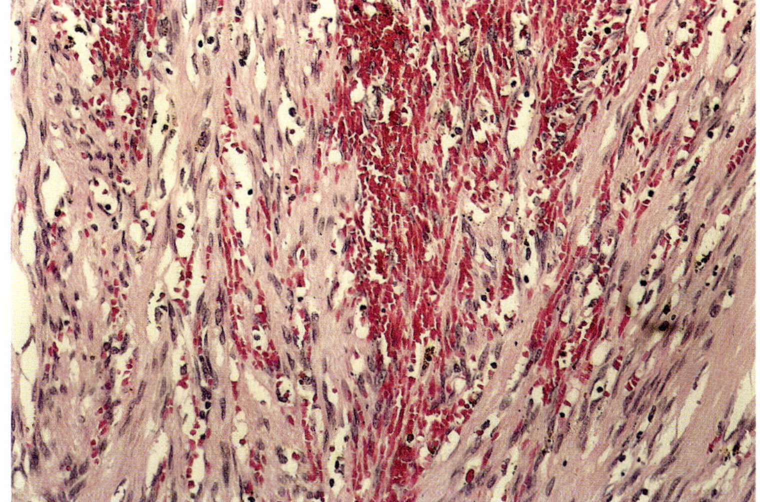

Intranodal hemorrhagic spindle cell tumor showing interlacing fascicles of spindle cells with sclerosis and hemorrhage.

FIGURE 28.5

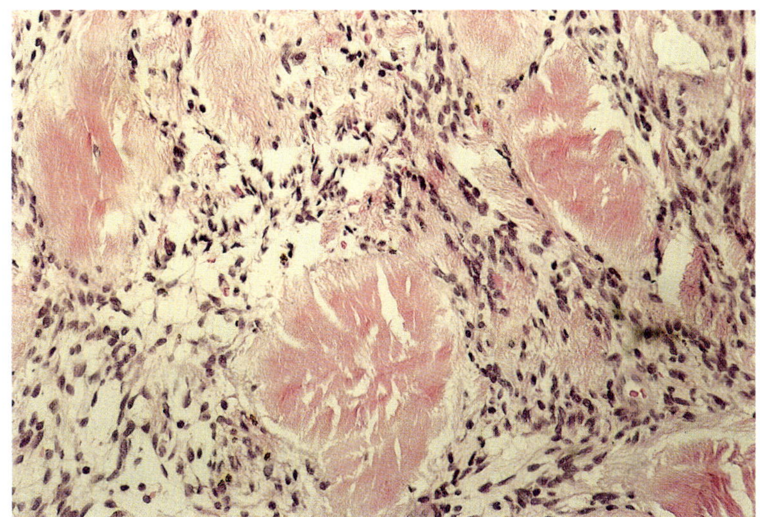

Intranodal hemorrhagic spindle cell tumor showing spindle cells and amianthoid fibers, stellate aggregates of eosinophilic fibrillar collagen and actin.

Differential Diagnosis

IHST should be distinguished from other spindle cell tumors which may involve lymph nodes. IHST may be confused with Schwannoma, the palisaded spindle cells and amianthoid fibers mimicking Antoni A and B areas and Verocay bodies. Misdiagnosis results from failure to appreciate the intranodal location of the lesion; careful inspection of IHST will usually reveal a characteristic rim of compressed, uninvolved lymph node. Immunohistochemical studies also permit distinction, since IHST are S100 negative.

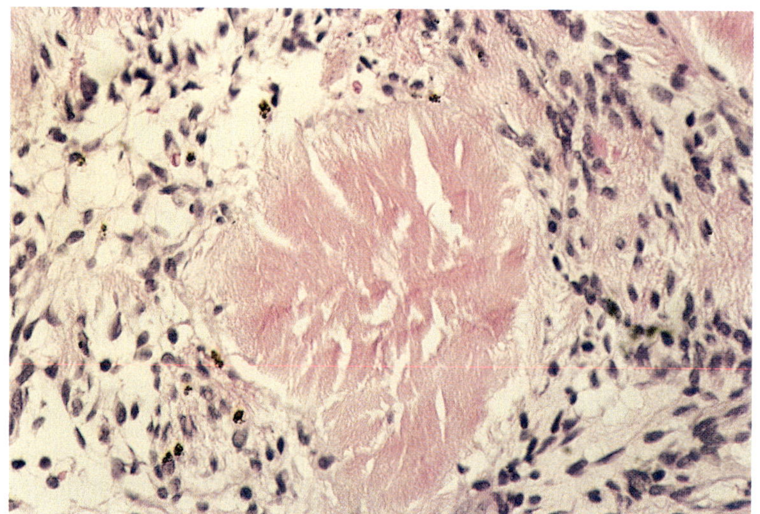

Intranodal hemorrhagic spindle cell tumor, higher magnification, showing detail of an amianthoid fiber.

IHST may also be confused with lymph node involvement by Kaposi's sarcoma, since
both contain foci of hemorrhage. The presence of amianthoid fibers and lack of vascular
spaces, as in Kaposi's sarcoma, permit distinction.

Course and Prognosis

IHST are treated by surgical excision. All cases reported to date have been benign,
without recurrence or metastases.

Smooth Muscle Proliferations

Smooth muscle proliferations involving the lymph nodes include hamartomatous proliferations (lymphangioleiomyomatosis, angiomyolipoma, angiomyomatous hamartoma),
benign transport or inclusion (lymph node leiomyomatosis), and true neoplasms (leiomyoma).

Hamartomatous Smooth Muscle Proliferations

Lymph node involvement in hamartomatous smooth muscle proliferation may occur as
part of a systemic hamartomatous syndrome (lymphangioleiomyomatosis of the lung,
angiomyolipoma of the kidney) or as a localized lymph node hamartoma (angiomyomatous hamartoma).

Lymphangioleiomyomatosis

Lymphangioleiomyomatosis (LL) occurs exclusively in women in the reproductive years
and is characterized by proliferation of smooth muscle and lymphatic channels in the

FIGURE
28.7

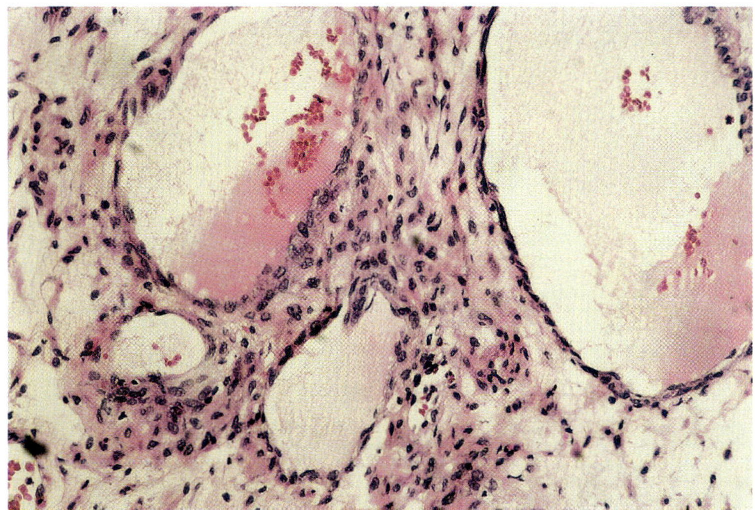

Lymphangioleiomyomatosis showing proliferation of smooth muscle and thin-walled lymphatic channels.

lungs and mediastinal and retroperitoneal lymph nodes. Rarely, isolated involvement of retroperitoneal lymph nodes occurs. Some patients with LL have associated stigmata of tuberous sclerosis. LL in lymph nodes is characterized by a predominantly sinusoidal proliferation of plump spindle cells, with clear to eosinophilic cytoplasm, separated by an anastomosing network of endothelial-lined channels (Fig. 28.7). The spindle cells characteristically stain for smooth muscle markers (smooth muscle actin and desmin) and the melanoma-associated antigen HMB-45 (Chan et al, 1993). Pulmonary involvement in LL is inexorably progressive with death from respiratory insufficiency. Involvement confined to retroperitoneal lymph nodes may have a better prognosis.

Angiomyolipoma

Angiomyolipoma (AL) occurs in both men and women, most frequently presenting as a renal mass. As in LL, associated stigmata of tuberous sclerosis may be present. AL is characterized by proliferation of thick-walled blood vessels, fat, and smooth muscle cells; the last may exhibit clear cell or epithelioid features and nuclear pleomorphism. As in LL, the smooth muscle cells stain for smooth muscle markers (smooth muscle actin and desmin) and HMB-45 (Chan et al, 1993). Involvement of retroperitoneal lymph nodes may occur in association with renal involvement. AL is benign; retroperitoneal lymph node involvement is considered evidence of multicentricity, rather than metastasis.

Angiomyomatous Hamartoma

Angiomyomatous hamartoma (AH) is a distinctive lesion occurring in inguinal lymph nodes (Chan et al, 1992). Most patients are men, presenting with long standing inguinal lymphadenopathy; edema of the ipsilateral lower extremity has been present in some patients. AH is characterized by proliferation of smooth muscle and fibrous tissue surrounding irregular vascular spaces (Figs. 28.8 and 28.9). Involvement extends from the

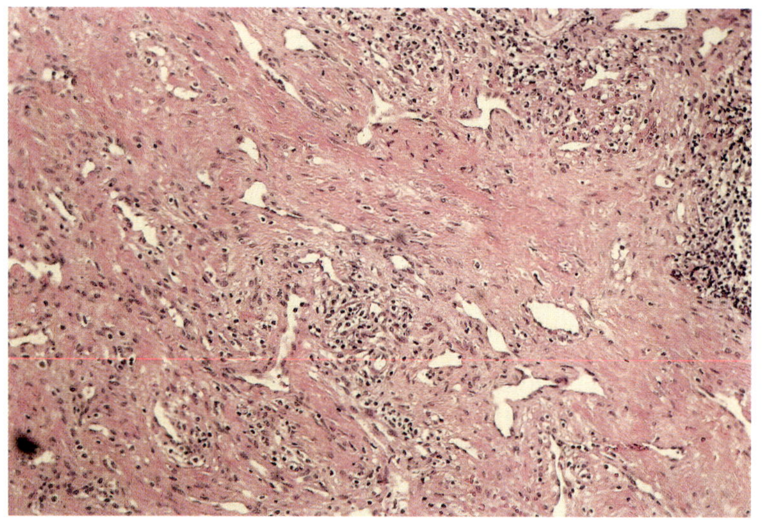

FIGURE
28.8

Angiomyomatous hamartoma of inguinal lymph node showing proliferation of smooth muscle and fibrous tissue around irregular vascular spaces.

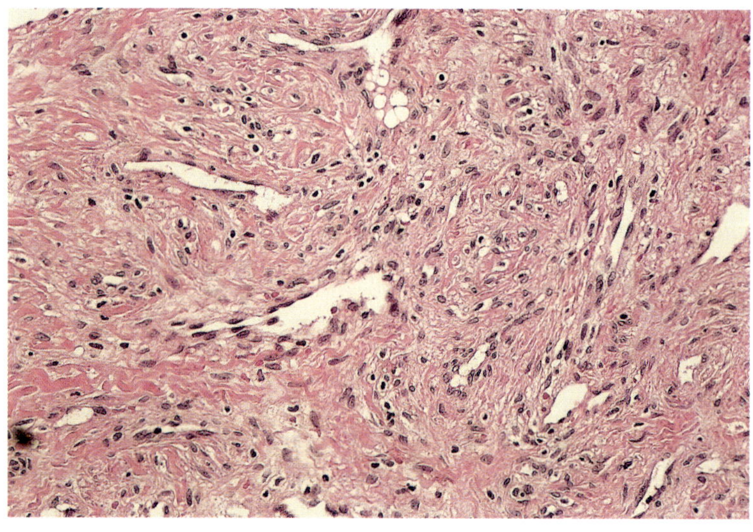

FIGURE
28.9

Angiomyomatous hamartoma of inguinal lymph node, higher magnification, showing characteristic irregular vascular spaces.

hilum into the lymph node parenchyma. In contrast to LL and AL, the smooth muscle cells are HMB-45 negative. AH is clinically benign.

Lymph Node Leiomyomatosis

Lymph node leiomyomatosis occurs predominantly in pelvic lymph nodes in women and is characterized by circumscribed nodules of cytologically bland smooth muscle cells (Figs. 28.10 and 28.11). The pathogenesis is obscure and may result from benign trans-

FIGURE
28.10

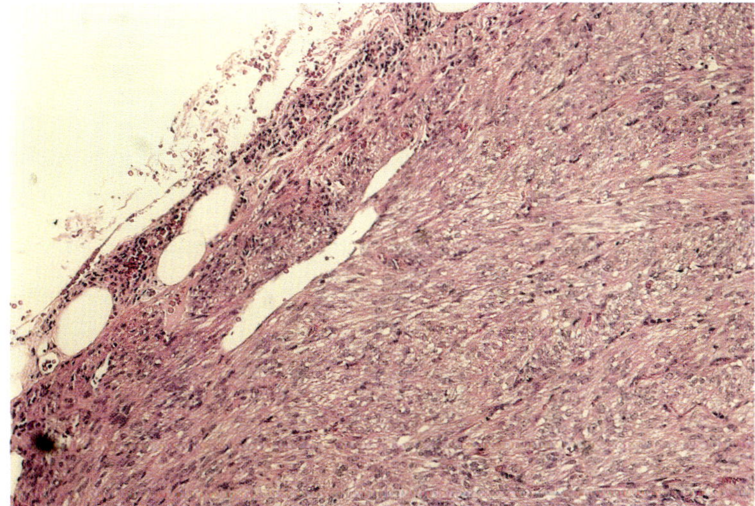

Leiomyomatosis of a pelvic lymph node in a woman showing nodular proliferation of smooth muscle cells.

FIGURE
28.11

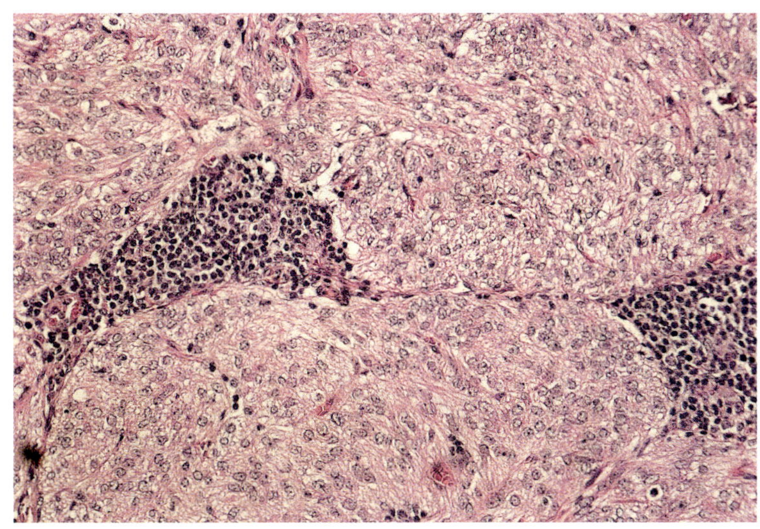

Leiomyomatosis of a pelvic lymph node in a woman, higher magnification, showing cytologically bland smooth muscle cells.

port of smooth muscle cells from an associated uterine leiomyoma (benign metastasizing leiomyoma), differentiation of subcoelomic mesenchyme, or metaplasia of Müllerian inclusions (Hsu et al, 1981).

Lymph Node Leiomyoma

True smooth muscle neoplasms of lymph nodes are extremely rare. A case of an intranodal leiomyoma in a patient with HIV infection has been reported (Starasoler et al,

1991). Smooth muscle neoplasms occur with increased frequency in patients with AIDS and are frequently associated with Epstein-Barr virus (McClain et al, 1995).

Vascular Proliferations

Vascular proliferations of lymph nodes arise from vascular or lymphatic endothelium and include Kaposi's sarcoma, vascular transformation of lymph node sinuses, hemangioma, lymphangioma, epithelioid vascular proliferations, and vascular proliferations in association with Castleman's disease.

Kaposi's Sarcoma

Kaposi's sarcoma (KS) is a spindle cell lesion of vascular origin with frequent multicentric involvement of the skin, lymph nodes, and visceral organs. Although the clonal origin of KS has been debated (Salahuddin et al, 1988), recent molecular evidence indicates that multicentric KS is a monoclonal neoplasm (Rabkin et al, 1997). KS is highly associated with a newly recognized herpesvirus, Kaposi's sarcoma–associated herpesvirus (KSHV), which is present in nearly all cases (Chang et al, 1994; Moore and Chang, 1996).

Clinical Features

KS occurs in classical, endemic (African and lymphadenopathic), post-transplantation, and epidemic (AIDS-related) forms. All forms of KS have been found to be associated with KSHV (Moore and Chang, 1996). KS may also develop in association with multicentric Castleman's disease, with or without associated HIV infection, a phenomenon which may be explained by the association of both disorders with KSHV (Soulier et al, 1995). KS typically presents with hemorrhagic cutaneous lesions. In classical KS, occurring in elderly men of Jewish or Mediterranean descent, involvement is typically confined to the lower extremities, and the clinical course is indolent; in other forms of the disease, including AIDS-related KS, lesions may be widely disseminated. Lymph node involvement in KS may occur in regional lymph nodes draining sites of cutaneous involvement or as a manifestation of disseminated disease. The endemic form of KS in African children frequently assumes a lymphadenopathic form, presenting as generalized lymphadenopathy in the absence of cutaneous involvement. KS, including classical KS, is associated with an increased incidence of malignant lymphoma (Safai et al, 1980). KSHV may be related to lymphoma in some cases (Strauchen et al, 1996).

Histopathology

Early lymph node involvement in KS is characterized by predominant involvement of the lymph node capsule and subcapsular and trabecular sinuses; more advanced cases are characterized by nodules of KS, which replace some or all of the lymph node parenchyma. The earliest lesion of KS is subtle and consists of thickening and increased cellularity of the lymph node capsule with a few spindle cells and plasma cells, irregular

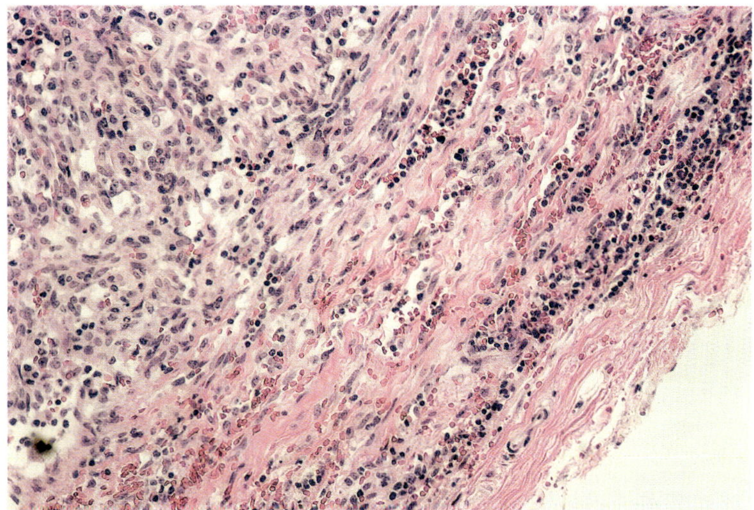

FIGURE 28.12

Kaposi's sarcoma, early lesion, showing thickening and hypercellularity of the lymph node capsule.

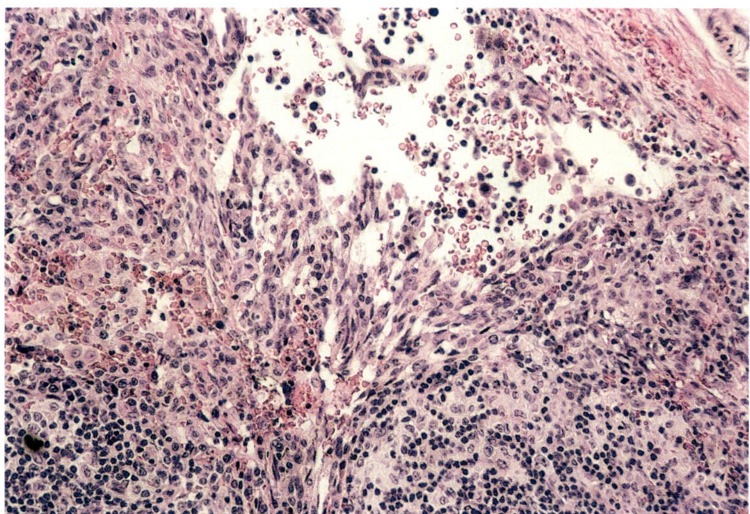

FIGURE 28.13

Kaposi's sarcoma, early lesion, showing proliferation of spindle cells within the subcapsular sinus.

vascular spaces, and hemosiderin deposition (Figs. 28.12 and 28.13). The well developed lesion of KS is characterized by proliferation of fascicles of spindle cells, with ovoid, hyperchromatic nuclei, eosinophilic cytoplasm, and slit-like intercellular spaces containing extravasated erythrocytes (Figs. 28.14 and 28.15). Scattered plasma cells and hemosiderin granules are frequently present. Fibrosis is characteristically absent. Well-formed vascular spaces and an angiomatous pattern may be present at the periphery of the lesions (Fig. 28.16). A characteristic feature of Kaposi's sarcoma is the presence of erythrocyte fragments and hyaline globules (Fukunga and Silverberg, 1991). The latter are intracellular, round, PAS-positive globules, smaller and more variable in size than

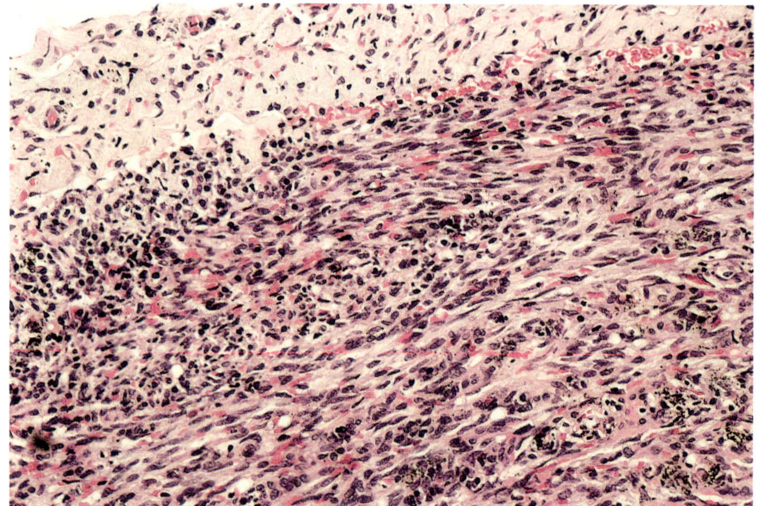

FIGURE
28.14

Kaposi's sarcoma, well-developed lesion, showing nodule composed of
fascicles of spindle cells.

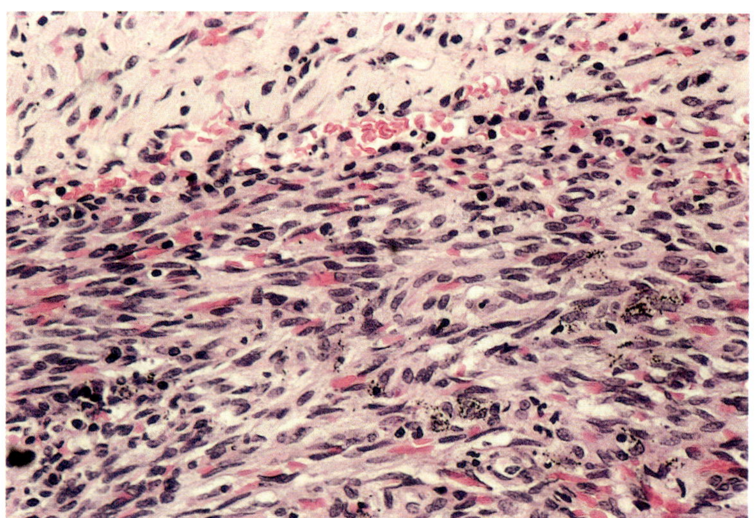

FIGURE
28.15

Kaposi's sarcoma, well-developed lesion, higher magnification, showing
fascicles of spindle cells with slit-like vascular spaces and extravasated
erythrocytes.

erythrocytes, which may be derived from degenerating erythrocytes (Fig. 28.17). Although seen rarely in other neoplasms, the presence of hyaline globules is of significant
diagnostic value in KS. The lymph node parenchyma in lymph nodes containing KS may
show changes resembling the multicentric form of Castleman's disease, with follicular
hyperplasia, hyalinized follicular centers, vascular proliferation, and plasmacytosis. Although it is unestablished whether these changes represent Castleman's disease or
Castleman's-like changes in association with KS or HIV infection, the presence of KSHV

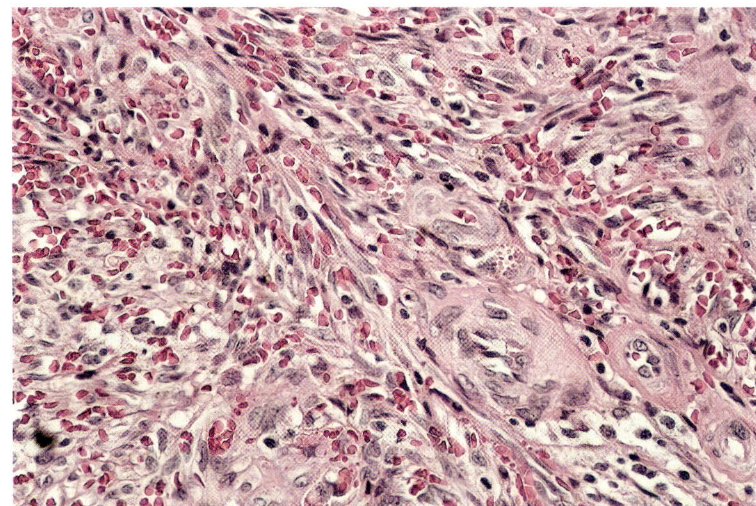

Kaposi's sarcoma showing spindle cells and vascular spaces lined by plump endothelial cells.

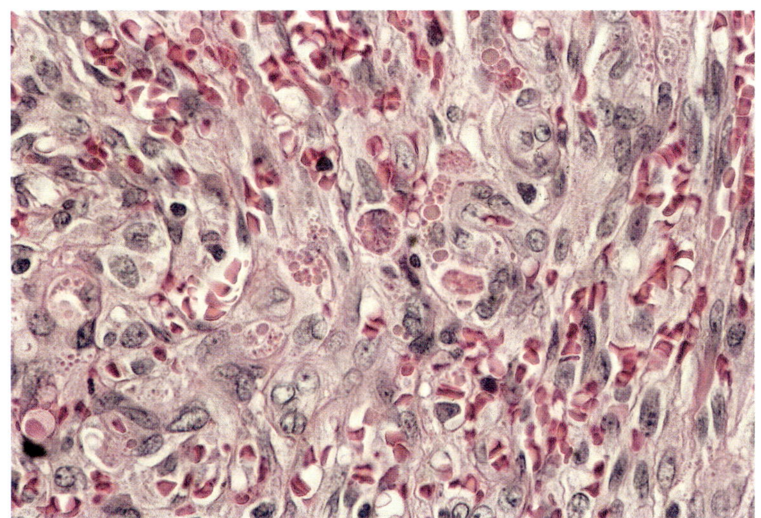

Kaposi's sarcoma showing intracellular hyaline globules.

in some cases of multicentric Castleman's disease suggests a close relation to KS (Soulier et al, 1995).

Immunopathology

The cell of origin of KS remains in dispute but is likely of vascular or lymphatic endothelial origin. The spindle cells of KS stain inconsistently for factor VIII–related antigen but are frequently positive for other endothelial markers, including *Ulex europaeus* lectin, CD31, and CD34.

Differential Diagnosis

KS must be distinguished from several benign spindle cell proliferations of lymph nodes which may mimic its appearance, including inflammatory pseudotumor (IPT), intranodal hemorrhagic spindle cell tumor (IHST), and vascular transformation of lymph node sinuses (VTLS). IPT and IHST are distinguishable from KS by their greater degree of fibrosis; the presence of vasculitis, involvement of perinodal soft tissue, and extensive involvement of the supporting structures in IPT, and the presence of "amianthoid fibers" in IHST are also helpful distinguishing features. VTLS, in contrast, may be difficult to distinguish from KS (see below). Fibrosis and well-formed vascular channels, with involvement confined to the lymph node sinuses, are features favoring VTLS (Chan et al, 1991).

Course and Prognosis

The course of KS is highly variable; classical KS is frequently indolent. Localized cutaneous lesions of KS are frequently treated with radiotherapy; disseminated KS is treated with chemotherapy.

Vascular Transformation of Lymph Node Sinuses

Vascular transformation of lymph node sinuses (VTLS, nodal angiomatosis) is a peculiar vascular proliferation of lymph nodes, in which the lymph node sinuses become replaced by vascular spaces, frequently accompanied by fibrosis. VTLS is as an incidental finding associated with venous obstruction but must be distinguished from KS and other lymph node vascular proliferations.

Clinical Features

VTLS is usually encountered in lymph nodes removed for other reasons, including adjacent mass or tumor, staging procedures, thrombosis of major vessels, draining the sites of hemangiomas, or in association with congestive heart failure or constrictive pericarditis (Chan et al, 1991). Occasional patients have presented with isolated lymphadenopathy; perinodal venous thrombosis is sometimes identified histologically (Chan et al, 1991). In some cases, the etiology is obscure.

Histopathology

VTLS is characterized by proliferation of endothelial cells and vascular spaces, which fill and expand the lymph node sinuses (Figs. 28.18 and 28.19). The proliferating cells are characteristically bland, ranging from plump spindle cells to flattened endothelial cells, and frequently associated with fibrosis. The vascular spaces may be rounded, cleft-like, or plexiform (Chan et al, 1991). A pattern of maturation may be present, with transition from central cellular areas to well-formed vascular spaces at the periphery (Fig. 28.20). Extravasated erythrocytes and, rarely, hyaline globules may be present (Chan et al, 1991). The intervening lymphoid tissue is frequently attenuated. Rarely, a

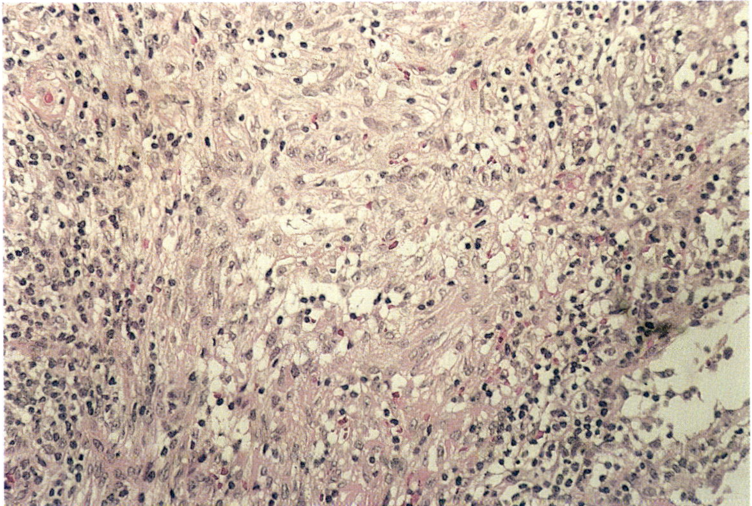

FIGURE 28.18

Vascular transformation of lymph node sinuses showing sinus filled with plump endothelial cells and spindle cells.

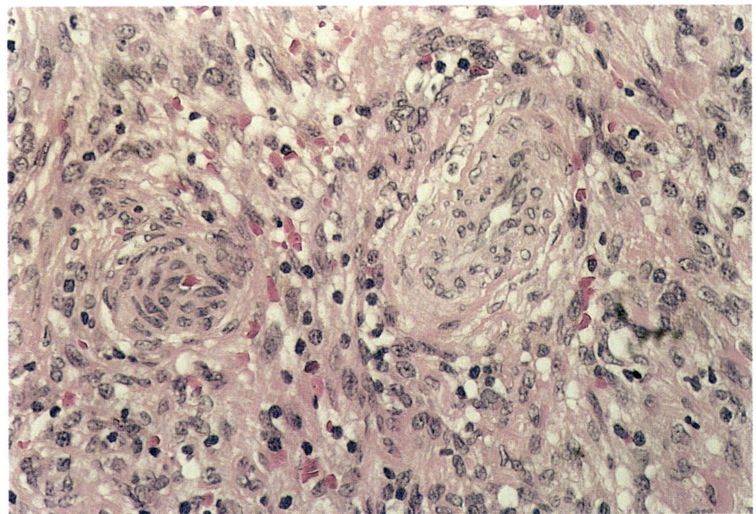

FIGURE 28.19

Vascular transformation of lymph node sinuses showing proliferation of plump spindle cells, mimicking the appearance of Kaposi's sarcoma.

striking nodular proliferation of spindled cells may occur in VTLS, particularly involving retroperitoneal lymph nodes (Cook et al, 1995).

Differential Diagnosis

VTLS may be confused with KS. Attention to the sinusoidal pattern of involvement, presence of fibrosis, maturation to well formed vascular spaces, and absence of fascicles in VTLS usually permits distinction. Hyaline globules, although rarely present in cases of VTLS, are frequently present in KS (Chan et al, 1991; Fukunga and Silverberg,

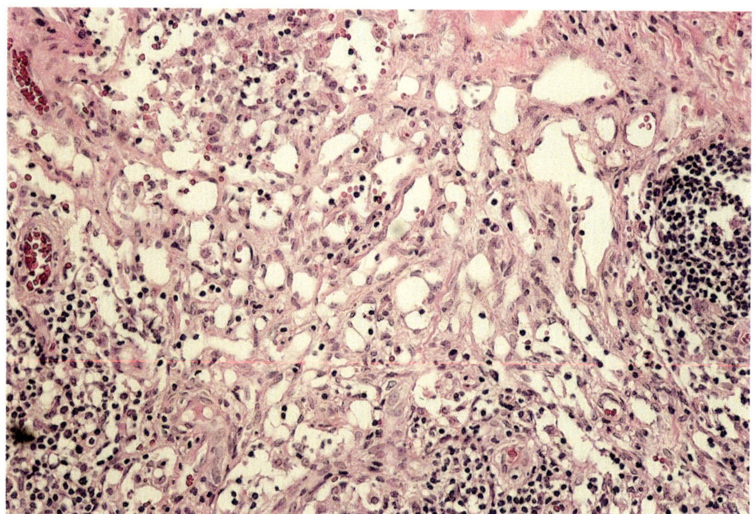

Vascular transformation of lymph node sinuses showing maturation to
well-formed capillary spaces.

1991). Inflammatory pseudotumor is distinguished by prominent involvement of the
lymph node supporting structures and perinodal soft tissue and the presence of numerous admixed inflammatory cells. Intranodal hemorrhagic spindle cell tumor is distinguished by predominant inguinal lymph node involvement, lack of sinusoidal pattern
and vascular spaces, and the presence of amianthoid fibers.

Course and Prognosis

VTLS is benign.

Hemangioma

Lymph node hemangiomas are usually encountered incidentally but occasionally present
as isolated lymphadenopathy. Lymph node hemangiomas consist of circumscribed
masses of vascular proliferation, usually arising from the hilus of the lymph node, with
partial or complete replacement of the lymph node parenchyma (Fig. 28.21). Lymph
node hemangiomas may be of any of the usual histologic types, including capillary,
cavernous, lobular or cellular (Chan et al, 1992). Lymph node hemangiomas are benign;
recurrence has not been reported.

Lymphangioma

Lymph node lymphangiomas occur in association with involvement of extranodal soft
tissue and consist of poorly circumscribed masses of dilated, cystic, endothelial-lined
spaces containing proteinaceous fluid and scattered small lymphocytes (Fig. 28.22). Aggregates of lymphocytes may be present in the fibrous septae separating the cystic
spaces. Lymphangiomas are benign lesions of likely hamartomatous origin.

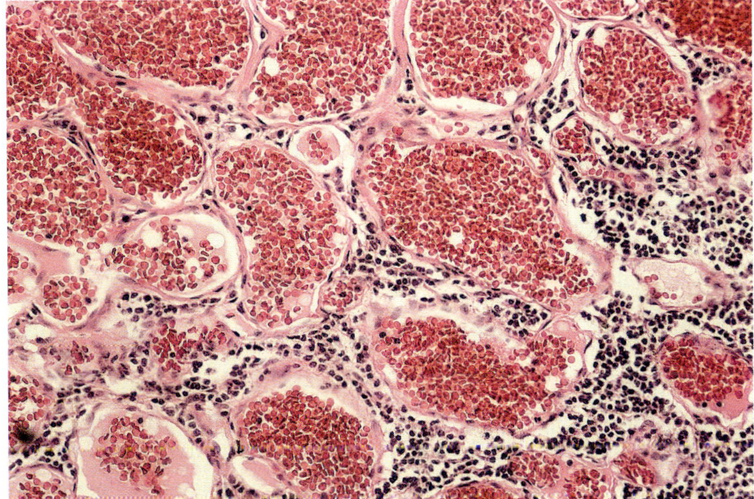

Lymph node hemangioma showing circumscribed mass of well-formed vascular spaces.

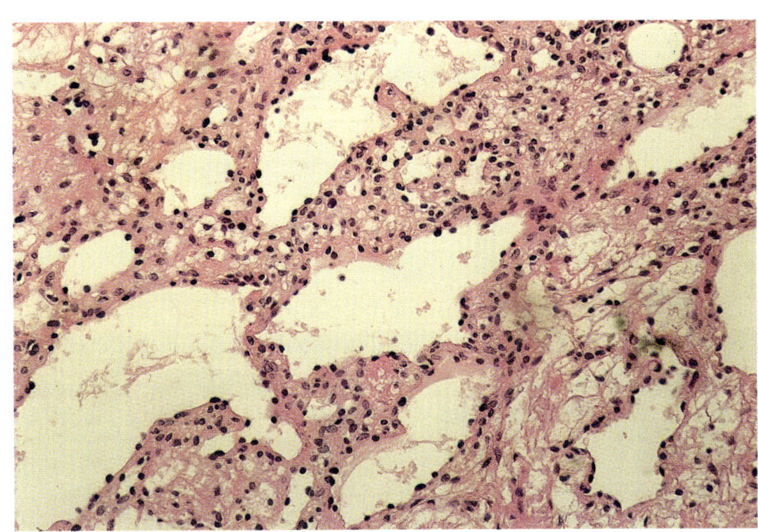

Lymph node lymphangioma showing irregular endothelial-lined spaces containing proteinaceous fluid.

Epithelioid Hemangioma and Hemangioendotheliomas

Lymph node involvement may occur in epithelioid hemangioma (angiolymphoid hyperplasia with eosinophilia) and in epithelioid hemangioendothelioma. Epithelioid hemangioma, characterized by well-formed vascular spaces, lined by plump, epithelioid endothelial cells, with or without an associated infiltrate of eosinophils and lymphocytes, has been frequently confused with Kimura's disease in the past (see Chapter 11). Epithelioid hemangioendothelioma, characterized by cords and strands of vacuolated endothelial cells in a hyaline or myxoid stroma, has been confused with metastatic carcinoma

(Chan et al, 1992). Immunohistochemical studies permit distinction. A distinctive form of hemangioendothelioma occurring in lymph nodes has been termed polymorphous hemangioendothelioma and is characterized by admixture of primitive solid and angiomatous vascular proliferation (Chan et al, 1992; Nascimento et al, 1997). Epithelioid hemangioma is benign; epithelioid and polymorphous hemangioendotheliomas are considered of borderline or low-grade malignancy.

Vascular Proliferations Associated With Castleman's Disease

The association of Kaposi's sarcoma with the multicentric form of Castleman's disease has already been discussed. In addition, the localized form of Castleman's disease has been associated with the development of a poorly characterized vascular neoplasm consisting of an admixture of spindle cells and irregular vascular channels (Gerald et al, 1990). An associated follicular dendritic cell tumor has been reported in one case (Chan et al, 1994). The vascular neoplasms associated with Castleman's disease have exhibited a range of biologic behavior, with metastases and death in two of seven patients in one series (Gerald et al, 1990). Castleman's disease may also occur in association with angiolipomatous hamartoma, a benign proliferation of fat and thick-walled blood vessels (Madero et al, 1986).

Lipomatous Proliferations

Fatty Infiltration

Fatty infiltration of lymph nodes (lymph node lipomatosis) is a frequent phenomenon in axillary and, occasionally, other lymph nodes. The central portion of the lymph node becomes replaced with mature adipose tissue, leaving a compressed crescent of lymph node at the periphery. The etiology of fatty infiltration is unestablished. Fatty infiltration is of no clinical significance but occasionally is the cause of isolated lymph node enlargement.

REFERENCES

Alguacil-Garcia A. Intranodal myofibroblastoma in a submandibular lymph node. A case report. Am J Clin Pathol 97:69–72, 1992.

Chan JKC, Warnke RA, Dorfman RF. Vascular transformation of sinuses in lymph nodes. A study of its morphologic spectrum and distinction from Kaposi's sarcoma. Am J Surg Pathol 15:732–743, 1991.

Chan JKC, Frizzera G, Fletcher CD, Rosai J. Primary vascular tumors of lymph nodes other than Kaposi's sarcoma: Analysis of 39 cases and delineation of two new entities. Am J Surg Pathol 16:335–350, 1992.

Chan JKC, Tsang WY, Pau MY, Tang MC, Pang SW,

Fletcher CD. Lymphangioleiomyomatosis and angiomyolipoma: Closely related entities characterized by hamartomatous proliferations of HMB-45–positive smooth muscle. Histopathology 22:445–455, 1993.

Chan JKC, Tsang WYW, Ng CS. Follicular dendritic cell tumor and vascular neoplasm complicating hyaline-vascular Castleman's disease. Am J Surg Pathol 18:517–525, 1994.

Chang Y, Cesarman E, Pessin MS, Lee F, Culpepper J, Knowles DM, Moore PS. Identification of herpesivirus-like DNA sequences in AIDS-associated Kaposi's sarcoma. Science 266:1865–1869, 1994).

Channer JL, Davies JD. Smooth muscle proliferation in the hilum of superficial lymph nodes. Virchows Arch (A) 406:261–270, 1985.

Chen KTK. Mycobacterial spindle cell pseudotumor of lymph nodes. Am J Surg Pathol 16:276–281, 1992.

Cook PD, Czerniak B, Chan JKC, Mackay B, Ordonez NG, Ayala AG, Rosai J. Nodular spindle-cell vascular transformation of lymph nodes. A benign process occurring predominantly in retroperitoneal lymph nodes draining carcinomas that can simulate Kaposi's sarcoma or metastatic tumor. Am J Surg Pathol 19:1010–1020, 1995.

Davis RE, Warnke RA, Dorfman RF. Inflammatory pseudotumor of lymph nodes. Additional observations and evidence for an inflammatory etiology. Am J Surg Pathol 15:744–756, 1991.

Facchetti F, De Wolf-Peeters C, De Wever I, Frizzera G. Inflammatory pseudotumor of lymph nodes: Immunohistochemical evidence for its fibrohistiocytic nature. Am J Pathol 137:281–289, 1990.

Fukunga M, Silverberg SG. Hyaline globules in Kaposi's sarcoma: A light microscopic and immunohistochemical study. Mod Pathol 4:187–190, 1991.

Gerald W, Kostianovsky W, Rosai J. Development of vascular neoplasia in Castleman's disease. Report of seven cases. Am J Surg Pathol 14:603–614, 1990.

Hsu YK, Rosenstein NB, Parmley TH, Woodruff JD, Elberfeld HT. Leiomyomatosis in pelvic lymph nodes. Obstet Gynecol 57:91s-93s, 1981.

Madero S, Onate JM, Garzon A. Giant lymph node hyperplasia in an angiolipomatous mediastinal mass. Arch Pathol Lab Med 110:853–855, 1986.

McClain KL, Leach CT, Jenson HB, Joshi VV, Pollock BH, Parmley RT, et al. Association of Epstein-Barr virus with leiomyosarcomas in young people with AIDS. N Engl J Med 332:12–18, 1995.

Moore PS, Chang Y. Detection of herpesvirus-like DNA sequences in Kaposi's sarcoma in patients with and without HIV infection. N Engl J Med 332:1181–1185, 1996.

Nascimento AG, Keeney GL, Sciot R, Fletcher CDM. Polymorphous hemangioendothelioma. A report of two cases, one affecting extranodal soft tissues, and review of the literature. Am J Surg Pathol 21:1083–1089, 1997.

Perrone T, De Wolf-Peeters C, Frizzera G. Inflammatory pseudotumor of lymph nodes. A distinctive pattern of nodal reaction. Am J Surg Pathol 12:351–361, 1988.

Rabkin CS, Janz S, Lashi A, Coleman AE, Musaba E, Liotta L, et al. Monoclonal origin of multicentric Kaposi's sarcoma lesions. N Engl J Med 336:988–993, 1997.

Safai B, Mike V, Giraldo G, Beth E, Good RA. Association of Kaposi's sarcoma with second primary malignancies: Possible etiopathogenic implications. Cancer 45:1472–1479, 1980.

Salahuddin SZ, Nakamura S, Biberfeld P, Kaplan MH, Markham PD, Larsson L, Gallo RC. Angiogenic properties of Kaposi's sarcoma-derived cells after long-term culture in vitro. Science 242:430–433, 1988.

Soulier J, Grollet L, Oksenhendler P, Cacoub P, Cazals-Hatem D, Babinet P, et al. Kaposi's sarcoma-associated herpesvirus-like DNA sequences in multicentric Castleman's disease. Blood 86:1276–1280, 1995.

Starasoler L, Vuitch F, Albores-Saavedra J. Intranodal leiomyoma. Another distinctive primary spindle cell neoplasm of lymph node. Am J Clin Pathol 95:858–862, 1991.

Strauchen JA, Hauser AD, Burstein D, Jimenez R, Moore PS, Chang Y. Body cavity-based malignant lymphoma containing Kaposi sarcoma-associated herpesvirus in an HIV-negative man with previous Kaposi sarcoma. Ann Intern Med 125:822–825, 1996.

Suster S, Rosai J. Intranodal hemorrhagic spindle cell tumor with "amianthoid" fibers. Report of six cases of a distinctive mesenchymal neoplasm of the inguinal region that simulates Kaposi's sarcoma. Am J Surg Pathol 13:347–357, 1989.

Weiss SE, Gnepp DR, Bratthauer GL. Palisaded myofibroblastoma. A benign mesenchymal tumor of lymph node. Am J Surg Pathol 13:341–346, 1989.

29

Lymph Node Inclusions

Lymph node inclusions refer to the presence in lymph nodes of heterologous elements normally not found in lymph nodes including a variety of epithelial, glandular, mesothelial, and nevus cell elements. Lymph node inclusions result from developmental abnormalities (embryologic rests), metaplasia of entrapped mesothelium, or benign transport of heterologous elements. Lymph node inclusions are generally not of clinical significance but must be carefully distinguished from metastatic tumors which they may closely resemble. Lymph node inclusions may rarely be the explanation for neoplasms of heterologous elements arising in lymph nodes (Shenoy et al, 1987).

Müllerian Inclusions

Inclusions of Müllerian epithelium are not infrequent in pelvic lymph nodes in women, occasionally occurring in extrapelvic and, rarely, supradiaphragmatic lymph nodes as well (Henley et al, 1995). Müllerian inclusions most likely arise by metaplasia of entrapped mesothelial cells; however, benign transport may also account for some cases. Müllerian inclusions are usually confined to the lymph node capsule and paracortex, but occasionally more extensive involvement occurs (Kheir et al, 1981). Müllerian inclusions typically consist of round or irregular, glandular, cystic, or papillary structures composed of ciliated columnar epithelium (Figs. 29.1 and 29.2). Müllerian inclusions are surrounded by a narrow zone of collagenous stroma or are "naked," surrounded by lymphoid tissue. The epithelium resembles that of endosalpingiosis or salpingitis isthmica nodosa, which may also be present (Shen et al, 1983). Müllerian inclusions may also contain endometrial, endocervical, or squamous epithelium; psammoma bodies may be present. Müllerian inclusions must be distinguished from metastatic adenocarcinoma. Müllerian inclusions characteristically exhibit little or no cytologic atypia or mitoses and, in contrast to metatstatic adenocarcinoma, destructive growth and desmoplasia are

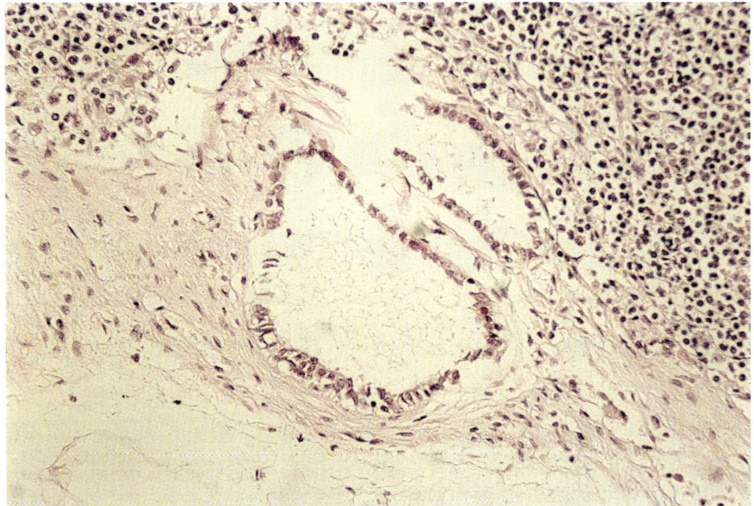

Müllerian inclusion showing glandular structure within capsule of a pelvic lymph node.

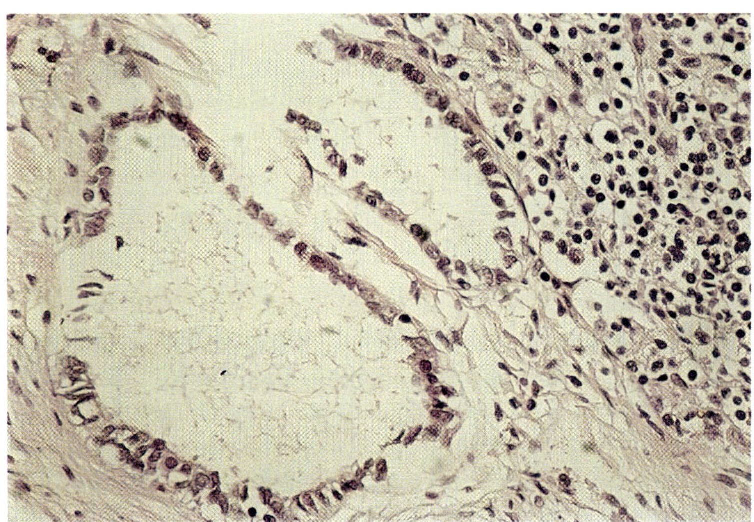

Müllerian inclusion, higher magnification, showing benign columnar epithelium surrounded by a zone of condensed stroma.

not a feature. Other conditions related to Müllerian inclusions include endometriosis, distinguished by the presence of endometrial stroma, frequently with evidence of old or recent hemorrhage, in addition to endometrial glands; leiomyomatosis, discussed in Chapter 28; and ectopic deciduosis, associated with pregnancy (Zaytsev and Taxy, 1987). The latter, characterized by subcapsular masses of large, polyhedral, pale to vacuolated cells, with prominent cell borders, may mimic metastatic squamous carcinoma; the lack of mitoses, keratinization, or desmoplasia permits distinction.

Mesothelial Inclusions

The presence of mesothelial cells in mediastinal and abdominal lymph node sinuses may cause confusion with metastatic carcinoma, morphologically and immunohistochemically (Brooks et al, 1990; Clement et al, 1996). Mesothelial cells reach mediastinal lymph nodes by drainage from inflamed pleural spaces and mimic the cytokeratin positivity of metastatic carcinoma; ultrastructural studies permit distinction (Brooks et al, 1990). Hyperplasia of mesothelial rests in abdominal lymph nodes may mimic metastatic papillary ovarian tumors (Clement et al, 1996).

Salivary Inclusions

Inclusions of salivary gland ducts and acini in cervical lymph nodes are not infrequent and are believed to have an embryologic basis; salivary inclusions are particularly frequent in juxtaparotid lymph nodes. The presence of benign salivary epithelium in lymph nodes may mimic the benign lymphoepithelial lesions of Sjögren's syndrome; hyperplasia of juxtaparotid lymph nodes with formation of epimyoepithelial islands, resembling those of Sjögren's syndrome, and lymphoepithelial cysts occurs frequently in patients with AIDS (Ryan et al, 1985). Lymph node salivary inclusions may also give rise to extraparotid salivary gland tumors, including Warthin's tumor and other benign and malignant ectopic salivary gland neoplasms (Luna and Monheit, 1988; Snyderman et al, 1986).

Thyroid Inclusions

The occurrence of benign thyroid follicles in cervical lymph nodes (lateral aberrant thyroid) and its relation to metastatic papillary thyroid carcinoma is controversial. Microscopically benign thyroid follicles are identified in fewer than 1% of cervical lymph nodes examined routinely (Gerard-Marchant and Caillou, 1981); but they are found in a higher proportion of extensively studied cases (Meyer and Steinberg, 1969). Some authors have expressed the view that the presence of thyroid follicles in cervical lymph nodes always indicates metastases from an occult papillary thyroid carcinoma. This view seems extreme. We accept the presence of a few subcapsular thyroid follicles (generally 20 or fewer) in a cervical lymph node as a benign inclusion, in the absence of cytologic atypia, papillary structures, or psammoma bodies. Lymph nodes extensively replaced by thyroid follicles, however, almost always indicate metastatic papillary thyroid carcinoma.

Mammary Inclusions

Epithelial inclusions of presumed mammary duct origin are occasionally identified in axillary lymph nodes (Fisher et al, 1994; Holdsworth et al, 1988). These may show changes reminiscent of fibrocystic disease of the breast, including cyst formation and squamous and apocrine metaplasia. The presence of myoepithelial cells and double-layered epithelium is helpful in distinction from metastatic adenocarcinoma. The occur-

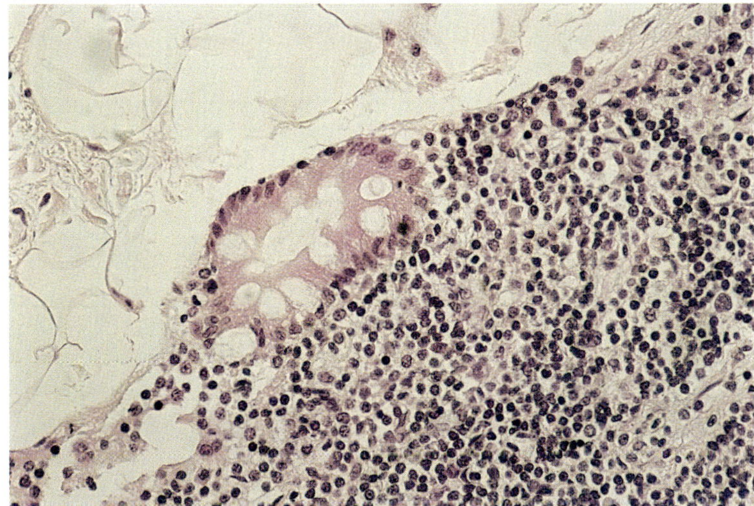

FIGURE 29.3

Inclusion of a benign colonic gland in a mesenteric lymph node following colonoscopic biopsies. Phenomenon is an example of benign transport.

rence of epithelial inclusion is a potential pitfall in the use of immunohistochemistry to detect micrometastases of breast carcinoma in axillary lymph node dissections. Malignant transformation of ectopic mammary epithelium in axillary lymph nodes has been reported but is a rare event (Walker and Fechner, 1982). Benign transport of intraductal papilloma of the breast to axillary lymph nodes has been described (Ackerman and Rosai, 1974).

Other Epithelial Inclusions

Glandular inclusions are rarely encountered in abdominal lymph nodes as a result of pancreatic heterotopia (Carr et al, 1987) or benign renal tubular inclusions containing Tamm-Horsfall protein in children with Wilms' tumor (Weeks et al, 1990). Benign transport of colonic glands to mesenteric lymph nodes has been reported following colonoscopic biopsy (Perrone, 1985), and we have seen a similar case (Fig. 29.3).

Nevus Cells

Benign nevus cell aggregates are encountered in 0.33–7.3% of lymph node dissections; the larger number reflects the incidence in patients undergoing lymph node resections for malignant melanoma (Bautista et al, 1994). Nevus cell aggregates are found predominantly in the capsules of superficial lymph nodes, including axillary, inguinal, and cervical lymph nodes. The nevus cells resemble those of common intradermal nevi, consisting of nests or strands of cytologically bland, round to ovoid cells, with round nuclei, inconspicuous nucleoli, moderately abundant eosinophilic to clear cytoplasm, and scant melanin pigment (Figs. 29.4 and 29.5). Mitoses and nuclear pleomorphism are absent. Melanocytic derivation is confirmed by the presence of melanosomes and S100 positi-

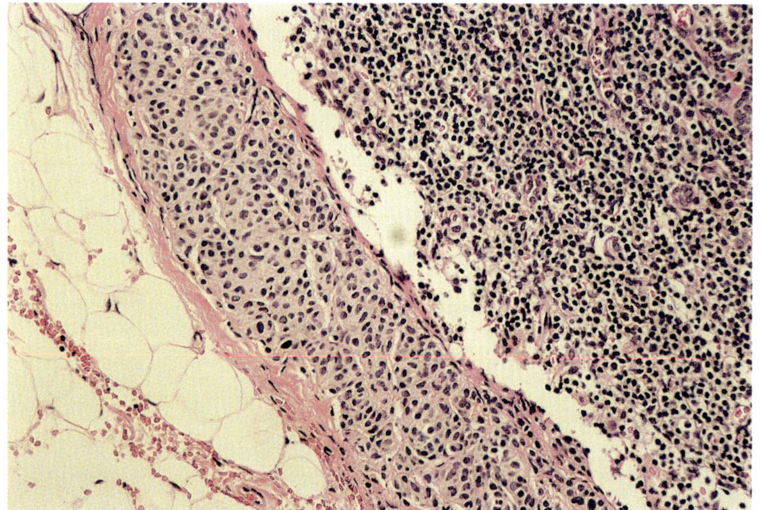

FIGURE 29.4

Nevus cell inclusion in the capsule of a lymph node.

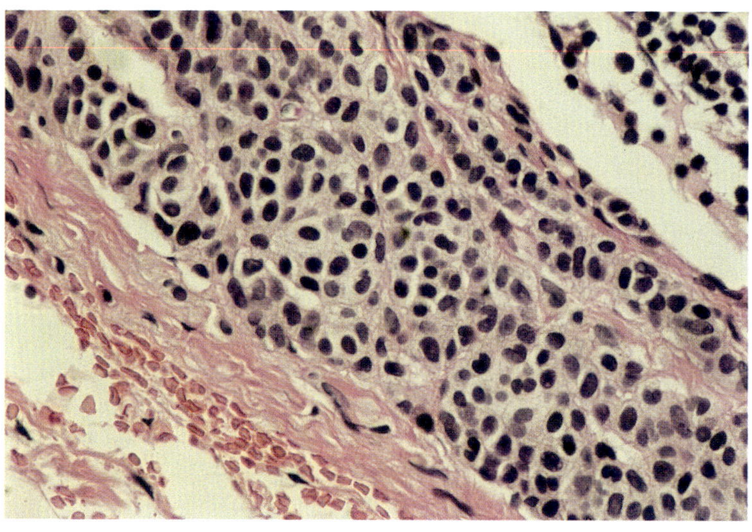

FIGURE 29.5

Nevus cell inclusion in the capsule of a lymph node, higher magnification, showing cytologically bland nevus cells with round to ovoid nuclei, inconspicuous nucleoli, and eosinophilic cytoplasm.

vity (Bautista et al, 1994). The presence of nevus cell aggregates in lymph nodes is most likely accounted for by arrested migration from the neural crest; however, benign transport from cutaneous nevi may also occur. Nevus cell aggregates in lymph nodes are not generally of clinical significance but must be distinguished from metastatic melanoma or carcinoma. Nevus cell aggregates in axillary lymph nodes may mimic the appearance of metastatic lobular breast carcinoma. The characteristic capsular location and, in difficult cases, immunohistochemical study for cytokeratin and S100 protein usually permit distinction. The occurrence of nevus cells in lymph nodes may account for some cases of malignant melanoma of unknown primary site (Shenoy et al, 1987). Blue nevi characterized by abundantly pigmented spindled or dendritic melanocytes also occur in the capsule of lymph nodes with or without simultaneous skin involvement (Epstein et al, 1984). Benign transport of cellular blue nevi to regional lymph nodes also occurs (Lambert and Brodkin, 1984).

REFERENCES

Ackerman LV, Rosai J. Surgical Pathology. 5th ed. St. Louis, C.V. Mosby, 1974.

Bautista NC, Cohen S, Anders KH. Benign melanocytic nevus cells in axillary lymph nodes. A prospective incidence and immunohistochemical study with literature review. Am J Clin Pathol 102:102–108, 1994.

Brooks JSJ, LiVolsi VA, Pietra GG. Mesothelial cell inclusions in mediastinal lymph nodes mimicking metastatic carcinoma. Am J Clin Pathol 93:741–748, 1990.

Carr RF, Tang CK, Carrozza MJ, Rodriguez FC. Unusual cystic epithelial choristoma in a celiac lymph node. Hum Pathol 18:866–869, 1987.

Clement PB, Young RH, Oliva E, Sumner HW, Scully RE. Hyperplastic mesothelial cells within abdominal lymph nodes: mimic of metastatic ovarian carcinoma and serous borderline tumor—A report of two cases associated with ovarian neoplasms. Mod Pathol 9:879–886, 1996.

Epstein JI, Erlandson RA, Rosin PP. Nodal blue nevi. A study of three cases. Am J Surg Pathol 8:907–915, 1984.

Fisher CJ, Hill S, Millis RR. Benign lymph node inclusions mimicking metastatic carcinoma. J Clin Pathol 47:245–247, 1994.

Gerard-Marchant R, Caillou B. Thyroid inclusions in cervical lymph nodes. Clin Endocrinol Metab 10:337–349, 1981.

Henley JD, Michael HB, English GW, Roth LM. Benign mullerian lymph node inclusions. An unsusual case with implications for pathogenesis and review of the literature. Arch Pathol Lab Med 119:841–844, 1995.

Holdsworth PJ, Hopkinson JM, Leveson SH. Benign axillary epithelial lymph node inclusions—A histological pitfall. Histopathology 13:226–228, 1988.

Kheir SM, Mann WJ, Wilkerson JA. Glandular inclusions in lymph nodes. The problem of extensive involvement and relationship to salpingitis. Am J Surg Pathol 5:353–359, 1981.

Lambert WC, Brodkin RH. Nodal and subcutaneous cellular blue nevi. A pseudometastasizing pseudomelanoma. Arch Dermatol 120:367–370, 1984.

Luna M, Monheit J. Salivary gland neoplasms arising in lymph nodes: A clinicopathologic analysis of 13 cases (abstract). Lab Invest 58:58a, 1988.

Meyer JS, Steinberg LS. Microscopically benign thyroid follicles in cervical lymph nodes. Serial section study of lymph node inclusions and entire thryroid gland in 5 cases. Cancer 24:302–311, 1969.

Perrone T. Embolization of benign colonic glands to mesenteric lymph nodes (letter). Am J Surg Pathol 9:538–541, 1985.

Ryan JR, Ioachim HL, Marmer J, Loubeau JM. Acquired immune deficiency syndrome-related lymphadenopathies presenting in salivary gland lymph nodes. Arch Otolaryngol 111:554–556, 1985.

Shen SC, Bansal M, Purrazzella R, Malviya V, Strauss L. Benign glandular inclusions in lymph nodes, endosalpingiosis, and salpingitis isthmicus nodosa in a young girl with clear cell adenocarcinoma of the cervix. Am J Surg Pathol 7:293–300, 1983.

Shenoy BV, Fort L, Benjamin SP. Malignant melanoma primary in lymph node. The case of the missing link. Am J Surg Pathol 11:140–146, 1987.

Snyderman C, Johnson JT, Barnes EL. Extraparotid Warthin's tumor. Otolaryngol Head Neck Surg 94:169–175, 1986.

Walker AN, Fechner RE. Papillary carcinoma arising from ectopic breast tissue in an axillary lymph node. Diagn Gynecol Obstet 4:141–145, 1982.

Weeks DA, Beckwith JB, Mierau GW. Benign nodal lesions mimicking metastases from pediatric renal neoplasms: a report of the National Wilms' Study Pathology Center. Hum Pathol 21:1239–1244, 1990.

Zaytsev P, Taxy JB. Pregnancy-associated ectopic decidua. Am J Surg Pathol 11:526–530, 1987.

30

Lymph Node Metastases

Lymph nodes are a frequent site of metastases of nonhematopoietic malignant tumors. Lymph node metastases occur most frequently in carcinoma and melanoma but also occur in some sarcomas, including epithelioid sarcoma, clear cell sarcoma, synovial sarcoma, and, occasionally, malignant fibrous histiocytoma (Enzinger and Weiss, 1995). Lymph node metastases are a manifestation of regional or systemic dissemination. Lymph node metastases may be diagnosed in lymph nodes removed for diagnostic evaluation in patients presenting with unexplained lymphadenopathy or in lymph nodes removed at staging or therapeutic lymphadenectomy in patients with a previously diagnosed malignant neoplasm. Recognition of lymph node metastases and distinction from malignant lymphoma is of major clinical importance because of differences in therapy and prognosis (Hainsworth and Greco, 1993).

Detection of Lymph Node Metastases

The pathologist is frequently called upon to examine lymph nodes removed at staging or therapeutic lymphadenectomy for the presence of lymph node metastases. Regional lymph node dissections are performed for a variety of malignant neoplasms, including squamous carcinoma of the head and neck, breast carcinoma, carcinoma of the gastrointestinal tract, testicular carcinoma, carcinomas of the prostate and bladder, carcinomas of the uterus and cervix, and cutaneous malignant melanoma. Routine lymph node dissections are rarely performed in cases of sarcoma because of the relatively low incidence of lymph node metastases (Enzinger and Weiss, 1995). The assessment of lymph node metastases is conventionally performed by histopathology. Identification of early lymph node metastases (micrometastases) is aided by the application of newer techniques, including immunohistochemistry (Ambrosch and Brinck, 1996; Cochran et al, 1988) and molecular biology (Brennan et al, 1995). Immunohistochemical detection of micrometastases by staining for the presence of cytokeratin- or EMA-positive cells in lymph nodes removed for carcinoma of the breast, colon, or head and neck, or of S100-positive cells in lymph nodes removed for malignant melanoma demonstrates the presence of positive cells in approximately 10% of cases which were negative by conventional histopathological assessment (Ambrosch and Brinck, 1996; Cochran et al, 1988). The clinical significance, however, of micrometastases is uncertain and may be dependent, in part, on other factors, such as tumor size (Rosen et al, 1981; Rosen and Obermann, 1993). Interpretation of immunohistochemical studies on lymph nodes is complicated by the presence of S100-positive interdigitating reticulum cells and cytokeratin-positive fibroblastic reticulum cells in normal and hyperplastic lymph nodes (Domagala et al, 1992; Gould et al 1995) and the occasional presence of cytokeratin-positive mesothelial cells in mediastinal lymph nodes (Brooks et al, 1990). Molecular assessment of micrometastases promises to be a sensitive and specific technique (Brennan et al, 1995). In squamous carcinoma of the head and neck, analysis of cervical lymph nodes for the presence of p53 gene mutations using the polymerase chain reaction demonstrated the presence of tumor cells in 21% of lymph nodes which were negative by histopathologic assessment (Brennan et al, 1995).

Histopathologic Assessment of Lymph Node Metastases

Lymph node metastases usually resemble the primary tumor from which they arose, but they may be more or less well differentiated. Some metastatic tumors present an unusually well differentiated appearance. Metastatic squamous carcinoma of the head and neck, for example, may present as a cystic mass, mimicking a branchial cleft cyst; indeed, most examples of squamous carcinoma arising in branchial cleft cysts are cystic lymph node metastases. Lymph node metastases are usually first evident histologically in the subcapsular sinus, where tumor cells entering the lymph node via the afferent lymphatic channels are first deposited (Fig. 30.1). Lymph node metastases eventually result in partial or complete effacement of the lymph node architecture; extensive lymph node involvement and invasion of extranodal soft tissue results in a confluent mass of "matted" lymph nodes, with discrete lymph nodes no longer recognizable. Occasionally, metastases remain confined to the lymph node sinuses, with preservation of the lymph node architecture, resulting in a histopathologic picture which may be confused with sinus histiocytosis; conversely, sinus histiocytosis may also rarely mimic metastatic signet ring cell adenocarcinoma (Gould et al, 1989).

Distinction from Malignant Lymphoma

Not infrequently, the pathologist is confronted with an undifferentiated malignant tumor in a lymph node. Distinction between lymph node metastases and malignant lymphoma is of major clinical importance because of differences in therapy and prognosis and the potential curability of some malignant lymphomas, even when advanced (Hainsworth and Greco, 1993). Metastases of poorly differentiated nonhematopoietic neoplasms, in general, have a poor prognosis; however, some specific subtypes may have a favorable response to specific therapy (Hainsworth et al, 1988; Richardson et al, 1981). Metastases

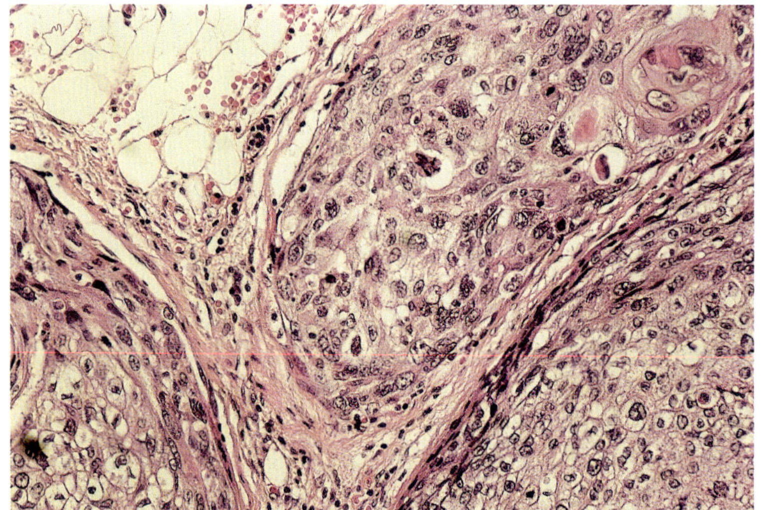

FIGURE
30.1

Metastatic squamous cell carcinoma showing involvement of the subcapsular sinus and afferent lymphatics.

of nonhematopoietic malignant neoplasms may mimic the histopathologic features of malignant lymphoma; conversely, some malignant lymphomas have histopathologic features, such as signet ring cells and sinusoidal involvement, which are frequently found in metastatic tumors. Metastatic carcinomas with prominent admixed inflammatory cells, such as giant cell carcinoma of the lung, squamous carcinoma of the head and neck, and nasopharyngeal carcinoma, may mimic Hodgkin's disease (Zarate-Osorno et al, 1992). Histopathologic features favoring a lymph node metastasis include an organoid or alveolar growth pattern, nesting of the tumor cells, cohesive growth pattern, the presence of spindled tumor cells, nuclear molding or extensive crush artifact. Nevertheless, each of these features may be seen in malignant lymphoma (Chan et al, 1990). Recognition of lymph node metastases is aided by application of histochemical stains (PAS with and without diastase digestion, melanin, reticulin) and ultrastructural studies. PAS-positive diastase-resistant mucin, PAS-positive diastase-sensitive glycogen, melanin, and an organoid pattern of reticulin fibers are features favoring a metastatic nonhematopoietic malignant neoplasm. Ultrastructural studies revealing evidence of epithelial (tonofilaments, desmosomes), neuroendocrine (neurosecretory granules), or melanocytic (melanosomes, premelanosomes) differentiation similarly favor a metastatic nonhematopoietic neoplasm.

Immunohistochemical Studies

Immunohistochemical studies have had a major impact on tumor pathology and are routinely applied to the distinction of lymph node metastases from malignant lymphoma (Table 30.1). Most, but not all, malignant lymphomas are positive for CD45RB (LCA) in deparaffinized tissue or frozen sections. Membranous staining for CD45RB is specific for hematolymphoid neoplasms and firmly establishes the hematolymphoid lineage of a malignant neoplasm. The absence of CD45RB staining, however, does not exclude the diagnosis of malignant lymphoma; lack of CD45RB staining may be due to poor antigen preservation in deparaffinized tissue or due to absence of CD45 expression in some lymphomas, particularly CD30-positive anaplastic large cell lymphomas. The presence of staining for cytokeratin, conversely, usually indicates an epithelial origin of a malignant neoplasm; however, CD30-positive anaplastic large cell lymphomas may also express cytokeratin (Gustmann et al, 1991). EMA is expressed on the cells of a variety of hematolymphoid neoplasms, including anaplastic large cell lymphomas, plasmacytomas, and nodular lymphocyte predominance Hodgkin's disease, as well as carcinomas, and is therefore of limited differential value. CD30 is consistently expressed on the cells of anaplastic large cell lymphoma and Hodgkin's disease and is rarely expressed on non-hematolymphoid neoplasms. CD30 staining has been reported in embryonal carcinoma and nasopharyngeal carcinoma, as has faint cytoplasmic staining in occasional salivary and pancreatic carcinomas and melanomas; CD30 staining alone, therefore, should not be used in distinguishing these neoplasms from anaplastic large cell lymphoma (Falini et al, 1995). CD15, expressed on the Reed-Sternberg cells of Hodgkin's disease and some peripheral T cell non-Hodgkin's lymphomas, is also expressed on many carcinomas (Sheibani et al, 1986). Application of a battery of immunohistochemical studies, therefore, is necessary for accurate diagnosis, and should include, at a minimum, CD45RB (LCA), cytokeratin (CAM5.2), CD30, and S100. In difficult or ambiguous cases, molecular studies for the presence of immunoglobulin or T cell antigen receptor gene rearrangements may be helpful; however, the absence of a gene rearrangement does not exclude a diagnosis of malignant lymphoma, since some lymphomas, particularly high-grade T cell lymphomas and anaplastic large cell lymphomas, may lack gene rearrangements (Kneba et al, 1991).

Table 30.1 Antibodies Useful in the Differential Diagnosis of Hematopoietic and Nonhematopoietic Malignant Neoplasms

Antibody	Hematopoietic Neoplasms	Nonhematopoietic Neoplasms
CD45RB (LCA)	Most (1)	None
CD15	Hodgkin's disease T cell lymphoma (some)	Adenocarcinoma
CD30	Anaplastic large cell lymphoma Hodgkin's disease	Embryonal carcinoma Nasopharyngeal carcinoma Melanoma (faint) Other carcinoma (faint)
Cytokeratin	Anaplastic large cell lymphoma	Carcinoma Melanoma, sarcoma (some)
EMA	Anaplastic large cell lymphoma LP Hodgkin's disease Plasmacytoma	Carcinoma Sarcoma (some)
S100 Protein	Interdigitating reticulum cell tumor Langerhans' cell histiocytosis True histiocytic lymphoma	Melanoma Carcinoma (some) Sarcoma (some)
013	Lymphoblastic lymphoma Lymphoblastic leukemia Thymocytes (in thymomas)	Ewing's tumor PNET

(1) Hodgkin's disease of classical type and anaplastic large cell lymphoma are frequently negative.

Differential Diagnosis of Lymph Node Metastases

Detailed consideration of the differential diagnosis of the neoplasms which may be metastatic to lymph nodes is beyond the scope of this volume, and the reader is referred to any textbook of surgical pathology. The differential diagnosis, however, of selected malignant neoplasms which frequently metastasize to lymph nodes and may be confused with malignant lymphoma will be considered.

Pediatric Round Cell Neoplasms

The round cell neoplasms of childhood classically include neuroblastoma, Ewing's tumor, primitive neuroectodermal tumor (PNET), Wilms' tumor, and embryonal rhabdomyosarcoma; to these may be added the intraabdominal desmoplastic round cell tumor, a tumor of uncertain histogenesis which shares histopathologic features of the round cell neoplasms (Gerald et al, 1991). Ewing's tumor and PNET share the t(11;22) chromosome translocation and are closely related tumors (Delattre et al, 1994). These round cell neoplasms of childhood must be distinguished from hematopoietic neoplasms, including lymphoblastic lymphoma, Burkitt's lymphoma, and acute lymphocytic leukemia, which are also prevalent in childhood. Histopathologic features are helpful in differential diagnosis. Neuroblastoma typically demonstrates neurofibrillary stroma and Homer-Wright rosettes, the latter consisting of a ring of nuclei surrounding a central mass of neurofibrillary material, composed ultrastructurally of axonal processes (Fig. 30.2); rosette-like structures and fibrillary material, however, are also rarely seen in lymphomas (Tsang et al, 1992). Ewing's tumor frequently demonstrates a lobular or filigree pattern, with empty-appearing nuclei with finely dispersed chromatin, inconspicuous nucleoli, and scant mitoses. Ewing's tumor is frequently positive for glycogen with the PAS stain and diastase digestion. Neuroblastomas and rhabdomyosarcomas may also be rich in glycogen; however, lymphomas are usually not. Immunohistochemical studies have proven particularly useful in the classification of the round cell neoplasms of childhood. Neuroblastomas are frequently positive for neuron specific enolase (NSE), neurofilament protein, and chromogranin; embryonal rhabdomyosarcomas are positive for desmin and myoglobin; Ewing's tumor is positive for vimentin; PNET and occasionally Ewing's tumor express neural markers (NSE, Leu 7, synaptophysin). Ewing's tumor and PNET consistently express the MIC2 protein (CD99) recognized by monoclonal antibody 013; 013 positivity is also observed in lymphoblastic lymphoma, acute lymphocytic leukemia, and thymocytes in the normal thymus and thymomas, and appears to correlate with TdT positivity (Robertson et al, 1997).

Malignant Melanoma

Metastases of malignant melanoma are notoriously variable in appearance and may be composed of spindle cells, spindle and epithelioid cells, epithelioid cells, or round cells, with varying degrees of pleomorphism (Fig. 30.3). Metastases of malignant melanoma are frequently amelanotic and may be confused with metastatic carcinoma, sarcoma, or lymphoma. Clues to the correct diagnosis include the presence of a focal organoid or nested pattern, prominent eosinophilic nucleoli, admixture of spindle and epithelioid cells, and nuclear pseudoinclusions, the latter consisting of invaginations of cytoplasm

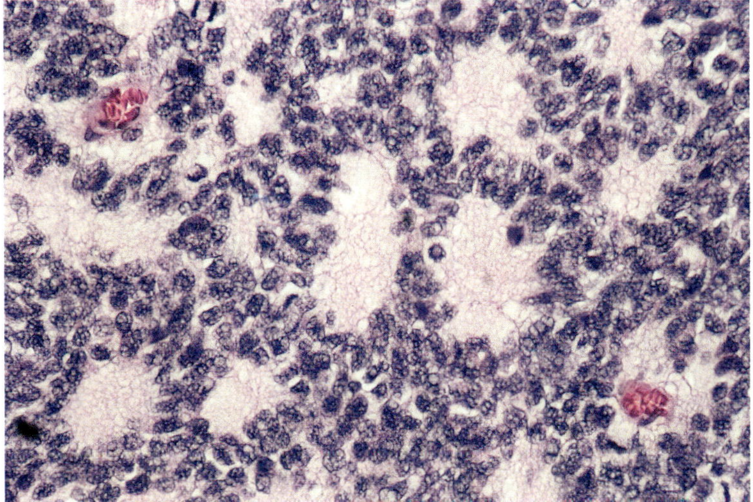

Metastatic neuroblastoma showing Homer-Wright rosettes.

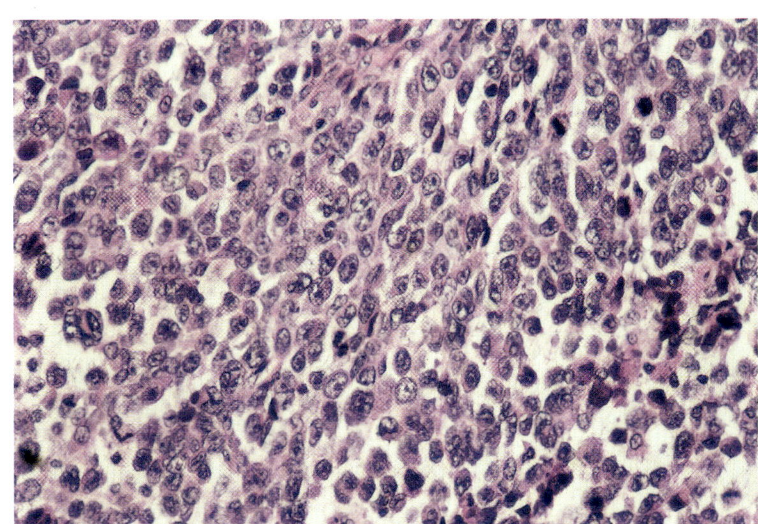

Metastatic malignant melanoma may exhibit an array of histologic patterns and mimic lymphoma, carcinoma, or sarcoma. Immunohistochemical studies for S100 protein and HMB45 are an important aid to diagnosis.

into the nucleus. Special studies aid in diagnosis. The melanin stain (Fontana-Masson) may be positive, even in cases without obvious pigment, and ultrastructural studies may reveal melanosomes or premelanosomes. Immunohistochemical studies are particularly useful in diagnosis. Melanomas are positive for S100 protein, usually demonstrating cytoplasmic and/or nuclear staining, and are frequently positive for the melanoma-associated antigen, HMB45. Melanomas are also positive for vimentin and, occasionally, for cytokeratin. S100 is not specific for melanoma, however, and S100 positivity is also

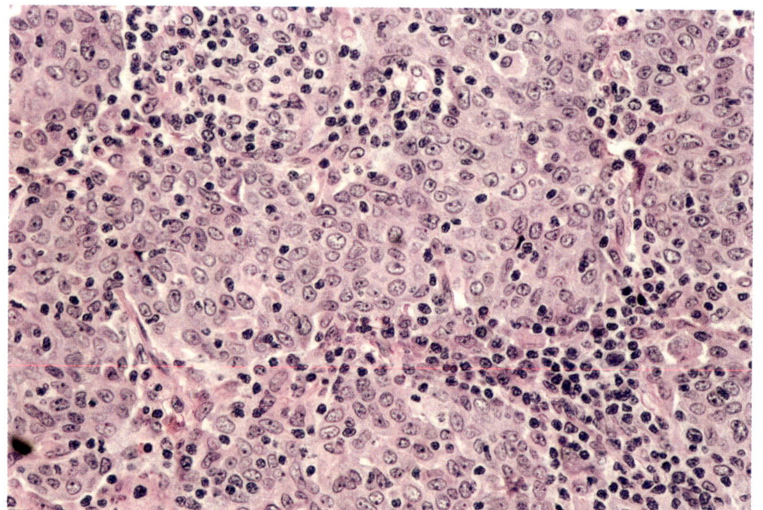

FIGURE
30.4

Metastatic nasopharyngeal carcinoma is composed of undifferentiated cells with a syncytial growth pattern, prominent nucleoli, and lymphoid stroma. Immunohistochemical studies are positive for cytokeratin.

seen in some carcinomas, sarcomas, and interdigitating reticulum cell tumors (Weiss et al, 1990).

Nasopharyngeal Carcinoma

Nasopharyngeal carcinoma (NPC) is a tumor of adults which occasionally also affects children and is particularly prevalent in the Far East. NPC is highly associated with Epstein-Barr virus, which can be demonstrated in the tumor cells of almost all cases. Patients with NPC frequently present with cervical lymphadenopathy due to lymph node metastases; the nasopharyngeal tumor is frequently clinically inapparent and the diagnosis is established on lymph node biopsy. Lymph node involvement in NPC is characterized by infiltration by sheets and clusters of large, undifferentiated-appearing cells with prominent eosinophilic nucleoli and a syncytial arrangement (Fig. 30.4); in some cases spindle cells predominate. The tumor cells are characteristically associated with an infiltrate of small lymphocytes and plasma cells (hence the previous designation of lymphoepithelioma for this tumor); in some cases eosinophils are prominent, mimicking Hodgkin's disease (Zarate-Osorno et al, 1992). Although NPC presents an undifferentiated light microscopic appearance, the tumor cells demonstrate evidence of squamous epithelial differentiation on ultrastructural and immunohistochemical studies. The tumor cells are positive for cytokeratin and EBV latent membrane protein; EBV genomes are also detected by molecular studies. Lymphoepithelioma-like carcinomas, occurring at sites outside the nasopharynx, including the lung and thymus, resemble NPC morphologically and are also associated with EBV (Leyvraz et al, 1985). NPC has been reported to express CD30 in some cases; CD30 staining alone, therefore, may not reliably distinguish NPC from anaplastic large cell lymphoma or Hodgkin's disease (Falini et al, 1995).

Neuroendocrine Carcinomas

Neuroendocrine carcinomas, including small cell lung carcinoma, large cell neuroendocrine carcinoma of the lung, small cell carcinoma of extrapulmonary sites, and Merkel cell carcinoma frequently present with lymph node metastases. Neuroendocrine carcinomas may present as metastatic disease, without an identifiable primary tumor (Hainsworth et al, 1988). Small cell carcinoma is most frequently encountered and usually arises in the lung but may also arise in a wide variety of extrapulmonary sites including the gastrointestinal tract, upper airways, salivary glands, thymus, uterus and cervix, bladder, and prostate (Ibrahim et al, 1984). Lymph node metastases of small cell carcinoma are characterized by hyperchromatic, round to ovoid or spindled cells, with scant cytoplasm, granular chromatin, and inconspicuous nucleoli (Fig. 30.5). The cells of small cell carcinoma are approximately two to four times the size of a small lymphocyte, or similar in size to the cells of large cell lymphoma. Histologic variants of small cell lung carcinoma include small cell carcinoma (formerly oat cell or lymphocyte-like and intermediate type), mixed small cell/large cell carcinoma, and combined small cell carcinoma, the latter containing squamous or adenocarcinomatous elements (Hirsch et al, 1988). An organoid pattern, nuclear molding, crush artifact, streaming of the nuclei, and perivascular deposition of hematoxylinophilic material (Azzopardi effect) are features which aid in distinction from malignant lymphoma. In difficult cases, and particularly in small, crushed biopsies, immunohistochemical studies are helpful. Small cell carcinomas are positive for cytokeratin, negative for CD45RB, and frequently express neuroendocrine markers, including NSE, chromogranin, and synaptophysin (Travis et al, 1991).

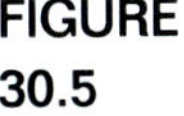

FIGURE 30.5

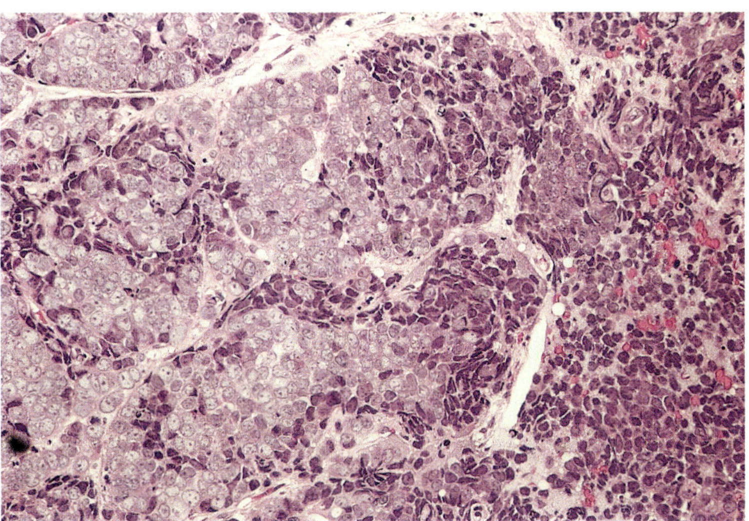

Metastatic small cell lung carcinoma is composed of hyperchromatic round to ovoid cells with granular chromatin, inconspicuous nucleoli, and scant cytoplasm. "Crush" artifact and streaming of the nuclei are frequent features.

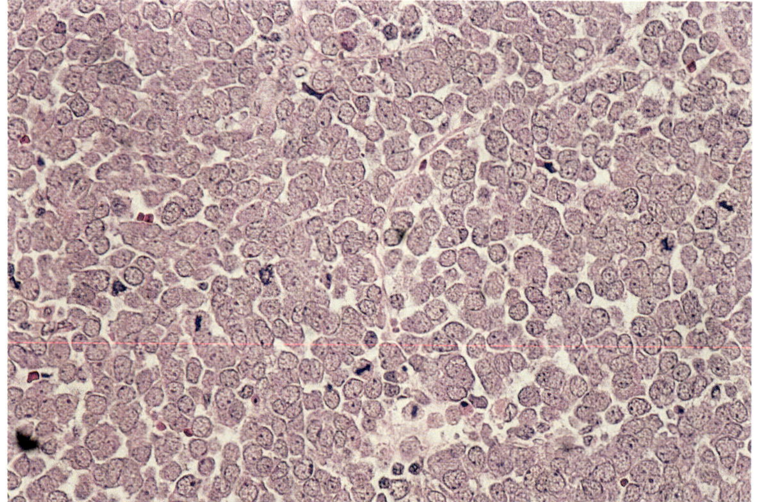

FIGURE
30.6

Metastatic Merkel cell carcinoma is composed of rounded cells with finely granular chromatin, scant cytoplasm, and numerous mitoses. An organoid pattern may be evident.

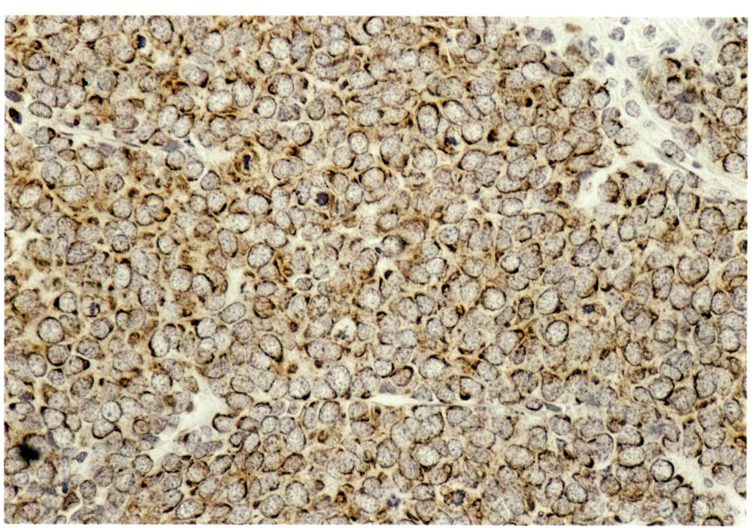

FIGURE
30.7

Metastatic Merkel cell carcinoma, stained for cytokeratin, showing dot-like paranuclear staining.

Merkel cell carcinoma, originally described as trabecular carcinoma, is a neuroendocrine carcinoma of the skin. Merkel cell carcinoma is characterized by a dermal or subcutaneous tumor composed of small, round cells, with finely granular chromatin, organoid arrangement, and numerous mitoses. Lymph node metastases occur frequently and are characterized by infiltrates of similar appearing cells (Fig. 30.6). Merkel cell carcinoma morphologically may mimic lymphoblastic lymphoma because of the fine chromatin and numerous mitoses, or metastatic small cell carcinoma. Immunohistochemical studies are helpful in recognition. Merkel cell carcinoma is characterized by expression of neuroendocrine markers, including NSE, neurofilament protein, and chromogranin, and by characteristic dot-like paranuclear staining for cytokeratin (Fig. 30.7). Merkel cell carcinoma may be distinguished from other small cell carcinomas by expression of cytokeratin 20 (Chan et al, 1997). Merkel cell carcinoma occasionally presents with lymph node involvement in the absence of a primary cutaneous tumor; primary lymph node origin has been considered in these cases (Eusebi et al, 1992).

Germ Cell Tumors

Germ cell tumors, including seminoma (germinoma) and embryonal carcinoma, arise in gonadal and extragonadal sites and may present with lymph node metastases. Germ cell origin of a poorly differentiated malignant tumor is suggested by midline (mediastinal or retroperitoneal) involvement, male sex, and elevation of serum β-human chorionic gonadotropin (HCG) or α-fetoprotein (Richardson et al, 1981). Seminomas are characterized by monomorphous large, round cells with abundant clear cytoplasm, prominent central nucleolus, and lymphocyte-rich or granulomatous stroma (Fig. 30.8). PAS stain with diastase digestion is positive for glycogen. Seminomas are negative or weakly positive for cytokeratin but strongly positive for placental alkaline phosphatase (PLAP). Embryonal carcinoma is characterized by pleomorphic cells with a sheet-like or papillary configuration. Embryonal carcinomas are positive for cytokeratin and frequently positive for CD30 (Falini et al, 1995). Metastatic germ cell tumors are particularly important to recognize because of their potential curability with platinum-based chemotherapy, even when advanced (Richardson et al, 1981).

Lobular Breast Carcinoma

Lobular breast carcinoma is characterized by small, round cells with a characteristically noncohesive Indian file growth pattern (Fig. 30.9). Variants of lobular carcinoma with signet ring cells, larger pleomorphic cells, and histiocytoid cells also occur (Rosen and Oberman, 1993). Lymph node metastases of lobular carcinoma may be histologically subtle because of the cytologic blandness of the cells or may be confused with malignant lymphoma because of the noncohesive growth pattern. Immunohistochemical studies are helpful in difficult cases. The cells of lobular carcinoma are positive for cytokeratin and, frequently, positive for BRST2 (GCDFP15), a breast-cancer-associated antigen, and estrogen receptor protein. Lymph node metastases of lobular carcinoma may be mimicked by signet ring cell sinus histiocytosis (Gould et al, 1989).

Metastatic Carcinoma of Unknown Primary Site

The pathologist is frequently confronted with the problem of identifying the primary site of a metastatic carcinoma in a patient with no known primary tumor. Although the prognosis of such patients is generally poor, some patients, including those with breast or prostate carcinoma, ovarian carcinoma, germ cell tumors, and neuroendocrine carcinomas, may respond to specific therapy (Hainsworth and Greco, 1993). Identification of

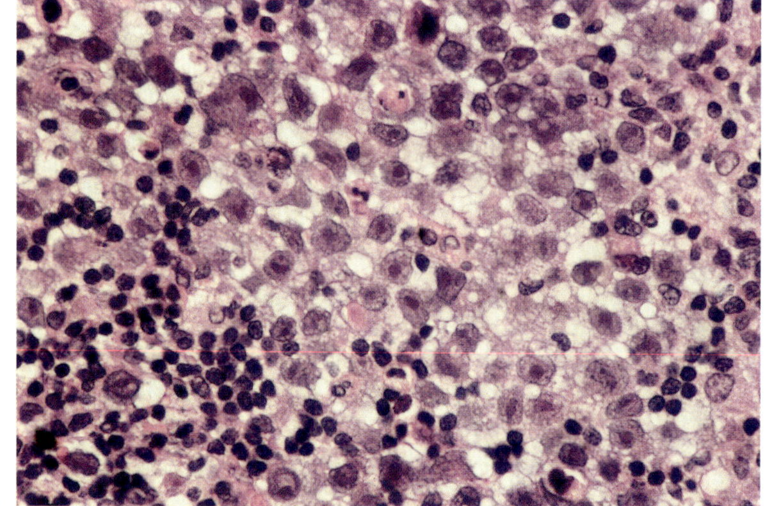

A

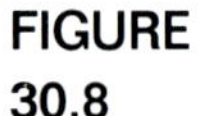

**FIGURE
30.8**

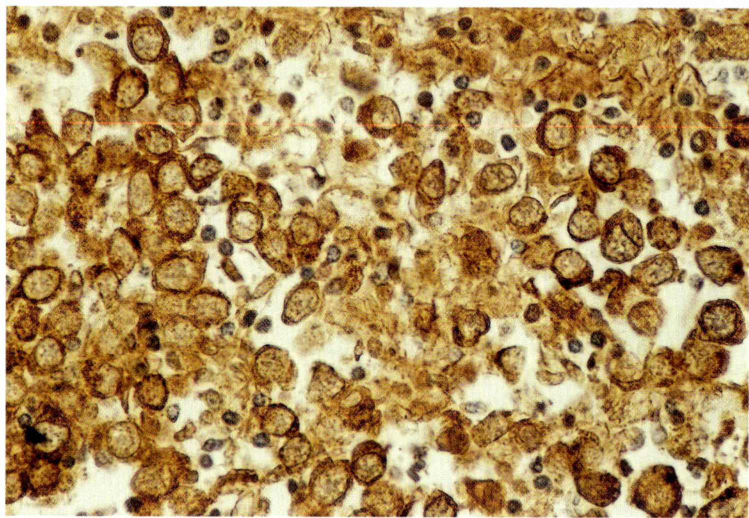

B

Metastatic seminoma showing large cells with abundant clear cytoplasm
and prominent central nucleoli (A). Tumor cells are positive for glycogen and for placental alkaline phosphatase (PLAP) (B); cytokeratin is
negative or weakly positive.

the primary site when possible—in particular, the exclusion of a potentially curable
tumor such as lymphoma or germ cell tumor—therefore, is clinically relevant. The site
and histology of metastases are potential clues to the primary tumor. Metastatic squamous carcinoma in cervical lymph nodes is frequently due to head and neck carcinoma.
Otolaryngologic evaluation with endoscopic biopsies may reveal a clinically inapparent
primary tumor; or, in the absence of a primary tumor, empiric neck dissection or radiation therapy may be undertaken, resulting in 30–50% disease-free survival (Hainsworth
and Greco, 1993). Similarly, metastatic squamous carcinoma in inguinal lymph nodes is

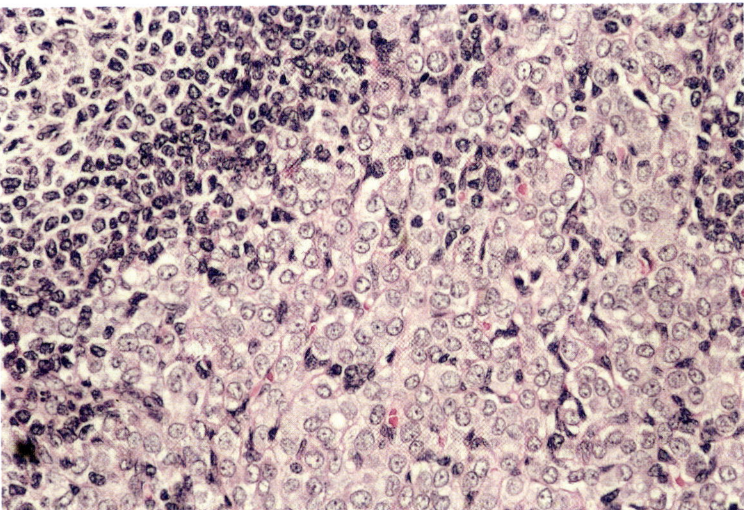

Metastatic lobular breast carcinoma showing noncohesive, cytologically bland cells. Metastatic lobular carcinoma cells may mimic reactive histiocytes or lymphoma cells. Immunohistochemical staining for cytokeratin is helpful in some cases.

FIGURE 30.9

frequently due to an anorectal or perineal primary and should be similarly approached. Metastatic adenocarcinoma in axillary lymph nodes in women frequently represents metastasis of an occult breast carcinoma. Mammography or empiric ipsilateral mastectomy may identify the primary tumor in the breast; carcinoma arising in ectopic breast tissue in axillary lymph nodes has also been rarely reported (Walker and Fechner, 1982). Axillary dissection with empiric ipsilateral mastectomy or breast irradiation yields results similar to that in women with known breast carcinoma of comparable stage (Ellerbroek et al, 1990). In patients with metastatic poorly differentiated carcinomas, the possibility of an extragonadal germ cell tumor (Richardson et al, 1981) or neuroendocrine carcinoma of unknown primary site (Hainsworth et al, 1988) should be considered; these tumors may respond favorably to specific therapy.

Immunohistochemical studies may aid in the identification of a primary tumor but are frequently disappointing, particularly in cases without histologic or clinical evidence narrowing the possible primary sites. Antibodies helpful in identifying the site of origin of metastases include carcinoembryonic antigen (CEA) in adenocarcinomas (canalicular staining is present in hepatocellular carcinoma); prostate-specific antigen (PSA) and prostatic acid phosphatase (PAP) in prostatic adenocarcinoma (PAP also stains some carcinoids); BRST2 (GCDFP15) in breast carcinomas (50–70% are positive, some sweat gland, salivary, and lung tumors are also stained); thyroglobulin in papillary and follicular thyroid carcinoma; calcitonin in medullary thyroid carcinoma; and α-fetoprotein (AFP), HCG, and placental alkaline phosphatase (PLAP) in germ cell tumors.

In many cases, despite intensive clinical and laboratory evaluation, the primary site remains undetermined (Hainsworth and Greco, 1993). The possibility that an unusual malignant tumor is primary in a lymph node, arising from either heterologous elements (Eusebi et al, 1992) or nonlymphoid cells (Weiss et al, 1990), must also be considered.

REFERENCES

Ambrosch P, Brinck U. Detection of nodal micrometastases in head and neck cancer by serial sectioning and immunostaining. Oncology 10:1221–1225, 1996.

Brennan JA, Mao L, Hruban RH, Boyle JO, Eby YJ, Kock WM, Goodman WN, Sidransky D. Molecular assessment of histopathological staging in squamous-cell carcinoma of the head and neck. N Engl J Med 332:429–435, 1995.

Brooks JJ, LiVolsi VA, Pietra GG. Mesothelial cell inclusions in mediastinal lymph nodes mimicking metastatic carcinoma. Am J Clin Pathol 93:741–748, 1990.

Chan JKC, Buchanan R, Fletcher CDM. Sarcomatoid variant of anaplastic large cell Ki-1 lymphoma. Am J Surg Pathol 14:983–988, 1990.

Chan JKC, Suster S, Wenig BM, Tsang WYW, Chan JBK, Lau ALW. Cytokeratin 20 immunoreactivity distinguishes Merkel cell (primary cutaneous neuroendocrine) carcinomas and salivary gland small cell carcinomas from small cell carcinomas of various sites. Am J Surg Pathol 21:226–234, 1997.

Cochran AJ, Wen DR, Morton DL. Occult tumor cells in the lymph nodes of patients with pathologicaly stage I malignant melanoma. An immunohistologic study. Am J Surg Pathol 12:612–618, 1988.

Delattre O, Zugman J, Melot T, Garau XS, Zucker J-M, Lenoir GM, et al. The Ewing family of tumors—A subgroup of small-round-cell-tumors defined by specific chimeric transcripts. N Engl J Med 331:294–299, 1994.

Domagala W, Bedner E, Chosia M, Weber K, Osborn M. Keratin-positive reticulum cells in fine needle aspirates and touch imprints of hyperplastic lymph nodes. A possible pitfall in the immunocytochemical diagnosis of metastatic carcinoma. Acta Cytol 36:241–245, 1992.

Ellerbroek N, Holmes F, Singletary E, Evans H, Oswald M, McNeese M. Treatment of patients with isolated axillary nodal metastases from an occult primary carcinoma consistent with breast origin. Cancer 66:1461–1467, 1990.

Enzinger FM, Weiss SW. Soft Tissue Tumors, 3rd ed. St. Louis, Mosby, 1995.

Eusebi V, Capella C, Cossu A, Rosai J. Neuroendocrine carcinoma within lymph nodes in the absence of a primary tumor with special reference to Merkel cell carcinoma. Am J Surg Pathol 16:658–666, 1992.

Falini B, Pileri S, Pizzolo G, Durkop H, Flenghi L, Stirpe F, Martelli MF, Stein H. CD30 (Ki-1) molecule: a new cytokine receptor of the tumor necrosis factor receptor superfamily as tool for diagnosis and immunotherapy. Blood 85:1–14, 1995.

Gerald WL, Miller HK, Battifora H, Miettinen M, Silva EG, Rosai J. Intra-abdominal desmoplastic small round cell tumor. Report of 19 cases of high-grade polyphenotypic malignancy affecting young individuals. Am J Surg Pathol 15:499–513, 1991.

Gould E, Perez J, Albores-Saavedra J, Legaspi A. Signet ring cell sinus histiocytosis. A previously unrecognized histologic condition mimicking metastatic adenocarcinoma in lymph nodes. Am J Clin Pathol 92:509–512, 1989.

Gould VE, Bloom KJ, Franke WW, Warren WH, Moll R. Increased numbers of cytokeratin-positive interstitial reticulum cells (CIRC) in reactive, inflammatory, and neoplastic lymphadenopathies: Hyperplasia or induced expression? Virchows Arch 425:617–629, 1995.

Gustmann C, Altsmannsberger M, Osborn M, Griesser H, Feller AC. Cytokeratin expression and vimentin content in large cell anaplastic lymphomas and other non-Hodgkin's lymphomas. Am J Pathol 138:1413–1422, 1991.

Hainsworth JD, Greco FA. Treatment of patients with cancer of an unknown primary site. N Engl J Med 329:257–263, 1993.

Hainsworth JD, Johnson DH, Greco FA. Poorly differentiated neuroendocrine carcinoma of unknown primay site. A newly recognized clinicopathologic entity. Ann Intern Med 109:364–371, 1988.

Hirsch FR, Matthews MJ, Aisner S, Campobasso O, Elema JD, Gazdar AF, et al. Histopathologic classification of small cell lung cancer. Changing concepts and terminology. Cancer 62:973–977, 1988.

Ibrahim NBN, Briggs JC, Corbishley CM. Extrapulmonray oat cell carcinoma. Cancer 54:1645–1661, 1984.

Kneba M, Bolz I, Bergholz M, Batge R, Nauck M, Nitsche R, Krieger G. Clinical characteristics of high-grade lymphomas with immune genes in germline configuration. Cancer 67:603–609, 1991.

Leyvraz S, Henle W, Chahinian AP, Perlmann C, Klein G, Gordon RE, Rosenblum M, Holland JF. Association of Epstein-Barr virus with thymic carcinoma. N Engl J Med 312:1296–1299, 1985.

Richardson RL, Schoumacher RA, Fer MF, Hande KR, Oldham RK, Greco FA. The unrecognized extragonadal germ cell cancer syndrome. Ann Intern Med 94:181–186, 1981.

Robertson PB, Neimann RS, Worapongpaiboon S, John K, Orazi A. 013 (CD99) positivity in hematologic proliferations correlates with TdT positivity. Mod Pathol 10:277–282, 1997.

Rosen PP, Oberman HA. Tumors of the mammary gland. In: Atlas of Tumor Pathology, Third series, Fascicle 7. Rosai J, Sobin LH, eds. Washington, D.C., Armed Forces Institute of Pathology, 1993.

Rosen PP, Saigo PE, Braun DW, Weathers E, Fracchia AA, Kinne DW. Axillary micro- and macrometastases in breast cancer: Prognostic significance of tumor size. Ann Surg 194:585–591, 1981.

Sheibani K, Battifora H, Burke JS, Rappaport H. Leu-M1 antigen in human neoplasms. An immunohistologic study of 400 cases. Am J Surg Pathol 10:227–236, 1986.

Travis WD, Linnoila I, Tsokos MG, Hitchcock CK,

Cutler GB, Nieman L, et al. Neuroendocrine tumors of the lung with proposed criteria for large-cell neuroendocrine carcinoma. An ultrastructural, immunohistochemical, and flow cytometric study of 35 cases. Am J Surg Pathol 15:529–553, 1991.

Tsang WY, Chan JK, Tang SK, Tse CC, Cheung MM. Large cell lymphoma with fibrillary matrix. Histopathology 20:80–82, 1992.

Walker AN, Fechner RE. Papillary carcinoma arising from ectopic breast tissue in an axillary lymph node. Diagn Gynecol Obstet 4:141–145, 1982.

Weiss LM, Berry GJ, Dorfman RF, Banks P, Kaiserling E, Curtis J, Rosai J, Warnke RA. Spindle cell neoplasms of lymph nodes of probable reticulum cell lineage. True reticulum cell sarcoma? Am J Surg Pathol 14:405–414, 1990.

Zarate-Osorno A, Jaffe ES, Medeiros LJ. Metastatic nasopharyngeal carcinoma initially presenting as cervical lymphadenopathy. A report of two cases that resembled Hodgkin's disease. Arch Pathol Lab Med 116:682, 1992.

Index